Roitt's
Essential
Immunology

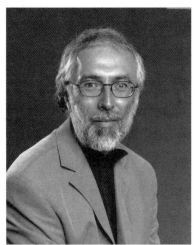

Peter J. Delves

Professor Delves obtained his PhD from the University of
London in 1986 and is a Professor of Immunology at UCL
(University College London). His research has focused on
molecular aspects of antigen recognition. He has authored and
edited a number of immunology books, and teaches the subject
at a broad range of levels.

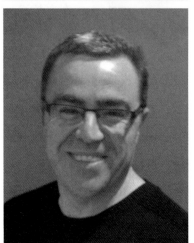

Seamus J. Martin

Professor Martin received his PhD from The National University
of Ireland in 1990 and trained as a post-doctoral fellow at
University College London (with Ivan Roitt) and The La Jolla
Institute for Allergy and Immunology, California, USA (with
Doug Green). Since 1999, he is the holder of the Smurfit Chair
of Medical Genetics at Trinity College Dublin and is also a
Science Foundation Ireland Principal Investigator. His research is
focused on various aspects of programmed cell death (apoptosis)
in the immune system and in cancer and he has received several
awards for his work in this area. He has previously edited two
books on apoptosis and was elected as a Member of The Royal
Irish Academy in 2006 and as a member of The European
Molecular Biology Organisation (EMBO) in 2009.

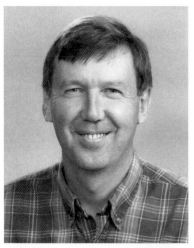

Dennis R. Burton

Professor Burton obtained his BA in Chemistry from the
University of Oxford in 1974 and his PhD in Physical
Biochemistry from the University of Lund in Sweden in 1978.
After a period at the University of Sheffield, he moved to the
Scripps Research Institute in La Jolla, California in 1989 where
he is Professor of Immunology and Molecular Biology. His
research interests include antibodies, antibody responses to
pathogens and vaccine design, particularly in relation to HIV.

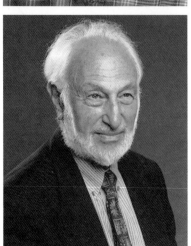

Ivan M. Roitt

Professor Roitt was born in 1927 and educated at King Edward's
School, Birmingham and Balliol College, Oxford. In 1956,
together with Deborah Doniach and Peter Campbell, he made
the classic discovery of thyroglobulin autoantibodies in
Hashimoto's thyroiditis which helped to open the whole concept
of a relationship between autoimmunity and human disease. The
work was extended to an intensive study of autoimmune
phenomena in pernicious anaemia and primary biliary cirrhosis.
In 1983 he was elected a Fellow of The Royal Society, and has
been elected to Honorary Membership of the Royal College of
Physicians and appointed Honorary Fellow of The Royal Society
of Medicine.

TWELFTH EDITION

Roitt's Essential Immunology

Peter J. Delves
PhD
Division of Infection and Immunity
UCL
London, UK

Seamus J. Martin
PhD, FTCD, MRIA
The Smurfit Institute of Genetics
Trinity College
Dublin, Ireland

Dennis R. Burton
PhD
Department of Immunology and Molecular Biology
The Scripps Research Institute
La Jolla, California, USA

Ivan M. Roitt
MA, DSc(Oxon), FRCPath, Hon FRCP (Lond), FRS
Centre for Investigative and Diagnostic Oncology
Middlesex University
London, UK

WILEY-BLACKWELL

A John Wiley & Sons, Ltd., Publication

This edition first published 2011 © 1971, 1974, 1977, 1980, 1984, 1988, 1991, 1994, 1997, 2001, 2006 by Peter J Delves, Seamus J. Martin, Dennis R. Burton, Ivan M. Roitt

Blackwell Publishing was acquired by John Wiley & Sons in February 2007. Blackwell's publishing program has been merged with Wiley's global Scientific, Technical and Medical business to form Wiley-Blackwell.

Registered office: John Wiley & Sons, Ltd, The Atrium, Southern Gate, Chichester, West Sussex, PO19 8SQ, UK

Editorial offices: 9600 Garsington Road, Oxford, OX4 2DQ, UK
   The Atrium, Southern Gate, Chichester, West Sussex, PO19 8SQ, UK
   111 River Street, Hoboken, NJ 07030-5774, USA

For details of our global editorial offices, for customer services and for information about how to apply for permission to reuse the copyright material in this book please see our website at www.wiley.com/wiley-blackwell

Library of Congress Cataloging-in-Publication Data

Roitt's essential immunology / Peter J. Delves ... [et al.]. – 12th ed.
      p. cm. – (Essentials ; 16)
   Rev. ed. of: Roitt's essential immunology / Ivan M. Roitt, Peter J. Delves.
   Includes bibliographical references and index.
   ISBN 978-1-4051-9683-3 (pbk.)
   1. Immunology.   I. Delves, Peter J.   II. Roitt, Ivan M. (Ivan Maurice) Roitt's essential immunology.   III. Title: Essential immunology.
   QR181.R57 2011
   616.07'9–dc22

                                   2010047392

A catalogue record for this book is available from the British Library.

Set in 10/12 pt Adobe Garamond Pro by Toppan Best-set Premedia Limited
Printed in Singapore by Ho Printing Singapore Pte Ltd
3   2012

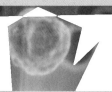

PART 1: Fundamentals of Immunology

PART 2: Applied Immunology

Acknowledgments

The input of the editorial team of Elizabeth Johnston, Laura Murphy and Cathryn Gates at Wiley-Blackwell and the project management of Ruth Swan is warmly acknowledged. We are much indebted to the co-editors of *Immunology*, J. Brostoff, D. Roth and D. Male, together with the publishers, Mosby, and the following individuals for permission to utilize or modify their figures: *J. Brostoff and A. Hall for figure 15.11; J. Horton for figure 11.19; and J. Taverne for figures 12.23 and 12.24.*

IMR would like to acknowledge the indefatigable secretarial assistance of Christine Griffin. DRB wishes to particularly acknowledge the invaluable contributions of Amandeep Gakhal, Erin Scherer, Rena Astronomo and Wendelien Oswald. He is grateful to Jenny Woof, Ann Feeney, Beatrice Hahn, Jim Marks, Don Mosier, Paul Sharp, Robyn Stanfield, James Stevens and Mario Stevenson for many very helpful comments. PJD would particularly like to thank Per Brandtzaeg, Volker Brinkmann, Greg Campbell, Peter Lydyard, Rand Swenson and Ulrich Wahn. SJM is indebted to Ed Lavelle, Sean Cullen, Cristina Munoz-Pinedo and all of the members of his laboratory for comments, suggestions and support. He would also like to thank Mia, Madeleine and Jamie for their support and indulgence.

Every effort has been made by the authors and the publisher to contact all the copyright holders to obtain their permission to reproduce copyright material. However, if any have been inadvertently overlooked, the publisher will be pleased to make the necessary arrangements at the first opportunity.

A number of scientists very generously provided illustrations for inclusion in this edition, and we have acknowledged our gratitude to them in the relevant figure legends.

Companion website

This book is accompanied by a companion website:

www.roitt.com

The website includes:

- Interactive MCQs and SBA questions for each chapter, with feedback on all answers selected

- Animations and videos showing key concepts

- Fully downloadable figures and illustrations, further reading and useful links

- Extracts from the *Encyclopaedia of Life Sciences*

- Podcasts to reinforce the key principles explained in the text: ideal for revision 'on the go'

Preface

Welcome to this new edition! When Ivan wrote the first edition some 40 years ago, he wanted to feel that he was chatting to the reader almost informally, rather than preaching, and it has been our intention to maintain this style. As a subject, immunology is exciting and dynamic and to persuade you that it is absolutely worthwhile for you to tackle this new edition we have made very extensive changes to update the previous edition. Accordingly, apart from the introduction of numerous new illustrations, we have:

- Expanded discussion of pathogen- and danger-associated molecular patterns (PAMPs & DAMPs)
- Introduced a new section on dendritic cells and their role in antigen processing including cross-presentation
- Updated sections on B-cell and NK receptors
- Enhanced discussion of lymphocyte trafficking
- Incorporated the latest findings on T-cell subsets, particularly Th17 and the diversity of regulatory T-cells
- Recorded newer information on NK and cytotoxic T-cell killing mechanisms
- Given more insight into the effects of aging on immune responses
- Carried out a major rewrite of the vaccine chapter with new emphasis on mechanisms of action of conventional and carbohydrate vaccines, and new approaches to vaccine development including reverse vaccinology, together with progress in malaria vaccines and adjuvant action
- Provided new information on novel genetic immunodeficiency defects, on the origin of AIDS and the ever-expanding plethora of AIDS drugs plus results from the latest HIV vaccine trials
- Clarified the recent findings on the cellular transformations leading to cancer, the manipulation of the immune system by tumors and the links between infection, inflammation and cancer
- Substantially rewritten the chapter on autoimmune diseases.

It is our fond expectation that you will enjoy and benefit from a reading of our offering.

Peter J. Delves
Seamus J. Martin
Dennis R. Burton
Ivan M. Roitt

Abbreviations

AAV	adeno-associated virus
Ab	antibody
AChR	acetylcholine receptor
ACT	adoptive cell transfer
ACTH	adrenocorticotropic hormone
ADA	adenosine deaminase
ADCC	antibody-dependent cellular cytotoxicity
AEP	asparagine endopeptidase
Ag	antigen
AID	activation-induced cytidine deaminase
AIDS	acquired immunodeficiency syndrome
AIRE	autoimmune regulator
ALBA	addressable laser bead assay
ANCA	antineutrophil cytoplasmic antibodies
APC	antigen-presenting cell
ARRE-1	antigen receptor response element-1
ARRE-2	antigen receptor response element-2
ART	antiretroviral therapy
ASFV	African swine fever virus
AZT	zidovudine (3′-azido-3′-deoxythymidine)
BAFF	B-cell-activating factor of the tumor necrosis factor family
B-cell	lymphocyte which matures in bone marrow
BCG	bacille Calmette–Guérin attenuated form of tuberculosis
BCR	B-cell receptor
BM	bone marrow
BSA	bovine serum albumin
BSE	bovine spongiform encephalopathy
Btk	Bruton's tyrosine kinase
BUDR	bromodeoxyuridine
C	complement
Cα(β/γ/δ)	constant part of TCR α(β/γ/δ) chain
CALLA	common acute lymphoblastic leukemia antigen
cAMP	cyclic adenosine monophosphate
CCP	complement control protein repeat
CD	cluster of differentiation
CDR	complementarity determining regions of Ig or TCR variable portion
CEA	carcinoembryonic antigen
CFA	complete Freund's adjuvant
cGMP	cyclic guanosine monophosphate
ChIP	chromatin immunoprecipitation
CHIP	chemotaxis inhibitory protein
$C_{H(L)}$	constant part of Ig heavy (light) chain
CLA	cutaneous lymphocyte antigen
CLIP	class II-associated invariant chain peptide
CMI	cell-mediated immunity
CML	cell-mediated lympholysis
CMV	cytomegalovirus
Cn	complement component "n"
$C\bar{n}$	activated complement component "n"
iCn	inactivated complement component "n"
Cna	small peptide derived by proteolytic activation of Cn
CpG	cytosine phosphate-guanosine dinucleotide motif
CR(n)	complement receptor "n"
CRP	C-reactive protein
CSF	cerebrospinal fluid
CSR	class switch recombination
CTLR	C-type lectin receptor
D gene	diversity minigene joining V and J segments to form variable region
DAF	decay accelerating factor
DAG	diacylglycerol
DAMP	danger-associated molecular pattern
DC	dendritic cells
DMARD	disease-modifying antirheumatic drug
DNP	dinitrophenyl
DTH	delayed-type hypersensitivity
DTP	diphtheria, tetanus, pertussis triple vaccine
EAE	experimental autoimmune (allergic) encephalomyelitis
EBV	Epstein–Barr virus
ELISA	enzyme-linked immunosorbent assay
EM	electron microscope
Eø	eosinophil
EPO	erythropoietin
ER	endoplasmic reticulum
ES	embryonic stem (cell)
ET	exfoliative toxins
F(B)	factor (B, etc.)
Fab	monovalent Ig antigen-binding fragment after papain digestion
F(ab′)₂	divalent antigen-binding fragment after pepsin digestion
FasL	Fas-ligand
FACS	fluorescence-activated cell sorter
Fc	Ig crystallisable-fragment originally; now non-Fab part of Ig
FcγR	receptor for IgG Fc fragment
FDC	follicular dendritic cell
flt-3	flk-2 ligand
(sc)Fv	(single chain) V_H–V_L antigen binding fragment
GADS	GRB2-related adapter protein
g.b.m.	glomerular basement membrane
G-CSF	granulocyte colony-stimulating factor

GEFs	guanine-nucleotide exchange factors
GM-CSF	granulocyte–macrophage colony-stimulating factor
gp$n$	n kDa glycoprotein
GRB2	growth factor receptor-binding protein 2
GSK3	glycogen synthase kinase 3
g.v.h.	graft versus host
H-2	the mouse major histocompatibility complex
H-2D/K/L (A/E)	main loci for classical class I (class II) murine MHC molecules
HAMA	human antimouse antibodies
HATA	human anti-toxin antibody
HBsAg	hepatitis B surface antigen
hCG	human chorionic gonadotropin
HCMV	human cytomegalovirus
HEL	hen egg lysozyme
HEV	high-walled endothelium of post capillary venule
HIV	human immunodeficiency virus
HLA	the human major histocompatibility complex
HLA-A/B/C (DP/DQ/DR)	main loci for classical class I (class II) human MHC molecules
HMG	high mobility group
HR	hypersensitive response
HRF	homologous restriction factor
HSA	heat-stable antigen
HSC	hematopoietic stem cell
hsp	heat-shock protein
5HT	5-hydroxytryptamine
HTLV	human T-cell leukemia virus
H-Y	male transplantation antigen
IBD	inflammatory bowel disease
ICAM-1	intercellular adhesion molecule-1
Id (αId)	idiotype (anti-idiotype)
IDC	interdigitating dendritic cells
IDDM	insulin-dependent diabetes mellitus
IDO	indoleamine 2,3-dioxygenase
IEL	intraepithelial lymphocyte
IFNα	α-interferon (also IFNβ, IFNγ)
IFR	interferon-regulated factor
Ig	immunoglobulin
IgG	immunoglobulin G (also IgM, IgA, IgD, IgE)
sIg	surface immunoglobulin
Ig-α/Ig-β	membrane peptide chains associated with sIg B-cell receptor
IgSF	immunoglobulin superfamily
IL-1	interleukin-1 (also IL-2, IL-3, etc.)
iNOS	inducible nitric oxide synthase
IP$_3$	inositol triphosphate
ISCOM	immunostimulating complex
ITAM	immunoreceptor tyrosine-based activation motif
ITIM	immunoreceptor tyrosine-based inhibitory motif
ITP	idiopathic thrombocytopenic purpura
IVIg	intravenous immunoglobulin
JAK	Janus kinases
J chain	polypeptide chain in IgA dimer and IgM
J gene	joining gene linking V or D segment to constant region
Ka(d)	association (dissociation) affinity constant (usually Ag–Ab reactions)
kDa	units of molecular mass in kilo Daltons
KIR	killer immunoglobulin-like receptors
KLH	keyhole limpet hemocyanin
LAK	lymphokine-activated killer cell
LAMP	lysosomal-associated membrane proteins
LAT	linker for activation of T cells
LATS	long-acting thyroid stimulator
LBP	LPS binding protein
LCM	lymphocytic choriomeningitis virus
Le$^{a/b/x}$	Lewis$^{a/b/x}$ blood group antigens
LFA-1	lymphocyte functional antigen-1
LGL	large granular lymphocyte
LHRH	luteinizing hormone releasing hormone
LIF	leukemia inhibiting factor
LRR	leucine-rich repeat
LT(B)	leukotriene (B etc.)
LPS	lipopolysaccharide (endotoxin)
Mφ	macrophage
mAb	monoclonal antibody
MAC	membrane attack complex
MAdCAM	mucosal addressin cell adhesion molecule
MALT	mucosa-associated lymphoid tissue
MAM	*Mycoplasma arthritidis* mitogen
MAP kinase	mitogen-activated protein kinase
MAPKKK	mitogen-associated protein kinase kinase kinase
MBL	mannose binding lectin
MBP	major basic protein of eosinophils (also myelin basic protein)
MCP	membrane cofactor protein (complement regulation)
MCP-1	monocyte chemotactic protein-1
M-CSF	macrophage colony-stimulating factor
MDP	muramyl dipeptide
MHC	major histocompatibility complex
MICA	MHC class I chain-related A chain
MIDAS	metal ion-dependent adhesion site
MIF	macrophage migration inhibitory factor
MIIC	MHC class II-enriched compartments
MLA	monophosphoryl lipid A
MLR	mixed lymphocyte reaction
MMTV	mouse mammary tumor virus
MRSA	methicillin-resistant *Staphylococcus aureus*
MS	multiple sclerosis
MSC	mesenchymal stem cell

MSH	melanocyte stimulating hormone
MTP	microsomal triglyceride-transfer protein
MuLV	murine leukemia virus
NADP	nicotinamide adenine dinucleotide phosphate
NAP	neutrophil activating peptide
NBT	nitroblue tetrazolium
NCF	neutrophil chemotactic factor
NFAT	nuclear factor of activated T-cells
NFκB	nuclear transcription factor
NK	natural killer cell
NLR	nod-like receptor
NO·	nitric oxide
NOD	Nonobese diabetic mouse
NZB	New Zealand Black mouse
NZB × W	New Zealand Black mouse × NZ White F1 hybrid
·O_2^-	superoxide anion
OD	optical density
ORF	open reading frame
OS	obese strain chicken
Ova	ovalbumin
PAF(-R)	platelet activating factor (-receptor)
PAGE	polyacrylamide gel electrophoresis
PAMP	pathogen-associated molecular pattern
PBSCs	peripheral blood stem cells
PCA	passive cutaneous anaphylaxis
PCR	polymerase chain reaction
PERV	porcine endogenous retroviruses
PG(E)	prostaglandin (E etc.)
PHA	phytohemagglutinin
phox	phagocyte oxidase
PI3K	phosphatidylinositol 3-kinase
PIAS	protein inhibitor of activated STAT
pIgR	poly-Ig receptor
PIP_2	phosphatidylinositol diphosphate
PKC	protein kinase C
PKR	RNA-dependent protein kinase
PLC	phospholipase C
PLCγ2	phospholipase Cγ2
PMN	polymorphonuclear neutrophil
PMT	photomultiplier tube
PNH	paroxysmal nocturnal hemoglobinuria
PPAR	peroxisome proliferator-activated receptor
PPD	purified protein derivative from *Mycobacterium tuberculosis*
PRR	pattern recognition receptors
PTFE	polytetrafluoroethylene
PTK	protein tyrosine kinase
PWM	pokeweed mitogen
RA	rheumatoid arthritis
RANTES	*r*egulated upon *a*ctivation *n*ormal *T*-cell *e*xpressed and *s*ecreted chemokine
RAST	radioallergosorbent test
RF	rheumatoid factor
Rh(D)	rhesus blood group (D)
RIP	rat insulin promoter
RLR	RIG-like helicase receptor
RNAi	RNA interference
ROI	reactive oxygen intermediates
RSS	recombination signal sequence
SAP	serum amyloid P
SAP	sphingolipid activator protein
SAR	systemic acquired resistance
SARS	severe acute respiratory syndrome
SARS-CoV	SARS-associated coronavirus
SC	Ig secretory component
SCF	stem cell factor
scFv	single chain variable region antibody fragment ($V_H + V_L$ joined by a flexible linker)
SCG	sodium cromoglycate
SCID	severe combined immunodeficiency
SDF	stromal-derived factor
SDS	sodium dodecyl sulfate
SDS-PAGE	sodium dodecyl sulfate–polyacrylamide gel electrophoresis
SEA(B etc.)	*Staphylococcus aureus* enterotoxin A (B etc.)
SEREX	serological analysis of recombinant cDNA expression libraries
siRNA	short-interfering RNA
SIV	Simian immunodeficiency virus
SLE	systemic lupus erythematosus
SLIT	sublingual allergen immunotherapy
SLP76	SH2-domain containing leukocyte protein of 76 kDa
SOCs	*s*uppressor of *c*ytokine *s*ignaling
SPE	streptococcal pyogenic exotoxins
SRID	single radial immunodiffusion
SSA	streptococcal superantigen
STAT	signal transducer and activator of transcription
TACI	transmembrane activator and calcium modulator and cyclophilin ligand [CAML] interactor
TAP	transporter associated with antigen processing
T-ALL	T-acute lymphoblastic leukemia
TB	tubercle bacillus
Tc	cytotoxic T-cell
T-cell	thymus-derived lymphocyte
TCF	T-cell factor
TCR1(2)	T-cell receptor with γ/δ chains (with α/β chains)
TdT	terminal deoxynucleotidyl transferase
TG-A-L	polylysine with polyalanyl side-chains randomly tipped with tyrosine and glutamic acid
TGFβ	transforming growth factor-β

Th(1/2/3/9/17)	T-helper cell (subset 1, 2, 3, 9 or 17)	Vα(β/γ/δ)	variable part of TCR α(β/γ/δ) chain
THF	thymic humoral factor	vCJD	variant Creutzfeldt–Jakob disease
Thp	T-helper precursor	VCP	valosin-containing protein
TLI	total lymphoid irradiation	*V* gene	variable region gene for immunoglobulin
TLR	Toll-like receptor		or T-cell receptor
TM	transmembrane	V$_H$	variable part of Ig heavy chain
TNF	tumor necrosis factor	VIP	vasoactive intestinal peptide
TNP	trinitrophenol	V$_L$	variable part of light chain
TPO	thrombopoietin	V$_{\kappa/\lambda}$	variable part of κ(λ) light chain
Treg	regulatory T-cell	VCAM	vascular cell adhesion molecule
Ts	suppressor T-cell	VEGF	vascular endothelial cell growth factor
TSAb	thyroid stimulating antibodies	VIMP	VCP-interacting membrane protein
TSE	transmissible spongiform encephalopathy	VLA	very late antigen
TSH(R)	thyroid stimulating hormone (receptor)	VLP	virus-like particle
TSLP	thymic stromal lymphopoietin	VNTR	variable number of tandem repeats
TSST	toxic shock syndrome toxin	VP1	virus-specific peptide 1
TUNEL	TdT-mediated dUTP (deoxyuridine triphosphate) nick end labeling	XL	X-linked
		ZAP-70	zeta chain associated protein of 70 kDa

How to get the best out of your textbook

Welcome to the new edition of *Roitt's Essential Immunology*. Over the next two pages you will be shown how to make the most of the learning features included in the textbook.

An interactive textbook ▶

For the first time, your textbook gives you free access to a Wiley DeskTop Edition – a digital, interactive version of this textbook. Your Wiley DeskTop Edition allows you to:

Search: Save time by finding terms and topics instantly in your book, your notes, even your whole library (once you've downloaded more textbooks)

Note and Highlight: Colour code highlights and make digital notes right in the text so you can find them quickly and easily

Organize: Keep books, notes and class materials organized in folders inside the application

Share: Exchange notes and highlights with friends, classmates and study groups.

Upgrade: Your textbook can be transferred when you need to change or upgrade computers

Link: Link directly from the page of your interactive textbook to all of the material contained on the companion website

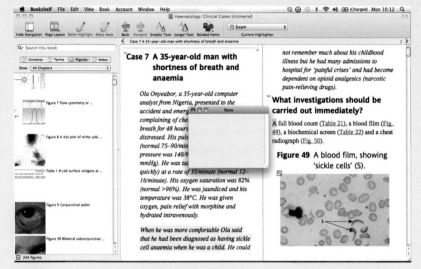

Simply find your unique Wiley desk top edition product code and carefully scratch away the top coating on the label on the front cover of this textbook and visit: **http://www.vitalsource.com/software/bookshelf/downloads/** to get started.

A companion website ▶

Your textbook is also accompanied by a FREE companion website that contains:

- Self-assessment material consisting of multiple choice questions and answers
- All of the illustrations and photographs contained in the book for use in assignments and presentations
- References and further reading suggestions

Log on to www.roitt.com to find out more.

Includes access to selected articles from the ELS ▼

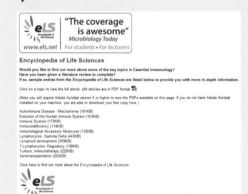

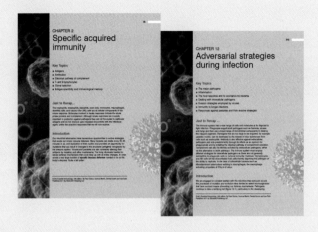

Features contained within your textbook

◀ Every chapter has its own chapter-opening page that offers a list of key topics contained within the chapter

Throughout your textbook you will find a series of icons outlining the learning features throughout the book:

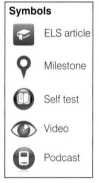

Throughout your book we'll point you to related resources available on the companion website using the following icons:	**Symbols**
	ELS article
Where you see the first icon, this indicates that a related article from the Encyclopaedia of Life Sciences (ELS) is available online, giving you more information on a key topic.	Milestone
	Self test
Milestone boxes indicate key developments in the field.	Video
	Podcast

Self-assessment multiple choice and single best answer questions and answers are available on the companion website: http://www.roitt.com, along with videos and animations showing key concepts.

You may also wish to use the short podcasts available online for revision, once you have read through the chapters.

You can access any of these features by clicking on the icon in your Desk Top Edition.

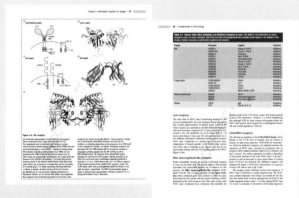

▲

Your textbook is full of useful photographs, illustrations and tables. The DeskTop Edition version of your textbook will allow you to copy and paste any photograph or illustration into assignments, presentations and your own notes. The photographs and illustrations are also available to download from the companion website. ▶

Cell guide

Throughout the illustrations, standard forms have been used for commonly-occurring cells and pathways. A key to these is given in the figure below.

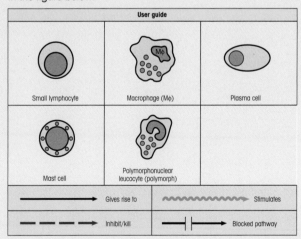

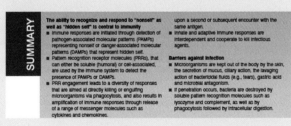

▲

A chapter summary which can be used for both study and revision purposes.

We hope you enjoy using your new textbook. Good luck with your studies!

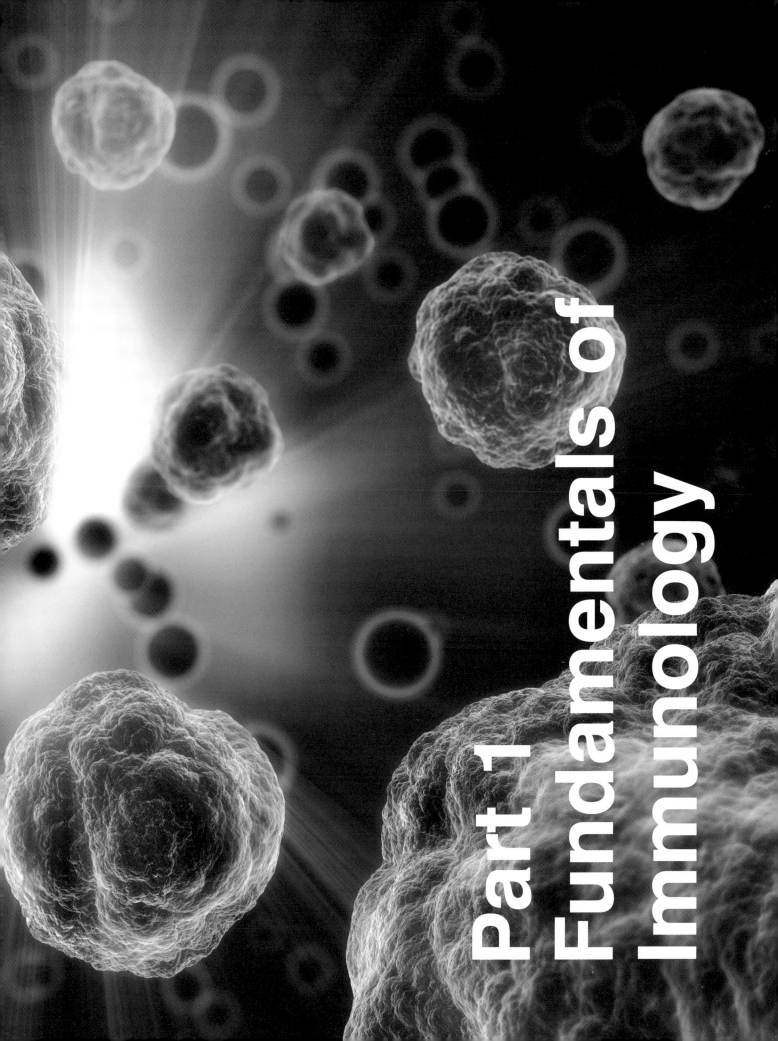

Part 1
Fundamentals of
Immunology

CHAPTER 1
Innate immunity

Key Topics

Introduction

We live in a potentially hostile world filled with a bewildering array of infectious agents (Figure 1.1) of diverse shape, size, composition and subversive character that would very happily use us as rich sanctuaries for propagating their "selfish genes" had we not also developed a series of defense mechanisms at least their equal in effectiveness and ingenuity (except in the case of many parasitic infections in which the situation is best described as an uneasy and often unsatisfactory truce). It is these defense mechanisms that can establish a state of immunity against infection (Latin *immunitas*, freedom from) and whose operation provides the basis for the delightful subject called "Immunology."

Aside from ill-understood constitutional factors that make one species innately susceptible and another resistant to certain infections, a number of relatively nonspecific antimicrobial systems (e.g. phagocytosis) have been recognized that are **innate** in the sense that they are not affected by prior contact with the infectious agent. We shall discuss these systems and examine how, in the state of **specific acquired immunity**, their effectiveness can be greatly increased.

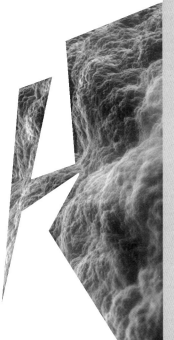
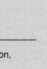

Roitt's Essential Immunology, Twelfth Edition. Peter J. Delves, Seamus J. Martin, Dennis R. Burton, Ivan M. Roitt.
© 2011 Peter J. Delves, Seamus J. Martin, Dennis R. Burton, Ivan M. Roitt. Published 2011 by Blackwell Publishing Ltd.

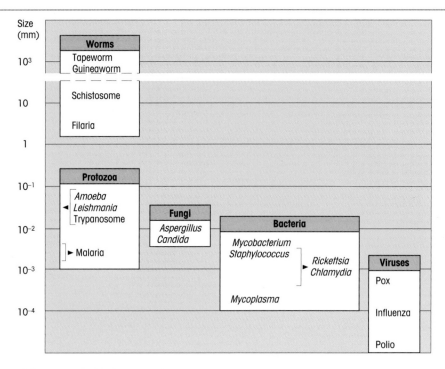

Figure 1.1. The formidable range of infectious agents that confronts the immune system.

Although not normally classified as such because of their lack of a cell wall, the mycoplasmas are included under bacteria for convenience. Fungi adopt many forms and approximate values for some of the smallest forms are given. ⌐►, range of sizes observed for the organism(s) indicated by the arrow; ◄⌐, the organisms listed have the size denoted by the arrow.

Knowing when to make an immune response

The ability to recognize and respond to foreign entities is central to the operation of the immune system

The vertebrate immune system is a conglomeration of cells and molecules that cooperate to protect us from infectious agents and also provides us with a surveillance system to monitor the integrity of host tissues. Although the immune system is quite elaborate, as we shall see, its function can be boiled down to two basic roles; **recognition** of foreign substances and organisms that have entered the body, and **removal** of such agents by a diverse repertoire of cells and molecules that act in concert to eliminate the potential threat. Thus, a major role of the immune system is to be able to determine what is foreign (what immunologists often call "nonself") from what is normally present in the body (i.e. self). The cells and molecules that comprise the innate immune system are preoccupied with detecting the presence of particular **molecular patterns** that are typically associated with infectious agents (Figure 1.2). Charlie Janeway dubbed such molecules **pathogen-associated molecular patterns** (**PAMPs**).

Tissue damage can also instigate an immune response

Aside from infection, there is a growing recognition that tissue damage, leading to nonphysiological cell death, can also provoke activation of the immune system (Figure 1.3). In this situation, the molecules that activate the immune system are derived from self but are not normally present within the extracellular space. Such molecules, for which Polly Matzinger coined the term "**danger signals**," are normally safely sequestered within healthy cells and only escape when a cell dies via an uncontrolled mode of cell death, called **necrosis** (see Videoclip 1). Necrosis is typically caused by tissue trauma, burns, certain toxins, as well as other non-physiological stimuli and is characterized by rapid swelling and rupture of the plasma membranes of damaged cells. This permits the release of multiple cellular constituents that don't normally escape from healthy cells.

The precise identity of the molecules that act as danger signals—now more commonly called **danger-associated molecular patterns** (**DAMPs**) or alarmins—is an area of active investigation at present but molecules such as HMGB1, a chromatin-binding protein, as well as the immunological messenger proteins interleukin-1α (IL-1α) and IL-33, repre-

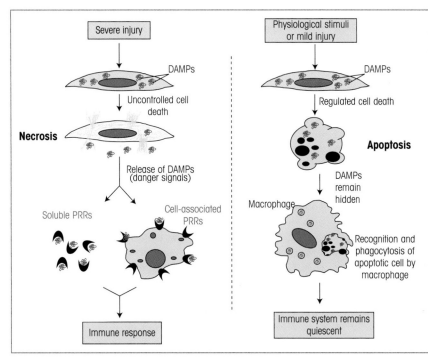

Figure 1.2. Pattern recognition receptors (PRRs) detect pathogen-associated molecular patterns (PAMPs) and initiate immune responses.

PRRs can be either soluble or cell-associated and can instigate a range of responses upon encountering their appropriate ligands.

Figure 1.3. Necrotic cells release danger-associated molecular patterns (DAMPs), whereas apoptotic cells typically do not.

Stimuli that induce necrosis frequently cause severe cellular damage, which leads to rapid cell rupture with consequent release of intracellular DAMPs. DAMPs can then engage cells of the immune system and can promote inflammation. On the other hand, because stimuli that initiate apoptosis are typically physiological and relatively mild, apoptotic cells do not rupture and their removal is coordinated by macrophages and other cells of the innate immune system, before release of DAMPs can occur. For this reason, apoptosis is not typically associated with activation of the immune system.

sent good candidates. It might seem surprising that the immune system can also be activated by self-derived molecules, however, this makes good sense when one considers that events leading to necrotic cell death are often rapidly followed or accompanied by infection. Furthermore, if a pathogen manages to evade direct detection by the immune system, its presence will be betrayed if it provokes necrosis within the tissue it has invaded.

Before moving on, we should also note that there is another mode of cell death that frequently occurs in the body that is both natural and highly controlled and is not associated with plasma membrane rupture and release of intracellular contents. This mode of cell death, called **apoptosis** (see Videoclip 2), is under complex molecular control and is used to eliminate cells that have reached the end of their natural lifespans. Apoptotic cells do not activate the immune system because cells dying in this manner display molecules on their plasma membranes (e.g. phosphatidylserine) that mark these cells out for removal through phagocytosis before they can rupture and release their intracellular contents. In this way, DAMPs remain hidden during apoptosis and such cells do not activate the immune system (Figure 1.3).

Pattern recognition receptors (PRRs) raise the alarm

To distinguish self-components from potentially dangerous microbial agents, our immune systems need to be able to discriminate between "noninfectious self and infectious nonself" as Janeway elegantly put it. Recognition of nonself entities is achieved by means of an array of **pattern recognition receptors and proteins** (collectively called pattern recognition molecules) that have evolved to detect conserved (i.e. not prone to mutation) components of infectious agents that are not normally present in the body (i.e. PAMPs).

In practice, PAMPs can be anything from carbohydrates that are not normally exposed in vertebrates, proteins only found in bacteria such as flagellin (a component of the bacterial flagellum that is used for swimming), double-stranded RNA that is typical of RNA viruses, as well as many other molecules that betray the presence of microbial agents. The cardinal rule is that a PAMP is not normally found in the body but is a common feature of many frequently encountered pathogens. Pattern recognition molecules also appear to be involved in the recognition of DAMPs released from necrotic cells.

Upon engagement of one or more of these pattern recognition molecules with an appropriate PAMP or DAMP, an immune response ensues (Figure 1.2). Fortunately, we have many ways in which an impending infection can be dealt with, and indeed it is a testament to the efficiency of our immune systems that the majority of us spend most of our lives relatively untroubled by infectious disease.

One way of dealing with unwelcome intruders involves the binding of soluble (humoral) pattern recognition molecules, such as **complement** (a series of molecules we will deal with later in this chapter), **mannose-binding lectin**, **C-reactive protein**, or **lysozyme**, to the infectious agent and this can lead directly to killing through destruction of microbial cell wall constituents and breaching of the plasma membrane due to the actions of such proteins. The latter humoral factors are also adept at coating microorganisms and enhancing their uptake and subsequent destruction by phagocytic cells. Other pattern recognition receptors are cell associated and engagement of such receptors can lead to **phagocytosis** of the microorganism followed by its destruction within phagocytic vesicles. Just as importantly, cellular PRR engagement also results in the activation of signal transduction pathways that culminate in the release of soluble messenger proteins (**cytokines**, **chemokines** and other molecules, see below) that mobilize other components of the immune system.

Cells of the immune system release messenger proteins that amplify immune responses

An important feature of the immune system is the ability of its constituent cells to communicate with each other upon

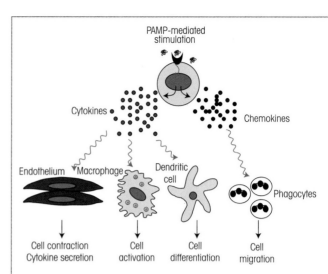

Figure 1.4. Cytokines and chemokines can have pleiotrophic effects.

Stimulation of cells of the innate immune system frequently leads to the production of inflammatory cytokines and chemokines that trigger responses from other cell types, as depicted. Note that the effects of chemokines and cytokines shown are not exhaustive.

encountering a pathogen. Although cells of the immune system are capable of releasing numerous biologically active molecules with diverse functions, two major categories of proteins—cytokines and chemokines—have particularly important roles in immunity. Cytokines are a diverse group of proteins that have pleiotropic effects, including the ability to activate other cells, induce differentiation and enhance microbicidal activity (Figure 1.4). Cytokines are commonly released by cells of the immune system in response to PAMPs and DAMPs, and this has the effect of altering the activation state and behaviour of other cells to galvanise them into joining the fight. Chemokines are also released upon encountering PAMPs/DAMPs and typically serve as **chemotactic factors**, helping to lay a trail that guides other cells of the immune system to the site of infection or tissue damage. Both types of messenger proteins act by diffusing away from the cells secreting them and binding to cells equipped with the appropriate plasma membrane receptors to receive such signals. Cytokines, chemokines and their respective receptors are discussed at length in Chapter 9.

Innate versus adaptive immunity

Three levels of immune defense

Before we get into the details, we will first take a look at how the immune system works in broad brushstrokes. The vertebrate immune system comprises three levels of defense (Figure 1.5). First, there is a **physical barrier** to infection that is provided by the skin on the outer surfaces of the body, along with the mucous secretions covering the epidermal layers of the

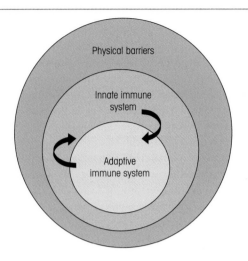

Figure 1.5. The vertebrate immune system comprises three levels of defense.

The physical barriers of the skin and mucosal surfaces comprise the first level of defense. Infectious agents that successfully penetrate the physical barriers are then engaged by the cells and soluble factors of the innate immune system. The innate immune system is also responsible for triggering activation of the adaptive immune system, as we will discuss later in this chapter. The cells and products of the adaptive immune system reinforce the defense mounted by the innate immune system.

inner surfaces of the respiratory, digestive and reproductive tracts. Any infectious agent attempting to gain entry to the body must first breach these surfaces that are largely impermeable to microorganisms; this is why cuts and scrapes that breach these physical barriers are often followed by infection. The second level of defense is provided by the **innate immune system**, a relatively broad-acting but highly effective defense layer that is largely preoccupied with trying to kill infectious agents from the moment they enter the body. The actions of the innate immune system are also responsible for alerting the cells that operate the third level of defense: the **adaptive (or acquired) immune system**. The latter cells represent the elite troops of the immune system and can launch an attack that has been specifically adapted to the nature of the infectious agent using sophisticated weapons such as antibodies.

Innate immune responses are immediate and relatively broad acting

Upon entry of a foreign entity into the body, the innate immune response occurs almost immediately. Innate immune responses do not improve upon frequent encounter with the same infectious agent. The innate immune system recognizes broadly conserved components of infectious agents, the aforementioned PAMPs, that are not normally present in the body. Upon detecting a PAMP, the innate immune system mounts an immediate attack on anything displaying such molecules by either engulfing such entities or through attacking them with

destructive enzymes, such as proteases or membrane attacking proteins (Figure 1.2). The clear intent is to bludgeon the unwanted intruder into submission as quickly as possible. This makes sense when one considers the prodigious rates of proliferation that bacteria can achieve—many bacterial species are capable of dividing every 20 minutes or so—particularly in the nutrient-rich environment our bodies provide. Key players in the innate immune response include **macrophages**, **neutrophils** and soluble bactericidal (i.e. bacterial killing) proteins such as **complement** and **lysozyme**. Although highly effective, innate immune responses are not always sufficient to completely deal with the threat, particularly if the infectious agent is well adapted to avoid the initial attack.

Adaptive immune responses are delayed but highly specific

Adaptive immune responses take longer to achieve functional significance, typically 4–5 days after the innate immune response, but are specifically tailored to the nature of the infectious agent (how this is achieved will be discussed at length in later chapters, but for now, let's not trouble ourselves with the details). Importantly, adaptive immune responses improve upon each encounter with a particular infectious agent, a feature called **immunological memory**, which underpins the concept of vaccination. The adaptive immune response is mediated primarily by **T- and B-lymphocytes** and these cells display specific receptors on their plasma membranes that can be tailored to recognize an almost limitless range of structures. By definition, molecules that are recognized by T- and B-lymphocytes are called **antigens**. Recognition of antigen by a lymphocyte triggers proliferation and differentiation of such cells and this has the effect of greatly increasing the numbers of lymphocytes capable of recognizing the particular antigen that triggered the response in the first place. This rapidly swells the ranks of lymphocytes capable of dealing with the infectious agent bearing the specific antigen and results in a **memory response** if the same antigen is encountered at some time in the future. We will look in detail at the receptors used by T- and B-cells to see antigen in Chapter 4.

Innate and adaptive immune responses are interdependent

The innate and adaptive immune systems work in tandem to identify and kill infectious agents (Figure 1.5). The innate immune system uses hard-wired (i.e. germline encoded, which means that such genes are passed in essentially identical form from parent to offspring) receptors and molecules that respond to **broad categories** of foreign molecules (i.e. PAMPs) that are commonly expressed on microorganisms. Because the receptors of the innate immune system are encoded by the germline, innate immune responses are quite similar between individuals of the same species. In contrast, the adaptive immune system uses randomly generated receptors that are **highly specific** for each infectious agent that the immune system comes into contact with. Therefore, adaptive immune responses are highly variable between individuals within a species and reflect the range of pathogens a particular individual has encountered.

Thus, when an infection occurs, **the innate immune system serves as a rapid reaction force** that deploys a range of relatively nonspecific weapons to eradicate the infectious agent, or at the very least to keep the infection contained. This gives time for the initially sluggish adaptive immune system to select and clonally expand cells with receptors that are capable of making a much more specific response that is uniquely tailored to the infectious agent. The adaptive immune response to an infectious agent reinforces and adds new weapons to the attack mounted by the innate immune system.

While it was once fashionable to view the innate immune system as somewhat crude and clumsy when compared to the relative sophistication of the adaptive immune system, an explosion of new discoveries over the past 5–10 years has revealed that the innate immune system is just as highly adapted and sophisticated as the adaptive immune system. Moreover, it has also become abundantly clear that **the adaptive immune system is highly dependent on cells of the innate immune system for the purposes of knowing when to respond, how to respond and for how long**. Exactly why this is so will be discussed later in this chapter, but for now let us consider the external barriers to infection in a little more detail.

External barriers against infection

As mentioned above, the simplest way to avoid infection is to prevent the microorganisms from gaining access to the body (Figure 1.6). When intact, the skin is impermeable to most infectious agents; when there is skin loss, as for example in burns, infection becomes a major problem. Additionally, most bacteria fail to survive for long on the skin because of the direct inhibitory effects of lactic acid and fatty acids in sweat and sebaceous secretions and the low pH that they generate. An exception is *Staphylococcus aureus*, which often infects the relatively vulnerable hair follicles and glands.

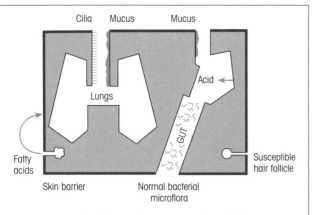

Figure 1.6. The first lines of defense against infection: protection at the external body surfaces.

Mucus, secreted by the membranes lining the inner surfaces of the body, acts as a protective barrier to block the adherence of bacteria to epithelial cells. Microbial and other foreign particles trapped within the adhesive mucus are removed by mechanical stratagems such as ciliary movement, coughing and sneezing. Among other mechanical factors that help protect the epithelial surfaces, one should also include the washing action of tears, saliva and urine. Many of the secreted body fluids contain bactericidal components, such as acid in gastric juice, spermine and zinc in semen, lactoperoxidase in milk and lysozyme in tears, nasal secretions and saliva.

A totally different mechanism is that of microbial antagonism associated with the normal bacterial flora of the body (i.e. commensal bacteria). This suppresses the growth of many potentially pathogenic bacteria and fungi at superficial sites by competition for essential nutrients or by production of inhibitory substances. To give one example, pathogen invasion is limited by lactic acid produced by particular species of commensal bacteria that metabolize glycogen secreted by the vaginal epithelium. When protective commensals are disturbed by antibiotics, susceptibility to opportunistic infections by *Candida* and *Clostridium difficile* is increased. Gut commensals may also produce colicins, a class of bactericidins that bind to the negatively charged surface of susceptible bacteria and insert a hydrophobic helical hairpin into the membrane; the molecule then undergoes a "Jekyll and Hyde" transformation to become completely hydrophobic and forms a voltage-dependent channel in the membrane that kills by destroying the cell's energy potential. Even at this level, survival is a tough game.

If microorganisms do penetrate the body, the innate immune system comes into play. Innate immunity involves two main defensive strategies to deal with a nascent infection: the destructive effect of soluble factors such as bactericidal enzymes and the mechanism of **phagocytosis**—literally "eating" by the cell (see Milestone 1.1). Before we discuss these strategies in more detail, let us first consider the stereotypical order of events that occur upon infection.

The beginnings of an immune response

A major player in the initiation of immune responses is the **macrophage**. These cells are relatively abundant in most tissues (approaching 10–15% of the total cell number in some areas of the body) and act as sentinels for infectious agent through an array of pathogen recognition receptors (PRRs) borne on their plasma membranes as well as other cellular compartments such as endosomes. Tissue macrophages are relatively quiescent cells, biding their time sampling the environment around them through continuous phagocytosis. However, upon entry of a microorganism that engages one or more of their PRRs (such as a Toll-like receptor or a NOD-like receptor), a startling transition occurs. Engagement of the PRR on the macrophage switches on a battery of genes that equip it to carry out a number of new functions.

📍 Milestone 1.1—Phagocytosis

The perceptive Russian zoologist, Elie Metchnikoff (1845–1916; Figure M1.1.1), recognized that certain specialized cells mediate defense against microbial infections (Figure M1.1.2), so fathering the whole concept of cellular immunity. He was intrigued by the motile cells of transparent starfish larvae and made the critical observation that, a few hours after the introduction of a rose thorn into these larvae, they became surrounded by these motile cells. A year later, in 1883, he observed that fungal spores can be attacked by the blood cells of *Daphnia*, a tiny metazoan that, also being transparent, can be studied directly under the microscope. He went on to extend his investigations to mammalian leukocytes, showing their ability to engulf microorganisms, a process that he termed **phagocytosis**.

Because he found this process to be even more effective in animals recovering from infection, he came to a somewhat polarized view that phagocytosis provided the main, if not the only, defense against infection. He went on to define the existence of two types of circulating phagocytes: the polymorphonuclear leukocyte, which he termed a "microphage," and the larger "macrophage."

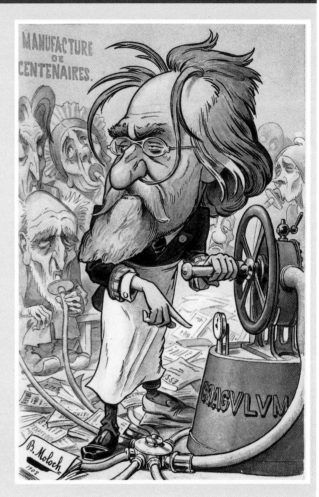

Figure M1.1.1. Caricature of Professor Metchnikoff. From *Chanteclair*, 1908, No. 4, p. 7. (Reproduction kindly provided by The Wellcome Institute Library, London, UK.)

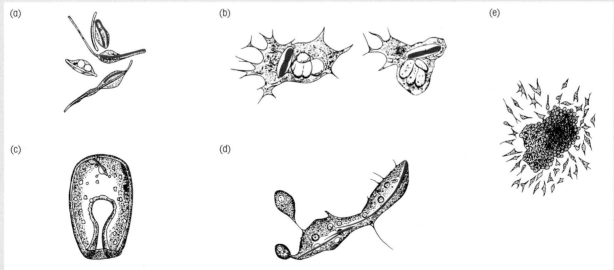

Figure M1.1.2. Reproductions of some of the illustrations in Metchnikoff's book, *Comparative Pathology of Inflammation* (1893). (a) Four leukocytes from the frog, enclosing anthrax bacilli; some are alive and unstained, others, which have been killed, have taken up the vesuvine dye and have been colored; (b) drawing of an anthrax bacillus, stained by vesuvine, in a leukocyte of the frog; the two figures represent two phases of movement of the same frog leukocyte which contains stained anthrax bacilli within its phagocytic vacuole; (c and d) a foreign body (colored) in a starfish larva surrounded by phagocytes that have fused to form a multinucleate plasmodium shown at higher power in (d); (e) this gives a feel for the dynamic attraction of the mobile mesenchymal phagocytes to a foreign intruder within a starfish larva.

First, the macrophage is put on a state of high alert (i.e. becomes activated) and is now better at engulfing and killing any microorganisms it encounters (this will be discussed in detail in the next section). Second, the macrophage begins to secrete cytokines and chemokines that have effects on nearby endothelial cells lining the blood capillaries; this makes the capillaries in this area more permeable than they would normally be. In turn, the increased vascular permeability permits two other things to happen. Plasma proteins that are normally largely restricted to blood can now invade the tissue at the point of infection and many of these proteins have microbicidal properties. A second consequence of increased vascular permeability is that another type of innate immune cell, the **neutrophil**, can now gain access to the site of infection. Neutrophils, like macrophages, are also adept at phagocytosis but are normally not permitted to enter tissues due to their potentially destructive behavior. Upon entry into an infected tissue, activated neutrophils proceed to attack and engulf any microorganisms they encounter with gusto. We will now deal with some of these events in more detail.

Pattern recognition receptors (PRRs) on phagocytic cells recognize and are activated by pathogen-associated molecular patterns (PAMPs)

Because the ability to discriminate friend from foe is of paramount importance for any self-respecting phagocyte, these cells are fairly bristling with receptors capable of recognizing diverse PAMPs. Several of these pattern recognition receptors are lectin-like and bind multivalently with considerable specificity to exposed microbial surface sugars with their characteristic rigid three-dimensional geometric configurations. They do not bind appreciably to the array of galactose or sialic acid groups that are commonly the penultimate and ultimate sugars that decorate mammalian surface polysaccharides so providing the molecular basis for discriminating between self and nonself

microbial cells. Other PRRs detect nucleic acids derived from bacterial and viral genomes by virtue of modifications not commonly found within vertebrate nucleic acids or conformations not normally found in the cytoplasm (e.g. double-stranded RNA). PRRs are a diverse group of receptors that can be subdivided into at least five distinct families (TLRs, CTLRs, NLRs, RLRs and scavenger receptors) based upon structural features. Multiple receptors also exist in each class with the result that in excess of 50 distinct PRRs may be expressed by a phagocyte at any given time. Because this topic is an area of active investigation at present, it is likely that many additional PRRs will be identified in the near future. Let us now look at the five known families of PRRs in more detail.

Toll-like receptors (TLRs)

A major subset of the PRRs belong to the class of so-called **Toll-like receptors (TLRs)** because of their similarity to the Toll receptor in the fruit fly, *Drosophila*, which in the adult triggers an intracellular cascade generating the expression of antimicrobial peptides in response to microbial infection. A series of cell surface TLRs acting as sensors for extracellular infections have been identified (Figure 1.7) that are activated by microbial elements such as peptidoglycan, lipoproteins, mycobacterial lipoarabinomannan, yeast zymosan, flagellin, as well as other pathogen-derived ligands.

Although many TLRs are displayed on the cell surface, some, such as TLR3 and TLR7/8/9 that are responsive to intracellular viral RNA and unmethylated bacterial DNA, are located in endosomes and become engaged upon encounter with phagocytosed material (Figure 1.7). Engagement of TLRs with their respective ligands drives activation of nuclear factor κB (NFκB) and several members of the interferon-regulated factor (IRF) family of transcription factors, depending on the specific TLR. Combinatorial activation of TLRs is also possible, for example TLR2 is capable of responding

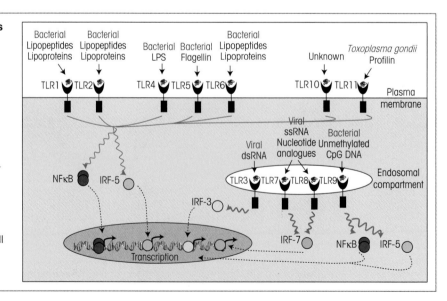

Figure 1.7. A family of Toll-like receptors (TLRs) act as sensors for pathogen-associated molecular patterns (PAMPs).

TLRs reside within plasma membrane or endosomal membrane compartments, as shown. Upon engagement of the TLR ectodomain with an appropriate PAMP (some examples are shown), signals are propagated into the cell that activate the nuclear factor κB (NFκB) and/or interferon-regulated factor (IRF) transcription factors, as shown. NFκB and IRF transcription factors then direct the expression of numerous anti-microbial gene products, such as cytokines and chemokines, as well as proteins that are involved in altering the activation state of the cell.

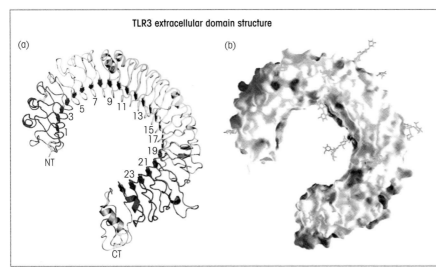

TLR3 extracellular domain structure

(a)

7 9 11
3 5 13
1 15
17
19
21
23
NT
CT

(b)

Figure 1.8. Toll-like receptor (TLR) structure.

TLR3 ectodomain structure. (a) Ribbon diagram of TLR3 ectodomain. Leucine-rich repeats (LRRs) are colored from blue to red beginning at LRR1 and proceeding to LRR23, as indicated. NT, N-terminus; CT, C-terminus. (b) Electrostatic potential surface shows positive (blue) and negative (red) charges at neutral pH. The *N*-linked glycans are shown as green ball-and-stick. (Reproduced from Bell J.K. *et al.* (2005) *Proceedings of the National Academy of Sciences USA* **102**, 10976–10980, with permission.)

to a wide diversity of PAMPs and typically functions within heterodimeric TLR2/TLR1 or TLR2/TLR6 complexes.

All TLRs have the same basic structural features, with multiple N-terminal leucine-rich repeats (LRRs) arranged in a horseshoe or crescent-shaped solenoid structure that acts as the PAMP-binding domain (Figure 1.8). Upon binding of a PAMP, TLRs transduce signals into the cell via C-terminal motifs called TIR domains which can recruit adaptor proteins within the cytoplasm (such as MyD88 or Mal) that possess similar TIR motifs. The latter adaptors propagate the signal downstream, culminating in activation of NFκB and IRF family transcription factors (Figures 1.7 and 1.9).

C-type lectin receptors (CTLRs)

Phagocytes also display another set of PRRs, the cell-bound **C-type (calcium-dependent) lectins**, of which the macrophage mannose receptor is an example. These transmembrane proteins possess multiple carbohydrate recognition domains whose engagement with their cognate microbial PAMPs generates an intracellular activation signal. The CTLR family is highly diverse and the ligands for many receptors in this category remain the subject of ongoing research.

NOD-like receptors (NLRs)

Turning now to the sensing of infectious agents that have succeeded in gaining access to the interior of a cell, microbial products can be recognized by the so-called NOD-like receptors. Unlike TLRs and CTLRs that reside within the plasma membrane or intracellular membrane compartments, NLRs are soluble proteins that reside in the cytoplasm where they also act as receptors for pathogen-derived molecular patterns. Although a diverse family of receptors, NLRs typically contain an N-terminal protein–protein interaction motif that enables these proteins to recruit proteases or kinases upon activation, followed by a central oligomerization domain and C-terminal leucine-rich repeats (LRRs) that appear to act as the sensor for

pathogen products. NLRs are thought to exist in an autoinhibited state with their N-terminal domains folded back upon their C-terminal LRRs, a conformation that prevents the N-terminal region from interacting with its binding partners in the cytoplasm. Activation of these receptors is most likely triggered through direct binding of a PAMP to the C-terminal LRRs which has the effect of disrupting the interaction between the N- and C-termini of the NLR and permits oligomerization into an complex that is now capable of recruiting either an NFκB-activating kinase (such as RIP-2) or members of the caspase family of proteases that can proteolytically process and activate the IL-1β precursor into the mature biologically active cytokine. The latter complex, called **the inflammasome**, is assembled in response to a number of PAMPs and is important for the production of IL-1β as well as IL-18.

RIG-like helicase receptors (RLRs)

The RIG-like helicases are a very recently discovered group of proteins that act as intracellular sensors for viral-derived products. Similar to the NLRs, RLRs are found in the cytoplasm and all appear to be activated in response to double-stranded RNA and are capable of directing the activation of NFκB and IRF3/4 that cooperatively induce antiviral type I interferons (IFNα and β).

Scavenger receptors

Scavenger receptors represent yet a further class of phagocytic receptors that recognize a variety of anionic polymers and acetylated low-density proteins. The role of the CD14 scavenger molecule in the handling of Gram-negative LPS (lipopolysaccharide endotoxin) merits some attention, as failure to do so can result in septic shock. The biologically reactive lipid A moiety of LPS is recognized by a plasma LPS-binding protein, and the complex that is captured by the CD14 scavenger molecule on the phagocytic cell then activates TLR4.

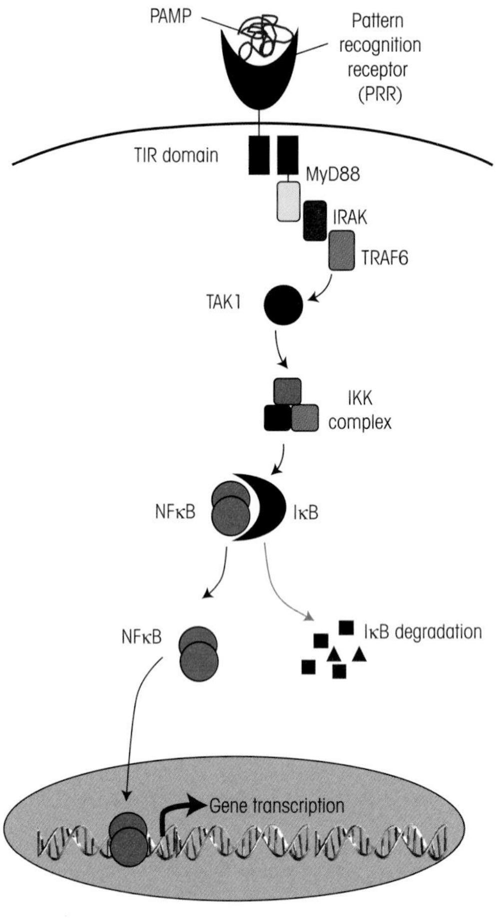

Figure 1.9. Toll-like receptors promote NFκB-dependent transcription through activation of the IκB kinase (IKK) complex.

Upon engagement of a TLR with its appropriate ligand, a series of adaptor proteins (as shown) are recruited to the TLR receptor *T*oll and *I*L-1 receptor-like (TIR) domain. Collectively, these proteins activate the IKK complex, which in turn phosphorylates the *I*nhibitor of NF*κB* (IκB), a protein that binds and tethers NFκB in the cytosol. IκB phosphorylation targets the latter for degradation, liberating NFκB which can then translocate into the nucleus and initiate transcription of multiple genes.

Pattern recognition receptor (PRR) engagement results in cell activation and pro-inflammatory cytokine production

Upon encountering ligands of any of the aforementioned PRRs, the end result is a switch in cell behavior from a quiescent state to an activated one. Activated macrophages and neutrophils are capable of phagocytosing particles that engage their PRRs and in this state they also release a range of cytokines and chemokines that amplify the immune response further.

As we have noted above, engagement of many of the above PPRs results in a signal transduction cascade culminating in activation of NFκB, a transcription factor that controls the expression of numerous immunologically important molecules such as cytokines and chemokines (Figures 1.7 and 1.9). In resting cells, NFκB is sequestered in the cytoplasm by its inhibitor IκB which masks a nuclear localization signal on the former. Upon binding of a PAMP to its cognate PRR, NFκB is liberated from IκB due to the actions of a kinase that phosphorylates IκB and promotes its destruction. NFκB is now free to translocate to the nucleus, seek out its target genes and initiate transcription (Figure 1.9).

Other transcription factor cascades, involving most notably the **interferon-regulated factors** (IRFs), are also activated downstream of the PRRs (Figure 1.7). Some of the most important inflammatory mediators synthesized and released in response to PRR engagement include the antiviral **interferons** (cf. p. 25), the small protein cytokines interleukin-1β (IL-1β), IL-6, IL-12, and tumor necrosis factor α (TNFα) (cf. p. 229), which activate other cells through binding to specific receptors, and chemokines, such as IL-8, which represent a subset of chemoattractant cytokines. Collectively, these molecules amplify the immune response further and have effects on the local blood capillaries that permit extravasation of neutrophils which come rushing into the tissue to assist the macrophage in dealing with the situation.

Dying cells also release molecules capable of engaging PRRs

As we have mentioned earlier, cells undergoing necrosis (but not apoptosis) are also capable of releasing molecules (i.e. DAMPs) that are capable of engaging PRRs (Figure 1.3). The identity of these molecules is only slowly emerging but includes HMGB1, members of the S100 calcium-binding protein family, HSP60 and the classical cytokines IL-1α and IL-33. Certain DAMPs appear to be able to bind to members of the TLR family (i.e. HMGB1 has been suggested to signal via TLR4), while others such as IL-1α and IL-33 bind to specific cell surface receptors that possess similar intracellular signaling motifs to the TLR receptors.

DAMPs are involved in amplifying immune responses to infectious agents that provoke cell death and also play a role in the phenomenon of **sterile injury**, where an immune response occurs in the absence of any discernable infectious agent (e.g. the bruising that occurs in response to a compression injury that doesn't breach the skin barrier represents an innate immune response). Indeed, Polly Matzinger has proposed that robust immune responses are only seen when nonself is detected in combination with tissue damage (i.e. a source of DAMPs). The thinking here is that the immune system does not need to respond if an infectious agent is not causing any harm. Thus, PAMPs and DAMPs may act synergistically to provoke more robust and effective immune responses than would occur in response to either alone.

Phagocytic cells engulf and kill microorganisms

Macrophages and neutrophils are dedicated "professional" phagocytes

The engulfment and digestion of microorganisms are assigned to two major cell types recognized by Elie Metchnikoff at the turn of the last century as microphages and macrophages.

The macrophage

These cells derive from bone marrow promonocytes that, after differentiation to blood monocytes (Figure 1.10a), finally settle in the tissues as mature macrophages where they constitute the **mononuclear phagocyte system** (Figure 1.11). They are present throughout the connective tissue and around the basement membrane of small blood vessels and are particularly concentrated in the lung (Figure 1.10h; alveolar macrophages), liver (Kupffer cells) and lining of spleen sinusoids and lymph node medullary sinuses where they are strategically placed to filter off foreign material. Other examples are mesangial cells in the kidney glomerulus, brain microglia and osteoclasts in bone. Unlike neutrophils, macrophages are long-lived cells with significant rough-surfaced endoplasmic reticulum and mitochondria and, whereas neutrophils provide the major defense against pyogenic (pus-forming) bacteria, as a rough generalization it may be said that macrophages are at their best in combating those bacteria (Figure 1.10g), viruses and protozoa that are capable of living within the cells of the host.

The polymorphonuclear neutrophil

This cell, the smaller of the two, shares a common hematopoietic stem cell precursor with the other formed elements of the blood and is the dominant white cell in the bloodstream. It is a non-dividing short-lived cell with a multilobed nucleus and an array of granules (Figure 1.12), which are virtually unstained by histologic dyes such as hematoxylin and eosin, unlike those structures in the closely related eosinophil and basophil (Figure 1.10c and 1.10i). These neutrophil granules are of two main types: (i) the **primary azurophil granule** that develops early (Figure 1.10e), has the typical lysosomal morphology and contains myeloperoxidase together with most of the nonoxidative antimicrobial effectors including defensins, bactericidal permeability increasing (BPI) protein and cathepsin G (Figure 1.12); and (ii) the peroxidase-negative **secondary specific granules** containing lactoferrin, much of the lysozyme, alkaline phosphatase (Figure 1.10d) and membrane-bound cytochrome b_{558} (Figure 1.12). The abundant glycogen stores can be utilized by glycolysis enabling the cells to function under anerobic conditions.

Microbes are engulfed by activated phagocytic cells

After adherence of the microbe to the surface of the neutrophil or macrophage through recognition of a PAMP (Figure 1.13.2),

the resulting signal (Figure 1.13.3) initiates the ingestion phase by activating an actin–myosin contractile system that extends pseudopods around the particle (Figures 1.13.4 and 1.14); as adjacent receptors sequentially attach to the surface of the microbe, the plasma membrane is pulled around the particle just like a "zipper" until it is completely enclosed in a vacuole (phagosome; Figures 1.13.5 and 1.14). Events are now moving smartly and, within 1 minute, the cytoplasmic granules fuse with the phagosome and discharge their contents around the imprisoned microorganism (Figures 1.13.7 and 1.15) which is subject to a formidable battery of microbicidal mechanisms.

There is an array of killing mechanisms

Killing by reactive oxygen intermediates

Trouble starts for the invader from the moment phagocytosis is initiated. There is a dramatic increase in activity of the hexose monophosphate shunt generating reduced nicotinamide adenine dinucleotide phosphate (NADPH). Electrons pass from the NADPH to a flavine adenine dinucleotide (FAD)-containing membrane flavoprotein and thence to a unique plasma membrane **cytochrome (cyt b_{558})**. This has the very low midpoint redox potential of −245 mV that allows it to reduce molecular oxygen directly to superoxide anion (Figure 1.16a). Thus the key reaction catalyzed by this NADPH oxidase, which initiates the formation of reactive oxygen intermediates (ROI), is:

$$NADPH + O_2 \rightarrow NADP^+ + \cdot O_2^-$$

$$(\text{superoxide anion}).$$

The superoxide anion undergoes conversion to hydrogen peroxide under the influence of superoxide dismutase, and subsequently to hydroxyl radicals ($\cdot OH$). Each of these products has remarkable chemical reactivity with a wide range of molecular targets, making them formidable microbicidal agents; $\cdot OH$ in particular is one of the most reactive free radicals known. Furthermore, the combination of peroxide, myeloperoxidase and halide ions constitutes a potent halogenating system capable of killing both bacteria and viruses (Figure 1.16a). Although H_2O_2 and the halogenated compounds are not as active as the free radicals, they are more stable and therefore diffuse further, making them toxic to microorganisms in the extracellular vicinity.

Killing by reactive nitrogen intermediates

Nitric oxide surfaced prominently as a physiologic mediator when it was shown to be identical with endothelium-derived relaxing factor. This has proved to be just one of its many roles (including the mediation of penile erection, would you believe it!), but of major interest in the present context is its formation by an inducible NO· synthase (iNOS) within most cells, but particularly macrophages and human neutrophils, thereby generating a powerful antimicrobial system (Figure 1.16b).

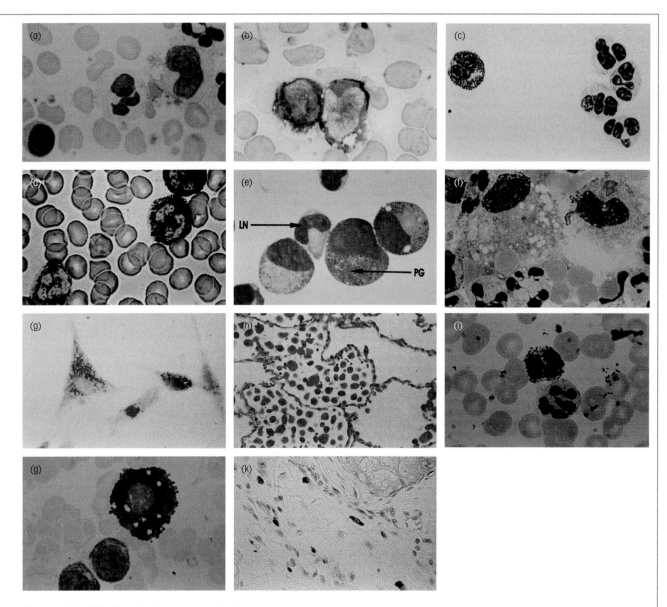

Figure 1.10. Cells involved in innate immunity.

(a) Monocyte, showing "horseshoe-shaped" nucleus and moderately abundant pale cytoplasm. Note the three multilobed polymorphonuclear neutrophils and the small lymphocyte (bottom left). Romanowsky stain. (b) Two monocytes stained for nonspecific esterase with α-naphthyl acetate. Note the vacuolated cytoplasm. The small cell with focal staining at the top is a T-lymphocyte. (c) Four polymorphonuclear neutrophils and one eosinophil. The multilobed nuclei and the cytoplasmic granules are clearly shown, those of the eosinophil being heavily stained. (d) Polymorphonuclear neutrophil showing cytoplasmic granules stained for alkaline phosphatase. (e) Early neutrophils in bone marrow. The primary azurophilic granules (PG), originally clustered near the nucleus, move towards the periphery where the neutrophil-specific granules are generated by the Golgi apparatus as the cell matures. The nucleus gradually becomes lobular (LN). Giemsa. (f) Inflammatory cells from the site of a brain hemorrhage showing the large active macrophage in the center with phagocytosed red cells and prominent vacuoles. To the right is a monocyte with horseshoe-shaped nucleus and cytoplasmic bilirubin crystals (hematoidin). Several multilobed neutrophils are clearly delineated. Giemsa. (g) Macrophages in monolayer cultures after phagocytosis of mycobacteria (stained red). Carbol-fuchsin counterstained with malachite green. (h) Numerous plump alveolar macrophages within air spaces in the lung. (i) Basophil with heavily staining granules compared with a neutrophil (below). (j) Mast cell from bone marrow. Round central nucleus surrounded by large darkly staining granules. Two small red cell precursors are shown at the bottom. Romanowsky stain. (k) Tissue mast cells in skin stained with toluidine blue. The intracellular granules are metachromatic and stain reddish purple. Note the clustering in relation to dermal capillaries. (The slides from which illustrations (a), (b), (d–f), (i) and (j) were reproduced were very kindly provided by Mr. M. Watts of the Department of Haematology, Middlesex Hospital Medical School; (c) was kindly supplied by Professor J.J. Owen; (g) by Professors P. Lydyard and G. Rook; (h) by Dr. Meryl Griffiths; and (k) by Professor N. Woolf.)

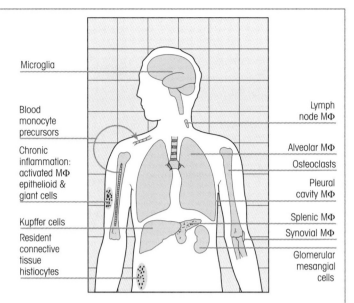

Figure 1.11. The mononuclear phagocyte system.

Promonocyte precursors in the bone marrow develop into circulating blood monocytes that eventually become distributed throughout the body as mature macrophages (Mφ) as shown. The other major phagocytic cell, the polymorphonuclear neutrophil, is largely confined to the bloodstream except when recruited into sites of acute inflammation.

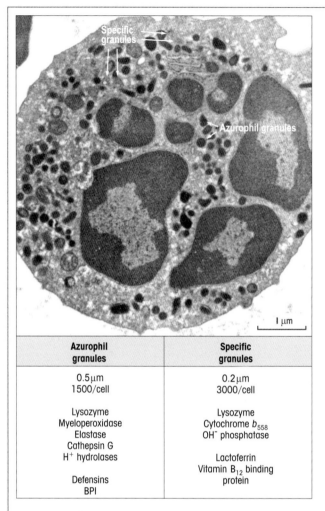

Azurophil granules	Specific granules
0.5 μm 1500/cell	0.2 μm 3000/cell
Lysozyme Myeloperoxidase Elastase Cathepsin G H⁺ hydrolases	Lysozyme Cytochrome b_{558} OH⁻ phosphatase
Defensins BPI	Lactoferrin Vitamin B_{12} binding protein

Figure 1.12. Ultrastructure of neutrophil.

The multilobed nucleus and two main types of cytoplasmic granules are well displayed. (Courtesy of Dr. D. McLaren.)

Whereas the NADPH oxidase is dedicated to the killing of extracellular organisms taken up by phagocytosis and cornered within the phagocytic vacuole, the NO· mechanism can operate against microbes that invade the cytosol; so, it is not surprising that the majority of nonphagocytic cells that may be infected by viruses and other parasites are endowed with an iNOS capability. The mechanism of action may be through degradation of the Fe–S prosthetic groups of certain electron transport enzymes, depletion of iron and production of toxic ·ONOO radicals. The *N-ramp* gene, linked with resistance to microbes such as bacille Calmette–Guérin (BCG), *Salmonella* and *Leishmania* that can live within an intracellular habitat, is now known to express a protein forming a transmembrane channel that may be involved in transporting NO· across lysosome membranes.

Killing by preformed antimicrobials (Figure 1.16c)

These molecules, contained within the neutrophil granules, contact the ingested microorganism when fusion with the phagosome occurs. The dismutation of superoxide consumes hydrogen ions and raises the pH of the vacuole gently, so allowing the family of cationic proteins and peptides to function optimally. The latter, known as **defensins**, are approximately 3.5–4 kDa and invariably rich in arginine, and reach incredibly high concentrations within the phagosome, of the order of 20–100 mg/ml. Like the bacterial colicins described

above, they have an amphipathic structure that allows them to insert into microbial membranes to form destabilizing voltage-regulated ion channels (who copied whom?). These antibiotic peptides, at concentrations of 10–100 μg/ml, act as disinfectants against a wide spectrum of Gram-positive and Gram-negative bacteria, many fungi and a number of enveloped viruses. Many exhibit remarkable selectivity for prokaryotic and eukaryotic microbes relative to host cells, partly dependent upon differential membrane lipid composition. One must be impressed by the ability of this surprisingly simple tool to discriminate large classes of nonself cells, i.e. microbes, from self.

As if this was not enough, further damage is inflicted on the bacterial membranes both by neutral protease (cathepsin G) action and by direct transfer to the microbial surface of BPI, which increases bacterial permeability. Low pH, lysozyme and lactoferrin constitute bactericidal or bacteriostatic factors

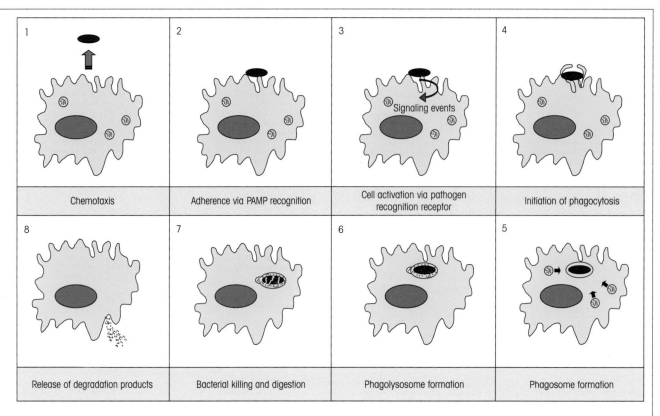

1	2	3	4
Chemotaxis	Adherence via PAMP recognition	Cell activation via pathogen recognition receptor	Initiation of phagocytosis

8	7	6	5
Release of degradation products	Bacterial killing and digestion	Phagolysosome formation	Phagosome formation

Figure 1.13. Phagocytosis and killing of a bacterium.

Stage 3/4, respiratory burst and activation of NADPH oxidase; stage 5, damage by reactive oxygen intermediates; stage 6/7, damage by peroxidase, cationic proteins, antibiotic peptide defensins, lysozyme and lactoferrin.

Figure 1.14. Adherence and phagocytosis.

(a) Phagocytosis of *Candida albicans* by a polymorphonuclear leukocyte (neutrophil). Adherence to the yeast wall surface mannan initiates enclosure of the fungal particle within arms of cytoplasm. Lysosomal granules are abundant but mitochondria are rare (×15000). (b) Phagocytosis of *C. albicans* by a monocyte showing near completion of phagosome formation (arrowed) around one organism and complete ingestion of two others (×5000). (Courtesy of Dr. H. Valdimarsson.)

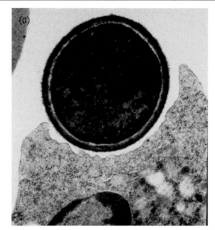
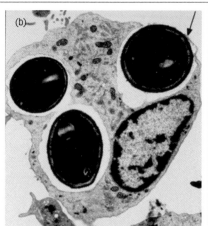

that are oxygen independent and can function under anerobic circumstances. Interestingly, lysozyme and lactoferrin are synergistic in their action. Finally, the killed organisms are digested by hydrolytic enzymes and the degradation products released to the exterior (Figure 1.13.8).

By now, the reader may be excused a little smugness as she or he shelters behind the impressive antimicrobial potential of the phagocytic cells. But there are snags to consider; our formidable array of weaponry is useless unless the phagocyte can: (i) "home onto" the microorganism; (ii) adhere to it; and (iii) respond by the membrane activation that initiates engulfment. Some bacteria do produce chemical substances, such as the peptide formyl.Met.Leu.Phe, which directionally attract leukocytes, a process known as **chemotaxis**; many organisms do

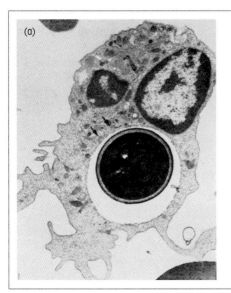
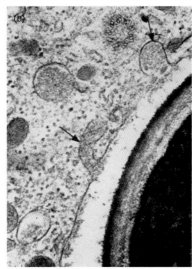

Figure 1.15. Phagolysosome formation.

(a) Neutrophil 30 minutes after ingestion of *C. albicans*. The cytoplasm is already partly degranulated and two lysosomal granules (arrowed) are fusing with the phagocytic vacuole. Two lobes of the nucleus are evident (×5000). (b) Higher magnification of (a) showing fusing granules discharging their contents into the phagocytic vacuole (arrowed) (×33 000). (Courtesy of Dr. H. Valdimarsson.)

adhere to the phagocyte surface and many do spontaneously provide the appropriate membrane initiation signal. However, our teeming microbial adversaries are continually mutating to produce new species that may outwit the defenses by doing none of these. What then? The body has solved these problems with the effortless ease that comes with a few million years of evolution by developing the **complement** system.

Complement facilitates phagocytosis and bacterial lysis

The complement system comprises a group of some 20 or so plasma proteins that becomes activated in a cascade-like manner upon binding to certain microbial polysaccharides that are not normally present in vertebrates, but are commonly found on bacterial membranes. Many of the complement factors are proteases that are initially produced as inactive precursors and become activated through the detection of PAMPs, with each protease activating the next in the chain. Complement activation can result in binding of complement to bacterial cell surfaces (called **opsonization** in immunological parlance), which can greatly enhance their uptake by phagocytes. Deposition of complement factors onto its surface can also result in **direct lysis** of a bacterium that has had the misfortune to trigger this cascade. Just as importantly, certain complement fragments that are produced as byproducts of complement activation can act as **chemotactic factors** to guide phagocytic cells (such as neutrophils and macrophages) to the hapless bacterium, resulting in its capture through phagocytosis. The latter complement factors can also **activate local mast cells** (which we will discuss in more detail shortly) to release molecules that help to recruit neutrophils and other cells of the immune system to the site of infection, through increasing the permeability of local blood vessels. Either way, complement activation spells trouble for our little bacterial foe. Due to the many pro-

teins involved, the complement system can initially appear daunting, but do keep in mind the overall objectives of enhancing phagocytosis, recruitment of other immune cells and direct lysis of microorganisms, as we proceed through the details.

Complement and its activation

The complement cascade, along with blood clotting, fibrinolysis and kinin formation, forms one of the triggered enzyme systems found in plasma. These systems characteristically produce a rapid, highly amplified response to a trigger stimulus mediated by a cascade phenomenon where the product of one reaction is the enzymic catalyst of the next.

Some of the complement components are designated by the letter "C" followed by a number that is related more to the chronology of its discovery than to its position in the reaction sequence. The most abundant and the most pivotal component is C3, which has a molecular weight of 195 kDa and is present in plasma at a concentration of around 1.2 mg/ml.

C3 undergoes slow spontaneous cleavage

Under normal circumstances, an internal thiolester bond in C3 (Figure 1.17) becomes activated spontaneously at a very slow rate, either through reaction with water or with trace amounts of a plasma proteolytic enzyme, to form a reactive intermediate, either the split product C3b, or a functionally similar molecule designated C3i or $C3(H_2O)$. In the presence of Mg^{2+} this can complex with another complement component, factor B, which then undergoes cleavage by a normal plasma enzyme (factor D) to generate $C3b\overline{Bb}$. Note that, conventionally, a bar over a complex denotes enzymic activity and that, on cleavage of a complement component, the larger product is generally given the suffix "b" and the smaller "a."

$C3b\overline{Bb}$ has an important new enzymic activity: it is a **C3 convertase** that can split C3 to give C3a and C3b. We will

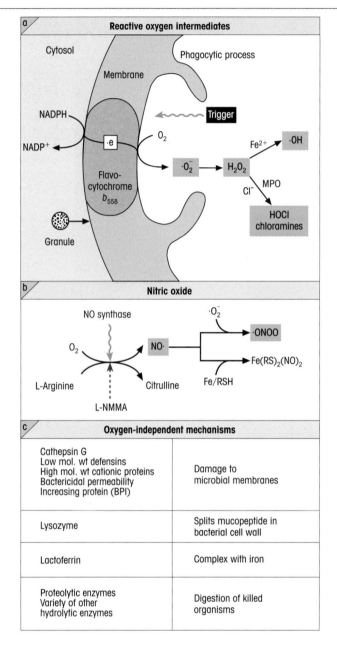

Figure 1.16. Microbicidal mechanisms of phagocytic cells.

(a) Production of reactive oxygen intermediates. Electrons from NADPH are transferred by the flavocytochrome oxidase enzyme to molecular oxygen to form the microbicidal molecular species shown in the orange boxes. (*For the more studious*—the phagocytosis triggering agent binds to a classic G-protein-linked seven transmembrane domain receptor that activates an intracellular guanosine triphosphate (GTP)-binding protein. This in turn activates an array of enzymes: phosphoinositol-3 kinase concerned in the cytoskeletal reorganization underlying chemotactic responses (p. 16), phospholipase-Cγ2 mediating events leading to lysosome degranulation and phosphorylation of p47 phox through activation of protein kinase C, and the MEK and MAP kinase systems (cf. Figure 8.8) that oversee the assembly of the NADPH oxidase. This is composed of the membrane cytochrome b_{558}, consisting of a p21 heme protein linked to gp91 with binding sites for NADPH and FAD on its intracellular aspect, to which phosphorylated p47 and p67 translocate from the cytosol on activation of the oxidase.) (b) Generation of nitric oxide. The enzyme, which structurally resembles the NADPH oxidase, can be inhibited by the arginine analog N-monomethyl-L-arginine (L-NMMA). The combination of NO· with superoxide anion yields the highly toxic peroxynitrite radical ·ONOO that cleaves on protonation to form reactive ·OH and NO_2 molecules. NO· can form mononuclear iron dithioldinitroso complexes leading to iron depletion and inhibition of several enzymes. (c) The basis of oxygen-independent antimicrobial systems.

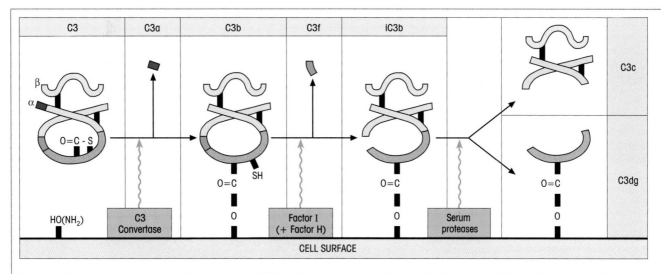

Figure 1.17. Structural basis for the cleavage of C3 by C3 convertase and its covalent binding to ·OH or ·NH$_2$ groups at the cell surface through exposure of the internal thiolester bonds.

Further cleavage leaves the progressively smaller fragments, C3dg and C3d, attached to the membrane. (Based essentially on

Law S.H.A. & Reid K.B.M. (1988) *Complement*, Figure 2.4. IRL Press, Oxford.)

shortly discuss the important biological consequences of C3 cleavage in relation to microbial defenses, but under normal conditions there must be some mechanism to restrain this process to a "tick-over" level as it can also give rise to more C3bBb, that is, we are dealing with a potentially runaway **positive-feedback loop** (Figure 1.18). As with all potentially explosive triggered cascades, there are powerful regulatory mechanisms.

C3b levels are normally tightly controlled

In solution, the C3bBb convertase is unstable and factor B is readily displaced by another component, factor H, to form C3bH, which is susceptible to attack by the C3b inactivator, factor I (Figure 1.18; further discussed on p. 373). The inactivated iC3b is biologically inactive and undergoes further degradation by proteases in the body fluids. Other regulatory mechanisms are discussed at a later stage (see p. 373).

C3 convertase is stabilized on microbial surfaces

A number of microorganisms can activate the C3bBb convertase to generate large amounts of C3 cleavage products **by stabilizing the enzyme on their (carbohydrate) surfaces**, thereby protecting the C3b from factor H. Another protein, properdin, acts subsequently on this bound convertase to stabilize it even further. As C3 is split by the surface membrane-bound enzyme to nascent C3b, it undergoes conformational change and its potentially reactive internal thiolester bond becomes exposed. As the half-life of nascent C3b is less than 100 microseconds, it can only diffuse a short distance before reacting covalently with local hydroxyl or amino groups available at the microbial cell surface (Figure 1.17). Each catalytic site thereby leads to the

clustering of large numbers of C3b molecules on the microorganism. This series of reactions leading to C3 breakdown provoked directly by microbes has been called **the alternative pathway** of complement activation (Figure 1.18).

The post-C3 pathway generates a membrane attack complex

Recruitment of a further C3b molecule into the C3bBb enzymic complex generates a C5 convertase that activates C5 by proteolytic cleavage releasing a small polypeptide, C5a, and leaving the large C5b fragment loosely bound to C3b. Sequential attachment of C6 and C7 to C5b forms a complex with a transient membrane-binding site and an affinity for the β-peptide chain of C8. The C8α chain sits in the membrane and directs the conformational changes in C9 that transform it into an amphipathic molecule capable of insertion into the lipid bilayer (cf. the colicins, p. 8) and polymerization to an annular **membrane attack complex** (MAC; Figures 1.19 and 2.4). This forms a transmembrane channel fully permeable to electrolytes and water, and due to the high internal colloid osmotic pressure of cells, there is a net influx of Na$^+$ and water frequently leading to lysis.

Complement has a range of defensive biological functions

These can be grouped conveniently under three headings:

1 **C3b adheres to complement receptors**
Phagocytic cells have receptors for C3b (CR1) and iC3b (CR3) that facilitate the adherence of C3b-coated microorganisms to the cell surface (discussed more fully on p. 323).

Figure 1.18. Microbial activation of the alternative complement pathway by stabilization of the C3 convertase (C3bBb), and its control by factors H and I.

When bound to the surface of a host cell or in the fluid phase, the C3b in the convertase is said to be "unprotected" in that its affinity for factor H is much greater than for factor B and is therefore susceptible to breakdown by factors H and I. On a microbial surface, C3b binds factor B more strongly than factor H and is therefore "protected" from or "stabilized" against cleavage—even more so when subsequently bound by properdin. Although in phylogenetic terms this is the oldest complement pathway, it was discovered after a separate pathway to be discussed in the next chapter, and so has the confusing designation "alternative." ⤳ represents an activation process. The horizontal bar above a component designates its activation.

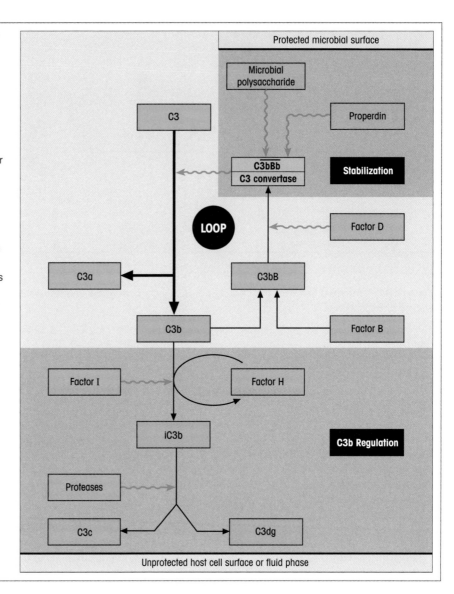

2 Biologically active fragments are released

C3a and C5a, the small peptides split from the parent molecules during complement activation, have several important actions. Both act directly on phagocytes, especially neutrophils, to stimulate the respiratory burst associated with the production of reactive oxygen intermediates and to enhance the expression of surface receptors for C3b and iC3b. Also, both are **anaphylatoxins** in that they are capable of triggering mediator release from mast cells (Figures 1.10k and 1.20) and their circulating counterpart, the basophil (Figure 1.10i), a phenomenon of such relevance to our present discussion that we have presented details of the mediators and their actions in Figure 1.21; note in particular the chemotactic properties of these mediators and their effects on blood vessels. In its own right, C3a is a chemoattractant for eosinophils whereas C5a is a potent neutrophil chemotactic agent and also has a striking ability to act directly on the capillary endothelium to produce vasodilatation and increased permeability, an effect that seems to be prolonged by leukotriene B$_4$ released from activated mast cells, neutrophils and macrophages.

3 The terminal complex can induce membrane lesions

As described above, the insertion of the membrane attack complex into a membrane may bring about cell lysis. Providentially, complement is relatively inefficient at lysing the cell membranes of the autologous host due to the presence of control proteins (cf. p. 373).

We can now put together an effectively orchestrated defensive scenario initiated by activation of the alternative complement pathway.

In the first act, C3bBb is stabilized on the surface of the microbe and cleaves large amounts of C3. The C3a fragment is released but C3b molecules bind copiously to the microbe. These activate the next step in the sequence to generate C5a and the membrane attack complex (although many organisms will be resistant to its action).

The inflammatory response

Inflammation is the term given to the series of events that surround an immune response and display a number of characteristic features including: local swelling (edema), redness (due to capillary dilation), pain and heat. These features are the collective consequence of the release of cytokines, chemokines, complement fragments and vasoactive amines from macrophages and mast cells upon the initial encounter with a pathogen. All of these inflammatory mediators help to recruit neutrophils as well as plasma proteins to the site of infection by inducing vasodilation of the blood vessels close to the site of infection and by acting as chemotactic factors for neutrophils circulating in blood. The extra cells and fluid that gather at the site of an infection (which contribute to the swelling seen), the increased redness of skin tone in the area and associated tenderness constitute the classic inflammatory reaction.

Mast cells and macrophages initiate inflammation

As we have already alluded to above, the macrophage plays a key role in the initiation of an inflammatory response through the secretion of cytokines and chemokines in response to engagement of its PRRs and through encounter with C3b-opsonized microbes (Figure 1.22). However, another innate immune cell, the **mast cell**, is instrumental in provoking increased permeability of blood vessels due to release of the contents of the numerous cytoplasmic granules that such cells possess (Figure 1.21). Mast cell granules contain, among other factors, copious amounts of the vasoactive amino acid histamine (Figure 1.21). Mast cell degranulation can be provoked by direct injury, in response to C3a and C5a complement components, encounter with PAMPs and through binding of specific antigen to a class of antibody (IgE) that binds avidly to mast cells via surface receptors (we will discuss antibody classes at length in Chapter 3). Histamine provokes dilation of post-capillary venules, activates the local endothelium and increases blood vessel permeability. Irritation of nerve endings is another consequence of histamine release and is responsible for the pain often associated with inflammation, an evolutionary adaptation that most likely encourages the host to protect the infected or injured area to minimize further damage.

The relaxation induced in arteriolar walls causes increased blood flow and dilatation of the small vessels, while contraction of capillary endothelial cells allows exudation of plasma proteins. Under the influence of the chemotaxins, neutrophils slow down and the surface adhesion molecules they are stimulated to express cause them to marginate to the walls of the capillaries where they pass through gaps between the endothelial cells (diapedesis) and move up the concentration gradient of chemotactic factors until they come face to face

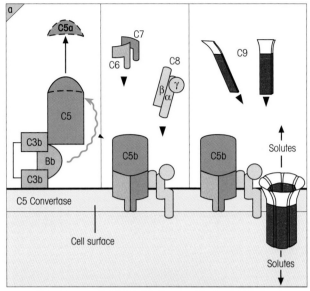
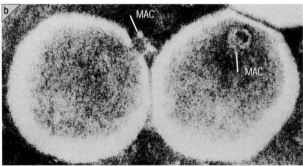

Figure 1.19. Post-C3 pathway generating C5a and the C5b–9 membrane attack complex (MAC).

(a) Cartoon of molecular assembly. The conformational change in C9 protein structure that converts it from a hydrophilic to an amphipathic molecule (bearing both hydrophobic and hydrophilic regions) can be interrupted by an antibody raised against linear peptides derived from C9; as the antibody does not react with the soluble or membrane-bound forms of the molecule, it must be detecting an intermediate structure transiently revealed in a deep-seated structural rearrangement. (b) Electron micrograph of a membrane C5b–9 complex incorporated into liposomal membranes clearly showing the annular structure. The cylindrical complex is seen from the side inserted into the membrane of the liposome on the left, and end-on in that on the right. Although in itself a rather splendid structure, formation of the annular C9 cylinder is probably not essential for cytotoxic perturbation of the target cell membrane, as this can be achieved by insertion of amphipathic C9 molecules in numbers too few to form a clearly defined MAC. (Courtesy of Professor J. Tranum-Jensen and Dr. S. Bhakdi.)

Figure 1.20. The mast cell.

(a) A resting cell with many membrane-bound granules containing preformed mediators. (b) A triggered mast cell. Note that the granules have released their contents and are morphologically altered, being larger and less electron dense. Although most of the altered granules remain within the circumference of the cell, they are open to the extracellular space. (Electron micrographs ×5400.) (Courtesy of Drs. D. Lawson, C. Fewtrell, B. Gomperts and M.C. Raff from (1975) *Journal of Experimental Medicine* **142**, 391.)

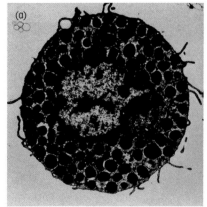 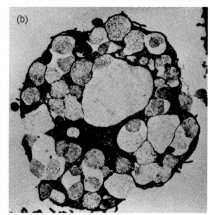

Figure 1.21. Mast cell triggering leading to release of mediators by two major pathways.

(i) Release of preformed mediators present in the granules; and (ii) the metabolism of arachidonic acid produced through activation of a phospholipase. Intracellular Ca^{2+} and cyclic AMP are central to the initiation of these events but details are still unclear. Mast cell triggering may occur through C3a, C5a and even by some microorganisms that can act directly on cell surface receptors. Mast cell heterogeneity is discussed on p. 395. ECF, eosinophil chemotactic factor; GM-CSF, granulocyte–macrophage colony-stimulating factor; NCF, neutrophil chemotactic factor; TNF, tumor necrosis factor. Chemotaxis refers to directed migration of granulocytes up the pathway concentration gradient of the mediator.

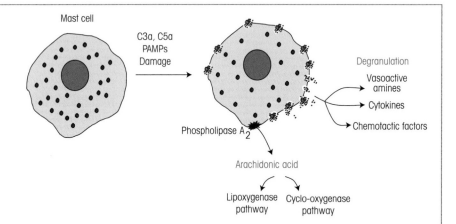

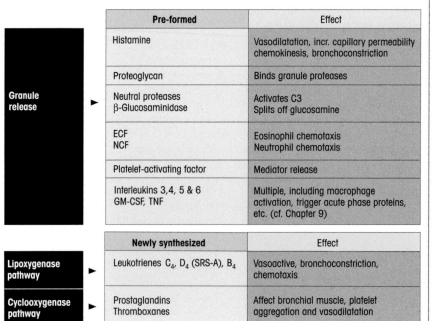

Pre-formed	Effect
Histamine	Vasodilatation, incr. capillary permeability chemokinesis, bronchoconstriction
Proteoglycan	Binds granule proteases
Neutral proteases β-Glucosaminidase	Activates C3 Splits off glucosamine
ECF NCF	Eosinophil chemotaxis Neutrophil chemotaxis
Platelet-activating factor	Mediator release
Interleukins 3,4, 5 & 6 GM-CSF, TNF	Multiple, including macrophage activation, trigger acute phase proteins, etc. (cf. Chapter 9)

Newly synthesized	Effect
Leukotrienes C_4, D_4 (SRS-A), B_4	Vasoactive, bronchoconstriction, chemotaxis
Prostaglandins Thromboxanes	Affect bronchial muscle, platelet aggregation and vasodilatation

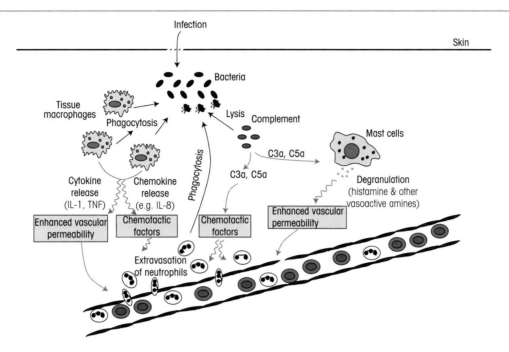

Figure 1.22. The acute inflammatory reaction.

Bacterial infection initiates a series of responses through activation of the alternative complement pathway, producing C3a and C5a, as well through stimulation of tissue-resident macrophages that detect bacterial-derived PAMPs. The C3b component of complement binds to bacteria, opsonizing the latter for more effective phagocytosis by macrophages and neutrophils. Complement activation can also lead to direct lysis of bacteria through assembly of membrane attack complexes. Activation of macrophages by PAMPs and complement components induces secretion of mediators (i.e. cytokines and chemokines) of the acute inflammatory response that increase vascular permeability and induce neutrophils to migrate from the blood into the tissue. C3a and C5a trigger mast cell activation and secretion of mediators that provoke capillary dilatation and exudation of plasma proteins. Attracted by C3a and C5a, as well as other factors, blood neutrophils stick to the adhesion molecules on the endothelial cell and use this to provide traction as they force their way between the cells, through the basement membrane (with the help of secreted elastase) and up the chemotactic gradient.

with the C3b-coated microbe. Adherence to the neutrophil C3b receptors then takes place, C3a and C5a (the byproducts of complement activation discussed above) at relatively high concentrations in the chemotactic gradient activate the respiratory burst and, hey presto, the slaughter of the last act can begin!

Humoral mechanisms provide a second defensive strategy

Microbicidal factors in secretions

Turning now to those defense systems that are mediated entirely by **soluble pattern recognition molecules** (Figure 1.2), we recollect that many microbes activate the complement system and may be lysed by the insertion of the membrane attack complex. The spread of infection may be limited by enzymes released through tissue injury that activate the clotting system. Of the soluble bactericidal substances elaborated by the body, perhaps the most abundant and widespread is the enzyme lysozyme, a muramidase that splits the exposed peptidoglycan wall of susceptible bacteria (cf. Figure 12.5).

Like the α-defensins of the neutrophil granules, the human β-defensins are peptides derived by proteolytic cleavage from larger precursors; they have β-sheet structures, 29–40 amino acids and three intramolecular disulfide bonds, although they differ from the α-defensins in the placement of their six cysteines. The main human β-defensin, hDB-1, is produced abundantly in the kidney, the female reproductive tract, the oral gingiva and especially the lung airways. As the word has it that we are all infected every day by tens of thousands of airborne bacteria, this must be an important defense mechanism. This being so, inhibition of hDB-1 and of a second pulmonary defensin, hDB-2, by high ionic strength could account for the susceptibility of cystic fibrosis patients to infection as they have an ion channel mutation that results in an elevated chloride concentration in airway surface fluids. Another airway antimicrobial active against Gram-negative and Gram-positive bacteria is LL-37, a 37-residue α-helical peptide released by proteolysis of a cathelicidin (cathepsin L-inhibitor) precursor.

This theme surfaces again in the stomach where a peptide split from lactoferrin by pepsin could provide the gastric and intestinal secretions with some antimicrobial policing. A rather longer two-domain peptide with 107 residues, termed secretory leukocyte protease inhibitor (SLPI), is found in many human secretions. The C-terminal domain is anti-protease but the N-terminal domain is distinctly unpleasant to metabolically active fungal cells and to various skin-associated microorganisms, which makes its production by human keratinocytes particularly appropriate. In passing, it is worth pointing out that many D-amino acid analogs of peptide antibiotics form left-handed helices that retain the ability to induce membrane ion channels and hence their antimicrobial powers and, given their resistance to catabolism within the body, should be attractive candidates for a new breed of synthetic antibiotics. Lastly, we may mention the two lung surfactant proteins SP-A and SP-D that, in conjunction with various lipids, lower the surface tension of the epithelial lining cells of the lung to keep the airways patent. They belong to a totally different structural group of molecules termed collectins (see below) that contribute to innate immunity through binding of their lectin-like domains to carbohydrates on microbes, and their collagenous stem to cognate receptors on phagocytic cells—thereby facilitating the ingestion and killing of the infectious agents.

Acute phase proteins increase in response to infection

A number of plasma proteins collectively termed acute phase proteins show a dramatic increase in concentration in response to early "alarm" mediators such as macrophage-derived interleukin-1 (IL-1) released as a result of infection or tissue injury. These include C-reactive protein (CRP), mannose-binding lectin (MBL) and serum amyloid P component (Table 1.1).

Table 1.1. Acute phase proteins.

Acute phase reactant	Role
Dramatic increases in concentration:	
C-reactive protein	Fixes complement, opsonizes
Mannose binding lectin	Fixes complement, opsonizes
α_1-Acid glycoprotein	Transport protein
Serum amyloid P component	Amyloid component precursor
Moderate increases in concentration:	
α_1-Protease inhibitors	Inhibit bacterial proteases
α_1-Antichymotrypsin	Inhibit bacterial proteases
C3, C9, factor B	Increase complement function
Ceruloplasmin	$\cdot O_2^-$ scavenger
Fibrinogen	Coagulation
Angiotensin	Blood pressure
Haptoglobin	Bind hemoglobin
Fibronectin	Cell attachment

Expression levels of the latter proteins can increase by as much as 1000-fold in response to pro-inflammatory cytokines such as IL-1 and IL-6. Other acute phase proteins showing a more modest rise in concentration include α_1-antichymotrypsin, fibrinogen, ceruloplasmin, C9 and factor B.

The acute phase proteins are a relatively diverse group of proteins belonging to several different families (including, but not limited to, the **pentraxin**, **collectin** and **ficolin** families) that have a number of functional effects in common. All of these proteins act as soluble pattern recognition molecules and are capable of binding directly to infectious agents to function as opsonins (i.e. "made ready for the table"), thereby enhancing uptake of microorganisms by macrophages and neutrophils. Many of these proteins also have the ability to activate complement and the assembly of a membrane attack complex. The ability to agglutinate microorganisms, thereby impeding their spread within the infected tissue, is another common theme. Some of these molecules can also form heterocomplexes that extend the range of PAMPs that can be detected.

These soluble pattern recognition molecules are frequently synthesized by activated macrophages upon stimulation of their pattern-recognition receptors, or are stored within neutrophil granules available for immediate release via degranulation in response to infection. The liver is another major source of many acute phase proteins that are released into the circulation as a result of the systemic effects of the major pro-inflammatory cytokines IL-1 and IL-6. Let us look at some examples further.

Pentraxins

Pentraxins (so called because these agents are made up of five identical subunits) constitute a superfamily of conserved proteins typified by a cyclic multimeric structure and a C-terminal 200 amino acid long pentraxin domain. CRP, serum amyloid P component (SAP) and pentraxin 3 are members of this family. Human CRP is composed of five identical polypeptide units noncovalently arranged as a cyclic pentamer around a calcium (Ca)-binding cavity, was the first pentraxin to be described, and is the prototypic acute phase response protein. Pentraxins have been around in the animal kingdom for some time, as a closely related homolog, limulin, is present in the hemolymph of the horseshoe crab, not exactly a close relative of *Homo sapiens*. A major property of CRP is its ability to bind in a Ca-dependent fashion, as a pattern recognition molecule, to a number of microorganisms that contain phosphorylcholine in their membranes, the complex having the useful property of activating complement (by the classical and not the alternative pathway with which we are at present familiar). This results in the deposition of C3b on the surface of the microbe that thus becomes opsonized for adherence to phagocytes.

SAP can complex with chondroitin sulfate, a cell matrix glycosaminoglycan, and subsequently bind lysosomal enzymes such as cathepsin B released within a focus of inflammation. The degraded SAP becomes a component of the amyloid fibrillar deposits that accompany chronic infections—it might even be a key initiator of amyloid deposition. SAP also binds several bacterial species via LPS and, similar to CRP, can also activate the classical complement pathway. CRP and SAP represent the main acute phase reactants in human and mouse, respectively.

Collectins

Nine members of the collectin family have been described in vertebrates to date, the most intensively studied of which is **mannose-binding lectin (MBL)**. MBL can react not only with mannose but several other sugars, so enabling it to bind with an exceptionally wide variety of Gram-negative and Gram-positive bacteria, yeasts, viruses and parasites; its subsequent ability to trigger the classical C3 convertase through two novel associated serine proteases (MASP-1 and MASP-2) is the basis of what is known as the **lectin pathway** of complement activation. (Please relax, we unravel the secrets of the classical and lectin pathways in the next chapter.)

MBL is a multiple of trimeric complexes, each unit of which contains a collagen-like region joined to a globular lectin-binding domain. This structure places it in the family of collectins (**col**lagen + **lectin**) that have the ability to recognize "foreign" carbohydrate patterns differing from "self" surface polysaccharides, normally terminal galactose and sialic acid groups, whereas the collagen region can bind to and activate phagocytic cells through complementary receptors on their surface. The collectins, especially MBL and the alveolar surfactant molecules SP-A and SP-D mentioned earlier, have many attributes that qualify them for a first-line role in innate immunity as soluble PRRs. These include the ability to differentiate self from nonself, to bind to a variety of microbes, to generate secondary effector mechanisms, and to be widely distributed throughout the body including mucosal secretions. They are of course the soluble counterparts to the cell surface C-type lectin PRRs described earlier.

Interest in the collectin conglutinin has intensified with the demonstration, first, that it is found in humans and not just in cows, and second, that it can bind to N-acetylglucosamine; being polyvalent, this implies an ability to coat bacteria with C3b by cross-linking the available sugar residue in the complement fragment with the bacterial proteoglycan. Although it is not clear whether conglutinin is a member of the acute phase protein family, we mention it here because it embellishes the general idea that the evolution of lectin-like molecules that bind to microbial rather than self polysaccharides, and which can then hitch themselves to the complement system or to phagocytic cells, has proved to be such a useful form of protection for the host.

Ficolins

These proteins are structurally and functionally related to collectins and can also recognize carbohydrate-based PAMPs on microorganisms to activate the lectin pathway of complement activation. Ficolins typically recognize N-acetylglucosamine residues in complex-type carbohydrates in addition to other ligands. Three ficolins have been identified in humans, ficolin-1, -2, -3 (also known as M-, L- and H-ficolin respectively), and a role as opsonins for the enhancement of phagocytosis has also been demonstrated for these proteins. Ficolins can also interact with CRP to widen the range of bacteria recognized by the latter and also to enhance complement-mediated killing. The range of bacterial structures recognized by ficolins and MBL are complementary and recognize different but overlapping bacterial species.

Interferons inhibit viral replication

Recall from our earlier discussion of pattern recognition receptors (PRRs) that engagement of many of these receptors by PAMPs results in the production of cytokines and chemokines that act to amplify immune responses by binding to cells in the vicinity. An important class of cytokines induced by viral as well as bacterial infection is the type I **interferons** (IFNα and IFNβ). These are a family of broad-spectrum antiviral agents present in birds, reptiles and fish as well as the higher animals, and first recognized by the phenomenon of viral interference in which an animal infected with one virus resists superinfection by a second unrelated virus. Different molecular forms of interferon have been identified, the genes for all of which have been isolated. There are at least 14 different α-interferons (IFNα) produced by leukocytes, while fibroblasts, and probably all cell types, synthesize IFNβ. We will keep a third type (IFNγ), which is not directly induced by viruses, up our sleeves for the moment.

Cells synthesize interferon when infected by a virus and secrete it into the extracellular fluid where it binds to specific receptors on uninfected neighboring cells. As we saw earlier, engagement of several members of the TLR family, as well as the RIG-like helicase receptors, with their cognate PAMPs results in the induction of members of the interferon-regulated factor (IRF) family of transcription factors (Figure 1.7). In combination with NFκB, another transcription factor activated by engagement of several of the PRRs, IRFs induce expression of type I interferons that are secreted and bind to cells in the vicinity. Long double-stranded RNA molecules, which are produced during the life cycle of most viruses, are particularly good inducers of interferons. The bound interferon now exerts its antiviral effect in the following way. At least two genes are thought to be derepressed in the interferon-binding cell allowing the synthesis of two new enzymes. The first, a protein kinase called **protein kinase R** (PKR), catalyzes the phosphorylation of a ribosomal protein and an initiation factor (eIF-2) necessary for protein synthesis. The net effect of this is to dramatically reduce protein translation as a means of reducing the efficiency of virus production. Another gene product induced by interferons, **oligoadenylate synthetase**, catalyzes the formation of a short polymer of adenylic acid which activates a latent endoribonuclease; this in turn degrades both viral and host mRNA. This is another clever adaptation that is designed to reduce the production of viral products. Another consequence of the downturn in protein synthesis is a reduction in the expression of major histocompatibility complex (MHC) proteins, making cells susceptible to the effects of **natural killer** cells (see below).

The net result is to establish a cordon of uninfectable cells around the site of virus infection so restraining its spread. The effectiveness of interferon *in vivo* may be inferred from experiments in which mice injected with an antiserum to murine interferons could be killed by several hundred times less virus than was needed to kill the controls. However, it must be presumed that interferon plays a significant role in the recovery from, as distinct from the prevention of, viral infections.

As a group, the interferons may prove to have a wider biological role than the control of viral infection. It will be clear, for example, that the induced enzymes described above would act to inhibit host cell division just as effectively as viral replication.

Natural killer cells

Thus far, we have dealt with situations that deal primarily with infectious agents that reside in the extracellular space. But what if an infectious agent manages to enter cells of the host, where they are protected from the attentions of the soluble PRRs (e.g. complement) and are also shielded from phagocytosis by macrophages and neutrophils. To deal with this situation, another type of immune cell has evolved—the natural killer (NK) cell—that is endowed with the ability to inspect host cells for signs of abnormal patterns of protein expression that may indicate that such cells might be harboring a virus. NK cells are also capable of killing cells that have suffered mutations and are on the way to malignant transformation into tumors. Note that although NK cells constitute a component of the innate response, under certain circumstances they exhibit immunological memory, a feature usually confined to adaptive responses.

Natural killer (NK) cells kill host cells that appear abnormal

NK cells are large granular leukocytes with a characteristic morphology. NK cells choose their victims on the basis of two major criteria. The first, termed **"missing self,"** relates to the fact that practically all nucleated cells in the body express molecules on their surface called **major histocompatibility complex (MHC)** proteins. The latter molecules have a very important role in activating cells of the adaptive immune system, which we will deal with later in this chapter, but for now, it is sufficient to know that a cell lacking MHC molecules is not a good proposition from the perspective of the immune system. NK cells exist as a countermeasure to such an eventuality and cells lacking the normal pattern of expression of MHC molecules are swiftly recognized and killed by NK cells. As we saw in the previous section dealing with interferons, one way

in which the expression of MHC molecules can be reduced is as a consequence of interferon responsive gene products that can interfere with protein translation within cells infected by viruses, or in the vicinity of such cells.

In addition to reduced or absent MHC expression, NK cells are also capable of inspecting cells for the expression of MHC-related molecules (called nonclassical MHC molecules) and other proteins that are not normally expressed on cells, but become so in response to certain stresses such as DNA damage. This scenario represents **"altered self"** and also results in such cells being singled out for the attentions of NK cells, culminating in swift execution. NK receptors have also been found to be capable of detecting certain viral proteins directly, such as hemagglutinin from the influenza virus, that qualifies such receptors as another class of PRRs. There are additional receptors on the surfaces of NK cells that enable these cells to recognize infected or transformed cells that we will discuss in Chapter 4. Clearly an NK is not a cell to get on the wrong side of.

NK cells kill target cells via two different pathways

Upon recognition of a target cell, through either of the mechanisms mentioned in the preceding section, the NK cell has two main weapons at its disposal, either of which is sufficient to kill a target cell within a matter of 30–60 minutes (see Videoclip 3). In both cases the target cell dies through switching on its own cell death machinery as a result of encounter with the NK cell; thus, NK killing represents a type of assisted cellular suicide. During NK-mediated killing, killer and target are brought into close apposition (Figure 1.23) as a result of detection of either missing self or altered self on the target cell. This can engage either the **death receptor pathway** or the **granule-dependent pathway** to apoptosis (Figure 1.24). We shall consider these in turn, although the outcomes are very similar.

Death receptor-dependent cell killing

Death receptors are a subset of the TNF receptor superfamily, which includes the receptors for Fas, TNF and TRAIL, and these molecules derive their name from the observation that ligation of such receptors with the appropriate ligand can result in death of the cell bearing the receptor (Figure 1.24). When this observation was first made, it was a fairly astonishing proposition as it suggested that a cell could be killed through the simple expedient of tickling a membrane receptor in the correct way. Clearly, this is a very different type of killing compared with that seen upon exposure of a cell to a toxic chemical or physical stress that can kill through disruption of normal cellular processes. Here we have a physiological receptor/ligand system that exists for the purpose of killing cells on demand—something it has to be said that the immune system does a lot of. Naturally, this sparked a lot of investigation directed towards understanding how ligation of Fas, TNF and related receptors culminates in cell death and this is now

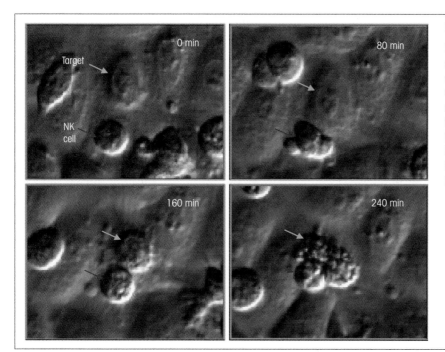

Figure 1.23. Cytotoxic lymphocyte killing.

In this time-lapse series, an NK cell (red arrows) is observed to come into close contact with a target cell (green arrows), which is rapidly followed by rounding up and vigorous membrane blebbing within the target cell as it undergoes apoptosis. The interval between each frame is 80 minutes. Figure kindly provided by Dr. Sean Cullen, Martin laboratory, Trinity College Dublin, Ireland.

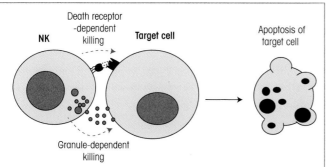

Figure 1.24. Natural killer (NK) cells can kill target cells by two major mechanisms: the death receptor and granule-dependent pathways.

In both cases, the target cell dies as a result of the activation of a battery of cytotoxic proteases within the target cell, called caspases. See Figure 1.25 for further details of the molecular mechanisms of killing in either case.

understood in fine detail as a consequence. Engagement of Fas or TNF receptors with their trimeric ligands results in the recruitment of a protease, called **caspase-8**, to the receptor complex that becomes activated as a result of receptor-induced aggregation of this protease that now undergoes autoactivation (Figure 1.25). Activation of caspase-8 at the receptor then results in propagation of the signaling cascade in two possible ways, either via proteolysis of Bid, which routes the signal through mitochondria, or by direct processing of other **effector caspases** (caspases-3 and -7) downstream. In each case, activation of the effector caspases culminates in death of the cell via apoptosis, which, as we mentioned earlier in this chapter, represents a programmed mode of cell death. NK cells can kill

target cells in a Fas ligand-dependent manner, but can also kill through the related TNF ligand to some extent.

Granule-dependent cell killing

NK cells also possess cytotoxic granules that contain a battery of serine proteases, called **granzymes**, as well as a pore-forming protein called **perforin**. Activation of the NK cell leads to polarization of granules between nucleus and target within minutes and extracellular release of their contents into the space between the two cells followed by target cell death. Polarization of the granules towards the target cell takes place as a result of the formation of a synapse between the killer and target that is composed of an adhesion molecule called LFA-1 and its cognate receptor ICAM-1.

Perforin bears some structural homology to C9; like that protein, but without any help other than from Ca^{2+} it can insert itself into the membrane of the target, apparently by binding to phosphorylcholine through its central amphipathic domain. It then polymerizes to form a transmembrane pore with an annular structure, comparable to the complement membrane attack complex (Figure 1.25). This pore then facilitates entry of the additional cytotoxic granule constituents, the granzymes, which do the actual killing. Perforin-deficient animals are severely compromised in terms of their ability to kill target cells, as the granule-dependent pathway no longer functions in the absence of a mechanism to deliver the granzymes into the target.

Granzymes kill through proteolysis of a variety of proteins within the target cell. Most of the killing potential resides in granzymes A and B, with the function of several additional granzymes (H, K and M in humans) still unclear. The mode of action of **granzyme B** is particularly well understood and

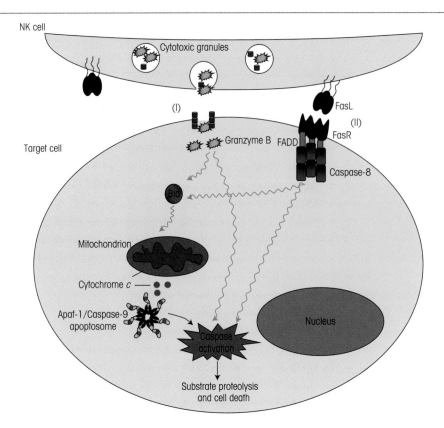

Figure 1.25. Signal transduction events involved in natural killer (NK) cell-mediated apoptosis.

NK cells can kill target cells by two major pathways (I) or (II) as shown. In the cytotoxic granule-dependent pathway (I), binding of the NK receptors to the surface of the virally infected cell triggers the extracellular release of perforin (a pore-forming protein) and granzymes (which are a diverse collection of proteases) from the NK cell cytotoxic granules; perforin polymerizes within the target cell membrane to form transmembrane channels that permit entry of granzymes into the target cell. Granzymes induce apoptotic cell death through activation of the caspase protease cascade, either by directly processing and activating caspases, or through release of cytochrome c from mitochondria that activates the "apoptosome" pathway to caspase activation. In the second pathway to cell death (called the death receptor pathway), membrane-bound Fas ligand (FasL) on the NK cell engages and trimerizes surface Fas receptors on the target cell. Engagement of Fas receptors recruits the adaptor protein FADD, followed by caspase-8, which then becomes activated at the receptor. Caspase-8 can then promote further caspase activation through directly processing other caspases, or via the mitochondrial apoptosome pathway similar to granzymes. In both pathways, the final common pathway to apoptosis occurs as a result of the activation of several "executioner caspases" that coordinate cell death through restricted proteolysis of hundreds of cellular proteins.

it has been found that this protease in essence mimics the action of caspase-8 in the death receptor pathway to apoptosis, as described above. Thus, upon entry into the target cell, granzyme B can initiate apoptosis by cleaving Bid or through directly processing and activating the downstream effector caspases (Figure 1.25). Both routes result in the activation of the effector caspases that coordinate the dismantling of the cell through restricted proteolysis of hundreds of key cellular proteins.

NK cell activity can be enhanced by PAMPs as well as type I interferons

We have already referred to the fact that macrophages display a range of receptors for PAMPs, an important subset of which are the TLRs. In a similar fashion, recent studies have also found that NK cells express a subset of the TLRs that are focused towards detecting PAMPs, such as double-stranded RNA, that are typically associated with viruses. TLR3, TLR7 and TLR8 all appear to be functional in NK cells and upon engagement of these receptors, NK cells become activated and their killing potential is enhanced. Interferon-α and interferon-β are also important activators of NK cells, the effects of which can increase the killing activity of such cells by up to 100-fold. This is a good example of cooperation between cells of the immune system, where cytokines produced by macrophages or other cells upon detection of a pathogen results in the activation of other cells, NK cells in the present context, that may be better adapted to dealing with the infectious threat.

Activated NK cells can amplify immune responses through production of IFNγ

Another consequence of the activation of NK cells is the production of another type of interferon, IFNγ, an important cytokine that has a set of activities distinct from that of IFNα and IFNβ. Macrophages respond to IFNγ by enhancing their microbicidal activities and also by producing other cytokines (such as IL-12) that have effects on cells of the adaptive immune system. Another effect of IFNγ is to enhance the **antigen presentation** function of dendritic cells, which is also important for activation of the adaptive immune system, a topic we shall deal with very shortly. This cytokine can also influence the type of adaptive immune response that is mounted by helping to polarize T-cells towards a particular response pattern; we shall discuss this issue at length in Chapter 9.

Dealing with large parasites

Because most infectious agents are physically much smaller than the average macrophage or neutrophil, phagocytosis of such agents is a sensible strategy for their removal. But what happens in situations where the invading organism hopelessly dwarfs the phagocytic cells of the immune system? A close cousin of the neutrophil, the eosinophil (Figure 1.10c), is important in such cases.

Eosinophils

Large parasites such as helminths cannot physically be phagocytosed and extracellular killing by eosinophils would seem to have evolved to help cope with this situation. These polymorphonuclear "cousins" of the neutrophil have distinctive granules that stain avidly with acid dyes (Figure 1.10c) and have a characteristic appearance in the electron microscope (see Figure 12.25). A major basic protein is localized in the core of the granules while an eosinophilic cationic protein together with a peroxidase have been identified in the granule matrix. Other enzymes include arylsulfatase B, phospholipase D and histaminase. They have surface receptors for C3b and on activation produce a particularly impressive respiratory burst with concomitant generation of active oxygen metabolites. Not satisfied with that, nature has also armed the cell with granule proteins capable of producing a transmembrane plug in the target membrane like C9 and the NK perforin. Quite a nasty cell.

Most helminths can activate the alternative complement pathway, but although resistant to C9 attack, their coating with C3b allows adherence of eosinophils through their C3b receptors. If this contact should lead to activation, the eosinophil will launch its extracellular attack, which includes the release of the major basic protein and especially the cationic protein which damages the parasite membrane.

The innate immune system instigates adaptive immunity

As we have seen throughout this chapter, any infectious agent that manages to enter the body faces a formidable array of defensive weapons ranging from macrophage- and neutrophil-mediated phagocytosis, to complement-mediated attack, membrane perforation by defensins and digestion by extracellular enzymes. As if all of this were not enough, the innate immune system also plays a critical role in initiating an immune response that is uniquely tailored to the ongoing infection. This is achieved by calling upon cells of the adaptive immune system and instructing these cells in the nature of the particular antigens that are giving cause for concern. This function, called **antigen presentation**, is carried out largely, but not exclusively, by a cell that has relatively recently come to the fore as being of critical importance as a conduit between the innate and adaptive immune systems: the **dendritic cell** (DC).

Dendritic cells, which were discovered by Steinman and Cohn in 1973, are produced primarily in the bone marrow and derive their name from the multiple long membrane projections or dendrites that these cells possess (Figure 1.26). These cells share a common progenitor with macrophages with the result that both macrophages and DCs have somewhat overlapping functions. DCs effectively grant permission for **T-cells** of the adaptive immune system to become involved in fighting an infection. They achieve this by providing such cells with **two signals** that are essential for a **naive T-cell** (i.e. one that has not previously been engaged in an immune response) to become activated and to undergo clonal expansion and differentiation to a fully fledged **effector T-cell** (i.e. capable of mounting immune responses). We will look at the role of the T-cell in the immune response in much greater detail in Chapter 9; for now it is sufficient to know that activated T-cells carry out a range of functions that reinforce the efforts of the adaptive immune system, by providing cytokines to help activate macrophages and attract neutrophils. Some T-cells also have functions very similar to NK cells and can detect and kill virally infected cells, while other T-cells assist in the production of antibodies, the functions of which we will deal with in the next chapter.

Dendritic cells provide a conduit between the innate and adaptive immune systems

Similar to macrophages, DCs migrate to the tissues where they reside in a quiescent state continuously sampling their environment by phagocytosis and pinocytosis. These cells have been given various names depending on the tissue they are found in; for example the DCs in the skin are called Langerhans' cells. DCs are equipped with a battery of TLRs and other PRRs and, similar to macrophages, perform a function as sentinels, waiting and watching for signs of infection or tissue damage (i.e. engagement of any of their PRRs). However, unlike the macrophage, DCs do not stand and fight upon PRR

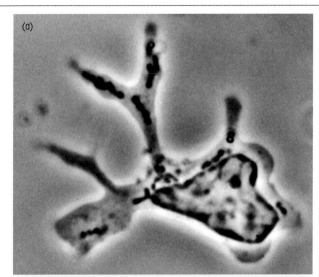

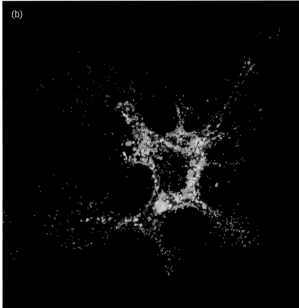

Figure 1.26. Dendritic cell morphology.

(a) Phase contrast image of an unstained dendritic cell with characteristic "dendron tree." (b) Confocal fluorescence microscopy image of a dendritic cell that has phagocytosed green fluorescent microparticles, followed by staining the plasma membrane with Alexa-594-conjugated wheat germ agglutinin (red) to decorate surface carbohydrate. The image in (a) was kindly provided by Dr. Ralph Steinman, The Rockefeller University, New York, USA and first published in "*Mononuclear phagocytes in immunity, infection, and pathology*" ed. R. van Furth, Blackwell Scientific (1975) p. 96. The image in (b) was kindly provided by Dr. Jim Harris and Dr. Ed Lavelle, Trinity College Dublin, Ireland.

engagement but rather take flight to the nearest lymph node (which acts as a kind of army barracks for lymphocytes) to carry out a special function, called **antigen presentation**, which awakens cells of the adaptive immune system (Figures 1.27 and 1.28). We will discuss this in much more detail in Chapter 5, but will quickly summarize events now as it is important that the reader is aware of the central role of DCs in adaptive immunity from the outset.

DCs present antigen to T-cells and provide co-stimulatory signals

Whereas cells of the innate immune system can directly sense nonself molecules using their panoply of PRRs, the T-lymphocytes of the adaptive immune system need to have antigen "presented" to them in a special format. Typically this involves protein antigens becoming internalized and broken down into small peptide fragments by an **antigen-presenting cell** (APC), such as a DC. Antigen presentation by the DC is achieved via a membrane complex called the **major histocompatibility complex** (MHC), which was originally discovered for its role in graft rejection (hence the unwieldy name). In essence, MHC molecules function as serving platforms for dismembered proteins and T-cells can only "see" antigen when presented within the cleft of an MHC molecule; this represents **signal 1** (Figure 1.28). T-cells inspect antigen presented on DCs using their membrane borne **T-cell receptors** (TCRs), which are specialized for the recognition of peptide–MHC complexes. Successful triggering of a TCR results in activation and the acquisition of various immune-related functions by the T-cell (see Chapters 8 and 9). Although DCs are the most efficient APCs for presenting antigen to T-cells, macrophages and B-cells can also perform this important function.

In addition to presenting antigen to T-cells in the correct format, DCs also give permission for T-cells to undergo clonal expansion by providing **co-stimulatory signals** in the form of the membrane ligands, B7-1 and B7-2 (also called CD80/CD86), that engage with CD28 on the surface of the T-cell; this represents **signal 2** (Figure 1.28).

Co-stimulation (i.e. signal 2) is not some afterthought on the part of the DC, for if it is absent the T-cell refuses to respond in the correct manner and will often kill itself through programmed cell death (apoptosis). Just to be sure that we are perfectly clear here, because this is critical for activation of the adaptive immune system, **naive T-cells require both signal 1 and 2 from an APC to become successfully activated.**

Engagement of PRRs equips DCs to provide co-stimulation

Because of the requirement for signals 1 and 2 for proper T-cell activation, knowing when to provide co-stimulation is a critical feature of the role of an APC. The astute reader will now be wondering how a DC knows when to provide co-stimulation, as this essentially dictates whether the adaptive immune system will be engaged or not.

(a)

Immature DC

Non-motile
MHC low
Highly phagocytic
B7 low (poorly co-stimulatory)

PAMPs
IL-1
TNF

Mature DC

Motile
MHC high
Poorly phagocytic
B7 high (co-stimulatory)

(b)

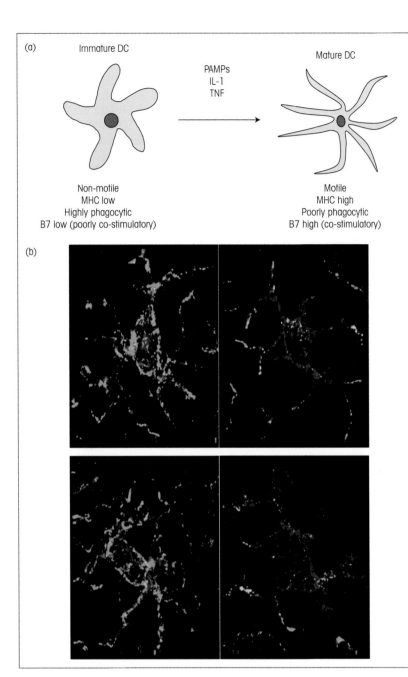

Figure 1.27. Dendritic cell maturation is induced by PAMPs and other signs of infection.

(a) Immature dendritic cells (DCs) undergo maturation and become equipped to present antigen and provide co-stimulatory signals upon activation by a pathogen-associated molecular patterns (PAMP) (or danger-associated molecular pattern (DAMP)), as this leads to a dramatic increase in the expression of surface MHC and B7 molecules on the DC. The expression of B7 family proteins is controlled by NFκB, which is activated downstream of many PRRs. Whereas immature DCs are relatively nonmotile, mature DCs are highly motile and migrate to secondary lymphoid tissues to present antigen to T-cells. (b) Mouse epidermal Langerhans' cells (i.e. DCs of the skin) were stained for langerin (green) and MHC class II (red) either before (left) or after maturation (right). Note that before DC maturation MHC class II (red) is present intracellularly, whereas after maturation it is readily detected on the cell surface. Part (b) courtesy of Dr. Ralph Steinman and Dr. Juliana Idoyaga, The Rockefeller University, New York, USA.

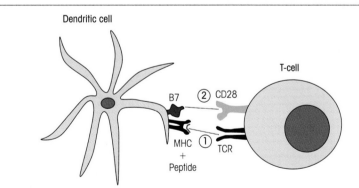

Figure 1.28. Dendritic cells (DCs) present antigen to T-cells of the adaptive immune system.

MHC molecules on DCs function as serving platforms for dismembered proteins (i.e. peptides). T-cells can only "see" antigen when presented within the cleft of an MHC molecule; this represents *signal 1*. In addition to presenting antigen to T-cells in the correct format, DCs also give permission for T-cells to undergo clonal expansion (i.e. proliferation to increase their numbers) by providing co-stimulatory signals in the form of the membrane ligands, B7-1 and B7-2 (also called CD80/CD86), that engage with CD28 on the surface of the T-cell; this represents *signal 2*.

Once again, PRRs provide the key to knowing when the immune system should respond or not. DCs only become equipped to provide co-stimulatory signals upon activation by a PAMP (or DAMP), as this leads to a dramatic increase in the expression of surface B7 molecules on the DC; the expression of B7 family proteins are also controlled by NFκB, which is activated downstream of many PRRs. DCs that present antigen acquired in the absence of PAMP-mediated stimula-tion are overwhelmingly likely to be presenting molecules derived from self and will therefore fail to provide the proper co-stimulatory signals required to activate naive T-cells (Figure 1.28).

The upshot of all of this is that the adaptive immune system is heavily reliant on cells of the innate immune system for the purposes of knowing when to initiate a response and what to respond to.

The ability to recognize and respond to "nonself" as well as "hidden self" is central to immunity
■ Immune responses are initiated through detection of pathogen-associated molecular patterns (PAMPs) representing nonself or danger-associated molecular patterns (DAMPs) that represent hidden self.
■ Pattern recognition receptor molecules (PRRs), which can be either soluble (humoral) or cell-associated, are used by the immune system to detect the presence of PAMPs or DAMPs.
■ PRR engagement leads to a diversity of responses that are aimed at directly killing or engulfing microorganisms via phagocytosis, and also results in amplification of immune responses through release of a range of messenger molecules such as cytokines and chemokines.

Three levels of immune defense operate in vertebrates
■ The skin and mucosal surfaces represent physical barriers to infection.
■ The innate immune system is comprised of a conglomeration of soluble factors and cells that detect and respond to infectious agents through binding to relatively nonspecific structures (PAMPs) common to many pathogens.
■ The adaptive immune system is comprised of T- and B-lymphocytes that recognize highly specific structures (antigens) on microorganisms via highly diverse membrane receptors that are generated randomly and are uniquely tailored to individual pathogens.
■ Innate immune responses to infection are rapid (minutes) whereas adaptive immune responses are delayed (days). Innate immune responses are broadly similar between individuals within a population and do not improve upon repeated exposure to infectious agents. Adaptive immune responses differ between individuals and improve upon a second or subsequent encounter with the same antigen.

■ Innate and adaptive immune responses are interdependent and cooperate to kill infectious agents.

Barriers against infection
■ Microorganisms are kept out of the body by the skin, the secretion of mucus, ciliary action, the lavaging action of bactericidal fluids (e.g. tears), gastric acid and microbial antagonism.
■ If penetration occurs, bacteria are destroyed by soluble pattern recognition molecules such as lysozyme and complement, as well as by phagocytosis followed by intracellular digestion.

Phagocytic cells recognize and kill microorganisms
■ The main phagocytic cells are polymorphonuclear neutrophils and macrophages.
■ The phagocytic cells use their membrane-localized pattern recognition receptors (PRRs) to recognize and adhere to pathogen-associated molecular patterns (PAMPs) on the microbe surface.
■ PRRs include Toll-like, C-type lectin, NOD-like, RIG-like and scavenger receptors.
■ PRR engagement leads to activation of phagocyte functions and to secretion of a range of cytokines and chemokines, many of which are expressed in an NFκB- and IRF-dependent manner.
■ Organisms adhering to the phagocyte surface activate the engulfment process and are taken inside the cell where they fuse with cytoplasmic granules.
■ A formidable array of microbicidal mechanisms then comes into play: the conversion of O_2 to reactive oxygen intermediates, the synthesis of nitric oxide and the release of multiple oxygen-independent factors from the granules.
■ Adherence to PRRs on dendritic cells initiates adaptive immune processes (see Chapter 2).

Complement facilitates phagocytosis and lysis of microorganisms

■ The complement system, a multicomponent triggered enzyme cascade, is used to attract phagocytic cells to the microbes and engulf them. Complement activation also leads to a membrane attack complex (MAC) that perforates microorganisms.

■ In what is known as the alternative complement pathway, the most abundant component, C3, is split by a convertase enzyme formed from its own cleavage product C3b and factor B and stabilized against breakdown caused by factors H and I, through association with the microbial surface. As it is formed, C3b becomes linked covalently to the microorganism and acts as an opsonin.

■ The next component, C5, is activated yielding a small peptide, C5a; the residual C5b binds to the surface and assembles the terminal components C6–9 into a membrane attack complex which is freely permeable to solutes and can lead to osmotic lysis.

■ C5a is a potent chemotactic agent for neutrophils and greatly increases capillary permeability.

■ C3a and C5a act on mast cells causing the release of further mediators, such as histamine, leukotriene B$_4$ and tumor necrosis factor (TNF), with effects on capillary permeability and adhesiveness, and neutrophil chemotaxis; they also activate neutrophils.

The inflammatory response

■ Inflammation is the term used to describe the series of events that surround an immune response and includes local swelling (due to recruitment of phagocytes and plasma proteins from blood), redness, pain and temperature elevation.

■ The products of activated mast cells and complement activation collectively promote inflammation.

■ Following the activation of complement with the ensuing attraction and stimulation of neutrophils, the activated phagocytes bind to the C3b-coated microbes by their surface C3b receptors and may then ingest them. The influx of polymorphs and the increase in vascular permeability constitute the potent antimicrobial **acute inflammatory response** (see Figure 2.18).

■ Inflammation can also be initiated by tissue macrophages that subserve a similar role to the mast cell, as signaling by bacterial toxins, C5a- or iC3b-coated bacteria adhering to surface complement receptors causes release of neutrophil chemotactic and activating factors.

Humoral mechanisms provide a second defensive strategy

■ A multitude of soluble pattern recognition molecules belonging to several protein families (e.g. pentraxins, collectins, ficolins) serve to detect conserved PAMPs on microorganisms. Mechanisms of action common to these soluble PRRs upon binding their targets include: opsonization, complement activation, enhanced phagocytic uptake and agglutination.

■ In addition to lysozyme, peptide defensins and the complement system, other humoral defenses involve the acute phase proteins, such as C-reactive and mannose-binding proteins, whose synthesis is greatly augmented by infection. Mannose-binding lectin generates a complement pathway that is distinct from the alternative pathway in its early reactions, as will be discussed in Chapter 2. It is a member of the collectin family that includes conglutinin and surfactants SP-A and SP-D, notable for their ability to distinguish microbial from "self" surface carbohydrate groups by their pattern recognition molecules.

■ Recovery from viral infections can be effected by the interferons that block viral replication.

Natural killer cells instruct abnormal or virally infected cells to commit suicide

■ NK cells can identify host cells that are expressing abnormal or altered patterns of proteins.

■ Upon selection of an appropriate target cell, NK cells can kill by engaging either the death receptor or cytotoxic granule pathway to apoptosis.

■ Both the death receptor and granule-dependent pathways to apoptosis involve activation of a group of proteases, called caspases, within the target cell that coordinate the internal dismantling of critical cellular structures, thereby killing the cell.

Dealing with large extracellular parasites

■ Large infectious agents that are physically too big to be readily phagocytosed by macrophages and neutrophils are treated to a bombardment with noxious enzymes by eosinophils.

■ Extracellular killing by C3b-bound eosinophils may be responsible for the failure of many large parasites to establish a foothold in potential hosts.

The innate immune system instigates adaptive immunity

■ Dendritic cells (DCs) provide a conduit between the innate and adaptive immune systems by presenting antigen to T-lymphocytes within lymph nodes.

■ Mature DCs present peptide fragments of antigens to T-cells via surface MHC molecules (signal 1) and also provide co-stimulatory signals via B7 family ligands (signal 2). Both signals are required for efficient T-cell activation.

■ PAMP-mediated stimulation of DCs triggers their maturation (i.e. the ability to efficiently present antigen and provide co-stimulation) and promotes their migration to lymph nodes.

FURTHER READING

Banchereau J. & Steinman R.M. (1998) Dendritic cells and the control of immunity. *Nature* **392**, 245–252.

Bottazzi B., Doni A., Garlanda C. & Mantovani A. (2010) An integrated view of humoral innate immunity: pentraxins as a paradigm. *Annual Review of Immunology* **28**, 157–183.

Creagh E.M. & O'Neill L.A. (2006) TLRs, NLRs and RLRs: a trinity of pathogen sensors that co-operate in innate immunity. *Trends in Immunology* **8**, 352–357.

Cullen S.P. & Martin S.J. (2008) Mechanisms of granule-dependent killing. *Cell Death & Differentiation* **15**, 251–262.

Delves P.J. & Roitt I.M. (2000) The immune system: first of two parts. *New England Journal of Medicine* **343**, 37–49.

Janeway C.A. Jr & Medzhitov R. (2002) Innate immune recognition. *Annual Review of Immunology* **20**, 197–216.

Matzinger P. (1994) Tolerance, danger, and the extended family. *Annual Review of Immunology* **12**, 991–1045.

Matzinger P. (2002) The danger model: a renewed sense of self. *Science* **296**, 301–305.

Medzhitov R. (2008) Origin and physiological roles of inflammation. *Nature* **454**, 428–35.

Meylan E., Tschopp J. & Karin M. (2006) Intracellular pattern recognition receptors in the host response. *Nature* **442**, 39–44.

Ricklin D. & Lambris J.D. (2007) Complement-targeted therapeutics. *Nature Biotechnology* **25**, 1265–1275.

Sayed B.A., Christy A., Quirion M.R. & Brown M.A. (2008) The master switch: the role of mast cells in autoimmunity and tolerance. *Annual Review of Immunology* **26**, 705–739.

Steinman R.M. & Idoyaga J. (2010) Features of the dendritic cell lineage. *Immunological Reviews* **234**, 5–17.

Tamura T., Yanai H., Savitsky D. & Taniguchi T. (2008) The IRF family transcription factors in immunity and oncogenesis. *Annual Review of Immunology* **26**, 535–584.

Taylor R.C., Cullen S.P. & Martin S.J. (2008) Apoptosis: controlled demolition at the cellular level. *Nature Reviews Molecular Cell Biology* **9**, 231–241.

 Now visit **www.roitt.com** to test yourself on this chapter.

CHAPTER 2
Specific acquired immunity

Key Topics

Just to Recap...

The neutrophils, eosinophils, basophils, mast cells, monocytes, macrophages, dendritic cells and natural killer (NK) cells are all cellular components of the innate response. Molecules involved in innate responses include the acute phase proteins and complement. Although innate responses are crucially important in protection against pathogens they are not fine-tuned to particular antigens and do not improve upon repeated encounters with the infectious agent, unlike the acquired responses that we will now explore.

Introduction

Our microbial adversaries have tremendous opportunities to evolve strategies that evade our innate immune defenses. Many bacteria can divide every 20–60 minutes or so, and replication of their nucleic acid provides an opportunity for mutations that can result in changes to the structures (antigens) recognized by the immune system. Viruses and parasites are also constantly altering their antigens by mutation and other mechanisms. The body obviously needed to devise defense mechanisms that could keep up with all these changes. In other words *a very large number* of **specific immune defenses** needed to be at the body's disposal. Quite a tall order!

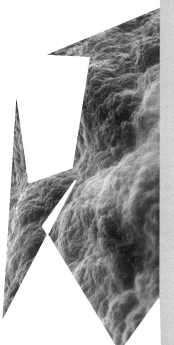

Roitt's Essential Immunology, Twelfth Edition. Peter J. Delves, Seamus J. Martin, Dennis R. Burton, Ivan M. Roitt.
© 2011 Peter J. Delves, Seamus J. Martin, Dennis R. Burton, Ivan M. Roitt. Published 2011 by Blackwell Publishing Ltd.

Antigens—"shapes" recognized by the immune system

The structures that are recognized by the specific acquired immune response are referred to as antigens. They possess a shape that is complementary to the antigen receptors on the cells of the immune system and to the secreted antibody molecules. Antigens can be proteins, carbohydrates, lipids, nucleic acids, small chemical groupings referred to as haptens, in fact virtually anything. The antigens may be a component of microorganisms, of larger infectious agents such as parasitic worms, of ingested substances such as foods, of inhaled substances such as pollens, of transplanted organs or tissues, or even our own body components ("self" antigens).

Antibody—a specific antigen recognition molecule

Evolutionary processes came up with what can only be described as a brilliant solution to the problem of recognizing an almost infinite diversity of antigens. This solution was to fashion a molecule that was capable not only of specifically recognizing the offending pathogen but also of recruiting various components of the immune response. *Voilà*, the antibody molecule!

Antibodies have two main parts, one called the variable region that is devoted to binding to the individual antigen (the antigen recognition function) and one called the constant region concerned with linking to complement, phagocytes, NK cells, and so forth (the effector function). Thus the body has to make hundreds of thousands, or even millions, of **antibody molecules with different antigen-recognition sites** but that all share the property of recruiting other elements of the immune response (Figure 2.1).

Antibody can activate the classical complement pathway

Human antibodies are divided into five main classes: immunoglobulin M (shortened to IgM), IgG, IgA, IgE, and IgD, which differ in the specialization of their effector "rear ends" for different biological functions. In Chapter 1 we discussed the antibody-independent alternative pathway of complement that relies upon microbial polysaccharides for its activation. However, the first complement pathway to be discovered, the **classical pathway**, required IgM or IgG antibody for its activation. Antibody of these two classes, when bound to antigen, will link to the first molecule in the classical pathway of complement , C1q, and trigger the latent proteolytic activity of the C1 complex (Figure 2.2).

A C1q is a hexamer arranged into a central collagen-like stem branching into six arms each tipped with an antibody-binding globular head. C1q is associated with two further subunits, C1r and C1s, in a Ca^{2+}-stabilized trimolecular complex (Figure 2.2). Both these molecules contain so-called sushi repeats of a 60-amino acid unit folded as a globular

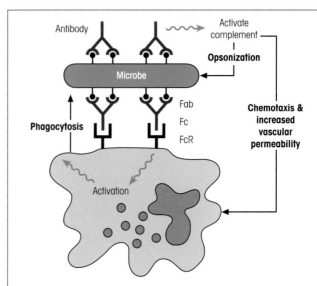

Figure 2.1. The antibody molecule links antigen to other components of the immune response.

The Fab (fragment antigen-binding) part of the antibody binds specific antigen on the microbe and varies from one antibody to another. The Fc (fragment crystallizable) part is identical for all antibodies of the same class/subclass and functionally activates complement (IgM and IgG antibodies, via the classical pathway) and phagocytic cells (IgG antibody, via binding to Fc receptors [FcR] on the surface of the phagocyte). Complement activation leads to opsonization of microbes to enhance their recognition by phagocytes (due to coating of the microbe with complement, which is recognized by complement receptors on the phagocyte [not shown, see Figure 12.10]). In addition, complement activation leads to chemotactic attraction of the phagocytes to the site of the infection and increased vascular permeability in order to facilitate their passage from the blood circulation to the tissues. Other activities of antibody not shown here include providing a link between killer cells (NK cells, eosinophils, etc) and the pathogen, a mechanism referred to as antibody-dependent cellular cytotoxicity (ADCC).

domain and often referred to as a complement control protein (CCP) repeat as it is a characteristic structural feature of several proteins involved in control of the complement system. The changes that occur in C1q upon binding the antigen–antibody complex bring about the autoactivation of proteolytic activity in C1r that then cleaves C1s. The activity of C1 is regulated by a C1-inhibitor (C1-Inh) that binds to $C1r_2$–$C1s_2$, causing them to dissociate from C1q and thus preventing the excessive activation of the classical pathway.

The next component in the pathway, C4 (unfortunately components were numbered before the sequence was established), now binds to the CCPs in C1s and is then cleaved enzymatically by $\overline{C1s}$. As expected in a multienzyme cascade, several molecules of C4 undergo cleavage, each releasing a small C4a fragment and revealing a nascent labile internal

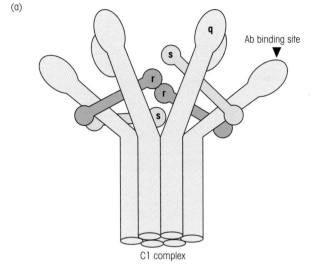

(a)

q

s

r

r

s

Ab binding site ▼

C1 complex

(b)

Microbe

Fab

Antibody

Fc

C1qrs

Figure 2.2. Activation of the classical complement pathway.

The first component, C1, of the classical pathway of complement activation is a complex composed of three subunits: C1q, C1r and C1s. (a) C1q forms a hexamer arranged in a "bunch of tulips"-like structure and is associated with the flexible rod-like Ca-dependent complex C1r$_2$–C1s$_2$, which interdigitates with the six arms of C1q. (b) Activation of the complement cascade by the classical pathway requires antibodies to be bound to antigen in order that the globular heads of the C1q hexamer can bind to the Fc part of at least two antibodies.

thiolester bond in the residual $\overline{\text{C4b}}$ (like that in C3, see Figure 1.17) that may then bind either to the antibody–C1 complex or the surface of the microbe itself. In the presence of Mg^{2+}, C2 can complex with the $\overline{\text{C4b}}$ to become a new substrate for the $\overline{\text{C1s}}$: the resulting product $\overline{\text{C4b2a}}$ now has the vital C3 convertase activity required to cleave C3 (Figure 2.3).

The classical pathway C3 convertase has the same specificity as the $\overline{\text{C3bBb}}$ generated by the alternative pathway. Activation of a single C1 complex can bring about the proteolysis of literally thousands of C3 molecules. The resulting C3b is added to $\overline{\text{C4b2a}}$ to make it into a C5 convertase, which generates C5a, with chemotactic and anaphylactic functions, and C5b, which forms the first component of the **membrane attack complex** (Figures 1.19 and 2.4). Just as the alternative pathway C3 convertase is controlled by factors H and I, so the breakdown of $\overline{\text{C4b2a}}$ is brought about by Factor I in the presence of either C4-binding protein (C4bp) or cell surface C3b receptor (CR1) acting as cofactors.

The lectin and classical complement pathways merge to generate the same C3 convertase

It is appropriate at this stage to recall the activation of complement by innate immune mechanisms involving mannose-binding lectin (MBL) (cf. p. 25). On complexing with a microbe, MBL binds and activates the latent proteolytic activity of the MBL-associated serine proteases, MASP-1 and 2, which structurally resemble C1r and C1s respectively.

In an analogous fashion to the C1qrs complex, MASP-1 and MASP-2 split C4 and C2 to generate the $\overline{\text{C4b2a}}$ C3 convertase.

Irrespective of whether activation occurs via the classical, lectin or alternative pathway, several biologically active complement components are generated that have important roles in the immune response (Figure 2.5).

Antibody can help phagocytosis

Microorganisms are sometimes able to resist phagocytosis. If small amounts of antibody are added the phagocyte springs into action. It does so through the recognition of two or more antibody molecules bound to the microbe, using specialized Fc receptors on the cell surface of the phagocyte (Figure 2.1).

A single antibody molecule complexed to the microorganism is not enough because it cannot cause the cross-linking of the Fc receptors on the phagocyte surface membrane that is required to activate the cell. There is a further consideration connected with what is often called the **bonus effect of multivalency**. For thermodynamic reasons, which will be touched on in Chapter 5, the association constant of ligands that use several rather than a single bond to react with receptors is increased geometrically rather than arithmetically. For example, three antibodies bound close together on a bacterium could be bound to a macrophage a thousand times more strongly than a single antibody molecule (Figure 2.6).

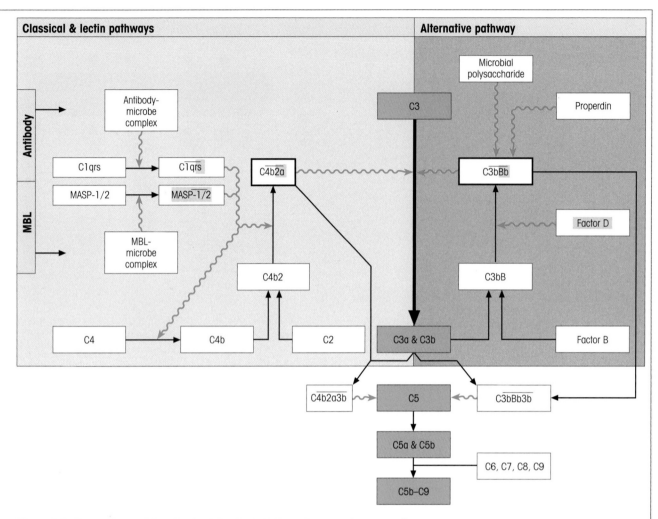

Figure 2.3. Comparison of the classical, lectin and alternative complement pathways.

The classical pathway is activated by antibody whereas the alternative and lectin pathways are not. The molecules with protease activity are highlighted in light blue. The key central event for all three pathways is the cleavage of C3 by C3 convertase (namely C4b2a for the classical and lectin pathways, C3bBb for the alternative pathway). Beware confusion with nomenclature; the large C2 fragment that forms the C3 convertase is designated as C2a, but to be consistent with C4b, C3b, and C5b, it would have been more logical to call it C2b. Note that C-reactive protein (p. 24), on binding to microbial phosphorylcholine, can also trigger the classical pathway. Mannose-binding lectin (MBL), when combined with microbial surface carbohydrate, associates with the MBL-associated serine proteases (MASP)-1 and -2 (p. 25), which split C4 and C2.

 ## Cellular basis of antibody production

Antibodies are made by lymphocytes

The majority of resting **lymphocytes** are small cells with a darkly staining nucleus due to condensed chromatin and relatively little cytoplasm containing the odd mitochondrion required for basic energy provision (Figures 2.7a and 2.8).

The central role of the small lymphocyte in the production of antibody was established largely by the work of James Gowans. He depleted rats of their lymphocytes by chronic drainage of lymph from the thoracic duct using an indwelling cannula, and showed that they had a grossly impaired ability to mount an antibody response to microbial challenge. The ability to form antibody could be restored by injecting thoracic duct lymphocytes obtained from another rat. The same effect could be obtained if, before injection, the thoracic duct T-cells were first incubated at 37°C for 24 hours under conditions that kill off large- and medium-sized cells and leave only the small lymphocytes. This experiment shows that the small lymphocyte is necessary for the **antibod**y response.

The small lymphocytes can be labeled if the donor rat is previously injected with radioactive tritiated [³H] thymidine; it then becomes possible to follow the fate of these lymphocytes

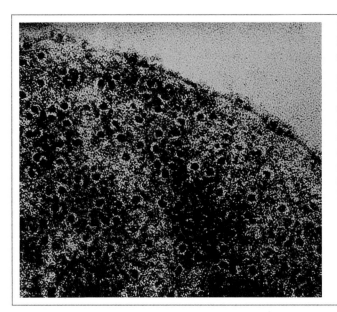

Figure 2.4. Multiple lesions in cell wall of *Escherichia coli* bacterium caused by interaction with IgM antibody and complement.

Each lesion is caused by a single IgM molecule and shows as a "dark pit" due to penetration by the "negative stain." This is somewhat of an illusion as in reality these "pits" are like volcano craters standing proud of the surface, and are each single membrane attack complexes. Comparable results may be obtained in the absence of antibody by using higher concentrations of complement as the cell wall endotoxin can activate the alternative pathway (×400 000). (Courtesy of R. Dourmashkin and J.H. Humphrey.)

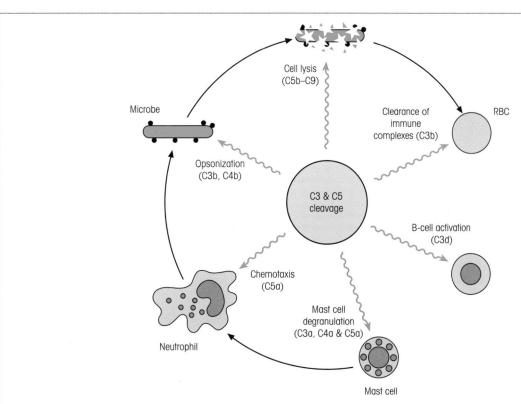

Figure 2.5. Activities generated by the triggering of the complement cascade.

Following the cleavage of C3 by C3 convertase and subsequently of C5 by C5 convertase, various biologically active complement components are generated. Certain cells of the immune system possess cell surface receptors for particular complement components, and microbial cell surfaces can become coated with complement. The functions that are generated work together to generate an effective immune response. Thus the release of inflammatory mediators from mast cells occurring in response to complement components C3a and C5a (and to a lesser extent C4a) leads to an increase in vascular permeability. This allows neutrophils to exit the circulation in response to an additional activity of C5a as a neutrophil chemoattractant. Microorganisms coated ("opsonized") with C3b and C4b are effectively phagocytosed by these neutrophils due to the phagocytes expressing complement receptors. Once C3b is deposited on the microbial surface, the terminal components (C5b–C9) of the complement system can assemble to form the membrane attack complex (MAC) with subsequent destruction of microorganisms. Because erythrocytes bear complement receptors they are able to bind antigens that are covered in complement, and these are rapidly transported to the spleen and liver for destruction. Complement component C3d acts to facilitate B-cell activation, either by providing co-stimulation via complement receptors on the B-cell or by mediating the retention of immune complexes on follicular dendritic cells, and thereby is involved in the generation of specific antibody against the microbe.

Figure 2.6. Binding of bacterium to phagocyte by multiple antibodies gives strong association forces and triggers phagocytosis by cross-linking the surface Fc receptors (FcR).

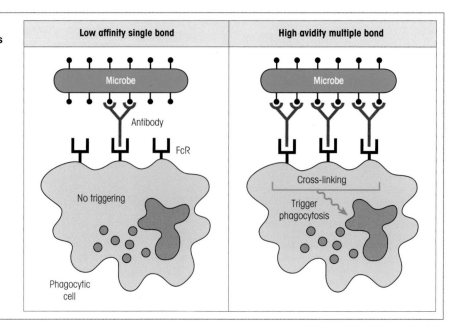

when transferred to another rat of the same strain that is then injected with microorganisms to produce an antibody response (Figure 2.9). After contact with the injected microbes, some of the transferred labeled lymphocytes develop into **plasma cells** (Figures 2.7d and 2.10) that can be shown to contain (Figure 2.7e) and secrete antibody.

Antigen selects those lymphocytes that possess the specific antibody

Lymphocytes come in two major varieties, **T-lymphocytes** (T-cells) and **B-lymphocytes** (B-cells). Although T-lymphocytes (so called because they differentiate in the thymus) have a variety of roles, it is only the B-lymphocytes (which differentiate in the bone marrow) that are able to make **antibody** to generate **humoral immunity**. Each B-cell is programmed to make one, and only one, specificity of antibody and it places a transmembrane version of these antibodies on its cell surface to act as receptors for the specific antigen. These antibodies can be detected by using fluorescent probes and, in Figure 2.7b, one can see the molecules of antibody on the surface of a human B-lymphocyte stained with a fluorescent rabbit antiserum raised against a preparation of human antibodies. Each B-lymphocyte has of the order of 10^5 antibody molecules, all of identical antigen specificity, on its surface.

When an antigen enters the body, it is confronted by a dazzling array of B-lymphocytes all bearing different antibodies each with its own individual recognition site. The antigen will only bind to those receptors with which it makes a good fit. B-lymphocytes whose receptors have bound antigen receive a triggering signal and develop into antibody-secreting plasma cells. As the B-lymphocytes are programmed to make only one specificity of antibody, the soluble version of the antibody molecule secreted by the plasma cell will recognize the same antigen

as the cell surface transmembrane version originally acting as the antigen receptor. In this way, antigen selects for the production of the antibodies that recognize it effectively (Figure 2.11). T-cells with a TCR of appropriate specificity are similarly selected, some of which are T-helper cells required in most cases to help B-cells proliferate and then differentiate into plasma cells.

The need for clonal expansion means humoral immunity must be acquired

Because we can make hundreds of thousands, maybe even millions, of different antibody molecules, it is not feasible for us to have too many lymphocytes producing each type of antibody; there just would not be enough room in the body to accommodate them. To compensate for this, lymphocytes that are triggered by contact with antigen undergo successive waves of proliferation to build up a large clone of plasma cells that will be making antibody of the kind for which the parent lymphocyte was programmed. By this system of **clonal selection**, large enough concentrations of specific antibody can be produced to combat infection effectively (Milestone 2.1; Figure 2.12). Clonal selection of T-lymphocytes similarly ensures that only cells of the appropriate specificity are induced to proliferate.

The importance of proliferation for the development of a significant antibody response is highlighted by the ability of antimitotic drugs to completely abolish antibody production to a given antigen stimulus.

Because it takes time for the proliferating clone to build up its numbers sufficiently, it is usually several days before antibodies are detectable in the serum following primary contact with antigen. The newly formed antibodies are a consequence of antigen exposure and it is for this reason that we speak of the **acquired (adaptive) immune response**.

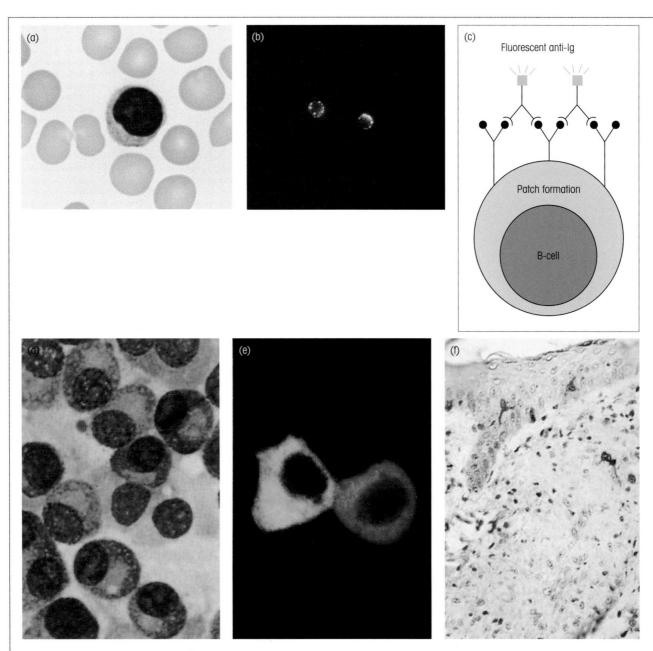

Figure 2.7. Cells involved in the acquired immune response.

(a) **Small lymphocyte**. Typical resting lymphocyte with a thin rim of cytoplasm. Condensed chromatin gives rise to heavy staining of the nucleus. Giemsa stain. (b) Immunofluorescence staining of **B-lymphocyte surface immunoglobulin** using fluorescein-conjugated (green) anti-Ig. Provided the reaction is carried out in the cold to prevent pinocytosis, the labeled antibody cannot penetrate to the interior of the viable lymphocytes and reacts only with surface components. Patches of aggregated surface Ig are seen that are beginning to form a cap in the right-hand lymphocyte. During cap formation, submembranous myosin becomes redistributed in association with the surface Ig. (c) Diagrammatic representation of the patch formation seen in (b). (d) **Plasma cells**. The nucleus is eccentric. The cytoplasm is strongly basophilic due to high RNA content. The juxtanuclear lightly stained zone corresponds with the Golgi region. May–Grünwald–Giemsa. (e) **Plasma cells** stained to show intracellular immunoglobulin using a fluorescein-labeled anti-IgG (green) and a rhodamine-conjugated anti-IgM (red). (f) **Langerhans' cells**, the interdigitating dendritic cells of the skin, in human epidermis in leprosy. They are increased in the subepidermal zone, possibly as a consequence of the disease process. Stained red by the immunoperoxidase method with antibodies against the calcium-binding protein S-100, present in (and thus a "marker" for) Langerhans' cells. (The photograph in (a) is reproduced from *Essential Haematology* 5th edn with kind permission from the authors A.V. Hoffbrand, J.E. Pettit & P.A.H. Moss; (b) by P. Lydyard; (d) and (e) by C. Grossi; and (f) by M. Ridley.)

Figure 2.8. Lymphocyte ultrastructure.

A **T-lymphocyte** with an indented nucleus containing condensed chromatin, sparse cytoplasm: single mitochondrion shown and many free ribosomes but otherwise few organelles (×13000). B-lymphocytes are essentially similar with slightly more cytoplasm and occasional elements of rough-surfaced endoplasmic reticulum. (Courtesy of A. Zicca.)

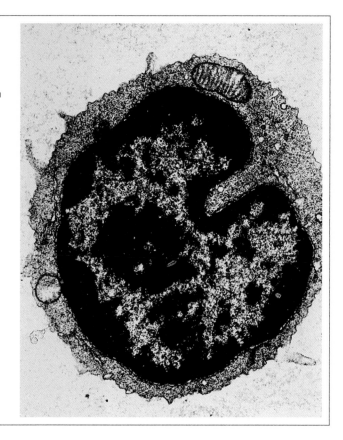

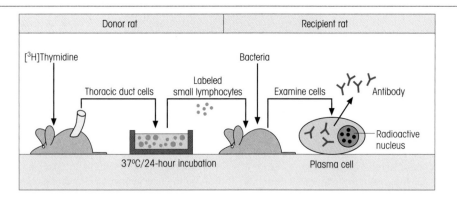

Figure 2.9. Small lymphocytes can become activated to differentiate into antibody-secreting plasma cells.

In this experimental system the lymphocytes in the donor rat are radioactively labeled *in vivo* with tritiated [³H]thymidine and then removed from the thoracic duct (an anatomic structure connecting the lymphatic and blood circulations and therefore a rich source of circulating lymphocytes, see Figure 7.4). Following incubation under certain *in vitro* conditions for 24 hours it is possible to obtain a lymphocyte population from which any already activated (and therefore larger) cells have been depleted. The remaining ³H-labeled small lymphocytes (which will have a diverse range of antigen specificities) are then transferred to a recipient rat, which is immunized with a strain of bacteria. Any small lymphocytes with specificity for this bacterial strain will become activated and some of these will be B-lymphocytes capable of differentiating into plasma cells. This observation is proved by the fact that cells of donor origin (i.e. with a radioactive nucleus shown by autoradiography) can also be shown to possess intracellular antibody revealed by staining with fluorescent probes (cf. Figure 2.7e) and to secrete antibody *in vitro*.

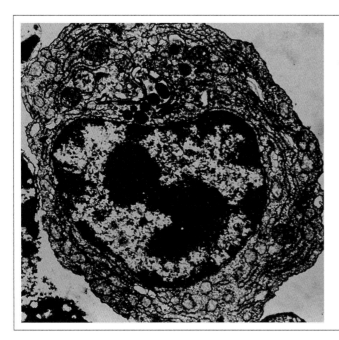

Figure 2.10. Plasma cell (×10 000).

Prominent rough-surfaced endoplasmic reticulum associated with the synthesis and secretion of Ig.

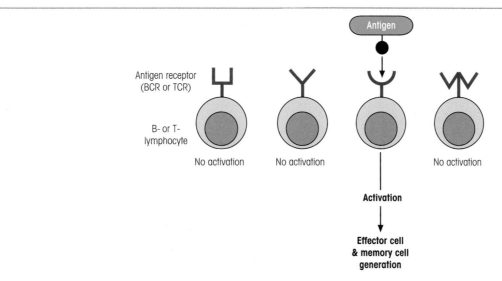

Figure 2.11. Antigen activates those lymphocytes with a complementary antigen receptor.

This process is referred to as clonal selection and ensures that only the relevant, antigen-specific, lymphocytes are triggered to produce the appropriate effector cells and memory cells. In the case of the antibody-producing B-lymphocytes they use a cell surface version of antibody, which directly binds native antigen, as the B-cell receptor (BCR). T-lymphocytes do not make antibody but also possess a cell surface antigen receptor, the T-cell receptor (TCR). Although for simplicity the TCR is shown directly recognizing antigen (just like the BCR of B-cells), in most cases the TCR has a rather more complicated recognition system in that it needs to see processed antigen fragments presented to it by MHC molecules (see Figures 2.15 and 2.16). Following their activation by antigen, B-cells can develop into antibody-secreting plasma cells or into memory B-cells. In contrast, the cells produced following the activation of T-lymphocytes will be helper, cytotoxic or regulatory effector T-cells, together with memory T-cells.

Milestone 2.1—Clonal Selection Theory

Antibody production according to Ehrlich

In 1894, well in advance of his time as usual, the remarkable Paul Ehrlich proposed the side-chain theory of antibody production. Each cell would make a large variety of surface receptors that bound foreign antigens by complementary shape "lock and key" fit. Exposure to antigen would provoke overproduction of receptors (antibodies), which would then be shed into the circulation (Figure M2.1.1).

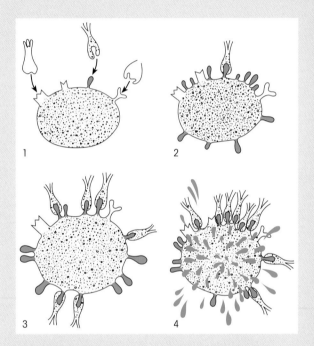

Figure M2.1.1. Ehrlich's side-chain theory of antibody production. (Reproduced from *Proceedings of the Royal Society B* (1900), **66**, 424.)

Template theories

Ehrlich's hypothesis implied that antibodies were preformed prior to antigen exposure. However, this view was difficult to accept when later work showed that antibodies could be formed to almost any organic structure synthesized in the chemist's laboratory (e.g. *m*-aminobenzene sulfonate; Figure 5.6) despite the fact that such molecules would never be encountered in the natural environment. Thus was born the idea that antibodies were synthesized by using the antigen as a template. Twenty years passed before this idea was "blown out of the water" by the observation that, after an antibody molecule is unfolded by guanidinium salts in the absence of antigen, it spontaneously refolds to regenerate its original specificity. It became clear that each antibody has a different amino acid sequence that governs its final folded shape and hence its ability to recognize antigen.

Selection theories

The wheel turns full circle and we once more live with the idea that, as different antibodies must be encoded by separate genes, the information for making these antibodies must pre-exist in the host DNA. In 1955, Nils Jerne perceived that this could form the basis for a selective theory of antibody production. He suggested that the complete antibody repertoire is expressed at a low level and that, when antigen enters the body, it selects its complementary antibody to form a complex that in some way provokes further synthesis of that particular antibody. But how?

Macfarlane Burnet now brilliantly conceived of a cellular basis for this selection process. Let each lymphocyte be programmed to make its own singular antibody that is inserted like an Ehrlich "side-chain" into its surface membrane. Antigen will now form the complex envisaged by Jerne, on the surface of the lymphocyte, and by triggering its activation and clonal proliferation, large amounts of the specific antibody will be synthesized (Figure 2.12). Bow graciously to that soothsayer Ehrlich, he came so close in 1894!

Acquired immunological memory

When we make an immune response to a given infectious agent, by definition that microorganism must exist in our environment and we are likely to meet it again. It would make sense then for the immune mechanisms alerted by the first contact with antigen to leave behind some memory system that would enable the response to any subsequent exposure to be faster and greater in magnitude.

Our experience of many common infections tells us that this must be so. We rarely suffer twice from such diseases as measles, mumps, chickenpox, whooping cough, and so forth. The first contact clearly imprints some information, imparts some **memory**, so that the body is effectively prepared to repel any later invasion by that organism and a state of immunity is established.

Secondary immune responses are better

By following the production of antibody and of effector T-cells on the first and second contacts with antigen, we can see the basis for the development of immunity. For example, when we inject a bacterial product such as tetanus toxoid into a rabbit, for the reasons already discussed, several days elapse before antibody production by B-cells can be detected in the blood; these antibodies reach a peak and then fall (e.g. Figure 2.13).

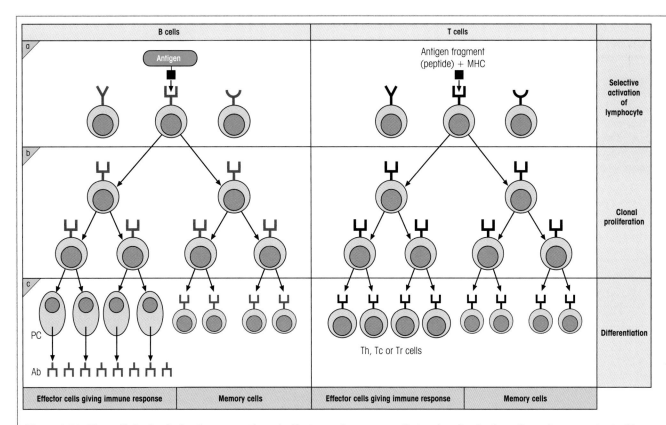

Figure 2.12. The cellular basis for the generation of effector and memory cells by clonal selection after primary contact with antigen.

(a) The lymphocyte (B- or T-cell) is selected by antigen and becomes activated. (b) It then undergoes repeated cell division (clonal proliferation) and the progeny give rise to an expanded population of antigen-specific cells. (c) A fraction of the progeny of the original antigen-reactive lymphocytes become memory cells whereas others differentiate into effector cells. In the case of B-lymphocytes the effector cells are the antibody-secreting plasma cells (PC), whereas for T-lymphocytes the effector cells may be T-helper cells (Th), cytotoxic T-cells (Tc) or regulatory T-cells (Tr).

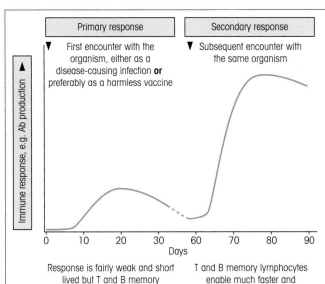

Figure 2.13. Primary and secondary response.

The first encounter with an antigen, for example on a pathogenic organism, elicits a primary immune response that is rather slow to get going because it takes a while for the naive lymphocytes to expand up to sufficient numbers. The response is not of great magnitude and fades relatively quickly. The response on the second contact with the same antigen is much more rapid and more intense. Memory cells generated during the primary response are both quantitatively and qualitatively superior to the naive lymphocytes, requiring fewer cycles of cell division before they develop into effectors. The generation of memory cells provides the basis for vaccination, where the immune response is primed by a relatively harmless form of the microbial antigen so that the immune system goes straight into making a secondary immune response upon the first encounter with the actual pathogen.

Figure 2.14. Memory for a primary response can be transferred by small lymphocytes.

Recipients are treated with a dose of X-rays that directly kill lymphocytes (highly sensitive to radiation) but only affect other body cells when they divide; the recipient thus permits the function of the donor cells to be followed. The reasons for the design of the experiment are given in the text.

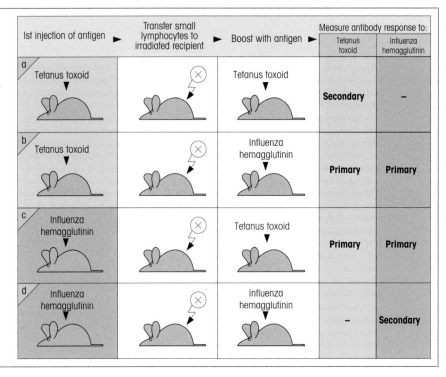

If we now allow the animal to rest and then give a second injection of toxoid, the course of events is dramatically altered. Within 2–3 days the antibody level in the blood rises steeply to reach much higher values than were observed in the **primary immune response**. This **secondary immune response** then is characterized by a more rapid and more abundant production of antibody resulting from the "tuning up" or priming of the antibody-forming system. T-lymphocytes similarly exhibit enhanced secondary responses, producing cells with improved helper or cytotoxic effector functions.

The fact that it is the lymphocytes that are responsible for immunological memory can be demonstrated by **adoptive transfer** of these cells to another animal, an experimental system frequently employed in immunology (cf. Figure 2.9). The immunological potential of the transferred cells is seen in a recipient treated with X-rays that destroy its own lymphocyte population; thus the recipient animal acts as a living "test tube" in which the activity of the transferred lymphocytes can be assessed *in vivo*. Small lymphocytes taken from an animal given a primary injection of antigen (for example, either tetanus toxoid or influenza hemagglutinin) and transferred to an irradiated host, which is then boosted with the same antigen, give a rapid, intense production of antibody characteristic of a secondary response (Figure 2.14 a and d). To exclude the possibility that the first antigen injection might exert a *nonspecific* stimulatory effect on the lymphocytes, "criss-cross" control animals are boosted by injection with a different antigen to that given for the primary injection. In these control animals only primary responses are seen to either antigen (Figure 2.14 b and c). We have explained the design of the experiment in detail to call attention to the need for careful selection of controls.

The higher response given by a primed lymphocyte population can be ascribed mainly to an expansion of the numbers of cells capable of being stimulated by the antigen (Figure 2.12), although we shall see later that there are some qualitative differences in these memory cells as well (pp. 254–8).

Acquired immunity has antigen specificity

Discrimination between different antigens

The establishment of memory or immunity to one microorganism does not confer protection against another unrelated microorganism. After an attack of measles we are immune to further infection but are susceptible to other agents such as the chickenpox or mumps viruses. Acquired immunity shows **specificity** and the immune system can differentiate specifically between the two organisms. A more formal experimental demonstration of this discriminatory power was seen in Figure 2.14 where priming with tetanus toxoid evoked memory for that antigen but not for influenza hemagglutinin and vice versa.

The basis for this lies of course in the ability of the recognition sites of the antibody molecules to distinguish between antigens; antibodies that react with the toxoid do not bind to influenza and, *mutatis mutandis* as they say, anti-influenza does not recognise the toxoid.

Discrimination between self and nonself

This ability to recognize one antigen and distinguish it from another goes even further. The individual must also recognize what is foreign, i.e. what is "nonself." The failure to discriminate between **self** and **nonself** could lead to the synthesis of antibodies directed against components of the subject's own body (**autoantibodies**), which might prove highly damaging. On purely theoretical grounds it seemed to Burnet and Fenner that the body must develop some mechanism whereby "self" and "nonself" could be distinguished, and they postulated that those circulating body components that were able to reach the developing lymphoid system in the perinatal period could in some way be "learnt" as "self." A permanent unresponsiveness or **tolerance** would then be created so that as immunological maturity was reached there would normally be an inability to respond to "self" components. Burnet argued that if, following clonal selection, each set of lymphocytes were making their own individual specific antibody, those cells programed to express antibodies reacting with circulating self components could be rendered unresponsive without affecting other lymphocytes specific for foreign antigens. In other words, self-reacting lymphocytes could be selectively suppressed or tolerized without undermining the ability of the host to respond immunologically to infectious agents. As we shall see in Chapter 11, these predictions have been amply verified, although we will learn that, as new lymphocytes differentiate throughout life, they will all go through this self-tolerizing screening process. However, self tolerance is not absolute and normally innocuous but potentially harmful anti-self lymphocytes exist in all of us.

Vaccination depends on acquired memory

Some 200 years ago, Edward Jenner carried out the remarkable studies that mark the beginning of immunology as a systematic subject. Noting the pretty pox-free skin of the milkmaids, he reasoned that deliberate exposure to the pox virus of the cow, which is not virulent for the human, might confer protection against the related human smallpox organism. Accordingly, he inoculated a small boy with cowpox and was delighted and presumably breathed a sigh of relief to observe that the boy was now protected against a subsequent exposure to smallpox (what would today's ethical committees have said about that?!). By injecting a harmless form of a disease organism, Jenner had utilized the specificity and memory of the acquired immune response to lay the foundations for modern **vaccination** (Latin *vacca*, cow).

The essential strategy is to prepare an *innocuous* form of the infectious organism or its toxins that still substantially retains the antigens responsible for establishing memory cells and protective immunity (Figure 2.13). This procedure can be done by using killed or live attenuated organisms, purified microbial components or chemically modified antigens.

Cell-mediated immunity protects against intracellular organisms

The term **cell-mediated immunity** is used to describe the responses of **T-cells**, particularly with respect to the ability of some types of T-helper cells to activate macrophages and the ability of cytotoxic T-lymphocytes to directly kill infected cells. Many microorganisms live inside host cells where it is impossible for humoral antibody to reach them. Obligate intracellular parasites like viruses have to replicate inside cells; facultative intracellular parasites like *Mycobacterium* and *Leishmania* can replicate within cells, particularly macrophages, but do not have to; they like the intracellular life because of the protection it affords. The T-cells are specialized to operate against cells bearing intracellular organisms. Their **T-cell receptor (TCR)** for antigen, which is different from the antibody molecule used by B-lymphocytes, does not directly recognize intact antigen. Instead it recognizes antigen that is first **processed** by the cell in which it is located and then subsequently **presented** to the T-cell. This rather more convoluted mechanism required for antigen recognition is necessary in order that the T-cell sees antigen in association with a cell, rather than non-cell-associated antigens such as extracellular bacteria that can be dealt with by antibody. Protein antigens within cells are chewed up by intracellular proteases to generate short **peptides**. These peptides then need to be taken to the cell surface in order for them to be recognized by the TCR on the T-cells. It is highly unlikely that, if unaccompanied, the peptides would stay on the cell surface. Without a transmembrane sequence they would simply fall off the surface of the cell and float away—not much use if the T-cell needs to identify the particular cell that is infected. An important group of molecules known as the **major histocompatibility complex (MHC)**, identified originally through their ability to evoke powerful transplantation reactions in other members of the same species, carry out the function of transporting the peptides to the cell surface and then displaying them to the TCR on T-cells. Most T-cells thus recognize **peptide + MHC** rather than the native antigen recognized by B-cells.

In general, cytotoxic T-cells recognize peptides presented by the **MHC class I** molecules that are present on virtually all nucleated cells in the body. In contrast, helper and regulatory T-cells usually recognize peptides presented by the **MHC class II** molecules that are, in addition to MHC class I molecules, present on so-called "professional antigen-presenting cells": the interdigitating dendritic cell, the macrophage and the B-lymphocyte. Naive (virgin) T-cells, i.e. those that have not previously encountered their antigen, must be introduced to the peptide antigen and MHC by interdigitating dendritic cells (Figures 2.7f and 7.16) before they can be initiated into the rites of a primary response. However, once primed, T-cells can be activated by peptide antigen and MHC present on the surface of macrophages (or B-cells) as we shall now see.

Figure 2.15. Intracellular killing of microorganisms by macrophages.

(1) An antigen peptide (§) derived from the intracellular microbes is complexed with cell surface class II MHC molecules (□). (2) The primed T-helper cell binds to this MHC–peptide complex using its T-cell receptor (TCR) and is triggered to release the cytokine γ-interferon (IFNγ). This process activates microbicidal mechanisms in the macrophage. (3) The infectious agent meets a timely death.

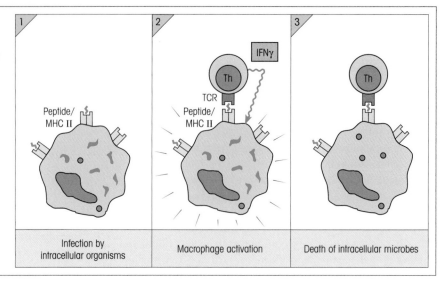

| Infection by intracellular organisms | Macrophage activation | Death of intracellular microbes |

Cytokine-producing T-cells help macrophages to kill intracellular parasites

Organisms that are able to survive inside macrophages do so through their ability to subvert the innate killing mechanisms of the phagocyte. Nonetheless, they mostly cannot prevent the macrophage from processing small antigenic fragments (possibly of organisms that have spontaneously died) and placing them on the host cell surface. The subpopulation of T-lymphocytes called **T-helper cells**, if primed to that antigen, will recognize and bind to the combination of antigen with **class II** MHC molecules on the macrophage surface and produce a variety of soluble factors termed **cytokines** that include the interleukins, IL-2, etc. (p. 229). Different cytokines can be made by various cell types and generally act at a short range on neighboring cells. Some T-cell cytokines help B-cells to make antibodies, while others such as γ-interferon (IFNγ) serve as **macrophage activating factors** that switch on the previously subverted microbicidal mechanisms of the macrophage and bring about the death of the intracellular microorganisms (Figure 2.15).

Virally infected cells can be killed by cytotoxic T-cells and by ADCC

We have already discussed the advantage to the host of killing virally infected cells before the virus begins to replicate and have seen that NK cells (p. 26) can carry out a cytotoxic function via their NK activating receptors (Figure 2.16a and Table 4.3). These receptors inherently have a limited range of specificities. However, NK cells also possess receptors for the constant (Fc) part of the antibody molecule (as discussed earlier with regard to phagocytic cells, p. 37). This situation enables their range of potential targets to be enormously expanded because the Fc receptors can recognize virus-specific antibody coating the target cell if any intact viral antigens are present on the surface of the infected cell. Thus antibodies will bring the NK

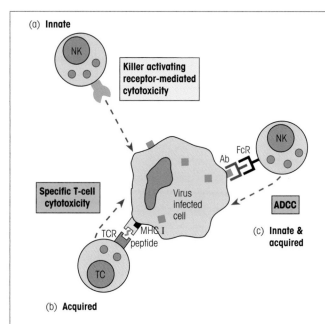

Figure 2.16. Killing virally infected cells.

(a) Destruction of infected cells by the natural killer (NK) cells of the innate response can follow their recognition by the killer activating receptors. (b) The cytotoxic T-cells of the acquired response recognise the infected target cell specifically through TCR recognition of virally derived peptides presented by MHC class I molecules. (c) In addition to the direct recognition by their killer activating receptors, NK cells possess Fc receptors and can therefore recognize any antibodies that are bound to any intact viral antigens present on the surface of infected cells. This is therefore an example of the innate and acquired responses working together to defeat the enemy and, in this case, is referred to as antibody-dependent cellular cytotoxicity (ADCC).

cell very close to the target by forming a bridge, and the NK cell being activated by the complexed antibody molecules is able to kill the virally infected cell by its extracellular mechanisms (Figure 2.16c). This system is termed **antibody-dependent cellular cytotoxic**ity (ADCC).

On the other hand, a **subset** of **T-cells with cytotoxic potential** also exists. Like the T-helpers, these cells have a very wide range of antigen specificities because they clonally express a large number of different TCRs similar to, but not identical with, the surface antibody on the B-lymphocytes. Again, each lymphocyte is programed to make only one receptor and, again like the T-helper cell, recognizes fragments of protein antigens (peptides) in association with a cell marker, in this case the **class I** MHC molecule (Figure 2.16b). Through this recognition of surface antigen, the cytotoxic cell comes into intimate contact with its target and administers the "kiss of apoptotic death." It also releases **IFNγ** that would help to reduce the spread of virus to adjacent cells, particularly in cases where the virus itself may prove to be a weak inducer of IFNα or β.

In an entirely analogous fashion to the B-cell, T-cells are selected and activated by combination with antigen, expanded by clonal proliferation and mature to give T-helpers, cytotoxic T-effectors or regulatory T-cells, together with an enlarged population of memory cells (Figure 2.12).

Thus both T- and B-cells provide **specific acquired immunity** with a variety of mechanisms, which in most cases operate to extend the range of effectiveness of innate immunity and confer the valuable advantage that a first infection prepares us to withstand further contact with the same microorganism. The defining characteristic of the acquired response is that it is mediated by **lymphocytes**, which in contrast to the cells of the innate response are highly **antigen-specific** and exhibit immunological **memory**. It is, however, worth noting two important points at this juncture. Firstly, the innate and acquired responses usually work together to defeat the pathogen and, secondly, that these two systems merge into one another with some cell types having characteristics that bridge both kinds of response.

Immunopathology

The immune system is clearly "a good thing," but like mercenary armies, it can turn to bite the hand that feeds it, and cause damage to the host (Figure 2.17).

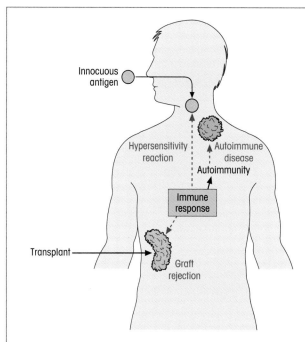

Figure 2.17. Inappropriate immune responses can produce damaging reactions such as the hypersensitivity response to inhaled otherwise innocuous antigens (allergens), the destruction of self tissue by autoimmune attack, and the rejection of tissue transplants.

Thus when there is an especially heightened response or persistent exposure to exogenous antigens, tissue damaging or **hypersensitivity** reactions may result. Examples are allergy to grass pollens, immune complex glomerulonephritis occurring after streptococcal infection, and chronic granulomas produced during tuberculosis or schistosomiasis.

In other cases, responses to autoantigens may arise through a breakdown in the mechanisms that control self tolerance, and a wide variety of **autoimmune diseases**, such as type 1 (insulin-dependent) diabetes and multiple sclerosis and many of the rheumatologic disorders, may result from an autoimmune attack.

Another immunopathologic reaction of some consequence is **transplant rejection**, in which the MHC antigens on the donor graft may well provoke a fierce reaction.

Antigen
- Antigens recognized by the immune system can be proteins, carbohydrates, lipids, or many other types of molecule.
- They have a conformation that is complementary to that of the antigen receptors on cells of the immune system and to the secreted antibody molecules.
- Components of foreign agents and also our own body components can act as antigens.

Antibody, the specific antigen-recognition molecule
- The antibody molecule evolved to attach to microorganisms and focus other components of the immune response into the infectious agent.
- The antibody binds to the antigen by its specific recognition site and its constant structure regions activate complement through the classical pathway (binding C1 and generating a C4b2a convertase to split C3) and phagocytes through their Fc receptors.

Figure 2.18. Production of a protective acute inflammatory reaction by microbes either: (i) through tissue injury (e.g. bacterial toxin) or direct activation of the alternative or lectin complement pathways, or (ii) by antibody-dependent triggering of the classical complement pathway or mast cell degranulation (a special class of antibody, IgE, does this).

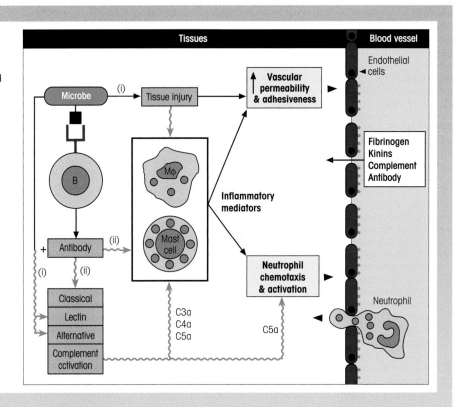

■ This route into the acute inflammatory reaction is enhanced by IgE antibodies that sensitize mast cells and by immune complexes that stimulate mediator release from tissue macrophages (Figure 2.18).

■ The innate immune reaction of mannose-binding lectin with microbes activates the MASP-1 and MASP-2 proteases, which join the classical complement pathway by splitting C4 and C2.

Cellular basis of antibody production

■ Antibodies are secreted by plasma cells derived from B-lymphocytes, each of which is programed to make antibody of a single specificity that is placed on the cell surface as a receptor for antigen.

■ Antigen binds to the B-cell bearing a complementary antibody, activates it, and causes clonal proliferation and finally differentiation into antibody-secreting plasma cells and memory B-cells. Thus the antigen brings about clonal selection of the cells making antibody to that particular antigen.

Acquired memory and vaccination

■ The increase in memory cells after priming means that the acquired secondary response is faster and greater, providing the basis for vaccination using a

harmless form of the infective agent for the initial encounter.

Acquired immunity has antigen specificity

■ Antibodies differentiate between antigens because recognition is based on molecular shape complementarity. Thus memory induced by one antigen will not extend to another unrelated antigen.

■ The immune system differentiates self components from foreign antigens by making immature self-reacting lymphocytes unresponsive through contact with the constantly present host molecules; lymphocytes reacting with foreign antigens are unaffected as (given that infection is usually a transient event) they normally only make contact after reaching maturity.

Cell-mediated immunity protects against intracellular organisms

■ Another class of lymphocyte, the T-cell, is concerned with control of intracellular infections. Like the B-cell, each T-cell has its individual antigen receptor (the TCR, which differs structurally from antibody) that recognizes antigen and the cell then undergoes clonal expansion to form effector and memory cells providing specific acquired immunity.

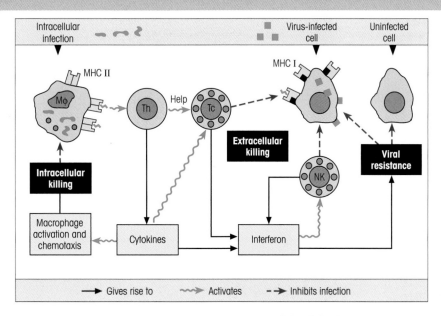

Figure 2.19. T-cells link with the innate immune system to resist intracellular infection.

Class I (⊔) and class II (⊔) major histocompatibility molecules are important for T-cell recognition of antigen. The T-helper cells (Th) cooperate in the development of cytotoxic T-cells (Tc) from precursors. The macrophage (Mφ) microbicidal mechanisms are switched on by macrophage activating cytokines. Interferon inhibits viral replication and stimulates natural killer (NK) cells that, together with Tc, kill virus-infected cells.

■ The T-cell recognizes processed antigens in association with molecules of the MHC. Naive T-cells are only stimulated to undergo a primary response by specialized dendritic antigen-presenting cells.

■ Primed T-helper cells, which see antigen as peptides with class II MHC on the surface of professional antigen-presenting cells (dendritic cells, macrophages and B-lymphocytes), release cytokines that in some cases can help B-cells to make antibody and in others activate macrophages and enable them to kill intracellular parasites.

■ Cytotoxic T-cells have the ability to recognize specific antigen peptides plus class I MHC on the surface of virally infected cells. The infected cells are then killed to prevent the virus replicating. T-cells also release γ-interferon, which can make surrounding cells resistant to viral spread (Figure 2.19).

■ The NK cells of the innate response can work together with the antibodies of the acquired response by recognizing antibody-coated virally infected cells

through their Fcγ receptors. They then kill the target by ADCC.

■ Although the innate mechanisms do not improve with repeated exposure to infection as do the acquired, they play a vital role as they are intimately linked to the acquired systems by **two different pathways** that all but **encapsulate the whole of immunology**. Antibody, complement and polymorphs (neutrophils, eosinophils, basophils and mast cells) give protection against most extracellular organisms, while T-cells, soluble cytokines, dendritic cells, macrophages and NK cells deal with intracellular infections (Figure 2.20).

Immunopathology
■ Immunopathologically mediated tissue damage to the host can occur as a result of:
■ inappropriate hypersensitivity reactions to exogenous antigens;
■ loss of tolerance to self giving rise to autoimmune disease;
■ reaction to foreign grafts.

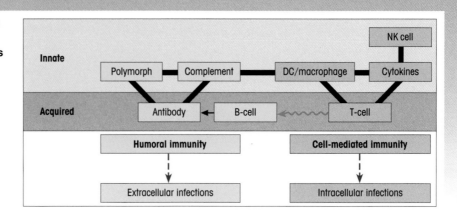

Figure 2.20. The two pathways linking innate and acquired immunity that provide the basis for humoral and cell-mediated immunity, respectively.

FURTHER READING

Berke G. & Clark W.R. (2007) *Killer lymphocytes*. Springer, Dordrecht, The Netherlands. 369 pp.

Borghesi L. & Milcarek C. (2007) Innate versus adaptive immunity: a paradigm past its prime? *Cancer Research* **67**, 3989–3993.

Carroll M.C. (2008) Complement and humoral immunity. *Vaccine* **26** Suppl 8:I28–33.

Cohn M., Mitchison N.A., Paul W.E., Silverstein A.M., Talmage D.W. & Weigert M. (2007) Reflections on the clonal-selection theory. *Nature Reviews Immunology* **7**, 823–830.

Lee H.K. & Iwasaki A. (2007) Innate control of adaptive immunity: dendritic cells and beyond. *Seminars in Immunology* **19**, 48–55.

Palm N.W. & Medzhitov R. (2009) Pattern recognition receptors and control of adaptive immunity. *Immunological Reviews* **227**, 221–233.

Ricklin D., Hajishengallis G., Yang K. & Lambris J.D. (2010) Complement: a key system for immune surveillance and homeostasis. *Nature Immunology* **11**, 785–797.

Silverstein A.M. (2009) *A History of Immunology*. 2nd edn. Academic Press, San Diego.

Sjöberg A.P., Trouw L.A. & Blom A.M. (2009) Complement activation and inhibition: a delicate balance. *Trends in Immunology* **30**, 83–90.

Now visit **www.roitt.com** to test yourself on this chapter.

CHAPTER 3
Antibodies

Key Topics

Just to Recap...

In order to resist the onslaught of a myriad of pathogens, we have evolved general mechanisms of defense (innate immunity) and mechanisms that are specific for a given pathogen (specific acquired or adaptive immunity). The latter mechanism, as its name implies, can be acquired and optimized through contact with the pathogen or through vaccination. The key players in specific immunity are antibodies and T-cells. In this chapter, we consider antibodies in some detail.

Introduction

In essence, antibody molecules carry out two principal functions in immune defense. The **first function** is to recognize and bind to foreign material (antigen). This generally means binding to molecular structures on the surface of the foreign material (antigenic determinants) that differ from molecular structures made by the cells of the host. These antigenic determinants are usually expressed in multiple copies on the foreign material, e.g. proteins or carbohydrates on a bacterial cell surface or envelope spikes on the surface of a virus. Antibodies of a single host can recognize a huge variety of different molecular structures—a human is capable of producing antibodies against billions of different molecular structures. This is described as antibody diversity and is necessary to respond to the huge diversity of molecular structures associated with (often highly mutable) pathogens.

The simple act of antibody binding may be sufficient to inactivate a pathogen or render a toxin harmless. For instance, antibody coating of a virus can prevent entry into target cells and thereby "neutralize" the virus. However, in many instances, a **second function** of the antibody molecule is deployed to trigger the elimination of foreign material. In molecular terms, this involves the binding

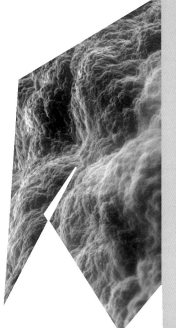

Roitt's Essential Immunology, Twelfth Edition. Peter J. Delves, Seamus J. Martin, Dennis R. Burton, Ivan M. Roitt.

Introduction (*Continued*)

of certain molecules (effector molecules) to antibody-coated foreign material to trigger complex elimination mechanisms, e.g. the complement system of proteins, phagocytosis by host immune cells such as neutrophils and macrophages, and antibody-dependent cellular cytotoxicity (ADCC) by NK cells. The powerful effector systems are generally triggered only by antibody molecules clustered together as on a foreign cell surface and not by free unliganded antibody. This is crucial considering the typically high serum concentrations of antibodies.

The division of labor

The requirements imposed on the antibody molecule by the two functions are in a sense quite opposite. The first function requires great antibody diversity. The second function requires that many different antibody molecules share common features, i.e. it is not practical for Nature to devise a different molecular solution for the problem of elimination of antigens for each different antibody molecule. The conflicting requirements are elegantly met by the antibody structure shown diagrammatically in Figure 3.1. The structure consists of three units. Two of the units are identical to one another and are involved in binding to antigen—the **Fab (fragment antigen binding)** arms of the molecule. These units contain regions of sequence that vary greatly from one antibody to another and

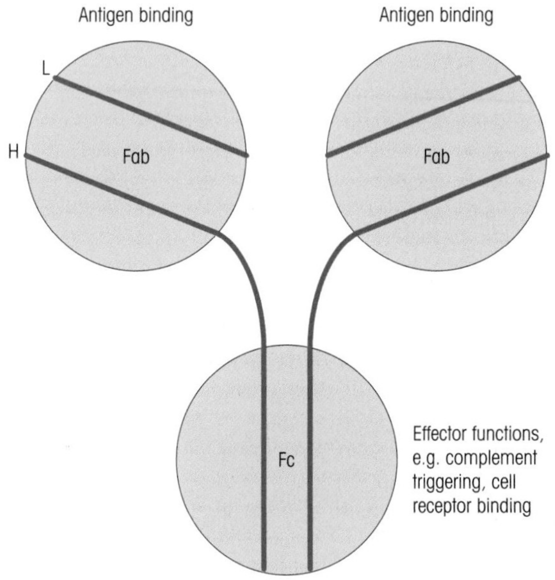

Figure 3.1. Simplified overall layout of the antibody molecule.

The structure consists of four polypeptide chains, two identical heavy (H) chains and two identical light (L) chains, arranged to span three structural units as shown. The two identical Fab units bind antigen and the third unit (Fc) binds effector molecules to trigger antigen elimination and to mediate functions such as maternal–fetal transport.

confer on a given antibody its unique binding specificity. The presence of two identical Fab arms enhances the binding of antibody to antigen in the typical situation where multiple copies of antigenic determinants are presented on foreign material. The third unit—**Fc (fragment crystallizable)** is involved in binding to effector molecules. As shown in Figure 3.1, the antibody molecule has a four-chain structure consisting of two identical heavy chains spanning Fab and Fc and two identical light chains associated only with Fab. The relationship between antigen binding, the different units and the four-chain structure of the antibody molecule were revealed by a series of key experiments summarized in Milestone 3.1.

Five classes of immunoglobulin

Antibodies are often referred to as **immunoglobulins** (immune proteins). There are five classes of antibodies or immunoglobulins termed immunoglobulin G (IgG), IgM, IgA, IgD and IgE. All these classes have the basic four-chain antibody structure but they differ in their heavy chains termed γ, μ, α, δ and ϵ, respectively. The differences are most pronounced in the Fc regions of the antibody classes and this leads to the triggering of different effector functions on binding to antigen, e.g. IgM recognition of antigen might lead to complement activation whereas IgE recognition (possibly of the same antigen) might lead to mast cell degranulation and anaphylaxis (increased vascular permeability and smooth muscle contraction). These differences are discussed in greater detail below. Structural differences also lead to differences in the polymerization state of the monomer unit shown in Figure 3.1. Thus, IgG and IgE are generally monomeric whereas IgM occurs as a pentamer. IgA occurs predominantly as a monomer in serum and as a dimer in seromucous secretions.

The major antibody in the serum is IgG and, as this is the best-understood antibody in terms of structure and function, we shall consider it first. The other antibody classes will be considered in relation to IgG.

The IgG molecule

In IgG, the Fab arms are linked to the Fc by an extended region of polypeptide chain known as the hinge. This region tends to be exposed and sensitive to attack by proteases that cleave the molecule in to its distinct functional units arranged around the

◉ Milestone 3.1—Four-polypeptide Structure of Immunoglobulin Monomers

Early studies showed the bulk of the antibody activity in serum to be in the slow electrophoretic fraction termed γ-globulin (subsequently immunoglobulin). The most abundant antibodies were divalent, i.e. had two combining sites for antigen and could thus form a precipitating complex (cf. Figure 6.24).

To Rodney Porter and Gerald Edelman must go the credit for unlocking the secrets of the basic structure of the immunoglobulin molecule. If the internal disulfide bonds are reduced, the component polypeptide chains still hang together by strong noncovalent attractions. However, if the reduced molecule is held under acid conditions, these attractive forces are lost as the chains become positively charged and can now be separated by gel filtration into larger so-called heavy chains of approximately 55000 Da (for IgG,

IgA and IgD) or 70000 Da (for IgM and IgE) and smaller light chains of about 24000 Da.

The clues to how the chains are assembled to form the IgG molecule came from selective cleavage using proteolytic enzymes. Papain destroyed the precipitating power of the intact molecule but produced two univalent Fab fragments still capable of binding to antigen (Fab—*fragment antigen binding*); the remaining fragment had no affinity for antigen and was termed Fc by Porter (*fragment crystallizable*). After digestion with pepsin a molecule called F(ab')₂ was isolated; it still precipitated antigen and so retained both binding sites, but the Fc portion was further degraded. The structural basis for these observations is clearly evident from Figure M3.1.1. In essence, with minor changes, all immunoglobulin molecules are constructed from one or more of the basic four-chain units.

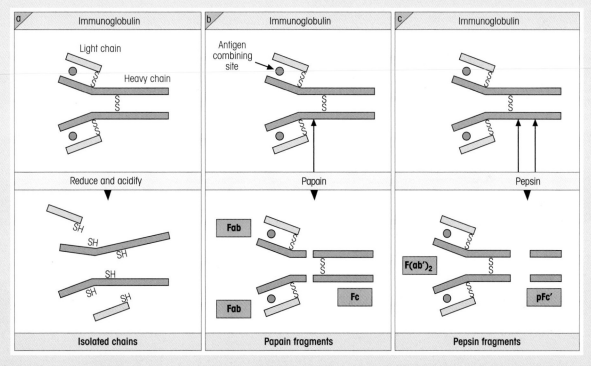

Figure M3.1.1. The antibody basic unit (IgG is represented), consisting of two identical heavy and two identical light chains held together by interchain disulfide bonds (a), can be broken down into its constituent polypeptide chains and to proteolytic fragments, the pepsin F(ab')₂ retaining two binding sites for antigen (c) and the papain Fab with one (b). After pepsin digestion the pFc' fragment representing the C-terminal half of the Fc region is formed and is held together by noncovalent bonds. The portion of the heavy chain in the Fab fragment is given the symbol Fd. The N-terminal residue is on the left for each chain.

four-chain structure (Milestone 3.1). This structure is represented in greater detail in Figure 3.2a. The light chains exist in two forms known as kappa (κ) and lambda (λ). In humans, κ chains are somewhat more prevalent than λ; in mice, λ chains are rare. The heavy chains can also be grouped into different forms or subclasses, the number depending upon the species under consideration. In humans there are four **subclasses** having heavy chains labeled γ1, γ2, γ3 and γ4 that give rise to

the IgG1, IgG2, IgG3 and IgG4 subclasses. In mice, there are again four subclasses denoted IgG1, IgG2a, IgG2b and IgG3. The subclasses—particularly in humans—have very similar primary sequences, the greatest differences being observed in the hinge region. The existence of subclasses is an important feature as they show marked differences in their ability to trigger effector functions. In a single molecule, the two heavy chains are generally identical as are the two light chains. The

Figure 3.2. The four-chain structure of IgG.

(a) Linear representation. Disulfide bridges link the two heavy chains and the light and heavy chains. A regular arrangement of intrachain disulfide bonds is also found. Fragments generated by proteolytic cleavage at the indicated sites are represented. (b) Domain representation. Each heavy chain (shaded dark) is folded into two domains in the Fab arms, forms a region of extended polypeptide chain in the hinge and is then folded into two domains in the Fc region. The light chain forms two domains associated only with a Fab arm. Domain pairing leads to close interaction of heavy and light chains in the Fab arms supplemented by a disulfide bridge. The two heavy chains are disulfide bridged in the hinge (the number of bridges depending on IgG subclass) and are in close domain-paired interaction at their carboxy-termini. (c) Domain nomenclature. The heavy chain is composed of V_H, C_H1, C_H2 and C_H3 domains. The light chain is composed of V_L and C_L domains. All the domains are paired except for the C_H2 domains, which have two branched N-linked carbohydrate chains interposed between them. Each domain has a molecular weight of approximately 12000 leading to a molecular weight of ~50000 for Fc and Fab and 150000 for the whole IgG molecule. Antigen recognition involves residues from the V_H and V_L domains, complement triggering the C_H2 domain, leukocyte Fc receptor binding the C_H2 domain and the neonatal Fc receptor the C_H2 and C_H3 domains (see text). (Adapted from Burton D.R. Structure and function of antibodies. (1987) In: *New Comprehensive Biochemistry, Vol. 17: Molecular Genetics of Immunoglobulin* F. Calabi & M.S. Neuberger (eds.). Elsevier, pp. 1–50.)

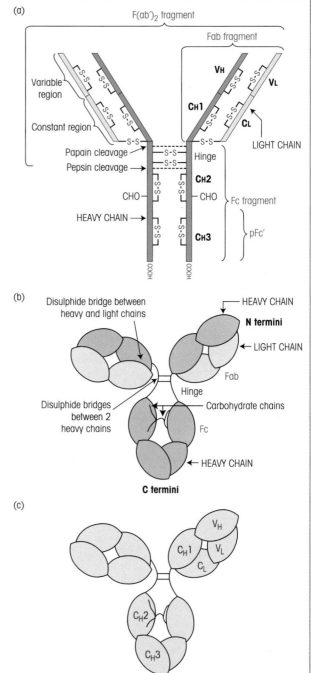

exception to the rule is provided by human IgG4, which can exchange heavy-light pairs between IgG4 molecules to produce hybrids. As the Fc parts of the exchanging molecules are identical the net effect is Fab arm exchange to generate IgG4 antibodies having two distinct Fab arms and dual specificity.

The amino acid sequences of heavy and light chains of antibodies have revealed much about their structure and function. However, obtaining the sequences of antibodies is much more challenging than for many other proteins because the population of antibodies in an individual is so incredibly het-

erogeneous. The opportunity to do this first came from the study of **myeloma proteins**. In the human disease known as multiple myeloma, one cell making one particular individual antibody divides over and over again in the uncontrolled way a cancer cell does, without regard for the overall requirement of the host. The patient then possesses enormous numbers of identical cells derived as a clone from the original cell and they all synthesize the same immunoglobulin—the myeloma protein—which appears in the serum, sometimes in very high concentrations. By purification of myeloma proteins, preparations of a single antibody for sequencing and many other applications can be obtained. An alternative route to single or **monoclonal antibodies** arrived with the development of **hybridoma technology**. Here, fusing individual antibody-forming cells with a B-cell tumor produces a constantly dividing clone of cells dedicated to making the one antibody. Finally, **recombinant antibody technologies**, developed most recently, provide an excellent source of monoclonal antibodies.

Sequence comparison of monoclonal IgG proteins indicates that the carboxy-terminal half of the light chain and roughly three-quarters of the heavy chain, again carboxy-terminal, show little sequence variation between different IgG molecules. By contrast, the amino-terminal regions of about 100 amino acid residues show considerable sequence variability in both chains. Within these variable regions there are relatively short sequences that show extreme variation and are designated hypervariable regions. There are three of these regions or "hot spots" on the light chain and three on the heavy chain. As the different IgGs in the comparison recognize different antigens, these **hypervariable regions** are expected to be associated with antigen recognition and indeed are often referred to as **complementarity determining regions (CDRs)**. The structural setting for the involvement of the hypervariable regions in antigen recognition and the genetic origins of the constant and variable regions will be discussed shortly.

The comparison of immunoglobulin sequences also reveals the organization of IgG into 12 homology regions or **domains** each possessing an internal disulfide bond. The basic domain structure is central to an understanding of the relation between structure and function in the antibody molecule and will shortly be taken up below. However, the structure in outline form is shown in Figure 3.2b,c. It is seen that the light chain consists of two domains, one corresponding to the variable sequence region discussed above and designated the V_L (variable-light) domain and the other corresponding to a constant region and designated the C_L (constant-light) domain. The IgG heavy chain consists of four domains, the V_H and C_H1 domains of the Fab arms being joined to the C_H2 and C_H3 domains of Fc via the hinge. Antigen binding is a combined property of the V_L and V_H domains at the extremities of the Fab arms and effector molecule binding a property of the C_H2 and/or C_H3 domains of Fc.

It is also clear (Figure 3.2b,c) that all of the domains except for C_H2 are in close lateral or "sideways" association with another domain: a phenomenon described as domain pairing. The C_H2 domains have two sugar chains interposed between them. The domains also exhibit weaker *cis*-interactions with neighboring domains on the same polypeptide chain.

Human IgG1 is shown in Figure 3.2 as a Y-shaped conformation with the Fab arms roughly in the same plane as the Fc. This is the classical view of the antibody molecule that has adorned countless meetings ads and appears in many company logos. In reality, this is likely just one of many shapes that the IgG molecule can adopt as it is very **flexible** as illustrated in Figure 3.3. It is believed that this flexibility may help IgG

function. Thus Fab–Fab flexibility gives the antibody a "variable reach" allowing it to grasp antigenic determinants of different spacings on a foreign cell surface or to form intricate immune complexes with a toxin (imagine a Y to T shape change). Fc–Fab flexibility may help antibodies in different environments, on foreign cells for example, to interact productively with common effector molecules. Figure 3.4 shows the complete structure of a human IgG1 antibody molecule determined by crystallography. The structure is quite removed from the classical symmetrical Y shape. The Fc is closer to one Fab arm than another and is rotated relative to the Fab arms. This

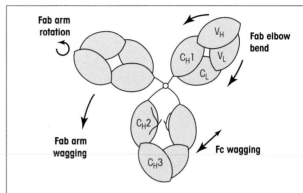

Figure 3.3. Modes of flexibility in the IgG molecule.

These modes have been described from electron microscopic studies (see Figure 3.10) and biophysical techniques in solution. Flexibility in structure probably facilitates flexibility in antigen recognition and effector function triggering.

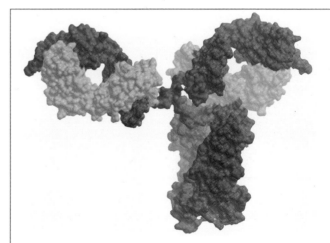

Figure 3.4. The structure of a human IgG molecule.

The heavy chains are shown in purple and the light chains in brown. Relative to the classical cartoon of an IgG molecule as a Y shape, this "snapshot" of the molecule finds the Fc (bottom) "side on" to the viewer and much closer to one Fab arm than the other. (Courtesy of Erica Ollmann Saphire.)

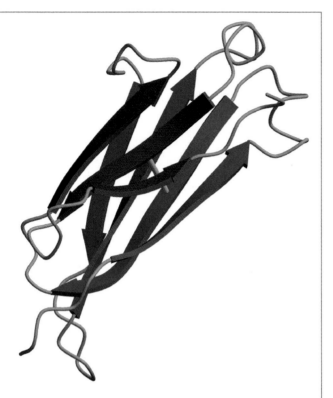

Figure 3.5. The immunoglobulin fold (constant domain).

An anti-parallel three-stranded β-sheet (red) interacts with a four-stranded sheet (blue). The arrangement is stabilized by a disulfide bond linking the two sheets. The β-strands are connected by helices, turns and other structures. A similar overall core structure is seen in all Ig-like domains but with some modifications such as extra β-strands or changes in how the edge strands pair with the β-sheets.

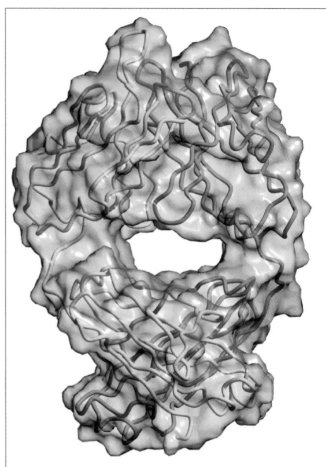

Figure 3.6. The structure of Fab.

The heavy chain is shown in green and the light chain in yellow. The V$_H$ and V$_L$ domains (top) are paired by contact between their five-strand faces and the C$_H$1 and C$_L$ domains between the four-strand faces. (Courtesy of Robyn Stanfield.)

is simply a "snapshot" of one of the many conformations that the antibody can adopt by virtue of its flexibility.

The structural organization of IgG into domains is clearly evident from Figures 3.2–3.4. Each of these domains has a common pattern of polypeptide chain folding (Figure 3.5). This pattern, the "immunoglobulin fold," consists of two twisted stacked β-sheets enclosing an internal volume of tightly packed hydrophobic residues. The arrangement is stabilized by an internal disulfide bond linking the two sheets in a central position (this internal bond is seen in Figure 3.2a). In a constant type Ig domain, one sheet has four and the other three anti-parallel β-strands. These strands are joined by bends or loops that generally show little secondary structure. Residues involved in the β-sheets tend to be conserved while there is a greater diversity of residues in the loops. The chain folding illustrated in Figure 3.5 is for a constant domain. The β-sheets of the variable domain are more distorted than those of the C domain and the V domain possesses an extra loop.

Structure of Fab fragment

The Fab fragment pairs V$_H$ and V$_L$ domains and C$_H$1 and C$_L$ domains (Figure 3.6). The V$_H$ and V$_L$ domains are paired by contact between the two respective three-strand β-sheet layers (red in Figure 3.5) whereas the C$_H$1 and C$_L$ domains are paired via the two four-strand layers (blue in Figure 3.5). The interacting faces of the domains are predominantly hydrophobic and the driving force for domain pairing is thus the removal of these residues from the aqueous environment. The arrangement is further stabilized by a disulfide bond between C$_H$1 and C$_L$ domains.

In contrast to the "sideways" interactions, the "longwise" or *cis* interactions between V$_H$ and C$_H$1 domains and between V$_L$ and C$_L$ domains are very limited and allow bending about the "elbows" between these domains. Elbow angles seen in crystal structures vary between about 117° and 249°.

The antibody combining site

Comparison of antibody sequence and structural data shows how antibodies are able to recognize an enormously diverse range of molecules. Sequence data shows that the variable domains have six hypervariable regions that display great variation in amino acids between different antibody molecules (Figure 3.7). Structural data of antibody–antigen complexes reveal that these hypervariable regions, or complementarity determining regions, come together in 3D space to form the antigen binding site, often also termed the **antibody combining site** (Figure 3.8). (Courtesy of Robyn Stanfield.)

Structure of Fc

For the Fc of IgG (Figure 3.9), the two C_H3 domains are classically paired whereas the two C_H2 domains show no close interaction, but have interposed between them two branched *N*-linked carbohydrate chains that have limited contact with one another. The carbohydrate chains are very heterogeneous. The C_H2 domains contain the binding sites for several important effector molecules, complement C1q and Fc receptors in particular, as shown. The neonatal Fc receptor, which is important in binding to IgG and maintaining its long half-life in serum, binds to a site formed between C_H2 and C_H3 domains. Protein A, much used in purifying IgGs, also binds to this site.

The hinge region and IgG subclasses

The term **"hinge"** arose from electron micrographs of rabbit IgG, which showed Fab arms assuming different angles relative to one another from nearly 0° (acute Y-shaped) to 180° (T-shaped). The Fab was specific for a small chemical group dinitrophenyl (DNP) that could be attached to either end of a hydrocarbon chain. As shown in Figures 3.10 and 3.11, different shapes were observed as the Fab arms linked together the bivalent antigen molecule using different Fab–Fab arm angles. Other biophysical techniques have demonstrated hinge flexibility in solution. The function of this flexibility has generally been seen as allowing divalent recognition of variably spaced antigenic determinants. The IgG class of antibody in humans exists as four subclasses and the biggest difference between the subclasses is in the nature and length of the hinge. IgG1 has been shown above. IgG3 has a hinge that if fully

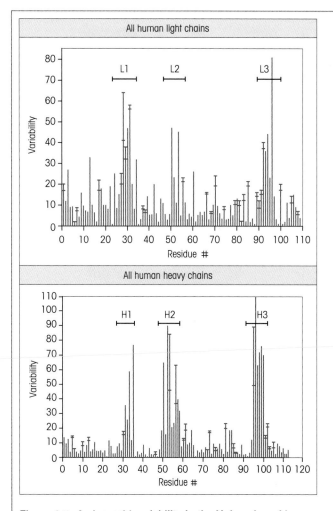

Figure 3.7. Amino acid variability in the V domains of human Ig heavy and light chains.

Variability, for a given position, is defined as the ratio of the number of different residues found at that position compared to the frequency of the most common amino acid. The complementarity determining regions (CDRs) are apparent as peaks in the plot and the frameworks as intervening regions of low variability. (After Dr. E.A. Kabat.)

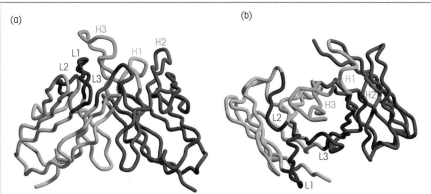

Figure 3.8. The proximity of complementarity determining regions (CDRs or variable loops) at the tip of the Fab arms creates the antibody combining site.

The V_H and V_L domains are shown from the side (a) and from above (b). The six CDRs (cf. Figure 3.7) are numbered 1–3 as belonging to the heavy (H) or light (L) chain. (Courtesy of Robyn Stanfield.)

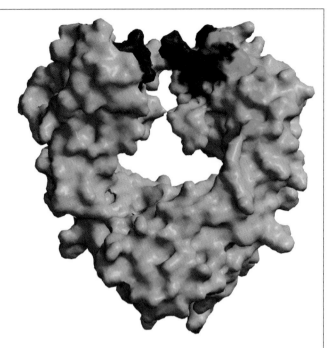

Figure 3.9. Structure of Fc of human IgG.

The C_H3 domains (bottom) are paired. The C_H2 domains are not and have two carbohydrate chains filling some of the space between them. Binding sites for the leukocyte FcγRIII receptor (red), complement C1q (green) and neonatal Fc receptor FcRn (yellow) are shown. The FcγRIII and FcRn sites were determined in crystallographic studies (Sondermann P. *et al.* (2000) *Nature* **406**, 267; Martin W.L. *et al.* (2001) *Molecular Cell* **7**, 867) and the C1q site by mutation analysis (Idusogie *et al.* (2000) *Journal of Immunology* **164**, 4178). (Courtesy of Robyn Stanfield.)

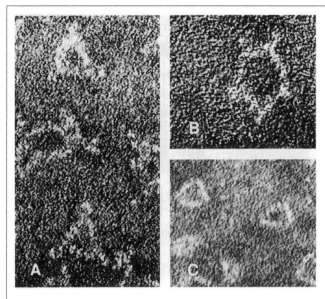

Figure 3.10. (a,b) Electron micrograph (×1 000 000) of complexes formed on mixing the divalent dinitrophenyl (DNP) hapten with rabbit anti-DNP antibodies. The "negative stain" phosphotungstic acid is an electron-dense solution that penetrates into the spaces between the protein molecules. Thus the protein stands out as a "light" structure in the electron beam. The hapten links together the Y-shaped antibody molecules to form trimers (a) and pentamers (b). The flexibility of the molecule at the hinge region is evident from the variation in angle of the arms of the "Y." (c) As in (a), but the trimers were formed using the F(ab')₂ antibody fragment from which the Fc structures have been digested by pepsin (×500 000). The trimers can be seen to lack the Fc projections at each corner evident in (A). (After Valentine R.C. & Green N.M. (1967) *Journal of Molecular Biology* **27**, 615; courtesy of Dr. Green and with the permission of Academic Press, New York.)

extended would be about twice the length of the Fc, thereby potentially placing the Fab arms far removed from the Fc. On the other hand, IgG2 and IgG4 have short compact hinges that probably lead to close approach of Fab and Fc. Interestingly, IgG1 and IgG3 are generally superior at mediating effector functions such as complement activation and ADCC relative to IgG2 and IgG4.

The structure and function of the immunoglobulin classes

The immunoglobulin classes (Table 3.1) fulfill different roles in immune defense and this can be correlated with differences in their structures as organized around the four-chain Ig domain arrangement (Figure 3.12). **IgG** is monomeric and the major antibody in serum and nonmucosal tissues, where it inactivates pathogens directly and through interaction with effector triggering molecules such as complement and Fc receptors. **IgM** is pentameric, is found in serum and is highly efficient at complement triggering. A monomeric form of IgM with a membrane-tethering sequence is the major antibody

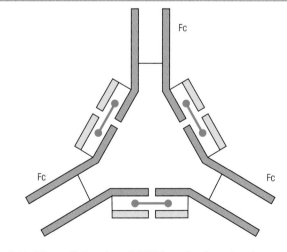

Figure 3.11. Three dinitrophenyl (DNP) antibody molecules held together as a trimer by the divalent antigen (●——●).

Compare Figure 3.10a. When the Fc fragments are first removed by pepsin, the corner pieces are no longer visible (Figure 3.10c).

Table 3.1. The human immunoglobulins.

Class (heavy chain designation)	Human subclasses	Principal molecular forms	Polypeptides	Primary location	Complement activation (pathway)
IgG (γ)	IgG1 IgG2 IgG3 IgG4	Monomer	γ2,L2	Serum (~12 mg/ml), tissues	IgG3 > IgG1 >> IgG2 >> IgG4 (classical)
IgA (α)	IgA1 IgA2	Monomer Dimer Secretory	α2, L2 (α2,L2)$_2$, J (α2, L2)$_2$, J, SC	Serum (~3 mg/ml): 90% monomer, 10% dimer Seromucous secretions, milk, colostrum, tears	Yes (mannose-binding lectin)
IgM (μ)		Pentamer	(μ2, L2)$_5$, J	Serum (~1.5 mg/ml)	Yes (classical)
IgE (ε)		Monomer	ε2, L2	Serum (0.05 μg/ml)	No
IgD (δ)		Monomer	δ2, L2	Serum (30 μg/ml)	No

receptor used by B lymphocytes to recognize antigen (cf. Figure 2.11). IgM differs from IgG in having an extra pair of constant domains instead of the hinge region. **IgA** exists in three soluble forms. Monomeric and small amounts of dimeric IgA (formed from two monomers linked by an extra polypeptide called J chain) are found in the serum where they can help link pathogens to effector cells via Fc receptors specific for IgA. Secretory IgA (see below) is formed of dimeric IgA and an extra protein known as secretory component and is crucial in protecting the mucosal surfaces of the body against attack by microorganisms. IgA exists as two subclasses in humans. IgA2 has a much shorter hinge than IgA1 and is more resistant to attack by bacterially secreted proteases. **IgE** is a monomeric antibody typically found at very low concentrations in serum. In fact most IgE is probably bound to IgE Fc receptors on mast cells. Antigen binding to IgE cross-links IgE Fc receptors and triggers an acute inflammatory reaction that can assist in immune defense. This can also lead to unwanted allergic symptoms for certain antigens (allergens). IgE, like IgM, has an extra pair of constant domains instead of the hinge region. Finally **IgD** is an antibody primarily found on the surface of B cells as an antigen receptor together with IgM, where it likely serves in the control of lymphocyte activation and suppression. It is monomeric and has a long hinge region.

The structures of the Fc regions of human IgA1 and IgE (C-terminal domains) have been determined and are compared with IgG1 in Figure 3.13. In all three cases, the penultimate domains are unpaired and have carbohydrate chains interposed between them.

Antibodies and complement

The clustering together of IgG molecules, typically on the surface of a pathogen such as a bacterium, leads to the binding of the complement C1 molecule via the hexavalent C1q subcomponent (cf. Figure 2.2). This triggers the classical pathway of complement and a number of processes that can lead to pathogen elimination. The subclasses of IgG trigger with different efficiencies. IgG1 and IgG3 trigger best; IgG2 is only triggered by antigens at high density such as carbohydrate antigens on a bacterium; and IgG4 does not trigger.

IgM triggers by a different mechanism. It is already "clustered" (pentameric) but occurs in an inactive form. Binding to multivalent antigen appears to alter the conformation of the IgM molecule to expose binding sites that allow C1q to bind and the classical pathway of complement to be triggered. Electron microscopy studies suggest the conformational change is a "star" to "staple" transition, in which the Fab arms move out of the plane of the Fc regions (Figure 3.14). IgM antibodies tend to be of low affinity as measured in a univalent interaction, e.g. binding of IgM to a soluble monomeric molecule or binding of an isolated Fab from an IgM to an antigen. However, their functional affinity (avidity) can be enhanced by multivalent antibody–antigen interaction (see p. 119) and it is precisely under such circumstances that they are most effective at activating complement.

Antibodies and human leukocyte Fc receptors

Specific human Fc receptors have been described for IgG, IgA and IgE (Table 3.2). The receptors differ in their specificities for antibody classes and subclasses, their affinities for different association states of antibodies (monomer versus associated antigen-complexed antibody), their distributions on different leukocyte cell types and their cellular signaling mechanisms. Most of the leukocyte Fc receptors are structurally related, having evolved as members of the Ig gene superfamily. Each comprises a unique ligand binding chain (α

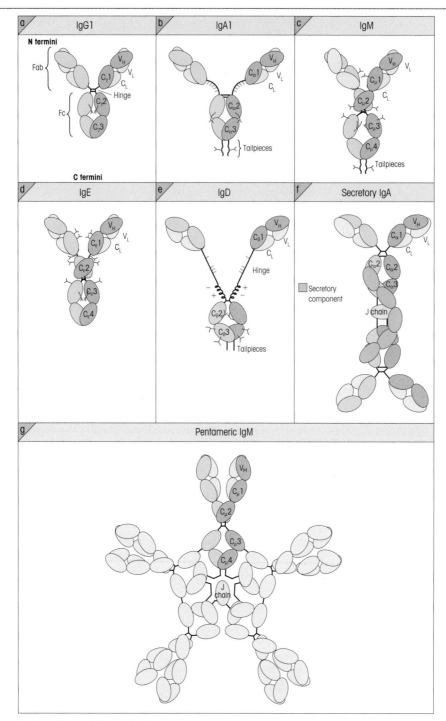

Figure 3.12. Schematic structures of the antibody classes.

The two heavy chains are shown in dark and pale blue (two colors to highlight chain pairing; the chains are identical) and the light chains in gray. *N*-linked carbohydrate chains (branched structures) are shown in blue and *O*-linked carbohydrates (linear structures) in green. The heavy chain domains are designated according to the class of the heavy chain, e.g. Cγ2 for the C_H2 domain of IgG, etc. For IgG, IgA and IgD, the Fc is connected to the Fab arms via a hinge region; for IgM and IgE an extra pair of domains replaces the hinge. IgA, IgM and IgD have tailpieces at the C termini of the heavy chains. IgA occurs in monomer and dimer forms. IgM occurs as a pentamer. (a) IgG1. The other human IgG subclasses (and IgGs of most other species) have this same basic structure but differ particularly in the nature and length of the hinge. (b) IgA1. The structure resembles IgG1 but with a relatively long hinge bearing *O*-linked sugar chains. The Fc also shows some differences from IgG1 (see Figure 3.13). In IgA2, the hinge is very short and, in the predominant allotype, the light chains are disulfide linked not to the heavy chain but to one another. (c) IgM monomeric unit. This representation relies greatly on comparison of the amino acid sequences of μ and γ heavy chains. (d) IgE. The molecule is similar to the monomeric unit of IgM. (e) IgD. The hinge can be divided into a region rich in charge (possibly helical) and one rich in *O*-linked sugars. The structure of the hinge may be much less extended in solution than represented schematically here. It is however very sensitive to proteolytic attack so that serum IgD is unstable. Mouse IgD has a structure very different to that of human IgD in contrast to the general similarity in structures for human and mouse Igs. (f) Secretory IgA (see also Figure 3.19). (g) Pentameric IgM. The molecule is represented as a planar star shape. One monomer unit is shown shaded as in (c). A minority of IgM units can also form a hexamer. For clarity the carbohydrate structures have been omitted in (f) and (g). The Fab arms can likely rotate out of the plane about their two-fold axis (see also Figure 3.14).

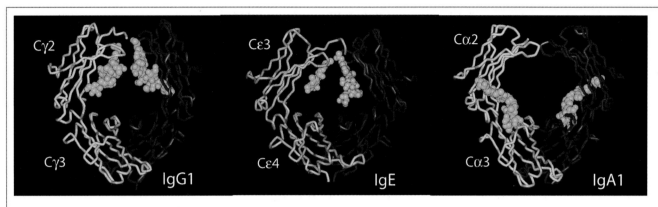

Figure 3.13. The structures of the Fc regions of human IgG1, IgE and IgA1.

The structures shown were determined by crystallographic analysis of Fcs in complex with Fc receptors. One heavy chain is shown in red, the other in yellow and the *N*-linked carbohydrate chains that are interposed between the penultimate domains are shown in blue. For IgE, the structure does not include the Cε2 domains, which form part of the Fc region of this antibody. For IgA1, the *N*-linked sugars are attached at a position quite distinct from that for IgG1 and IgE. Also the tips of the Cα2 domain are joined by a disulfide bridge. (Courtesy of Jenny Woof; after Woof J.M. & Burton D.R. (2004) *Nature Reviews Immunology* **4**, 89–99.)

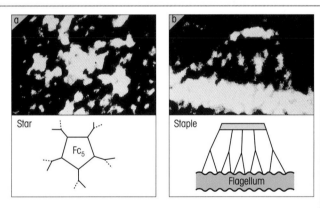

Figure 3.14. Structural changes in IgM associated with complement activation.

(a) The "star" conformation. EM of an uncomplexed IgM protein shows a "star-shaped" conformation (cf. Figure 3.12g). (b) The "staple" conformation. EM of a specific sheep IgM bound to a *Salmonella paratyphi* flagellum as antigen suggests that the five F(ab′)₂ units and Cμ2 domains have been dislocated relative to the plane of the Fcs to produce a "staple" or "crab-like" conformation. Complement C1 is activated on binding to antigen-complexed IgM (staple), but interacts only very weakly, yielding no significant activation, with free IgM (star), implying that the dislocation process plays an important role in complement activation. It is suggested that movement of the Fabs exposes a C1q binding site on the Cμ3 domains of IgM. This is supported by observations that an Fc5 molecule, obtained by papain digestion of IgM, can activate complement directly in the absence of antigen. (Electron micrographs are negatively stained preparations of magnification ×2.10⁶, i.e. 1 mm represents 0.5 nm; kindly provided by Drs. A. Feinstein and E.A. Munn.)

chain), which is often complexed via its transmembrane region with a dimer of the common FcRγ chain. The latter plays a key role in the **signaling functions** of many of the receptors. FcRγ chains carry immunoreceptor tyrosine-based activation motifs (ITAMs) in their cytoplasmic regions, critical for initiation of activatory signals. Some receptor α chains carry their own ITAMs in their cytoplasmic regions, while others bear the immunoreceptor tyrosine-based inhibitory motifs (ITIMs).

For IgG, three different classes of human leukocyte FcγRs have been characterized, most with several variant forms. In addition, the neonatal Fc receptor FcRn also binds IgG and will be dealt with later. **FcγRI** (CD64) is characterized by its high affinity for monomeric IgG. It is also unusual in that it has three extracellular Ig-like domains in its ligand-binding chain, while all other Fc receptors have two. FcγRI is constitutively expressed on monocytes, macrophages and dendritic cells, and is induced on neutrophils and eosinophils following their activation by IFNγ and G-CSF (*g*ranulocyte *c*olony-*s*timulating *f*actor). Conversely, FcγRI can be downregulated in response to IL-4 and IL-13. Structurally, it consists of an IgG-binding α chain and a γ chain homodimer containing ITAMs. It binds monomeric IgG avidly to the surface of the cell thus sensitizing it for subsequent encounter with antigen. Its main roles are probably in facilitating phagocytosis, antigen presentation and in mediating extracellular killing of target cells coated with IgG antibody, a process referred to as *a*ntibody-*d*ependent *c*ellular *c*ytotoxicity (ADCC; p. 48).

FcγRII (CD32) binds very weakly to monomeric IgG but with considerably enhanced affinity to associated IgG as in immune complexes or on an antibody-coated target cell. Therefore cells bearing FcγRII are able to bind antibody-coated

Table 3.2. Human leukocyte Fc receptors. (From Woof J.M. & Burton D.R. (2004) *Nature Reviews Immunology* **4**, 89.)

MW (kDa)	FcγRI (CD64)	FcγRII (CD32)				FcγRIII (CD16)		FcεRI	FcεRII (CD23)		FcαRI (CD89)
	50–70	40				50–80		45–65	45–50		50–70
Major isoforms expressed	FcγRIa	FcγRIIa		FcγRIIb	FcγRIIc	FcγRIIIa	FcγRIIIb	FcεRI	FcεRIIa	FcεRIIb	FcαRIa
Allotypes		LR	HR				NA1 and NA2				
Specificity for human Ig*	IgG1 = 3 > 4 IgG2 doesn't bind	IgG3 ≥ 1 = 2 IgG4 doesn't bind	IgG3 ≥ 1 >>> 2 IgG4 doesn't bind	IgG3 ≥ 1 >> 2 > 4	ND	ND	IgG1 = 3 >>> 2 = 4	IgE	IgE		Serum IgA1 = 2, SIgA1 = SIgA2
Affinity for monomer Ig (M^{-1})	High (10^8–10^9)	Low ($<10^7$)	Low ($<10^7$)	Low ($<10^7$)	Low ($<10^7$)	Medium (10^7)	Low ($<10^7$)	Very high (10^{10})	Low ($<10^7$)		Medium (10^7)
Signaling motif	γ chain ITAM	α chain ITAM		α chain ITIM	α chain ITAM	γ chain ITAM	No signaling motif. Anchored in membrane via glycan phosphatidylinositol (GPI) linkage	γ chain ITAM β chain also present but role unclear	C-type lectin	C-type lectin	γ chain ITAM
Cellular distribution	Monocytes, macrophages, DC, neutrophils (IFNγstim), eosinophils (IFNγstim)	Monocytes, macrophages, neutrophils, platelets, Langerhans cells		Monocytes, macrophages, B-cells	Monocytes, macrophages, neutrophils, B-cells	Macrophages, NK cells, γδ T-cells, some monocytes	Neutrophils, eosinophils (IFNγstim)	Mast cells, basophils, Langerhans cells, activated monocytes	B-cells	B-cells, T-cells, monocytes, eosinophils, macrophages	Neutrophils, monocytes, some macrophages, eosinophils, Kupffer cells, some DC

*Relative affinities of various ligands for each receptor are indicated in decreasing order starting with the isotype with highest affinity. Arrowheads and equal signs are used to show the differences in affinity.

targets in the presence of high serum concentrations of monomeric IgG. Unlike the single isoform of FcγRI, there are multiple expressed isoforms of FcγRII that collectively are present on the surface of most types of leukocyte (Table 3.2). The binding of IgG complexes to FcγRII triggers phagocytic cells and may provoke thrombosis through their reaction with platelets. FcγRIIa are activating receptors expressed on phagocytes that mediate phagocytosis and ADCC. In contrast, FcγRIIb are inhibitory receptors that have cytoplasmic domains containing ITIMs and their occupation leads to *downregulation* of cellular responsiveness. FcγRIIb occurs as two isoforms generated by alternative splicing. FcγRIIb1 present on B-cells crosslinks *B-c*ell *r*eceptors (BCR) and transmits an inhibitory signal to inactivate the B cell with a negative-feedback effect on antibody production. FcγRIIb2 is expressed on phagocytes where it efficiently mediates endocytosis leading to antigen presentation.

FcγRIII (CD16) also binds rather poorly to monomer IgG but has low to medium affinity for aggregated IgG. The two *FcγRIII* genes encode the isoforms FcγRIIIa and FcγRIIIb that have a medium and low affinity for IgG, respectively. FcγRIIIa is found on most types of leukocyte, whereas FcγRIIIb is restricted mainly to neutrophils and is unique amongst the Fc receptors in being attached to the cell membrane by a glycosylphosphatidylinositol (GPI) anchor rather than a transmembrane segment. FcγRIIIa is known to be associated with the γ chain signaling dimer on monocytes and macrophages, and with either ζ and/or γ chain signaling molecules in NK cells, and its expression is upregulated by transforming growth factor β (TGFβ) and downregulated by IL-4. With respect to their functions, FcγRIIIa is largely responsible for mediating ADCC by NK cells and the clearance of immune complexes from the circulation by macrophages. For example, the clearance of IgG-coated erythrocytes from the blood of chimpanzees was essentially inhibited by the monovalent Fab fragment of a monoclonal anti-FcγRIII. FcγRIIIb cross-linking stimulates the production of superoxide by neutrophils.

For IgE, two different FcγRs have been described. The binding of IgE to its receptor **FcεRI** is characterized by the remarkable high affinity of the interaction, reflecting a very slow dissociation rate (the half-life of the complex is ~20 hours). FcεRI is a complex comprising a ligand-binding α chain structurally related to those of FcγR, a β chain, and the FcRγ chain dimer. Contact with antigen leads to degranulation

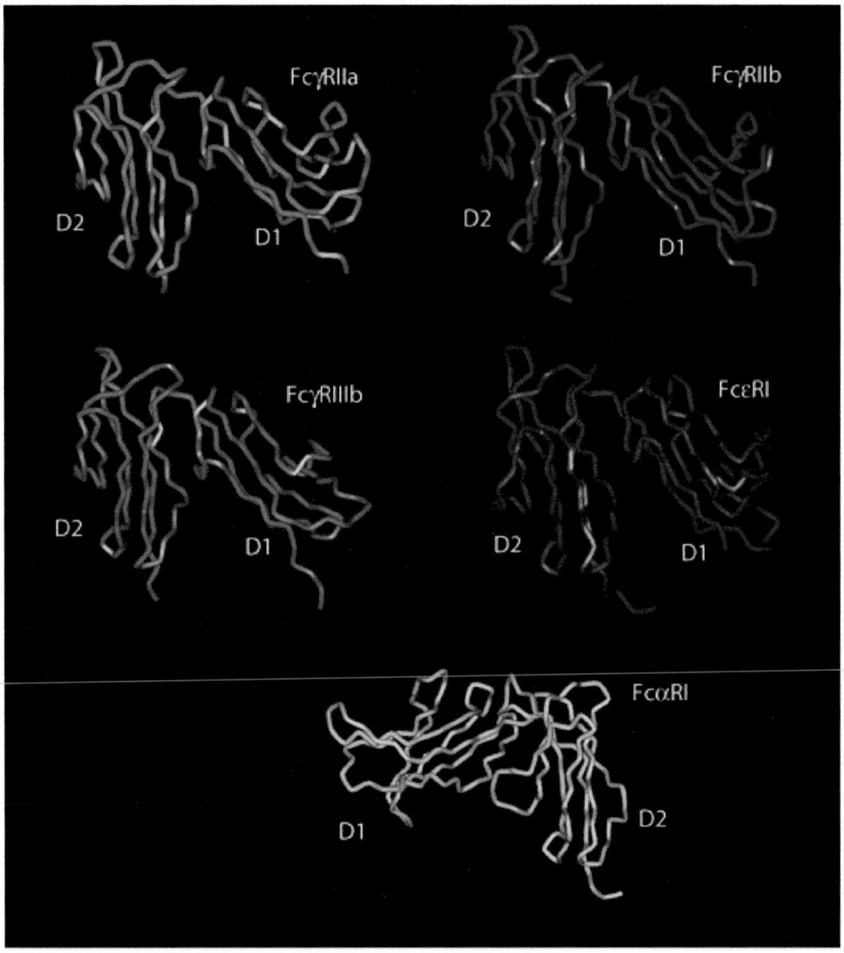

Figure 3.15. Structures of human leukocyte Fc receptors.

In each case, a similar view of the receptor is shown, in its uncomplexed state. D1, membrane distal; D2, membrane proximal domain. For the FcγRs and FcεRI, the Fc binding site is present at the "top" of the D2 domain. For FcαRI, the D1–D2 domain arrangement is reversed and the Fc interaction site is present at the top of the D1 domain. (Courtesy of Jenny Woof.)

of the mast cells with release of preformed vasoactive amines and cytokines, and the synthesis of a variety of inflammatory mediators derived from arachidonic acid (cf. Figure 1.21). This process is responsible for the symptoms of hay fever and of extrinsic asthma when patients with atopic allergy come into contact with the allergen, e.g. grass pollen. The main *physiological* role of IgE would appear to be protection of anatomical sites susceptible to trauma and pathogen entry by local recruitment of plasma factors and effector cells through the **triggering of an acute inflammatory reaction**. Infectious agents penetrating the IgA defenses would combine with specific IgE on the mast cell surface and trigger the release of vasoactive agents and factors chemotactic for polymorphs, so leading to an influx of plasma IgG, complement, neutrophils and eosinophils. In such a context, the ability of eosinophils to damage IgG-coated helminths and the generous IgE response to such parasites would constitute an effective defense.

The low affinity IgE receptor **FcεRII** (CD23) is a C-type (calcium-dependent) lectin. It is present on many different types of hematopoietic cells (Table 3.2). Its primary function appears to be in the regulation of IgE synthesis by B-cells, with a stimulatory role at low concentrations of IgE and an inhibitory role at high concentrations. It can also facilitate phagocytosis of IgE opsonized antigens.

For IgA, **FcαRI** (CD89), is the only well characterized Fc receptor. Its ligand-binding α chain is structurally related to those of the FcγRs and FcεRI but represents a more distantly related member of the family. In fact, it shares closer homology with members of a family including natural killer cell immunoglobulin-like receptors (KIRs), leukocyte Ig-like receptors (LIR/LILR/ILTs) and the platelet-specific collagen receptor (GPVI). FcαRI is present on monocytes, macrophages, neutrophils, eosinophils and Kupffer cells. The cross-linking of FcαRI by antigen can activate endocytosis, phagocytosis, inflammatory mediator release and ADCC. Expression of FcαRI on monocytes is strongly upregulated by bacterial polysaccharide.

Crystal structures are available for FcγRIIa, FcγRIIb, FcγRIIIb, FcεRI and FcαRI (Figure 3.15). In all cases, the structures represent the two Ig-like extracellular domains of the receptor α chain, termed D1 (N-terminal, membrane distal) and D2 (C-terminal, membrane proximal). No structure is yet available for the cytoplasmic portions of any receptor. The extracellular regions of FcγRIIa/b, FcγRIII and FcεRI are seen to share the same overall structure and are so similar that they can be readily superimposed. Despite the basic sequence similarity between FcαRI and these receptors, the IgA receptor turns out to have a strikingly different structure. While the two individual domains of the FcαRI extracellular portion fold up in a similar manner to those of the other receptors, the arrangement of the domains relative to each other is very different. The domains are rotated through ~180° from the positions adopted in the other Fc receptors, essentially inverting the D1–D2 orientations.

Crystallographic studies of antibody–Fc receptor complexes have revealed how antibodies interact with leukocyte Fc receptors (Figure 3.16). For the IgG–FcγRIII interaction, the D2 membrane-proximal domain of FcγRIII interacts with the top of the C_H2 domains and the bottom of the hinge. This requires the antibody to adopt a "dislocated" conformation in which the Fab arms are rotated out of the plane of the Fc. One consequence of this mode of interaction, recognized many years ago, is that it promotes close approach of the target cell membrane (upwards on the page) to the effector cell membrane. This may favor effector cell activity against the target cell. Given the similarities between FcγRI, FcγRII and FcγRIII, it is likely that all three FcRs share a common mode of binding to IgG. Indeed, this mode of binding seems also to be shared by IgE binding to the FcεRI receptor although the Cε2–Cε3 domain linker region replaces the hinge contribution to receptor binding. By contrast, IgA binds to the FcαRI receptor at a site between Cα2 and Cα3 domains. This mode of binding permits an IgA:FcR stoichiometry of 2:1 whereas the stoichiometry for IgG and IgE in the above complexes is 1:1. The significance of these differences in the modes of binding is not understood at this time.

Antibodies and the neonatal Fc receptor

An important Fc receptor for IgG is the neonatal receptor, FcRn. This receptor mediates **transport of IgG from mother to child** across the placenta (Figure 3.17). Such antibody, surviving for some time in the blood of the newborn child, is believed to be important in directly protecting the child from pathogens. Furthermore, the presence of maternal antibody has been proposed to help the development of cellular immunity in the young child by attenuating pathogen challenge rather than stopping it completely. FcRn may also be important in transporting maternal IgG from mother's milk across the intestinal cells of the young infant to the blood. Equally, FcRn is crucial in **maintaining the long half-life of IgG in serum** in adults and children. The receptor binds IgG in acidic vesicles (pH < 6.5) protecting the molecule from degradation, and then releasing the IgG at the higher pH of 7.4 in blood.

Structural studies have revealed the molecular basis for FcRn activity. FcRn is unlike leukocyte Fc receptors and instead has structural similarity to MHC class I molecules. It is a heterodimer composed of a β_2-microglobulin chain noncovalently attached to a membrane-bound chain that includes three extracellular domains. One of these domains, including a carbohydrate chain, together with β_2-microglobulin interacts with a site between the C_H2 and C_H3 domains of Fc (Figure 3.18). The interaction includes three salt bridges made to histidine (His) residues on IgG that are positively charged at pH < 6.5. At higher pH, the His residues lose their positive charges, the FcRn–IgG interaction is weakened and IgG dissociates.

Secretory IgA

IgA appears selectively in the seromucous secretions, such as saliva, tears, nasal fluids, sweat, colostrum, milk, and secretions of the lung, genitourinary and gastrointestinal tracts, where it defends the exposed external surfaces of the body against attack by microorganisms. This is an important function as approximately 40 mg of secretory IgA/kg body weight is transported daily through the human intestinal crypt epithelium to the mucosal surface as compared with a *total* daily production of IgG of 30 mg/kg.

The IgA is synthesized locally by plasma cells and dimerized intracellularly together with a cysteine-rich polypeptide called J chain, of molecular weight 15 000. Dimeric IgA binds strongly to a receptor for polymeric Ig (**poly-Ig receptor, pIgR**, which also binds polymeric IgM) present in the membrane of mucosal epithelial cells. The complex is then actively endocytosed, transported across the cytoplasm and secreted into the external body fluids after cleavage of the pIgR peptide chain. The fragment of the receptor remaining bound to the IgA is termed secretory component and the whole molecule, **secretory IgA** (Figure 3.19).

Isotypes, allotypes and idiotypes: antibody variants

The variability of antibodies is often conveniently divided into three types. **Isotypes** are variants present in all healthy members of a species: immunoglobulin classes and subclasses are examples of isotypic variation involving the constant region of the heavy chain. **Allotypes** are variants that are inherited as alternatives (alleles) and therefore not all healthy members of a species inherit a particular allotype. Allotypes occur mostly as variants of heavy-chain constant-region genes, in man in all four IgG subclasses, IgA2 and IgM. The nomenclature of human immunoglobulin allotypes is based on the isotype on which it is found (e.g. G1m defines allotypes on an IgG1 heavy chain, Km defines allotypes on κ light chains) followed by an accepted WHO numbering system.

The variable region of an antibody can act as an antigen, and the unique determinants of this region that distinguish it from most other antibodies of that species are termed its

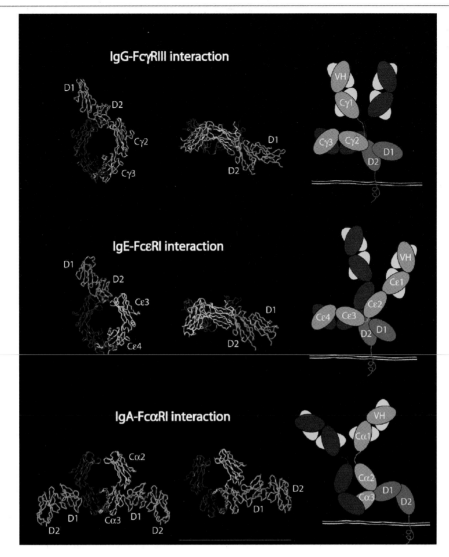

Figure 3.16. Structures of antibody–leukocyte Fc receptor interactions.

The left-hand side and middle columns show views of the crystal structures of the complexes of the FcRs with their respective Fc ligands. The extracellular domains of the receptors are shown in blue while one heavy chain of each Fc region is shown in red and the other in gold. In the left hand column, each Fc region is viewed face on. The similarity between the IgG–FcγRIII and IgE–FcεRI interaction is striking while the IgA–FcαRI interaction is quite different in terms of the sites involved and the stoichiometry. The middle column shows a view where the D2 domains of each of the receptors are positioned so that their C-termini face downwards. Here the Fc regions of IgG and IgE are seen in a horizontal position from the side. For the IgA interaction only one receptor molecule is shown. The right-hand column shows a schematic representation of the receptors and their intact ligands from the same viewpoint as the images in the middle column. Light chains are shown in pale yellow. The necessity for dislocation of IgG and IgE to allow positioning of the Fab tips away from the receptor-bearing cell surface is apparent. (Courtesy of Jenny Woof.)

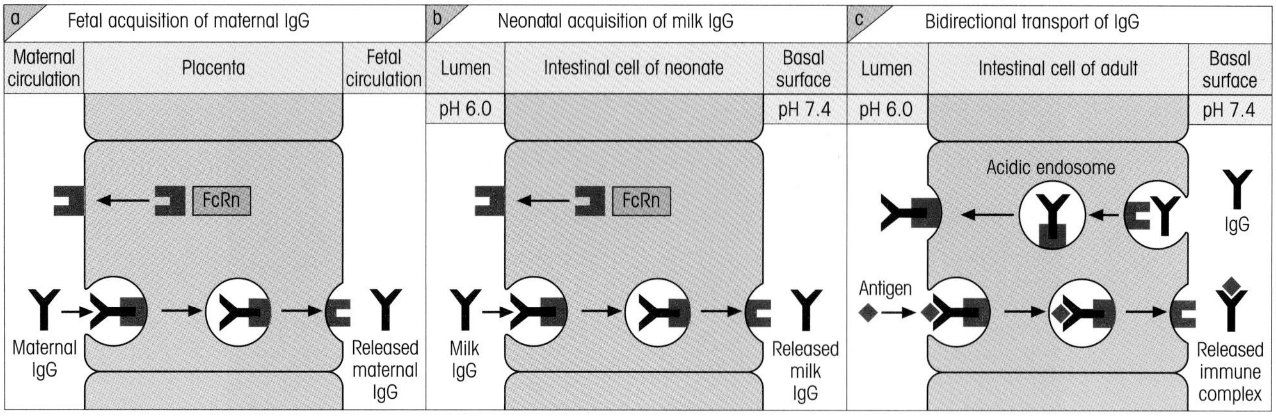

Figure 3.17. Function of the neonatal receptor for IgG (FcRn) on epithelial cells.

(a) The FcRn receptor is present in the placenta where it fulfills the important task of transferring maternal IgG to the fetal circulation. This will provide protection prior to the generation of immunocompetence in the fetus. Furthermore, it is self-evident that any infectious agent that might reach the fetus *in utero* will have had to have passed through the mother first, and the fetus will rely upon the mother's immune system to have produced IgG with appropriate binding specificities. This maternal IgG also provides protection for the neonate, because it takes some weeks following birth before the transferred IgG is eventually all catabolized. (b) It has been clearly demonstrated in rodents, although remains speculative in humans, that there is epithelial transport of IgG from maternal milk across the intestinal cells of the newborn. IgG binds to FcRn at pH 6.0, is taken into the cell within a clathrin-coated vesicle and released at the pH of the basal surface. The directional movement of IgG is achieved by the asymmetric pH effect on Ig–receptor interaction. Knockout mice lacking FcRn are incapable of acquiring maternal Ig as neonates. Furthermore, they have a grossly shortened IgG half-life, consistent with the role of FcRn as a protective receptor that prevents degradation of IgG and then recycles it to the circulation. The IgG half-life is unusually long compared with that of IgA and IgM and this enables the response to antigen to be sustained for many months following infection. (c) An additional role of FcRn may be as a bidirectional shuttle receptor. IgG binding on the nonluminal side of the epithelial cell may occur, following endocytosis, within the more favorable pH of acidic endosomes. This receptor may thus provide a mechanism for mucosal immunosurveillance, traveling back and forth across the epithelial cell, delivering IgG to the intestinal lumen and then returning the same antibodies in the form of immune complexes for the stimulation of B-cells by follicular dendritic cells.

idiotypic determinants. The **idiotype** of an antibody, therefore, consists of a set of idiotypic determinants that individually are called idiotopes. Polyclonal anti-idiotypic antibodies generally recognize a set of idiotopes whilst a monoclonal anti-idiotype recognizes a single idiotope. Idiotypes are usually specific to an individual antibody clone (private idiotypes) but are sometimes shared between different antibody clones (public, recurrent or cross-reacting idiotypes). An anti-idiotype may react with determinants distant from the antigen binding site, it may fit the binding site and express the image of the antigen or it may react with determinants close to the binding site and interfere with antigen binding. Sequencing of an anti-idiotypic antibody generated against an antibody specific for the polypeptide GAT antigen in mice revealed a CDR3 with an amino acid sequence identical to that of the antigen epitope, i.e. the anti-idiotype contains a true image of the antigen but this is probably the exception rather than the rule.

Genetics of antibody diversity and function

Antibody genes are produced by somatic recombination

The immunoglobulin repertoire is encoded for by multiple germline gene segments that undergo somatic diversification in developing B-cells. Hence, although the basic components needed to generate an immunoglobulin repertoire are inherited, an individual's mature antibody repertoire is essentially formed during their lifetime by alteration of the inherited germline genes.

The first evidence that immunoglobulin genes rearrange by **somatic recombination** was reported by Hozumi and Tonegawa in 1976 (Milestone 3.2). Because somatic recombination involves rearrangement of DNA in somatic, in contrast to gamete cells, the newly recombined genes are not inherited.

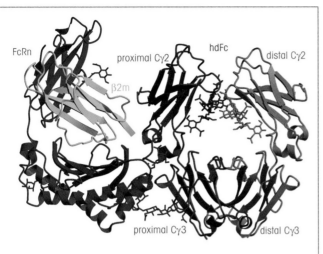

Figure 3.18. Structure of the rat neonatal Fc receptor binding to the Fc of IgG.

A heterodimeric Fc (hdFc) is shown with the FcRn binding chain in red and the nonbinding chain in orange. The orange chain has been mutated at several positions to eliminate FcRn binding. If the normal homodimeric molecule is used then oligomeric ribbon structures are created in which FcRn dimers are bridged by Fcs thereby preventing crystallization. The three domains of FcRn are shown in dark blue (two are close together at the bottom of the picture in this view) and β_2-microglobulin in light blue. A portion of the α_2 domain, an N-linked carbohydrate attached to this domain and the C-terminus of β_2-microglobulin form the FcRn side of the interaction site. Residues at the C_H2/C_H3 domain interface form the Fc side of the interaction site. (After Martin W.L. *et al.* (2001) *Molecular Cell* **7**, 867.)

As a result, the primary immunoglobulin repertoire will differ slightly from one individual to the next, and will be further modified during an individual's lifetime by their exposure to different antigens.

The immunoglobulin variable gene segments and loci

The variable light and heavy chain loci in humans contain multiple gene segments, which are joined, using somatic recombination, to produce the final V region exon. The human heavy chain variable region is constructed from the joining of three gene segments, **V (variable), D (diversity), and J (joining)**, whereas the light chain variable gene is constructed by the joining of two gene segments, V and J. There are multiple V, D and J segments at the heavy chain and light chain loci, as illustrated in Figure 3.20.

The human V_H genes have been mapped to chromosome 14, although orphan IgH genes have also been identified on chromosomes 15 and 16. The human V_H locus is highly polymorphic, and may have evolved through the repeated duplication, deletion and recombination of DNA. Polymorphisms found within the germline repertoire are due to the insertion or deletion of gene segments or the occurrence of different alleles of the same segment. A number of pseudogenes, ranging from those that are more conserved and contain a few point mutations to those that are more divergent with extensive mutations, are also present in immunoglobulin loci. There are approximately 100 human V_H genes, which can be grouped

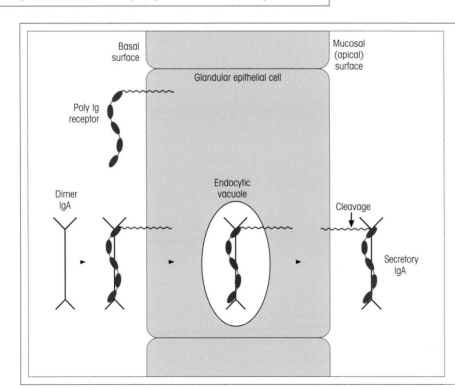

Figure 3.19. IgA secretion at the mucosal surface.

The mucosal cell synthesizes a receptor for polymeric Ig (pIgR) that is inserted into the basal membrane. Dimeric IgA binds to this receptor and is transported via an endocytic vacuole to the apical surface. Cleavage of the receptor releases secretory IgA still attached to part of the receptor termed the secretory component. Note how the receptor cleavage introduces an asymmetry, which drives the transport of IgA dimers to the mucosal surface (in quite the opposite direction to the transcytosis of milk IgG in Figure 3.17).

into seven families based on sequence homology, and these families can be further grouped into three clans. Members of a given family show approximately 80% sequence homology at the nucleotide level. The functional heavy chain repertoire is formed from approximately 50 functional V_H genes, 27 D_H genes and six J_H genes. The human lambda locus maps to chromosome 22, with approximately 33–36 functional V_λ genes and five functional J_λ gene segments. The V_λ genes can be grouped into 10 families, which are further divided into seven clans. The human kappa locus on chromosome 2 is composed of a total of approximately 34–40 functional V_κ genes and five functional J_κ genes. However, the kappa locus contains a large duplication of most of the V_κ genes, and most of the V_κ genes in this distal cluster, although functional are seldom used.

The immunoglobulin loci also contain regulatory elements (Figure 3.21), such as a conserved octamer motif and TATA box in the promoter regions. Leader sequences are also found upstream of the variable segments, and enhancer elements are also present within the loci to facilitate productive transcription.

V(D)J recombination and combinatorial diversity

The joining of these gene segments, illustrated in Figure 3.22, is known as **V(D)J recombination**. V(D)J recombination is a highly regulated and ordered event. The light chain exon is constructed from a single V-to-J gene segment join. However, at the heavy chain locus, a D-segment is first joined to a J-segment, and then the V-segment is joined to the combined

◉ Milestone 3.2—The 1987 Nobel Prize in Physiology or Medicine

Susumu Tonegawa was awarded the 1987 Nobel Prize in Physiology or Medicine for "his discovery of the genetic principle for generation of antibody diversity." In his 1976 paper, Tonegawa used Southern blot analysis of restriction enzyme digested DNA from lymphoid and nonlymphoid cells to show that the immunoglobulin variable and constant genes are distant from each other in the germline genome. Embryo DNA showed two components when hybridized to RNA probes

specific for: (i) both variable and constant regions; and (ii) only the constant region, whereas both probes localized to a single band when hybridized to DNA from an antibody-producing plasmacytoma cell. He proposed that the differential hybridization patterns could be explained if the variable and constant genes were distant from each other in germline DNA, but came together to encode the complete immunoglobulin gene during lymphocyte differentiation.

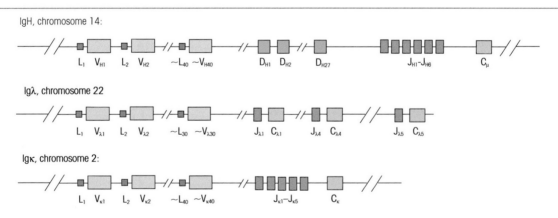

Figure 3.20. The human immunoglobulin loci.

Schematics of the human heavy chain (top) and light chain lambda (middle) and kappa (bottom) loci are shown. The human heavy chain locus on chromosome 14 consists of approximately 38–46 functional V_H genes, 27 D_H genes and six J_H genes, which are organized into clusters upstream of the constant regions. The human lambda locus on chromosome 22 consists of

approximately 30 functional V_λ genes and five functional J_λ gene segments, with each J segment followed by a constant segment. The human kappa locus on chromosome 2 consists of 34–40 functional V_κ genes and five functional J_κ genes, with the J segments clustered upstream of the constant region. L, leader sequence.

DJ sequence. The rearranged DNA is transcribed, the RNA transcript is spliced to bring together the V region exon and the C-region exon, and lastly the spliced mRNA is translated to produce the final immunoglobulin protein.

Numerous unique immunoglobulin genes can be made by joining different combinations of the V, D and J segments at the heavy and light chain loci. The creation of diversity in the immunoglobulin repertoire through this joining of various gene segments is known as **combinatorial diversity**. Additional diversity is created by the pairing of different heavy chains with different lambda or kappa light chains. For example, the potential heavy chain repertoire is approximately $50\,V_H \times 27\,D_H \times$

$6\,J_H = 8.1 \times 10^3$ different combinations. Similarly, there are approximately 165 ($33\,V_\lambda \times 5\,J_\lambda$) and 200 ($40\,V_\kappa \times 5\,J_\kappa$) different combinations, for a total of 365 light chain combinations. If we consider that each heavy chain could potentially pair with each light chain, then the diversity of the immunoglobulin repertoire is quite large, on the order of 3.10^6 possible combinations. Additional diversity is also generated during gene segment recombination and by somatic hypermutation, as explained in the following sections. In this manner, although the number of germline gene segments appears limited in size, an incredibly diverse immunoglobulin repertoire can be generated.

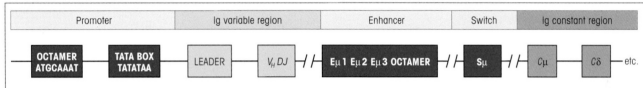

Figure 3.21. Regulatory elements of immunoglobulin loci.

Each *VDJ* segment encoding the variable region is associated with a leader sequence. Closely upstream is the TATA box of the promoter, which binds RNA polymerase II and the octamer motif that is one of a number of short sequences that bind transacting regulatory transcription factors. The *V region* promoters are relatively inactive and only association with enhancers, which are also composites of short sequence motifs capable of binding nuclear proteins, will increase the transcription rate to levels typical of actively secreting B-cells. The enhancers are near to the regions that control switching from one Ig class constant region to another, e.g. IgM to IgG (Figure 3.27). Primary transcripts are initiated 20 nucleotides downstream of the TATA box and extend beyond the end of the constant region. These are spliced, cleaved at the 3′ end and polyadenylated to generate the translatable mRNA.

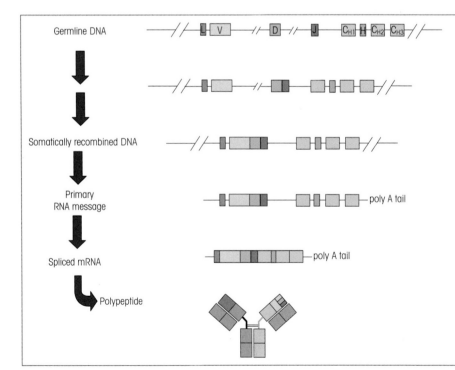

Figure 3.22. Overview of V(D)J recombination.

Diversity (D) and joining (J) gene segments in the germline DNA are joined together through somatic recombination at the heavy chain locus. The variable (V) gene segment is then joined to the recombined D-J gene, to produce the fully recombined heavy chain exon. At the light chain loci, somatic recombination occurs with V and J segments only. The recombined DNA is transcribed, and the primary RNA transcript is then spliced, bringing together the variable and constant regions. The spliced mRNA molecule is translated to produce the immunoglobulin protein. The contribution of the different gene segments to the polypeptide sequence is illustrated for one of the heavy chains. H, hinge.

Recombination signal sequences

The **recombination signal sequence** (RSS) helps to guide recombination between appropriate gene segments. The RSS (Figure 3.23) is a noncoding sequence that flanks coding gene segments. It is made up of a conserved heptamer and nonamer sequences, which are separated by an unconserved 12- or 23-nucleotide spacer. Efficient recombination occurs between segments with a 12-nucleotide spacer and a 23-nucleotide spacer. This **"12/23" rule** helps make certain that appropriate gene segments are joined together.

At the V_H locus, the V and J segments are flanked by RSSs with a 23-nucleotide spacer, whereas the D segments are flanked by RSSs with a 12-nucleotide spacer. At light chain loci, the V_κ segments are flanked by RSSs with 12-nucleotide spacers, J_κ segments are flanked by RSSs with 23-nucleotide spacers, and this arrangement is reversed in the lambda locus.

The recombinase machinery

The V(D)J recombinase is a complex of enzymes that mediates somatic recombination of immunoglobulin gene segments (Figure 3.24). The gene products of recombination-activating genes 1 and 2, RAG-1 and RAG-2, are lymphocyte-specific enzymes essential for V(D)J recombination. In the initial steps of V(D)J recombination, the RAG complex binds the recombination signal sequences and, in association with high mobility group (HMG) proteins that are involved in DNA bending, the two recombination signal sequences are brought together.

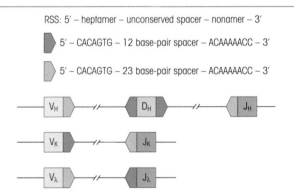

Figure 3.23. The recombination signal sequence.

The recombination signal sequence (RSS) is made up of conserved heptamer and nonamer sequences, separated by an unconserved 12- or 23-nucleotide spacer. Efficient recombination occurs between segments with a 12-nucleotide spacer and a 23-nucleotide spacer. RSSs with 23-nucleotide spacers flank the V and J segments of the heavy chain locus, the J segments of the kappa locus and the V segments of the lambda locus, whereas RSSs with 12-nucleotide spacers flank the D segments of the heavy chain locus, the V segments of the kappa locus and the J segments of the lambda locus.

In contrast to the lymphoid-specific RAG enzymes, HMG proteins are ubiquitously expressed.

Next, a single-stranded nick is introduced between the 5'-heptameric end of the recombination signal sequence and the coding segment. This nick results in a free 3' OH group, which attacks the opposite, anti-parallel DNA strand in a transesterification reaction. This attack gives rise to a double-stranded DNA break that leads to the formation of covalently sealed hairpins at the two coding ends and the formation of blunt signal ends. At this stage a post-cleavage complex is formed, in which the RAG recombinase remains associated with the DNA ends.

The DNA break is finally repaired by non-homologous end-joining machinery. The recombination signal sequences are joined precisely to generate the signal joint. By contrast, nucleotides can be lost or added during repair of the coding ends (Figure 3.25). **Junctional diversity** is the diversification of variable region exons due to this imprecise joining of the coding ends.

First, a small number of nucleotides are often deleted from the coding end by an unknown exonuclease. Also, junctional diversity involves the potential addition of two types of nucleotides, **P-nucleotides** and **N-nucleotides**. The palindromic sequences that result from the asymmetric cleavage and template mediated fill-in of the coding hairpins are referred to as P-nucleotides. N-nucleotides are generated by the nontemplated addition of nucleotides to the coding ends, which is mediated by the enzyme terminal deoxynucleotidyl transferase (TdT). Although P- and N- nucleotides and deletion of the coding end and nucleotides serve to greatly diversify the immunoglobulin repertoire, the addition of these nucleotides may also result in the generation of receptor genes that are out of frame.

Similar to the RAG recombinase complex, the **DNA repair machinery** works as a protein complex. However, unlike the RAG recombinase, the nonhomologous end-joining proteins are ubiquitously expressed. In the first steps of DNA repair, the Ku70 and Ku80 proteins form a heterodimer that bind the broken DNA ends. The Ku complex recruits the catalytic subunit of DNA-dependent protein kinase, DNA-PKcs, a serine-threonine protein kinase. The activated DNA-PKcs then recruits and phosphorylates XRCC4 and Artemis. Artemis is an endonuclease that opens the hairpin coding ends. Finally, DNA ligase IV binds XRCC4 to form an end-ligation complex, and this complex mediates the final ligation and fill-in steps needed to form the coding and signal joints.

Regulating V(D)J recombination

V(D)J recombination and the recombinase machinery must be carefully regulated to avoid wreaking havoc on the cellular genome. For instance, aberrant V(D)J recombination is implicated in certain B-cell lymphomas. V(D)J recombination is largely regulated by controlling expression of the recombination machinery and the accessibility of gene segments and

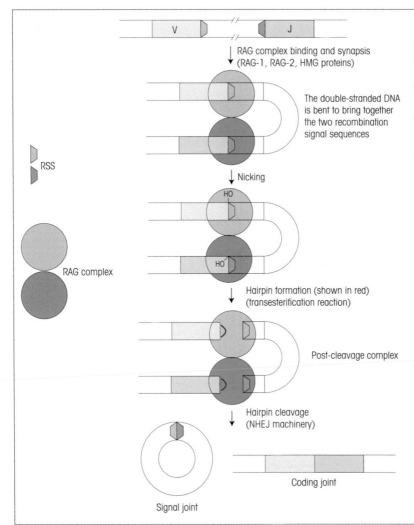

Figure 3.24. The V(D)J recombinase.

In the initial steps of V(D)J recombination, the RAG-1 and RAG-2 proteins associate with the recombination signal sequences. A single-stranded nick is then introduced between the 5′-heptameric end of the recombination signal sequence and the coding segment, giving rise to a free 3′-OH group that mediates a transesterification reaction. This reaction leads to the formation of DNA hairpins at the coding ends. Hairpin cleavage and resolution of the post-cleavage complex by nonhomologous end-joining (NHEJ) proteins results in the formation of separate coding and signal joints, in the final steps of V(D)J recombination.

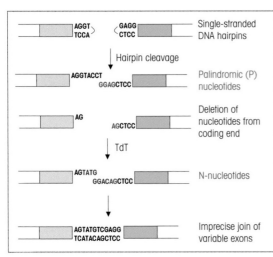

Figure 3.25. Junctional diversity further diversifies the immune repertoire.

The immunoglobulin repertoire is further diversified during cleavage and resolution of the coding-end hairpins by deletion of a variable number of coding end nucleotides, the addition of N-nucleotides by terminal deoxynucleotidyl transferase (TdT), and palindromic (P) nucleotides that arise due to template-mediated fill-in of the asymmetrically cleaved coding hairpins. TdT randomly adds nucleotides to the DNA ends (N-nucleotides), and the single-stranded ends pair, possibly but not necessarily, through complementary nucleotides (TG on top strand and AC on bottom strand). Exonuclease trimming, to remove unpaired nucleotides, and the DNA-repair machinery act to repair the DNA joint.

nearby enhancers and promoters. As previously mentioned, RAG-1 and RAG-2 activity is specific to lymphoid cells, and further regulation is imposed by downregulating RAG activity during appropriate stages of B-cell development. Differential accessibility of gene segments to the recombinase machinery, which can be achieved by altering chromatin structure, also plays a role in making certain that appropriate gene segments are recombined in an appropriate order. *Cis*-acting transcriptional control elements, such as enhancers and promoters, also help regulate recombination. Although it is not a hard and fast rule, transcription from certain regulatory elements seems to correlate with rearrangement of the adjacent genes. This **sterile**, or nonproductive, **transcription** may somehow help target required proteins or modulate gene accessibility. Finally, in addition to directing recombination between appropriate gene segments, the precise sequences of the RSS itself, as well as the sequences of the gene segments themselves, can influence the efficiency of the recombination reaction.

Somatic hypermutation

Following antigen activation, the variable regions of immunoglobulin heavy and light chains are further diversified by somatic hypermutation. **Somatic hypermutation** involves the introduction of nontemplated point mutations into V regions of rapidly proliferating B-cells in the germinal centers of lymphoid follicles. Antigen-driven somatic hypermutation of variable immunoglobulin genes can result in an increase in binding affinity of the B-cell receptor for its cognate ligand. As B-cells with higher affinity immunoglobulins can more successfully compete for limited amounts of antigen present, an increase in the average affinity of the antibodies produced during an immune response is observed. This increase in the average affinity of immunoglobulins is known as **affinity maturation**.

Somatic hypermutation occurs at a high rate, thought to be on the order of about 1×10^{-3} mutations per base-pair per generation, which is approximately 10^6 times higher than the mutation rate of cellular housekeeping genes. There is a bias for transition mutations, and the "mutation hotspots" in variable regions map to RGWY motifs (R = purine, Y = pyrimidine, W = A or T). The exact mechanisms by which mutations are introduced and preferentially targeted to appropriate V regions, while constant regions of the immunoglobulin loci remain protected, is not clearly understood and is the subject of current research. Transcription through the target V region seems required, but is not necessarily sufficient, for somatic hypermutation. Additionally, the enzyme **activation-induced cytidine deaminase (AID)** has been demonstrated to be essential for both somatic hypermutation and class-switch recombination.

AID is a cytidine deaminase capable of carrying out targeted deamination of C to U, and shows strong homology with the RNA-editing enzyme APOBEC-1. Two current hypotheses have been proposed to explain the mechanism by which AID acts, one favoring RNA editing while the second favors DNA

deamination. It is possible that AID recognizes and acts on an mRNA precursor, or more likely that AID directly deaminates DNA to produce U : G mismatches. The exact mechanism by which AID can differentially regulate somatic hypermutation and class switch recombination is currently being studied, and may depend on interactions of specific cofactors with specific domains of AID.

Therefore, diversity within the immunoglobulin repertoire is generated by: (i) the combinatorial joining of gene segments; (ii) junctional diversity; (iii) combinatorial pairing of heavy and light chains; and (iv) somatic hypermutation of V regions.

Gene conversion and repertoire diversification

Although mice and humans use combinatorial and junctional diversity as a mechanism to generate a diverse repertoire, in many species, including birds, cattle, swine, sheep, horses and rabbits, V(D)J recombination results in assembly and expression of a single functional gene. Repertoire diversification is then achieved by **gene conversion**, a process in which pseudo-V genes are used as templates to be copied into the assembled variable region exon. Further diversification may be achieved by somatic hypermutation.

The process of gene conversion was originally identified in chickens, in which immature B-cells have the same variable region exon. During B-cell development in the bursa of Fabricius, rapidly proliferating B-cells undergo gene conversion to diversify the immunoglobulin repertoire (Figure 3.26). Stretches of sequences from germline variable region pseudogenes, located upstream of the functional V genes, are introduced into the V_L and V_H regions. This process takes place in the ileal Peyer's patches of cattle, swine and horses, and in the appendix of rabbits. These gut-associated lymphoid tissues are the mammalian equivalent of the bursa in these species.

Class switch recombination

Antigen-stimulated IgM expressing B-cells in germinal centers of secondary lymphoid organs, such as the spleen and lymph nodes, undergo class switch recombination. **Class switch recombination (CSR)** allows the IgH constant region exon of a given antibody to be exchanged for an alternative exon, giving rise to the expression of antibodies with the same antigen specificity but of differing isotypes, and therefore of differing effector functions as described above. CSR occurs through a deletional DNA recombination event at the IgH locus (Figure 3.27), which has been extensively studied in mice. Constant region exons for IgD, IgG, IgE, and IgA isotypes are located downstream of the IgM (Cμ) exon, and CSR occurs between **switch** or **S regions.** S regions are repetitive sequences, which are often G-rich on the nontemplate strand, that are found upstream of each C_H exon. Breaks are introduced into the DNA of two S regions and fusion of the S regions leads to a rearranged C_H locus, in which the variable exon is joined to an exon for a new constant region. The DNA between the two

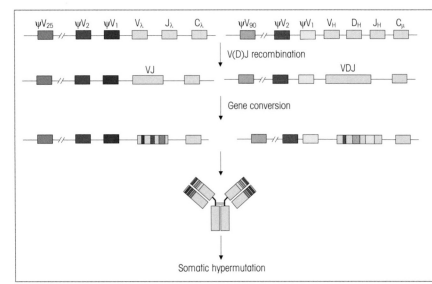

Figure 3.26. Immunoglobulin diversification using gene conversion.

V(D)J recombination in chicken B-cells results in assembly of a single variable region exon. In the process of gene conversion, sequences of pseudogenes, located upstream of the functional gene segments, are copied into the recombined variable exons at the light and heavy chain loci in rapidly proliferating B-cells in the bursa of Fabricius. This results in a diversified antibody repertoire.

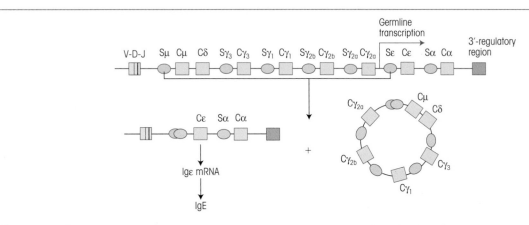

Figure 3.27. Class switch recombination allows expression of different antibody isotypes.

Class switch recombination involves DNA recombination at repetitive sequences termed switch or S regions, and is illustrated here for an IgM to IgE switch, at the mouse heavy chain locus. Switching to an IgE isotype begins with germline transcription from the promoter upstream of the constant region exon and recombination between the Sμ and Sε regions. This DNA recombination reaction brings the IgE constant region exon downstream of the variable region exon. The remaining switch regions and constant region exons are deleted and form an episomal circle. Transcription of the rearranged DNA yields IgE mRNA, which can be translated to give rise to the IgE immunoglobulin protein.

switch regions is excised and forms an episomal circle. Finally, alternative splicing of the primary RNA transcript generated from the rearranged DNA gives rise to either membrane-bound or secreted forms of the immunoglobulin.

Prior to recombination between switch regions, transcription is initiated from a promoter found upstream of an exon that precedes all C_H genes capable of undergoing CSR, the intervening (I) exon. These germline transcripts include I, S and C region exons, and do not appear to code for any functional protein. However, this germline transcription is required,

although not sufficient, to stimulate CSR. The precise mechanism responsible for CSR is the subject of current study, but work indicates that AID, described previously to be involved in somatic hypermutation, helps mediate CSR, along with some components of the nonhomologous end-joining pathway and several other DNA repair pathways. The joining of S regions may be mediated by association with transcriptional promoters, enhancers, chromatin factors, DNA repair proteins, AID-associated factors or by interactions involving S region sequences themselves.

Antibody structure and function

- Antibodies recognize foreign material and trigger its elimination.
- They are Y- or T-shaped molecules in which the arms of the molecule (Fab) recognize foreign material and the stem (Fc) interacts with immune molecules that lead to the elimination of the antibody-decorated foreign material.
- Antibodies are based on a four-chain structure consisting of two identical heavy chains and two identical light chains.
- The N-terminal parts of the heavy chains and the light chains form the two identical Fab arms that are linked to the Fc stem of the molecule consisting of the C-terminal parts of the heavy chains.
- The extremities of the Fab arms consist of regions of variable amino acid sequences that are involved in binding antigen and thereby give each antibody its unique specificity. The human antibody repertoire is vast, allowing the recognition of essentially any molecular shape.
- The Fc stem of the molecule has a more conserved sequence and is involved in binding effector molecules such as complement and Fc receptors.
- Differences in the Fc regions lead to different classes and subclasses of antibodies or immunoglobulins (Igs).
- There are five different classes of Ig—IgG, IgM, IgA, IgD and IgE—that fulfill different roles in immune protection. They also have different polymerization states.
- The structure of antibodies is organized into domains based on a β-sheet arrangement called the immunoglobulin fold.
- For IgG, the Fab arms, consisting of two variable domains and two constant domains, are linked via a flexible hinge region to the Fc, which consists of four constant domains.
- Flexibility is an important feature of antibody structure allowing interaction with antigens and effector molecules in a variety of environments.

Antibody interaction with effector molecules

- IgG triggers complement by binding C1q when clustered on an antigen such as a pathogen. IgM is already multivalent but, on binding antigen, it undergoes a conformational change to bind C1q.
- Leukocyte receptors have been described for IgG, IgA and IgE that, on binding antigen-associated antibody, trigger effector mechanisms such as phagocytosis, antibody-dependent cellular cytoxicity and acute inflammatory responses. Interaction between antibody and Fc receptors can also be immunoregulatory.
- The structures of IgG Fc receptors and the mast cell IgE Fc receptor and the mode of interaction of the receptors with Ig appear to be quite similar. The IgA receptor has however a distinct structure and mode of interaction with IgA.
- IgG interacts with the neonatal receptor FcRn to promote transport of IgG from mother to child and to maintain the long half-life of IgG in serum.

Overview of the Ig classes

- IgG is monomeric and the major antibody in serum and nonmucosal tissues, where it inactivates pathogens directly and through interaction with triggering molecules such as complement and Fc receptors.
- IgA exists mainly as a monomer in plasma, but in the seromucous secretions, where it is the major Ig concerned in the defense of the external body surfaces, it is present as a dimer linked to a secretory component.
- IgM is most commonly a pentameric molecule although a minor fraction is hexameric. It is essentially intravascular and is produced early in the immune response. Because of its high valency it is a very effective bacterial agglutinator and mediator of complement-dependent cytolysis and is therefore a powerful first-line defense against bacteremia.

- IgD is largely present on the lymphocyte and functions together with IgM as the antigen receptor on naive B-cells.
- IgE binds very tightly to mast cells and contact with antigen leads to local recruitment of antimicrobial agents through degranulation of the mast cells and release of inflammatory mediators. IgE is of importance in certain parasitic infections and is responsible for the symptoms of atopic allergy.

The generation of antibody diversity
- The antibody repertoire of an individual is generated through somatic recombination events from a limited set of germline gene segments.
- The human heavy chain variable region is generated by joining of V_H, D and J gene segments and the light chain variable regions (κ and λ) by joining of V_L and J segments. Joining is imprecise, leading to the generation of further diversity.
- Still further diversification results from somatic mutation events targeted to the variable regions. Somatic mutation and selection allows affinity maturation of antibodies.
- Some species use gene conversion rather than combinatorial and junctional diversity to achieve antibody diversification.
- Class switch recombination events allow the same antibody specificity (variable regions) to be associated with different antibody classes and subclasses (constant regions) and therefore with different functions.

FURTHER READING

Arakawa H. & Buerstedde J. (2004) Immunoglobulin gene conversion: insights from bursal B cells and the DT40 cell line. *Developmental Dynamics* **229**, 458–464.

Carroll M.C. (2008) Complement and humoral immunity. *Vaccine* **26**, I28–I33.

Chan A.C. & Carter P.J. (2010) Therapeutic antibodies for autoimmunity and inflammation. *Nature Reviews Immunology* **10**, 301–316.

Di Noia J.M. & Neuberger M.S. (2007) Molecular mechanisms of antibody somatic hypermutation. *Annual Review of Biochemistry* **76**, 1–22.

Hozumi N. & Tonegawa S. (1976) Evidence for somatic rearrangement of immunoglobulin genes coding for variable and constant regions. *Proceedings of the National Academy of Sciences of the USA* **73**, 3628–3632.

Hudson P.J. & Souriau C. (2003) Engineered antibodies. *Nature Medicine* **9**, 129–134.

IMGT database: http://imgt.cines.fr

Jung D. & Alt F.W. (2004) Unraveling V(D)J recombination: insights into gene regulation. *Cell* **116**, 299–311.

Maizels N. (2005) Immunoglobulin gene diversification. *Annual Review of Genetics* **39**, 23–46.

Maki R., Traunecker, A., Sakano, H., Roeder, W. & Tonegawa, S. (1980) Exon shuffling generates an immunoglobulin heavy chain gene. *Proceedings of the National Academy of Sciences of the USA* **77**, 2138–2142.

Martin W.L., West A.P. Jr, Gan L. & Bjorkman P.J. (2001) Crystal structure at 2.8 Å of an FcRn/heterodimeric Fc complex: mechanism of pH-dependent binding. *Molecular Cell* **7**, 867–877.

Matsuda F. & Honjo T. (1996) Organization of the human immunoglobulin heavy-chain locus. *Advances in Immunology* **62**, 1–29.

McCormack W.T., Tjoelker L.W. & Thompson C.B. (1991) Avian B-cell development: generation of an immunoglobulin repertoire by gene conversion. *Annual Review of Immunology* **9**, 219–241.

Metzger H. (2004) The high affinity receptor for IgE, FcεRI. *Novartis Foundation Symposium* **257**, 51–59.

Min I.M. & Selsing E. (2005) Antibody class switch recombination: roles for switch sequences and mismatch repair proteins. *Advances in Immunology* **87**, 297–328.

Nemazee D. (2006) Receptor editing in lymphocyte development and central tolerance. *Nature Reviews Immunology* **6**, 728–740.

Neuberger M.S. (2008) Antibody diversification by somatic mutation: from Burnet onwards. *Immunology and Cell Biology* **86**, 124–132.

Nimmerjahn F. & Ravetch J.V. (2008) Fcgamma receptors as regulators of immune responses. *Nature Reviews Immunology* **8**, 34–47.

Padlan E.A. (1994) Anatomy of the antibody molecule. *Molecular Immunology* **31**, 169–217.

Padlan E.A. (1996) X-ray crystallography of antibodies. *Advances in Protein Chemistry* **49**, 57–133.

Parren P.W. & Burton D.R. (2001) The antiviral activity of antibodies *in vitro* and *in vivo*. *Advances in Immunology* **77**, 195–262.

Peled J.U., Kuang F.L., Iglesias-Ussel M.D., Roa S., Kalis S.L., Goodman M.F. & Scharff M.D. (2008) The biochemistry of somatic hypermutation. *Annual Review of Immunology* **26**, 481–511.

Perlot T. & Alt F.W. (2008) *Cis*-regulatory elements and epigenetic changes control genomic rearrangements of the IgH locus. *Advances in Immunology* **99**, 1–32.

Roth D.B. (2003) Restraining the V(D)J recombinase. *Nature Reviews Immunology* **3**, 656–666.

Schroeder H.W. Jr. & Cavacini L. (2010) Structure and function of immunoglobulins. *Journal of Allergy and Clinical Immunology* **125**, S41–S52.

Swanson P.C. (2004) The bounty of RAGs: recombination signal complexes and complex outcomes. *Immunological Reviews* **200**, 90–114.

Ward E.S. (2004) Acquiring maternal immunoglobulin; different receptors, similar functions. *Immunity* **20**, 507–508.

Woof J.M. & Burton D.R. (2004) Human antibody-Fc receptor interactions illuminated by crystal structures. *Nature Reviews Immunology* **4**, 89–99.

Woof J.M. & Kerr M.A. (2006) The function of immunoglobulin A in immunity. *Journal of Pathology* **208**, 270–282.

Yoo E.M. & Morrison S.L. (2005) IgA: an immune glycoprotein. *Clinical Immunology* **116**, 3–10.

Zachau H.G. (2000) The immunoglobulin kappa gene families of human and mouse: a cottage industry approach. *Biological Chemistry* **381**, 951–954.

Now visit **www.roitt.com** to test yourself on this chapter.

CHAPTER 4
Membrane receptors for antigen

Key Topics

Just to Recap...

Upon maturation by exposure to PAMPs, dendritic cells (DCs) of the innate immune system initiate adaptive immune responses through **presentation of peptides to T-cells** within the context of MHC molecules. MHC molecules function as peptide-binding "billboards" adapted to displaying protein fragments for inspection by T-cell receptors. In response to an appropriate peptide–MHC combination (signal 1) and co-stimulatory B7 molecules (signal 2) presented by the DC, T-cells become activated and undergo clonal expansion and differentiation to mature effector cells. B-cells, on the other hand, do not require antigen to be presented to them and are capable of directly responding to soluble or particulate antigens through their membrane-bound immunoglobulins (i.e. the B-cell receptor). Thus, the requirements for recognition of antigen by T- and B-cells are quite different. Nonetheless, successful engagement of a T- or B-cell receptor empowers the responding lymphocyte to undergo clonal expansion to produce numerous identical daughter cells capable of recognizing the same antigen. Thus, recognition of antigen by T- or B-cells is a critically important step in the initiation of adaptive immune responses. In Chapter 1 we learned that NK cells can detect differences in the normal patterns of expression of MHC class I molecules. Because the latter are normally expressed on virtually all cells in the body, their absence is taken as a sign of danger lurking within. Here, we will look in more detail at the membrane receptors for antigen and how the incredible diversity that is displayed by such receptors is acquired. We will also explore the nature of MHC and MHC-like proteins and their central role as an interface between cells of the body and the cells of the immune system.

Roitt's Essential Immunology, Twelfth Edition. Peter J. Delves, Seamus J. Martin, Dennis R. Burton, Ivan M. Roitt.
© 2011 Peter J. Delves, Seamus J. Martin, Dennis R. Burton, Ivan M. Roitt. Published 2011 by Blackwell Publishing Ltd.

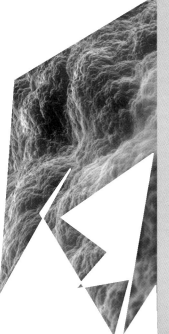

Introduction

The interaction of lymphocytes with antigen takes place through binding to specialized cell surface antigen-specific receptors functioning as recognition units. In the case of B-cells, the situation is straightforward as membrane-bound immunoglobulin serves as the receptor for antigen (Figure 4.1a). T-cells use distinct antigen receptors, which are also expressed at the plasma membrane, but T-cell receptors (TCRs) differ from B-cell receptors (BCRs) in a very fundamental way; TCRs cannot recognize free antigen as immunoglobulin can. The majority of T-cells can only recognize antigen when presented within the peptide-binding groove of an MHC molecule (Figure 4.1b). While this may seem rather cumbersome, a major advantage that T-cells have over their B-cell brethren is that they can inspect antigens that are largely confined within cells and are therefore inaccessible to Ig. In this chapter we will see that MHC molecules come in two major flavors, called MHC class I and class II, respectively. The major difference between these two major classes is in the cellular compartments they acquire their peptide cargoes from. **MHC class I molecules present peptides that come largely from intracellular sources**, while class II molecules acquire peptides from extracellular sources. There are other differences too, such as structural and tissue expression differences, but the major consequence of the separate locations that the different MHC classes acquire their peptides from is that recognition of a peptide loaded onto a MHC class I molecule will result in killing of that cell, whereas recognition of a peptide within a class II molecule mostly triggers a positive, even helpful, response. This is because a nonself peptide that is being made within a cell (and consequently presented on MHC class I) clearly signifies an intracellular infection and the most effective way to deal with this is to kill the infected cell. However, presentation of a nonself peptide that has been acquired from outside the cell (through phagocytosis), denotes an extracellular infection that will not be resolved by killing the cell that is raising the alarm. Indeed, things are set up in such a way that the only cells capable of presenting peptides on MHC class II molecules are cells that have a role in immunity. In contrast, practically all cells express MHC class I. Another leukocyte class, natural killer (NK) cells, can also detect trouble brewing within. NK cells possess their own unique receptors that check for appropriate levels of MHC class I molecules, as these are normally expressed on practically all nucleated cells within the body; NK receptors can also detect signs of abnormality such as increases in the expression of stress proteins by cells. Here we will focus mainly on the structural aspects of these various receptor types.

Figure 4.1. B-cells and T-cells "see" antigen in fundamentally different ways.

(a) In the case of B-cells, membrane-bound immunoglobulin serves as the B-cell receptor (BCR) for antigen. (b) T-cells use distinct antigen receptors, which are also expressed at the plasma membrane, but T-cell receptors (TCRs) cannot recognize free antigen as immunoglobulin can. The majority of T-cells can only recognize antigen when presented within the peptide-binding groove of an MHC molecule. Productive stimulation of the BCR or TCR results in activation of the receptor-bearing lymphocyte, followed by clonal expansion and differentiation to effector cells.

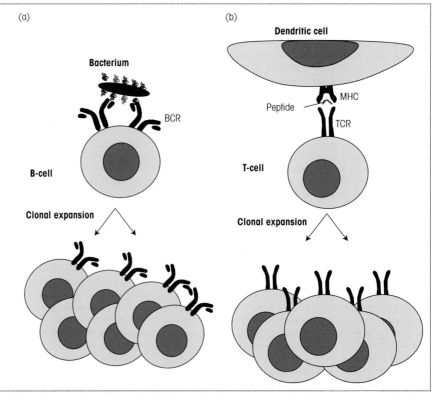

The B-cell surface receptor for antigen (BCR)

The B-cell displays a transmembrane immunoglobulin on its surface

In Chapter 2 we discussed the cunning system by which an antigen can be led inexorably to its doom by activating B-cells that are capable of making antibodies complementary in shape to itself through interacting with a copy of the antibody molecule on the lymphocyte surface. It will be recalled that binding of antigen to membrane antibody can activate the B-cell and cause it to proliferate followed by maturation into a clone of plasma cells secreting antibody specific for the inciting antigen (Figure 4.1a).

Immunofluorescence staining of live B-cells with labeled anti-immunoglobulin (anti-Ig) (e.g. Figure 2.6b) reveals the earliest membrane Ig to be of the IgM class. Each individual B-cell is committed to the production of just one antibody specificity and so transcribes its individual rearranged *VJCκ* (or *λ*) and *VDJCμ* genes. Ig can be either secreted or displayed on the B-cell surface through **differential splicing** of the pre-mRNA transcript encoding a particular immunoglobulin. The initial nuclear μ chain RNA transcript includes sequences coding for **hydrophobic transmembrane regions** that enable the IgM to sit in the membrane where it acts as the BCR, but if these are spliced out, the antibody molecules can be secreted in a soluble form (Figure 4.2).

As the B-cell matures, it coexpresses a BCR utilizing surface IgD of the same specificity. This surface IgM surface IgD B-cell phenotype is abundant in the mantle zone lymphocytes of

secondary lymphoid follicles (cf. Figure 7.8d) and is achieved by differential splicing of a single transcript containing VDJ, Cμ and Cδ segments producing either membrane IgM or IgD (Figure 4.3). As the B-cell matures further, other isotypes such as IgG may be utilized in the BCR (cf. p. 302).

Surface immunoglobulin is complexed with associated membrane proteins

Because secreted immunoglobulin is no longer physically connected to the B-cell that generated it, there is no way for the B-cell to know when the secreted Ig has found its target antigen. In the case of membrane-anchored immunoglobulin however, there is a direct link between antibody and the cell making it and this can be exploited to instruct the B-cell to scale-up production. As any budding industrialist knows, one way of increasing production is to open up more manufacturing plants, and another is to increase the rate of productivity in each one. When faced with the prospect of a sudden increase in demand for their particular product, B-cells do both of these things, through clonal expansion and differentiation to plasma cells. So how does the BCR spur the B-cell into action upon encounter with antigen?

Unlike many plasma membrane receptors that boast all manner of signaling motifs within their cytoplasmic tails, the corresponding tail region of a membrane-anchored IgM is a miserable three amino acids long. In no way could this accommodate the structural motifs required for interaction with the adaptor proteins, intracellular protein kinases or phosphatases that typically initiate signal transduction cascades. With some difficulty, it should be said, it eventually proved possible to

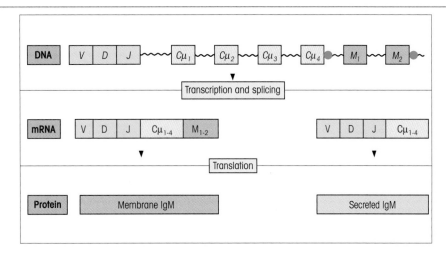

Figure 4.2. Splicing mechanism for the switch from the membrane to the secreted form of IgM.

Alternative processing determines whether a secreted or membrane-bound form of the μ heavy chain is produced. If transcription termination or cleavage occurs in the intron between $C\mu_4$ and M_1, the $C\mu_4$ poly-A addition signal (AAUAAA) is used and the secreted form is produced. If transcription continues through the membrane exons, then $C\mu4$ can be spliced to the *M* sequences resulting in the M_2 poly-A addition signal being utilized. The hydrophobic sequence encoded by the exons M_1 and M_2 then anchors the receptor IgM to the membrane. For simplicity, the leader sequence has been omitted. ∿ = introns.

Figure 4.3. Surface membrane IgM and IgD receptors of identical specificity appear on the same cell through differential splicing of the composite primary RNA transcript (leader sequences again omitted for simplicity).

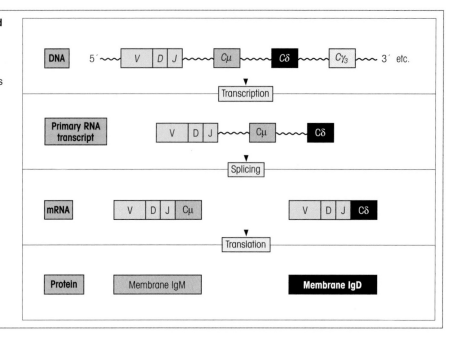

Figure 4.4. Model of B-cell receptor (BCR) complex.

The Ig-α/Ig-β heterodimer is encoded by the B-cell-specific genes *mb-1* and *B29*, respectively. Two of these heterodimers are shown with the Ig-α associating with the membrane-spanning region of the IgM μ chain. The Ig-like extracellular domains are colored blue. Each tyrosine (Y)-containing box possesses a sequence of general structure Tyr.X_2.Leu.X_7.Tyr.X_2.Ile (where X is not a conserved residue), referred to as the immunoreceptor tyrosine-based activation motif (ITAM). On activation of the B-cell, these ITAM sequences act as signal transducers through their ability to associate with and be phosphorylated by a series of tyrosine kinases. Note that whilst a light chain is illustrated for the surface IgM, some B-cells utilize a λ light chain.

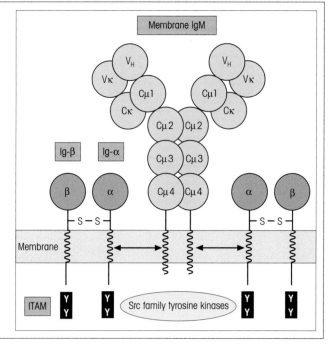

isolate a disulfide-linked heterodimer, **Ig-α (CD79a) and Ig-β (CD79b)**, which copurifies with membrane Ig and is responsible for transmitting signals from the BCR to the cell interior (Figure 4.4). Both Ig-α and Ig-β have an extracellular immunoglobulin-type domain, but it is their C-terminal cytoplasmic domains that are obligatory for signaling and which become phosphorylated upon cross-linking of the BCR by antigen (Figure 4.5), an event also associated with rapid Ca^{2+} mobilization.

Ig-α and Ig-β each contain a single **ITAM (*i*mmunorecep-tor *t*yrosine-based *a*ctivation *m*otif)** within their cytoplasmic tails and this motif contains two precisely spaced tyrosine residues that are central to their signaling role (Figures 4.4 and 4.5). Engagement of the BCR with antigen leads to rapid phosphorylation of the tyrosines within each ITAM, by kinases associated with the BCR, and this has the effect of creating binding sites for proteins that have an affinity for phosphorylated tyrosine residues. In this case, a protein kinase called

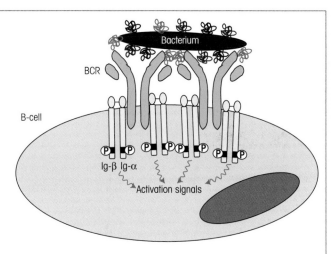

Figure 4.5. B-cell receptor clustering drives activation.

Activation of the BCR complex through antigen engagement results in signal propagation as a consequence of phosphorylation of the intracellular ITAMs within the Ig-α/Ig-β heterodimer.

Syk becomes associated with the phosphorylated Ig-α/-β heterodimer and is instrumental in coordinating events that culminate in entry of the activated B-cell into the cell cycle to commence clonal expansion. We will revisit this topic in Chapter 8 where the details of the BCR signal transduction cascade will be elaborated upon in greater detail (see p. 220).

Specific antigen drives formation of B-cell-receptor microclusters

Recent studies suggest that many of the BCRs do not freely diffuse within the plasma membrane with their associated Ig-α/β heterodimers, but are confirmed within specific zones by the underlying actin cytoskeleton. The actin cytoskeleton does not make contact with the BCR directly but corrals the receptor into confinement zones through interaction with membrane ezrin. There is a good reason for this confinement, as this appears to be required to prevent spontaneous formation of **BCR microclusters**, as these appear to be the structures that are capable of transmitting signals into the B-cell that represents an activation stimulus. BCR microclusters are made up of 50–500 BCR molecules and have been visualized on the surface of B-cells using advanced microscopy techniques. Indeed, mere depolymerization of the actin cytoskeleton appears to be sufficient to permit weak B-cell activation signals to occur spontaneously, without any requirement for antigen; suggesting that cytoskeleton-based confinement is necessary and acts as a "safety catch" on BCR triggering. Indeed, weak background or "tonic" BCR signals appear to be necessary for B-cell development, as interference with this situation results in death of developing B-cells. Presumably a small fraction of the BCR pool that is freely diffusible within the plasma membrane provides this tonic signaling.

B-cell activation appears to require that many BCRs become dislodged from their confinement zones to become recruited into microclusters, an event that very recent evidence suggests is achieved through antigen-induced conformational changes within the antibody constant region that permits self-association within the membrane. More effective BCR stimulation is also achieved through **cross-linking of the BCR with its co-receptor complex**, which is discussed below. B-cell activation through BCR stimulation alone is possible, but the former tends to lead to low affinity IgM production and is far less preferable to co-stimulation via the BCR co-receptor complex.

There is also a growing appreciation that while B-cells can be stimulated by soluble antigen, **the primary form of antigen that triggers B-cell activation *in vivo* is predominantly localized to membrane surfaces**. The most likely source of membrane-localized antigen are the follicular dendritic cells that are resident within lymph nodes and are specialized at capturing complement-decorated antigen complexes that diffuse into these lymphoid tissues. Interaction between a B-cell and membrane-immobilized antigen provides the opportunity for the B-cell membrane to spread along the opposing antigen-bearing membrane, gathering sufficient antigen to trigger B-cell microcluster formation and activate the B-cell.

In addition to providing an optimal activation stimulus, there might be another reason why B-cells are keen to engage as many BCRs as possible with specific antigen. This is because **activated B-cells require help**, in the form of cytokines and CD40 receptor stimulation, from T-helper cells, to undergo class switching and somatic hypermutation. This help is only forthcoming if the B-cell can present antigen to T-cells in the context of MHC class II molecules. Thus, the more antigen captured by a stimulated B-cell, the more efficient it will be in subsequently acquiring T-cell help. Thus, spreading along an antigen-coated surface facilitates engagement of many BCRs with antigen, which can then be internalized by the B-cell to be processed and presented to T-helper cells. We will revisit the issue of T-cell–B-cell interactions in Chapters 8 and 9 when we will look at these events in more detail.

The B-cell co-receptor complex synergises with the BCR to activate B-cells

We have already made reference to the two-signal model for activation of naive T-cells. Similarly, **B-cells also require two signals** (with some exceptions) to become productively activated and this most likely represents a safeguard to limit the production of autoantibodies. Indeed, as we will discuss in more detail in Chapter 8, there are actually two distinct types of co-stimulation a B-cell needs to receive, at different times, for truly optimum activation and subsequent class switching and affinity maturation. One form of co-stimulation takes place at the point of initial encounter of the BCR with its cognate antigen and is provided by the **B-cell co-receptor complex** that is capable of engaging with molecules such as complement that may be decorating the same surface (e.g. on a bacterium)

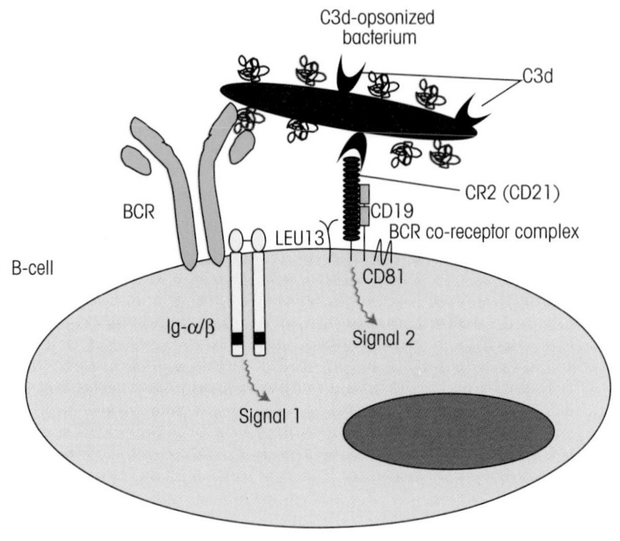

Figure 4.6. The B-cell co-receptor complex synergizes with the BCR to activate B-cells.

The B-cell coreceptor complex is composed of four components: CD19, CD21 (complement receptor type 2, CR2), CD81 (TAPA-1) and CD225 (LEU13, interferon-induced transmembrane protein 1, see also Figure 8.19). Because CR2 is a receptor for the C3d breakdown product of complement, its presence within the BCR co-receptor complex enables complement to synergise with the BCR, thereby enhancing B-cell activation signals.

The T-cell surface receptor for antigen (TCR)

As alluded to earlier, T-cells interact with antigen in a manner that is quite distinct from the way in which B-cells do; the receptors that most T-cells are equipped with cannot directly engage soluble antigens but instead "see" fragments of antigen that are immobilized within a narrow groove on the surface of MHC molecules (Figure 4.1b). As we shall discuss in detail in Chapter 5, MHC molecules bind to short 10–20 amino acid long peptide fragments that represent "quality control" samples of the proteins a cell is expressing at any given time, or what it has internalized through phagocytosis, depending on the type of MHC molecule. In this way, T-cells can effectively inspect what is going on, antigenically speaking, within a cell at any given moment by surveying the range of peptides being presented within MHC molecules. Another major difference between B- and T-cell receptors is that T-cells cannot secrete their receptor molecules in the way that B-cells can switch production of Ig from a membrane-bound form to a secreted form. These differences aside, **T-cell receptors** are structurally quite similar to antibody as they are also built from modules that are based upon the immunoglobulin fold.

Before we explore the structural aspects of T-cell receptors, please keep in mind that the practical function of these receptors is to enable a T-cell to probe the surfaces of cells looking for nonself peptides. If a T-cell finds a peptide–MHC combination that is a good match for its T-cell receptor (TCR) it will become activated, undergo clonal expansion, and differentiate to a mature effector T-cell capable of joining the fight against the infectious agent generating these nonself peptides. In practice, such an eventuality is a very low probability event because, as we shall see, TCRs are generated in such a way as to produce an enormous variety of these receptors, each with their own exquisite specificity for a particular peptide–MHC combination. Moreover, because the majority of peptides presented on MHC molecules at any one time will be derived from self (unless the antigen-presenting cell is infected with a microorganism), this further reduces the probability of a T-cell encountering a perfect nonself peptide-MHC combination to trigger a response.

The receptor for antigen is a transmembrane heterodimer

Identification of the TCR proved more difficult than initially anticipated (Milestone 4.1), but eventually the receptor was found to be a membrane-bound molecule composed of two disulfide-linked chains, α and β. Each chain folds into two Ig-like domains, one having a relatively invariant structure and the other exhibiting a high degree of variability, so that the αβ TCR has a structure really quite closely resembling an Ig Fab fragment. This analogy stretches even further—each of the two variable regions has three hypervariable regions (or complementarity-determining regions, CDRs) that X-ray

displaying the specific antigen recognized by the BCR (Figure 4.6). The other form of co-stimulation required by B-cells takes place after the initial encounter with antigen and is provided by T-cells in the form of membrane-associated **CD40 ligand** that engages with surface CD40 on the B-cell. We will discuss CD40L-dependent co-stimulation in Chapter 8, as this is not required for initial activation but is very important for class switching and somatic hypermutation.

The B-cell coreceptor complex (Figure 4.6) is composed of four components: CD19, CD21 (complement receptor type 2, CR2), CD81 (TAPA-1) and LEU13 (interferon-induced transmembrane protein 1). CR2 is a receptor for the C3d breakdown product of complement and its presence within the BCR coreceptor complex enables complement to synergise with the BCR, thereby enhancing cross-linking, which drives microcluster formation. Thus, in situations in which a bacterium has activated complement and is coated with the products of complement activation, when it is subsequently captured by the BCR on a B-cell there is now an opportunity for CR2 within the BCR coreceptor complex to bind C3d on the bacterium. This effectively means that the B-cell now receives two signals simultaneously. Signal one comes via the BCR and signal two via the coreceptor complex.

○ Milestone 4.1—The T-cell Receptor

As T-lymphocytes respond by activation and proliferation when they contact antigen presented by cells such as macrophages, it seemed reasonable to postulate that they do so by receptors on their surface. In any case, it would be difficult to fit T-cells into the clonal selection club if they lacked such receptors. Guided by Occam's razor (the law of parsimony, which contends that it is the aim of science to present the facts of nature in the simplest and most economical conceptual formulations), most investigators plumped for the hypothesis that nature would not indulge in the extravagance of evolving two utterly separate molecular recognition species for B- and T-cells, and many fruitless years were spent looking for the "Holy Grail" of the T-cell receptor with anti-immunoglobulin serums or monoclonal antibodies (cf. p. 143). Success only came when a monoclonal antibody directed to the idiotype of a T-cell was used to block the response to antigen. This was identified by its ability to block one individual T-cell clone out

of a large number, and it was correctly assumed that the structure permitting this selectivity would be the combining site for antigen on the T-cell receptor. Immunoprecipitation with this antibody brought down a disulfide-linked heterodimer composed of 40–44 kDa subunits (Figure M4.1.1).

The other approach went directly for the genes, arguing as follows. The T-cell receptor should be an integral membrane protein not present in B-cells. Hence, T-cell polysomal mRNA from the endoplasmic reticulum, which should provide an abundant source of the appropriate transcript, was used to prepare cDNA from which genes common to B- and T-cells were subtracted by hybridization to B-cell mRNA. The resulting T-specific clones were used to probe for a T-cell gene that is rearranged in all functionally mature T-cells but is in its germline configuration in all other cell types (Figure M4.1.2). In such a way were the genes encoding the β-subunit of the T-cell receptor uncovered.

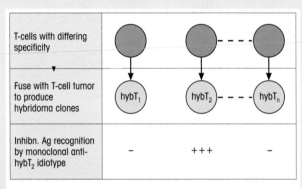

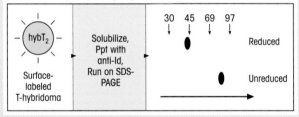

Figure M4.1.1. Antibody (Ab) to T-cell receptor (anti-idiotype) blocks antigen (Ag) recognition.

(Based on Haskins K., Kubo R., White J., Pigeon M., Kappler J. & Marrack P. (1983) *Journal of Experimental Medicine* **157**, 1149; simplified a little.)

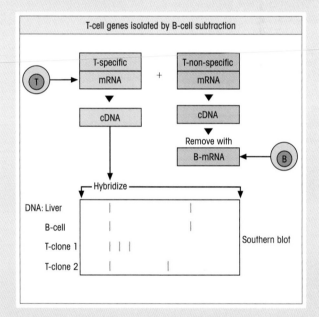

Figure M4.1.2. Isolation of T-cell receptor genes.

DNA fragments of differing sizes, produced by a restriction enzyme, are separated by electrophoresis and probed with the T-cell gene. The T-cells show rearrangement of one of the two germline genes found in liver or B-cells. (Based on Hendrick S.M., Cohen D.I., Nielsen E.A. & Davis M.M. (1984) *Nature* **308**, 149.)

diffraction data have defined as incorporating the amino acids that make contact with the peptide–major histocompatibility complex (MHC) ligand. Plasticity of the CDR loops is an important factor enabling TCRs to mould around structurally diverse peptide–MHC combinations. Although the manner in which the TCR makes contact with peptide–MHC is still not fully understood, it appears that in some TCRs CDRs 1 and 2 of the TCR bear much of the responsibility for making contact with the MHC molecule itself, while CDR3 makes contact with the peptide; however in other TCRs the reverse is true. Whatever CDRs bear the responsibility for contacting MHC versus peptide, it is clear that these are the recognition components of the receptor and so it follows that it is here that much of the variability is seen between TCRs, as we shall discuss later.

Both α and β chains are required for antigen specificity as shown by transfection of the T-receptor genes from a cytotoxic T-cell clone specific for fluorescein to another clone of a different specificity; when it expressed the new α and β genes, the transfected clone acquired the ability to lyse the fluoresceinated target cells. Another type of experiment utilized T-cell hybridomas formed by fusing single antigen-specific T-cells with T-cell tumors to achieve "immortality." One hybridoma recognizing chicken ovalbumin, presented by a macrophage, gave rise spontaneously to two variants, one of which lost the chromosome encoding the α chain, and the other, the β chain. Neither variant recognized antigen but, when they were physically fused together, each supplied the complementary receptor chain, and reactivity with antigen was restored.

CD4 and CD8 molecules act as co-receptors for TCRs

In addition to the TCR, the majority of peripheral T-cells also express one or other of the membrane proteins **CD4** or **CD8** that act as co-receptors for MHC molecules (Figure 4.7). CD4 is a single chain polypeptide containing four Ig-like domains packed tightly together to form an extended rod that projects from the T-cell surface. The cytoplasmic tail of the CD4 molecule is important for TCR signaling as this region is constitutively bound by a protein tyrosine kinase, **Lck**, that initiates the signal transduction cascade that follows upon encounter of a T-cell with antigen (Figure 4.8). CD8 plays a similar role to CD4, as it also binds Lck and recruits this kinase to the TCR complex, but is structurally quite distinct; CD8 is a disulfide-linked heterodimer of α and β chains, each of which contains a single Ig-like domain connected to an extended and heavily glycosylated polypeptide projecting from the T-cell surface (Figure 4.7).

CD4 and CD8 molecules play important roles in antigen recognition by T-cells as these molecules dictate whether a T-cell can recognize antigen presented by MHC molecules that obtain their peptide antigens primarily from intracellular (**MHC class I**), or extracellular (**MHC class II**), sources. This has major functional implications for the T-cell, as those lymphocytes that become activated upon encounter with antigen presented within MHC class I molecules (CD8+ T-cells) invariably become cytotoxic T-cells, and those that are activated by peptides presented by MHC class II molecules (CD4+ T-cells) become helper T-cells (see Figure 8.1).

There are two classes of T-cell receptors

Not long after the breakthrough in identifying the αβ TCR, reports came of the existence of a second type of receptor composed of γ and δ chains. As it appears earlier in thymic ontogeny, the γδ receptor is sometimes referred to as **TCR1** and the αβ receptor as **TCR2** (cf. p. 293).

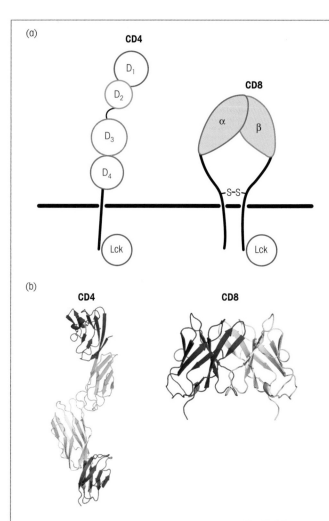

Figure 4.7. CD4 and CD8 act as co-receptors for MHC molecules and define functional subsets of T-cells.

(a) Schematic representation of CD4 and CD8 molecules. CD4 is composed of four Ig-like domains (D$_1$ to D$_4$, as indicated) and projects from the T-cell surface to interact with MHC class II molecules. CD8 is a disulfide-linked heterodimer composed of Ig-like α and β subunits connected to a heavily glycosylated rod-like region that extends from the plasma membrane. CD8 interacts with MHC class I molecules. The cytoplasmic tails of CD4 and CD8 are associated with the tyrosine kinase Lck. (b) Ribbon diagram representations of the extracellular portions of CD4 and CD8. The Ig-like domains (D$_1$ to D$_4$) of CD4 are colored blue, green, yellow and red respectively. A CD8 homodimer of two α subunits is shown. (Structures were kindly provided by Dr. Dan Leahy and are based upon coordinates reported in Leahy D. *et al.* (1992) *Cell* **68**, 1145 and in Wu H. *et al.* (1997) *Nature* **387**, 527.)

γδ cells make up only 1–5% of the T-cells that circulate in blood and peripheral organs of most adult animals; however these cells are much more common in epithelial-rich tissues such as the skin, intestine, reproductive tract and the lungs where they can comprise almost 50% of the T-cell population.

It cannot be denied that γδ T-cells are somewhat of an oddity among T-cells; unlike αβ T-cells, γδ cells do not appear to require antigen to be presented within the context of MHC molecules and are thought to be able to recognize soluble antigen akin to B-cells. Perhaps because of this lack of dependence on MHC for antigen presentation, the majority of γδ T-cells do not express either of the MHC co-receptors, CD4 or CD8 (Table 4.1).

The mechanism of antigen recognition by γδ T-cells is still somewhat mysterious but these cells are known to be able to interact with MHC-related molecules, such as the mouse T10 and T22 proteins, in a manner that does not require antigen. Because the latter MHC-like molecules are upregulated upon activation of αβ T-cells, this has led to the view that γδ T-cells may have an important immunoregulatory function; by becoming activated by molecules that appear on activated T-cells, γδ T-cells may help to regulate immune responses in a positive or negative manner. γδ T-cells can also recognize pathogen-derived lipids, organic phosphoesters, nucleotide conjugates and other nonpeptide ligands.

Certain γδ T-cells (the Vγ1 Vδ1 subset, which are enriched in epithelial tissues) also share some of the same recognition features of NK cells of the innate immune system, as they can both recognize the MHC class I-like proteins MICA and MICB, which do not function as antigen-presenting molecules. Rather, MICA and MICB are typically present at low levels on epithelial tissues but are upregulated in response to cellular stress, including heat shock and DNA damage. Infection with cytomegalovirus or *Mycobacterium tuberculosis* is also capable of inducing the surface appearance of these primitive MHC-like molecules and other stress-inducible γδ T-cell ligands are almost certain to exist. As we shall see later in this chapter, MICA and MICB are also used by NK cells as activation ligands, although in this case a very different receptor is responsible.

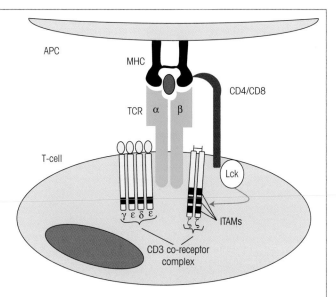

Figure 4.8. The T-cell receptor (TCR) complex, assisted by CD4 or CD8 receptors, recognizes peptide antigen in the context of MHC molecules.

TCR activation signals are propagated via the CD3 co-receptor complex, which is made up of CD3 γ, ε, δ and ζ chains. Co-clustering of CD4 or CD8, which are constitutively associated with the Lck kinase, with the TCR complex facilitates Lck-initiated signal propagation through phosphorylation of immunoreceptor tyrosine-based activation motifs (ITAMs) within the CD3 ζ chain.

The encoding of T-cell receptors is similar to that of immunoglobulins

The gene segments encoding the TCR β chains follow a broadly similar arrangement of *V*, *D*, *J* and constant segments to that described for the immunoglobulins (Figure 4.9). In a parallel fashion, as an immunocompetent T-cell is formed, rearrangement of *V*, *D* and *J* genes occurs to form a continuous *VDJ* sequence. The firmest evidence that B- and T-cells use similar recombination mechanisms comes from mice with severe combined immunodeficiency (SCID) that have a single autosomal

Table 4.1. Comparison between αβ and γδ T-cells.

Characteristic	αβ T-cells	γδ T-cells
Antigen receptor	αβ TCR + CD3 complex	γδ TCR + CD3 complex
Form of antigen recognized	MHC + peptide	MHC-like molecules plus nonprotein ligands
CD4/CD8 expression	Yes	Mainly no
Frequency in blood	60–75%	1–5%
MHC restricted	Yes	Mostly no
Function	Help for lymphocyte and macrophage activation Cytotoxic killing	Immunoregulatory function? Cytotoxic activity

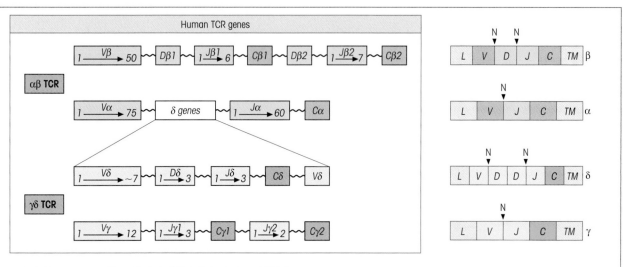

Figure 4.9. Genes encoding αβ and γδ T-cell receptors (TCRs).

Genes encoding the δ chains lie between the Vα and Jα clusters and some V segments in this region can be used in either δ or α chains, i.e. as either Vα or Vδ. TCR genes rearrange in a manner analogous to that seen with immunoglobulin genes, including

N-region diversity at the V(D)J junctions. One of the Vδ genes is found downstream (3′) of the Cδ gene and rearranges by an inversional mechanism.

recessive defect preventing successful recombination of V, D and J segments (cf. p. 71). Homozygous mutants fail to develop immunocompetent B- and T-cells and identical sequence defects in VDJ joint formation are seen in both pre-B- and pre-T-cell lines.

Looking first at the β chain cluster, one of the two Dβ genes rearranges next to one of the Jβ genes. Note that, because of the way the genes are organized, the first Dβ gene, Dβ₁, can utilize any of the 13 Jβ genes, but Dβ₂ can only choose from the seven Jβ₂ genes (Figure 4.9). Next, one of the 50 or so Vβ genes is rearranged to the preformed DβJβ segment. **Variability in junction formation** and the **random insertion of nucleotides** to create N-region diversity either side of the D segment mirror the same phenomenon seen with Ig gene rearrangements. Sequence analysis emphasizes the analogy with the antibody molecule; each V segment contains two hypervariable regions, while the **DJ** junctional sequence provides the **very hypervariable** CDR3 structure, making a total of six potential complementarity determining regions for antigen binding in each TCR (Figure 4.10). As in the synthesis of antibody, the intron between VDJ and C is spliced out of the mRNA before translation with the restriction that rearrangements involving genes in the Dβ₂Jβ₂ cluster can only link to Cβ₂.

All the other chains of the TCRs are encoded by genes formed through similar translocations. The α chain gene pool lacks D segments but possesses a prodigious number of J segments. The number of Vγ and Vδ genes is small in comparison with Vα and Vβ. Like the α chain pool, the β chain cluster has no D segments. The awkward location of the δ locus embedded within the α gene cluster results in T-cells that have undergone Vα–Jα combination having no δ genes on the

rearranged chromosome; in other words, the δ genes are completely excised.

The CD3 complex is an integral part of the T-cell receptor

The T-cell antigen recognition complex and its B-cell counterpart can be likened to army scouts whose job is to let the main battalion know when the enemy has been sighted. When the TCR "sights the enemy," i.e. ligates antigen, it relays a signal through an associated complex of transmembrane polypeptides (**CD3**) to the interior of the T-lymphocyte, instructing it to awaken from its slumbering G0 state and do something useful—like becoming an effector cell. In all immunocompetent T-cells, the TCR is noncovalently but still intimately linked with CD3 in a complex that, as current wisdom has it, may contain two heterodimeric TCR αβ or γδ recognition units closely apposed to one molecule of the invariant CD3 polypeptide chains γ and δ, two molecules of CD3ε, plus the disulfide-linked ζ–ζ dimer. The total complex therefore has the structure TCR₂-CD3γδε₂-ζ₂ (Figures 4.8 and 4.10b).

Similar to the BCR-associated Ig–α/β heterodimer, the CD3 chains also contain one or more ITAMs and these motifs, once again, are instrumental in the propagation of activation signals into the lymphocyte. Upon encounter of the TCR with peptide–MHC, the ITAMs within the CD3 complex become phosphorylated at tyrosine residues; these then act as a platform for the recruitment of a veritable multitude of phosphotyrosine-binding proteins that further disseminate the signal throughout the T-cell. It is here that the role of the CD4 and CD8 co-receptors becomes apparent; phosphorylation of

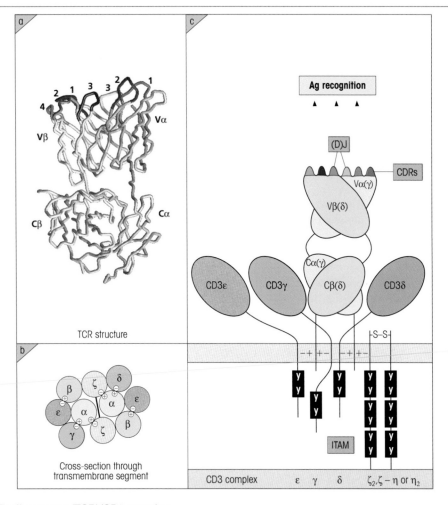

Figure 4.10. The T-cell receptor (TCR)/CD3 complex.

The TCR resembles the immunoglobulin Fab antigen-binding fragment in structure. The variable and constant segments of the TCR α and β chains (VαCα/VβCβ), and of the corresponding γ and δ chains of the γδ TCR, belong structurally to the immunoglobulin-type domain family. (a) In the model the α chain CDRs are colored magenta (CDR1), purple (CDR2) and yellow (CDR3), whilst the β chain CDRs are cyan (CDR1), navy blue (CDR2) and green (CDR3). The fourth hypervariable region of the β chain (CDR4), which constitutes part of the binding site for some superantigens, is colored orange. (Reproduced from Garcia K. *et al.* (1998) *Science* **279**, 1166; with permission.) The TCR α and β CDR3 loops encoded by *(D)J* genes are both short; the TCR γ CDR3 is also short with a narrow length distribution, but the δ loop is long with a broad length distribution, resembling the Ig light and heavy chain CDR3s, respectively. (b) The TCRs may be expressed in pairs linked to the CD3 complex. Negative charges on transmembrane segments of the invariant chains of the CD3 complex contact the opposite charges on the TCR Cα and Cβ chains conceivably as depicted. (c) The cytoplasmic domains of the CD3 peptide chains contain *i*mmunoreceptor *t*yrosine-based *a*ctivation *m*otifs (ITAM; cf. BCR, Figure 4.4) that contact src protein tyrosine kinases. Try not to confuse the TCR γδ and the CD3 γδ chains.

the ITAMs within the CD3 ζ (zeta) chain is accomplished by the Lck tyrosine kinase that, you may recall, is associated with the cytoplasmic tails of CD4 and CD8 (Figures 4.7 and 4.8). In mice, either or both of the ζ chains can be replaced by a splice variant from the ζ gene termed η. The ζ chain also associates with the FcγRIIIA receptor in natural killer (NK) cells where it functions as part of the signal transduction mechanism in that context also. We shall discuss TCR-initiated signal transduction in much greater detail in Chapter 8.

The generation of diversity for antigen recognition

We know that the immune system has to be capable of recognizing virtually any pathogen that has arisen or might arise. The awesome genetic solution to this problem of anticipating an unpredictable future involves the generation of millions of different specific antigen receptors, probably vastly more than the lifetime needs of the individual. As this greatly exceeds the estimated number of 25 000–30 000 genes in the human body, there are some clever ways to generate all this diversity, particularly as the total number of V, D, J and C genes in an individual human coding for antibodies and TCRs is only around 400. Let's revisit the genetics of antibody diversity, and explore the enormous similarities, and occasional differences, seen with the mechanisms employed to generate TCR diversity.

Intrachain amplification of diversity

Random VDJ combination increases diversity geometrically

We saw in Chapter 3 that, just as we can use a relatively small number of different building units in a child's construction set such as LEGO® to create a rich variety of architectural masterpieces, so the individual receptor gene segments can be viewed as building blocks to fashion a multiplicity of antigen specific receptors for both B- and T-cells. The immunoglobulin light chain variable regions are created from V and J segments, and the heavy chain variable regions from V, D and J segments.

Likewise, for both the αβ and γδ T-cell receptors the variable region of one of the chains (α or γ) is encoded by a V and a J segment, whereas the variable region of the other chain (β or δ) is additionally encoded by a D segment. As for immunoglobulin genes, the enzymes RAG-1 and RAG-2 recognize recombination signal sequences (RSSs) adjacent to the coding sequences of the TCR V, D and J gene segments. The RSSs again consist of conserved heptamers and nonamers separated by spacers of either 12 or 23 base-pairs (cf. p. 72) and are found at the 3′ side of each V segment, on both the 5′ and 3′ sides of each D segment, and at the 5′ of each J segment. Incorporation of a D segment is always included in the rearrangement; Vβ cannot join directly to Jβ, nor Vδ directly to Jδ. To see how sequence diversity is generated for TCR, let us take the αβ TCR as an example (Table 4.2). Although the precise number of gene segments varies from one individual to another, there are typically around 75 Vα gene segments and 60 Jα gene segments. If there were entirely **random joining** of any one V to any one J segment, we would have the possibility of generating 4500 VJ combinations (75 × 60). Regarding

Table 4.2. Calculations of human V gene diversity. It is known that the precise number of gene segments varies from one individual to another, perhaps 40 or so in the case of the V_H genes for example, so that these calculations represent "typical" numbers. The number of specificities generated by straightforward random combination of germline segments is calculated. These will be increased by the further mechanisms listed: *minimal assumption of approximately 10 variants for chains lacking D segments and 100 for chains with D segments. The calculation for the T-cell receptor β chain requires further explanation. The first of the two D segments, $D\beta_1$, can combine with 50 V genes and with all 13 $J\beta_1$ and $J\beta_2$ genes. $D\beta_2$ behaves similarly but can only combine with the seven downstream $J\beta_2$ genes.

	γδTCR (TCR1) γ	γδTCR (TCR1) δ	αβTCR (TCR2) α	αβTCR (TCR2) β	Ig H	Ig L κ	Ig L λ
V gene segments	12	~8	75	50	40	40	30
D gene segments	—	3	—	1,1	27	—	—
J gene segments	3,2	3	60	6,7	6	5	5
Random combinatorial joining	V × J	V × D × J	V × J	V × D × J	V × D × J	V × J	V × J
(without junctional diversity)	12 × 5	8 × 3 × 3	75 × 60	50(13 + 7)	40 × 27 × 6	40 × 5	30 × 4
Total	60	72	4500	1000	6480	200	150
Combinatorial heterodimers	60 × 72		4500 × 1000		6480 × 200		6480 × 150
Total (rounded)	4.3 × 10³		4.5 × 10⁶		1.3 × 10⁶		1.0 × 10⁶
Other mechanisms: Ds in 3 reading frames, junctional diversity, N region insertion; × 10³	4.3 × 10⁶		4.5 × 10⁹		1.3 × 10⁹		1.0 × 10⁹
Somatic mutation	–		–		+++		+++

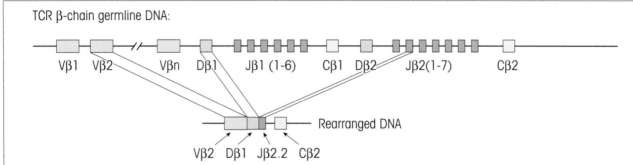

TCR β-chain germline DNA:

Vβ1 Vβ2   Vβn Dβ1   Jβ1 (1-6)   Cβ1 Dβ2 Jβ2(1-7)   Cβ2

Rearranged DNA

Vβ2 Dβ1 Jβ2.2 Cβ2

Figure 4.11. Rearrangement of the T-cell receptor β-chain gene locus.

In this example Dβ1 has rearranged to Jβ2.2, and then the *Vβ2* gene selected out of the 50 or so (Vβn) Vβ genes. If the same V and D segments had been used, but this time Jβ1.4 had been employed, then the Cβ1 gene segment would have been utilized instead of Cβ2.

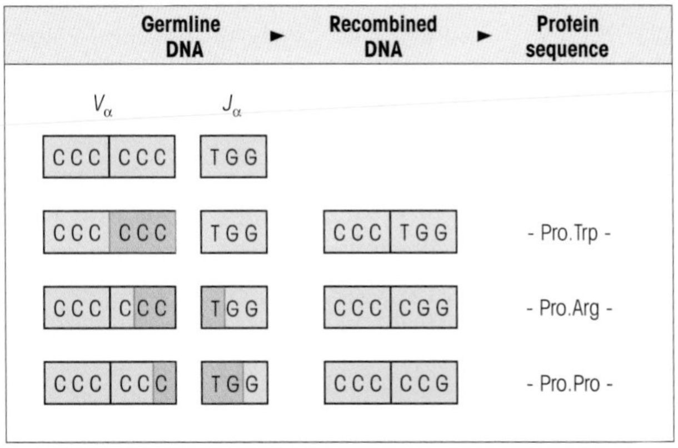

Germline DNA	Recombined DNA	Protein sequence
V_α J_α		
CCC CCC TGG		
CCC CCC TGG	CCC TGG	- Pro.Trp -
CCC CCC TGG	CCC CGG	- Pro.Arg -
CCC CCC TGG	CCC CCG	- Pro.Pro -

Figure 4.12. Junctional diversity between a TCR Vα and Jα germline segment producing three variant protein sequences.

The nucleotide triplet that is spliced out is colored the darker blue. For TCR β chain and Ig heavy chain genes junctional diversity can apply to V, D and J segments.

to just 200, they produce a vast number of different α and β variable regions by **geometric recombination** of the basic elements. But, as with immunoglobulin gene rearrangement, that is only the beginning.

Playing with the junctions

Another ploy to squeeze more variation out of the germline repertoire that is used by both the T-cell receptor and the immunoglobulin genes (cf. Figure 3.25) involves variable boundary recombinations of V, D and J to produce different junctional sequences (Figure 4.12).

As discussed in Chapter 3, further diversity results from the generation of palindromic sequences (P-elements) arising from the formation of hairpin structures during the recombination process and from the insertion of nucleotides at the N region between the V, D and J segments, a process associated with the expression of terminal deoxynucleotidyl transferase. While these mechanisms add nucleotides to the sequence, yet more diversity can be created by nucleases chewing away at the exposed strand ends to remove nucleotides. These maneuvers again greatly increase the repertoire, especially important for the TCR γ and δ genes, which are otherwise rather limited in number.

Additional mechanisms relate specifically to the *D*-region sequence: particularly in the case of the TCR δ genes, where the *D* segment can be read in three different reading frames and two *D* segments can join together, such *DD* combinations produce a longer third complementarity determining region (CDR3) than is found in other TCR or antibody molecules.

As the CDR3 in the various receptor chains is essentially composed of the regions between the *V(D)J* segments, where junctional diversity mechanisms can introduce a very high degree of amino acid variability, one can see why it is that this hypervariable loop usually contributes the most to determining the fine antigen-binding specificity of these molecules.

the TCR β-chain, there are approximately 50 Vβ genes that lie upstream of two clusters of DβJβ genes, each of which is associated with a Cβ gene (Figure 4.11). The first cluster, which associated with C1, has a single β1 gene and 6 Jβ1 genes, whereas the second cluster associated with Cβ2 again has a single Dβ gene (Dβ2) with 7 Jβ2 genes. The *Dβ1* segment can combine with any of the 50 *Vβ* genes and with any of the 13 *Jβ1* and *Jβ2* genes (Figure 4.11). β2 behaves similarly but can only combine with one of the seven downstream *Jβ2* genes. This provides 1000 different possible VDJ combinations for the TCR β-chain. Therefore, although the TCR α and β chain V, D and *J* genes add up arithmetically

Receptor editing

Recent observations have established that lymphocytes are not necessarily stuck with the antigen receptor they initially make; if they don't like it they can change it. The replacement of an undesired receptor with one that has more acceptable characteristics is referred to as receptor editing. This process has been described for both immunoglobulins and for TCR, allowing the replacement of either nonfunctional rearrangements or autoreactive specificities. Furthermore, receptor editing in the periphery may rescue low affinity B-cells from apoptotic cell death by replacing a low affinity receptor with a selectable one of higher affinity. That this does indeed occur in the periphery is strongly supported by the finding that mature B-cells in germinal centers can express RAG-1 and RAG-2 that mediate the rearrangement process.

But how does this receptor editing work? Well, in the case of the receptor chains that lack *D* gene segments, namely the immunoglobulin light chain and the TCR α chain, a secondary rearrangement may occur by a *V* gene segment upstream of the previously rearranged *VJ* segment recombining to a 3′ *J* gene sequence, both of these segments having intact RSSs that are compatible (Figure 4.13a). However, for immunoglobulin heavy chains and TCR β chains the process of *VDJ* rearrangement deletes all of the *D* segment-associated RSSs (Figure 4.13b). Because V_H and J_H both have 23 base-pair spacers in their RSSs, they cannot recombine: that would break the 12/23 rule. This apparent obstacle to receptor editing of these chains may be overcome by the presence of a sequence near the 3′ end of the *V* coding sequences that can function as a surrogate RSS, such that the new *V* segment would simply replace the previously rearranged *V*, maintaining the same *D* and *J* sequence (Figure 4.13b). This is probably a relatively inefficient process and receptor editing may therefore occur more readily in immunoglobulin light chains and TCR α chains than in immunoglobulin heavy chains and TCR β chains. Indeed, it has been suggested that the TCR α chain may undergo a series of rearrangements, continuously deleting previously functionally rearranged *VJ* segments until a selectable TCR is produced.

Recognition of the correct genomic regions by the RAG recombinase

A question that is only now being resolved is how the RAG-1/RAG-2 recombinase selects the correct genomic regions to target for recombination. Clearly it would be disastrous were this complex able to access DNA randomly leaving double-stranded breaks in its wake. One mechanism of protection is to induce RAG expression only where and when it is needed, but doesn't explain how the RAG complex is targeted only to Ig and TCR loci in the cells in which it is expressed. This puzzle is explained by observations that suggest that **alterations to histones**—the proteins upon which DNA is packaged—flag particular loci for binding of the RAG complex. Recent studies have shown that histone H3 that has been modified by tri-methylation on lysine at position 4 (H3K4me3) acts as a binding site for RAG-2. Thus, genomic regions that are poised for VDJ recombination are located close to H3K4me3 histone "marks." Consistent with this idea, experimental ablation of H3K4me3 marks results in greatly impaired V(D)J recombination. But the H3K4me3 mark is found at many more sites throughout the genome than there are antigen receptor loci, so how does the RAG-1/RAG-2 complex find the correct sites? The answer seem to be that the specificity of RAG-1 for RSS sites, combined with that of RAG-2 for H3K4me3 chromatin marks may act as a clamp that guides the recombinase to the right locations. Binding of the RAG complex to the H3K4me3 mark may also activate the recombinase activity of RAG-1 through an allosteric mechanism, increasing the catalytic activity of the complex when it has been positioned at the correct location.

Interchain amplification

The immune system took an ingenious step forward when two different types of chain were utilized for the recognition molecules because the combination produces not only a larger combining site with potentially greater affinity, but also new variability. Heavy–light chain pairing amongst immunoglobulins appears to be largely random and therefore two B-cells can employ the same heavy chain but different light chains. This route to producing antibodies of differing specificity is easily seen *in vitro* where shuffling different recombinant light chains against the same heavy chain can be used to either fine tune, or sometimes even alter, the specificity of the final antibody. In general, the available evidence suggests that *in vivo* the major contribution to diversity and specificity comes from the heavy chain, perhaps not unrelated to the fact that the heavy chain CDR3 gets off to a head start in the race for diversity being, as it is, encoded by the junctions between three gene segments: *V*, *D* and *J*.

This random association between TCR γ and δ chains, TCR α and β chains, and Ig heavy and light chains yields a further geometric increase in diversity. From Table 4.2 it can be seen that approximately 230 functional TCR and 153 functional Ig germline segments can give rise to 4.5 million and 2.3 million different combinations, respectively, by straightforward associations *without* taking into account all of the fancy junctional mechanisms described above. Hats off to evolution!

Somatic hypermutation

As discussed in Chapter 3, there is inescapable evidence that immunoglobulin *V*-region genes can undergo significant **somatic hypermutation**. Analysis of 18 murine λ myelomas revealed 12 with identical structure, four showing just one amino acid change, one with two changes and one with four changes, all within the hypervariable regions and indicative of somatic hypermutation of the single mouse λ germline gene. In another study, following immunization with pneumococcal

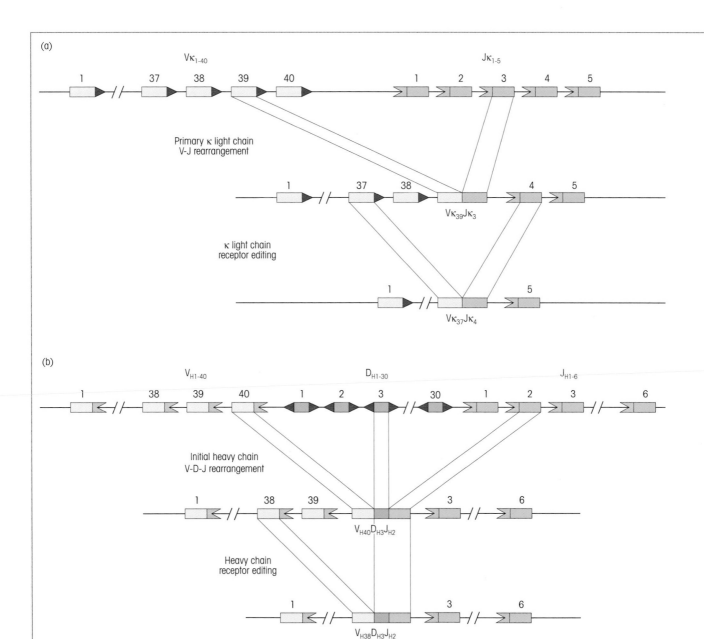

Figure 4.13. Receptor editing.

(a) For immunoglobulin light chain or TCR α chain the recombination signal sequences (RSSs; heptamer–nonamer motifs) at the 3′ end of each variable (V) segment and the 5′ of each joining (J) segment are compatible with each other and therefore an entirely new rearrangement can potentially occur as shown. This would result in a receptor with a different light chain variable sequence (in this example $Vk_{37}Jk_4$ replacing $Vk_{39}Jk_3$) together with the original heavy chain. (b) With respect to the immunoglobulin heavy chain or TCR β chain the organization of the heptamer–nonamer sequences in the RSS precludes a V segment directly recombining with the J segment. This is the so-called 12/23 rule whereby the heptamer–nonamer sequences associated with a 23 base pair spacer (colored violet) can only base-pair with heptamer–nonamer sequences containing a 12 base-pair spacer (colored red). The heavy chain V and J both have an RSS with a 23 base-pair spacer and so this is a nonstarter. Furthermore, all the unrearranged D segments have been deleted so that there are no 12 base-pair spacers remaining. This apparent bar to secondary rearrangement is probably overcome by the presence of an RSS-like sequence near the 3′ end of the V gene coding sequences, so that only the V gene segment is replaced (in the example shown, the sequence $V_{H38}D_{H3}J_{H2}$ replaces $V_{H40}D_{H3}J_{H2}$).

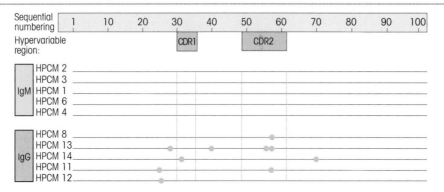

Figure 4.14. Mutations in a germline gene.

The amino acid sequences of the V_H regions of five IgM and five IgG monoclonal phosphorylcholine antibodies generated during an antipneumococcal response in a single mouse are compared with the primary structure of the T15 germline sequence. A line indicates identity with the T15 prototype and an orange circle a single amino acid difference. Mutations have only occurred in the IgG molecules and are seen in both hypervariable and framework segments. (After Gearhart P.J. (1982) *Immunology Today* **3**, 107.) While in some other studies somatic hypermutation has been seen in IgM antibodies, the amount of mutation usually greatly increases following class switching.

antigen, a single germline T15 V_H gene gave rise by mutation to several different V_H genes all encoding phosphorylcholine antibodies (Figure 4.14).

A number of features of this somatic diversification phenomenon are worth revisiting. The mutations are the result of single nucleotide substitutions, they are restricted to the variable as distinct from the constant region and occur in both framework and hypervariable regions. The mutation rate is remarkably high, approximately 1×10^{-3} per base-pair per generation, which is approximately a million times higher than for other mammalian genes. In addition, the mutational mechanism is bound up in some way with class switch recombination as the enzyme **activation-induced cytidine deaminase** (AID) is required for both processes and hypermutation is more frequent in IgG and IgA than in IgM antibodies, affecting both heavy (Figure 4.14) and light chains. However, V_H genes are on average more mutated than V_L genes. This might be a consequence of receptor editing acting more frequently on light chains, as this would have the effect of wiping the slate clean with respect to light chain V gene mutations whilst maintaining already accumulated heavy chain V gene point mutations.

As we outlined in Chapter 3, AID initiates both class switch recombination as well as somatic hypermutation through deaminating deoxy-cytidine within certain DNA hotspots that are characterized by the presence of WRC sequences (W = A or T, R = purine, and C is the deoxy-cytidine that becomes deaminated). Although the target of AID was initially thought to be RNA, more recent evidence suggests that this enzyme works directly on DNA, although RNA editing is not ruled out. Deamination of deoxy-cytidine changes this base to a deoxy-uracil that would normally be repaired by mismatch repair enzymes but, for reasons that are not yet fully understood, can result in removal of the mis-matched uracil that generates a gap that is filled in by an error-prone polymerase to generate a point mutation at this position and can also mutate surrounding bases. It remains unclear how AID is targeted to the correct locations within V regions of rearranged Ig genes, to ensure that mutations are not inadvertently introduced at other loci, but similar to the RAG recombinase, this might involve specific histone modifications. Hyperacetylated versions of histones H3 and H4 appear to be more abundant in mutating V regions than in the C regions of Ig genes. This observation, coupled with observations that AID is recruited to actively transcribing Ig genes by proteins that bind to CAGGTG sequences found in all Ig transcriptional enhancers, suggests a possible mechanism. Thus, the combination of the CAGGTG sequence motif, coupled with the modified histones discussed above, may position AID at the correct locations from which to operate.

Somatic hypermutation does not appear to add significantly to the repertoire available in the early phases of the primary response, but occurs during the generation of memory and is responsible for tuning the response towards higher affinity.

Recently, data have been put forward suggesting that there is yet another mechanism for creating further diversity. This involves the insertion or deletion of short stretches of nucleotides within the immunoglobulin *V* gene sequence of both heavy and light chains. This mechanism would have an intermediate effect on antigen recognition, being more dramatic than single point mutation, but considerably more subtle than receptor editing. In one study, a *reverse transcriptase-polymerase chain reaction* (RT-PCR) was employed to amplify the expressed V_H and V_L genes from 365 IgG⁺ B-cells and it was shown that 6.5% of the cells contained nucleotide insertions or deletions. The transcripts were left in-frame and no stop codons were introduced by these modifications. The percentage of cells containing these alterations is likely to be an underestimate. All the insertions and deletions were in, or near to, CDR1 and/or CDR2. N-region diversity of the CDR3 meant that it was not possible to analyse the third hypervariable region for insertions/deletions of this type and therefore these would be missed in the analysis. The fact that the alterations were associated with CDRs does suggest that the B-cells had been subjected to selection by antigen. It was also notable that the insertions/deletions occurred at known hot spots for somatic point mutation, and the same error-prone DNA polymerase responsible for somatic hypermutation may also be involved here. The sequences were often a duplication of an adjacent sequence in the case of insertions or a deletion of a known repeated sequence. This type of modification may, like receptor editing, play a major role in eliminating autoreactivity and also in enhancing antibody affinity.

T-cell receptor genes, on the other hand, **do not generally undergo somatic hypermutation**. It has been argued that this would be a useful safety measure as T-cells are positively selected in the thymus for weak reactions with self MHC (cf. p. 297), so that mutations could readily lead to the emergence of high affinity autoreactive receptors and autoimmunity.

One may ask how it is that this array of germline genes is protected from genetic drift. With a library of 390 or so functional *V*, *D* and *J* genes, selection would act only weakly on any single gene that had been functionally crippled by mutation and this implies that a major part of the library could be lost before evolutionary forces operated. One idea is that each subfamily of related *V* genes contains a prototype coding for an antibody indispensable for protection against some common pathogen, so that mutation in this gene would put the host at a disadvantage and would therefore be selected against. If any of the other closely related genes in its set became defective through mutation, this indispensable gene could repair them by gene conversion, a mechanism in which it will be remembered that two genes interact in such a way that the nucleotide sequence of part or all of one becomes identical to that of the other. Although gene conversion has been invoked to account for the diversification of MHC genes, it can also act on other families of genes to maintain a degree of sequence homogeneity. Certainly it is used extensively by, for example, chickens and rabbits, in order to generate immunoglobulin diversity. In the rabbit only a single germline *V_H* gene is rearranged in the majority of B-cells; this then becomes a substrate for gene conversion by one of the large number of *V_H* pseudogenes. There are also large numbers of *V_H* pseudogenes and orphan genes (genes located outside the gene locus, often on a completely different chromosome) in humans that actually outnumber the functional genes, although there is no evidence to date that these are used in gene conversion processes.

NK receptors

Natural killer (NK) cells are a population of leukocytes that, like T- and B-cells, employ receptors that can provoke their activation, the consequences of which are the secretion of cytokines, most notably IFNγ, and the delivery of signals to their target cells via Fas ligand or cytotoxic granules that are capable of killing the cell that provided the activation signal (Figures 1.24 and 1.25; see also Videoclip 3). However, in addition to **activating NK receptors**, NK cells also possess receptors that can inhibit their function. As we shall see, **inhibitory NK cell receptors** are critical to the correct functioning of these cells as these receptors are what prevent NK cells from indiscriminately attacking healthy host tissue. Let us dwell on this for a moment because this is quite a different set-up to the one that prevails with T- and B-cells. A T- or B-lymphocyte has a single type of receptor that either recognizes antigen or it doesn't. NK cells have two types of receptor: activating receptors that trigger cytotoxic activity upon recognition of ligands that should not be present on the target cell, and inhibitory receptors that restrain NK killing by recognizing ligands that ought to be present. Thus, NK cell killing can be triggered by two different situations; either the appearance of ligands for the activating receptors or the disappearance of ligands for the inhibitory receptors. Of course, both things can happen at once, but one is sufficient.

We have already discussed NK cell-mediated killing in some detail in Chapter 1 (p. 26), here we will focus on how these cells select their targets as a consequence of alterations to the normal pattern of expression of cell surface molecules, such as **classical MHC class I** molecules, that can occur during viral infection. NK cells can also attack cells that have normal expression levels of classical MHC class I but have upregulated **nonclassical MHC class-I** related molecules due to cell stress or DNA damage.

NK cells express diverse "hard-wired" receptors

Unlike the antigen receptors of T- and B-lymphocytes, NK receptors are "hard-wired" and do not undergo VDJ recombination to generate diversity. As a consequence, NK cell receptor diversity is achieved through gene duplication and divergence and, in this respect, resembles the pattern recognition receptors we discussed in Chapter 1. Thus, NK receptors are a somewhat confusing ragbag of structurally disparate molecules that share the common functional property of being able to survey cells for normal patterns of expression of MHC and MHC-related molecules. NK cells, unlike αβ T-cells, are not **MHC-restricted** in the sense that they do not see antigen only when presented within the groove of MHC class I or MHC class II molecules. On the contrary, one of the main functions of NK cells is to patrol the body looking for cells that have lost expression of the normally ubiquitous classical MHC class I molecules; a situation that is known as **"missing-self" recognition** (Figure 4.15). Such abnormal cells are usually either malignant or infected with a microorganism that interferes with class I expression.

We saw in Chapter 1 that many pathogens activate pattern recognition receptors (PRRs) such as Toll-like receptors that

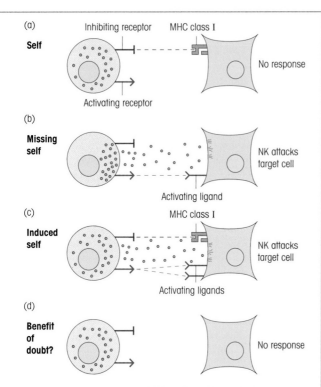

Figure 4.15. Natural killer (NK) cell-mediated killing and the "missing-self" hypothesis.

(a) Upon encounter with a normal autologous MHC class I-expressing cell, NK inhibitory receptors are engaged and activating NK receptors remain unoccupied because no activating ligands are expressed on the target cell. The NK cell does not become activated in this situation. (b) Loss of MHC class I expression ("missing-self"), as well as expression of one or more ligands for activating NK receptors, provokes NK-mediated attack of the cell via NK cytotoxic granules. (c) Upon encountering a target cell expressing MHC class I, but also expressing one or more ligands for activating NK receptors ("induced-self", cf. p. 99), the outcome will be determined by the relative strength of the inhibitory and activating signals received by the NK cell. (d) In some cases, cells may not express MHC class I molecules or activating ligands and may be ignored by NK cells possibly due to expression of alternative ligands for inhibitory NK receptors.

induce transcription of interferon-regulated factors that direct the transcription of type I interferons (IFNα and IFNβ). PRRs, such as TLR3, TLR7–9 and the RIG-like helicases, that reside within intracellular compartments are particularly attuned to inducing the expression of type I interferons (see Figure 1.7). Such PRRs typically detect long single or double-stranded RNA molecules that are characteristically produced by many viruses. One of the downstream consequences of interferon secretion is the cessation of protein synthesis and consequent downregulation of, amongst other things, MHC class I molecules. Thus, detection of pathogen-associated molecular patterns (PAMPs) from intracellular viruses or other

intracellular pathogens can render such cells vulnerable to NK cell-mediated attack. Which is exactly the point? Many intracellular pathogens also directly interfere with the expression or surface exposure of MHC class I molecules as a strategy to evade detection by CD8-positive T-cells that survey such molecules for the presence of nonself peptides.

Because of the central role that MHC class I molecules play in presenting peptides derived from intracellular pathogens to the immune system, it is relatively easy to understand why these molecules may attract the unwelcome attentions of viruses or other uninvited guests planning to gatecrash their cellular hosts. It is probably for this reason that NK cells co-evolved alongside MHC-restricted T-cells to ensure that pathogens, or other conditions that may interfere with MHC class I expression and hence antigen presentation to αβ T-cells, are given short shrift. Cells that end up in this unfortunate position are likely to soon find themselves looking down the barrel of an activated NK cell. Such an encounter typically results in death of the errant cell as a result of attack by cytotoxic granules, containing a battery of proteases and other destructive enzymes released by the activated NK cell.

NK receptors can be activating or inhibitory

NK cells play an important role in the ongoing battle against viral infection and tumor development and carry out their task using two sets of receptors; activating receptors, which recognize molecules that are upregulated on stressed or infected cells, and inhibitory receptors that recognize MHC class I molecules, or MHC-related molecules that monitor the correct expression classical MHC class I molecules. It is the balance between inhibitory and activating stimuli that will dictate whether NK-mediated killing will occur (Figure 4.15).

Several structurally distinct families of NK receptors have been identified: including the **C-type lectin receptors (CTLRs)** and the **Ig-like receptors**. Both receptor types include inhibitory and activating receptors (Table 4.3). Those that are inhibitory contain **ITIMs (immunoreceptor tyrosine-based inhibitory motifs)** within their cytoplasmic tails that exert an inhibitory function within the cell by recruiting phosphatases, such as **SHP-1**, that can antagonize signal transduction events that would otherwise lead to release of NK cytotoxic granules or cytokines (Figure 4.16). Activating receptors, on the other hand, are associated with accessory proteins, such as **DAP-12**, that contain positively acting ITAMs within their cytoplasmic tails that can promote events leading to NK-mediated attack. Upon engagement with their cognate ligands (MHC class I molecules), inhibitory receptors suppress signals that would otherwise lead to NK cell activation. Cells that lack MHC class I molecules are therefore unable to engage the inhibitory receptors and are likely to suffer the consequences (Figure 4.15).

NK receptors are highly diverse and, as this is an area of active investigation, we will make some necessary generalizations.

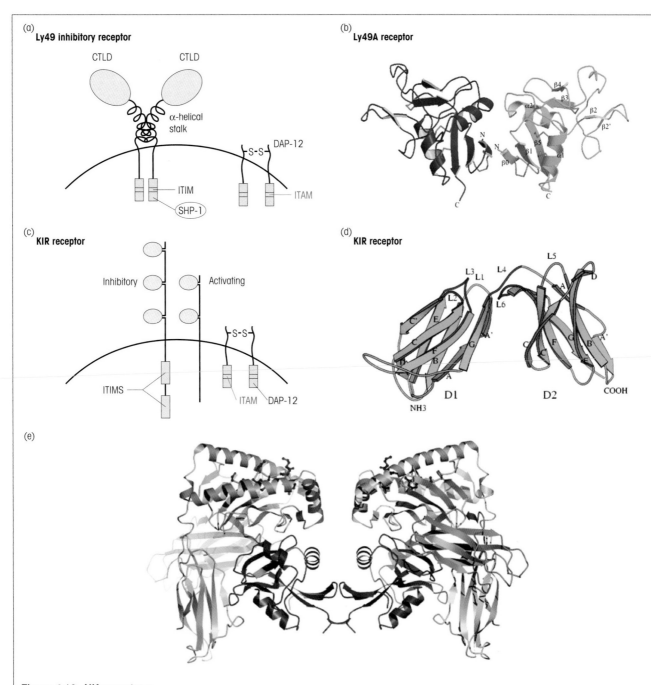

Figure 4.16. NK receptors.

(a) Schematic representation of an inhibitory Ly49 receptor dimer composed of two C-type lectin domains (CTLD). The cytoplasmic tails of inhibitory Ly49 receptors contain *i*mmunoreceptor *t*yrosine-based *i*nhibitory *m*otifs (ITIMs) that can recruit phosphatases, such as SHP-1, capable of antagonizing NK activation. Activating Ly49 receptors lack ITIMs and can associate with ITAM-containing accessory proteins such as DAP-12 that can promote NK cell activation. (b) C-type lectin-like domain of the Ly49 NK cell receptors. The three-dimensional structure shown is the dimeric Ly49A (Protein Data Bank entry code 1QO3), the monomer A is colored blue and the monomer B is colored green. For clarity, secondary structural elements α-helices, β-strands, disulfide bonds and N and C termini are labeled only on one monomer. (Kindly provided by Dr. Nazzareno Dimasi.) (c) The human KIRs (*k*iller *i*mmunoglobulin-like *r*eceptors) are functionally equivalent to the murine Ly49

receptors but remain structurally distinct. These receptors contain two or three Ig-like extracellular domains and can also be inhibitory or activating depending on the presence of an ITIM motif in their cytoplasmic domains, as shown. Activating receptors can associate with the ITAM-bearing DAP-12 accessory complex to propagate activating signals into the NK cell that result in NK-mediated attack. (d) Structure of the extracellular Ig-like domains (D1 and D2) of a KIR receptor. (Kindly provided by Dr. Peter Sun and based upon coordinates originally published in Boyington J.C. *et al.* (2000) *Nature* **405**, 537.) (e) Ribbon diagram of the crystal structure of the Ly49C/H-2K^b complex. Ly49C, the H-2K^b heavy chain, and β$_2$-microglobulin (β$_2$M) are shown in red, gold and green, respectively. The MHC-bound peptide (gray) is drawn in ball-and-stick representation. (Kindly provided by Dr. Lu Deng and Professor Roy A. Mariuzza.)

Table 4.3. Natural killer (NK) activating and inhibitory receptors in man. This table is not exhaustive as some receptors have not been included. Note that the killer immunoglobulin-like receptor (KIR) family is not utilized in the mouse, instead numerous Ly49 family receptors are present.

Family	Receptor	Ligand	Function
KIR	KIR2DL1	Group 2 HLA-C	Inhibitory
	KIR2DL2/3	Group 1 HLA-C	Inhibitory
	KIR2DL5	Unknown	Inhibitory
	KIR3DL1	Bw4, HLA-B	Inhibitory
	KIR3DL2	HLA-A3/HLA-A11	Inhibitory
	KIR2DS1	Group 2 HLA-C	Activating
	KIR2DS2	Group 1 HLA-C	Activating
	KIR3DS1	Bw4, HLA-B	Activating
	KIR2DS3	Unknown	Activating
	KIR2DS4	HLA-Cw4	Activating
	KIR2DS5	Unknown	Activating
	KIR2DL4	HLA-G	Activating
C-type lectin	CD94:NKG2A	HLA-E	Inhibitory
	NKR-P1A	LLT1	Inhibitory
	CD94:NKG2C	HLA-E	Activating
	CD94:NKG2E	HLA-E	Activating
	NKG2D	MICA, MICB, ULBP	Activating
Natural cytotoxicity	NKp30	BAT-3	Activating
	NKp44	Viral haemagglutinin	Activating
	NKp48	Viral haemagglutinin	Activating
Others	CD18	IgG	Activating
	ILT2	HLA-A, B, C, G	Inhibitory

Ly49 receptors

The main class of MHC class I-monitoring receptors in the mouse is represented by the Ly49 multigene family of receptors that contains approximately 23 distinct genes; Ly49A to W. These receptors are expressed as disulfide-linked homodimers, with each monomer composed of a C-type lectin domain connected to the cell membrane via an α-helical stalk of ~40 amino acids (Figure 4.16a); each NK cell expresses from one to four different Ly49 genes. Individual Ly49 receptors recognize MHC class I molecules in a manner that is, in most cases, independent of bound peptide. Ly49 dimers make contact with MHC class I molecules at two distinct sites that do not significantly overlap with the TCR binding area on the MHC (Figure 4.16e).

Killer immunoglobulin-like receptors

Rather remarkably, humans do not use Ly49-based receptors to carry out the same task, but instead employ a functionally equivalent, but structurally distinct, set of receptors for this purpose, the **killer immunoglobulin-like receptors** (KIRs; Figure 4.16c,d). This is a good example of **convergent evolution** where unrelated genes have evolved to fulfill the same functional role. By contrast with the mode of binding to MHC displayed by the Ly49 receptors, the KIRs make contact with MHC class I molecules in an orientation that resembles the

docking mode of the TCR where contact with bound peptide is part of the interaction. However, it is worth emphasizing that although KIRs do make contact with peptide within the MHC class I groove, these receptors do not distinguish between self and nonself peptides as TCRs do.

CD94/NKG2 receptors

NK cells also use members of the **CD94/NKG2 family**, which belong to the CTLR class of receptor, that are present in human, rat and mouse genomes. CD94/NKG2A heterodimers, which are inhibitory receptors, can indirectly monitor the expression of MHC class I proteins by interacting with an invariant MHC-related molecule called HLA-E (human) and Qa1[b] (mouse), the surface expression of which is dependent on the proper synthesis of the main MHC class I A, B and C proteins as will be discussed in more detail below. If normal levels of HLA-E are detected, the inhibitory receptors will suppress NK attack. CD94/NKG2 heterodimers are expressed on most NK cells as well as $\gamma\delta$ T-cells.

This receptor system indirectly monitors the expression of MHC class I molecules in a rather ingenious way. The MHC class I-related molecules HLA-E/Qa1[b] are notable for the fact that they mainly bind invariant peptides that are found in the leader sequences (amino acids 3–11) of the classical MHC class I A, B and C molecules. In the absence of the leader sequences from these peptides, HLA-E and Qa1[b] are not expressed on the cell surface, thereby triggering NK attack. Because many microbial agents, particularly viruses, antagonize the expression of MHC class I molecules, monitoring the expression level of such molecules is a neat way of indirectly detecting that all is not well.

Another member of this receptor family, NKG2D, does not associate with CD94 and instead forms NKG2D/NKG2D homodimers, which are activating receptors. NKG2D homodimers recognize the MHC-related proteins, **MHC class I chain-related A chain (MICA)** and the related **MICB**, as well as UL16 binding proteins in human and the homologous H60/RAE-1/MULT-1 proteins in mice. These ligands become upregulated in damaged or stressed cells as will be elaborated upon below.

Natural cytotoxicity receptors

Additional NK receptors, which belong to the Ig-like class, are the **natural cytotoxicity receptors**, which include NKp30, NKp44 and NKp46, all of which are activating receptors. The ligands for these receptors remain unclear but there is some evidence that they can detect certain viral products, such as hemagglutinin of influenza virus or Sendai virus and may also be sensitive to altered patterns of heparan sulphate on the surfaces of tumors. BAT-3 (HLA-B associated transcript-3) a protein that has been implicated in DNA damage response pathways has also recently been implicated as a ligand for NKp30.

CD16 Fc receptors

Another example of an activating NK receptor is CD16, the low-affinity Fc receptor for IgG that is responsible for *a*ntibody-*d*ependent *c*ellular *c*ytotoxicity (ADCC, cf. p. 48). In this case, the receptor ligand is IgG bound to antigen present on a target cell, which is clearly an abnormal situation.

Cell stress and DNA damage responses can activate NK cells

Cellular stress, such as heat shock, is also a matter for concern for cells of the immune system as this can also be caused by infection, or alternatively, such cells may be undergoing malignant transformation. The HLA-E/Qa1 system, which as we discussed earlier is involved in monitoring the ongoing expression of MHC class I proteins, is also involved in attracting the attentions of NK cells in the context of cell stress. In response to diverse forms of cellular stress, heat-shock proteins such as HSP-60 are induced and peptides derived from the HSP-60 leader peptide can displace MHC class I-derived peptides from the HLA-E peptide binding cleft. Although HLA-E/HSP-60 peptide complexes are trafficked to the cell surface, they are no longer recognized by CD94/NKG2 heterodimers, which results in NK activation due to "missing self."

In addition to recognizing "missing-self," NK cells also use their receptors to directly recognize pathogen components or nonclassical MHC class I-like proteins, such as MICA and MICB, which are normally poorly expressed on normal healthy cells. MICA, and related ligands, have a complex pattern of expression but are often upregulated on transformed or infected cells and this may be sufficient to activate NK receptors that are capable of delivering activating signals; a phenomenon that has been termed **"induced-self" recognition** (Figure 4.15). Upon ligation, the activating receptors signal the NK cell to kill the target cell and/or to secrete cytokines. The potentially anarchic situation in which the NK cells would attack all cells in the body is normally prevented due to the recognition of MHC class I by the inhibitory receptors. Thus, normal patterns of MHC class I expression suppress NK killing, whereas the presence of abnormal patterns of self molecules induce NK activation. It is the relative intensity of these signals that determines whether an attack will occur.

Recent studies also suggest that checkpoint kinases, such as Chk1, that are involved in the **DNA damage response** can induce expression of a variety of activating ligands for NKG2 receptors, when a cell is damaged by γ-irradiation, or after treatment with DNA-damaging drugs. This suggests that cells that have suffered DNA damage may, in addition to activating their DNA repair machinery, also upregulate NK receptor ligands to alert the immune system. This makes perfect sense, as such cells are dangerous as they have the potential to escape normal growth controls and form a tumor due to faulty or incomplete DNA repair. Indeed, tumor surveillance is thought to be one of the major roles of NK cells, a topic we will revisit again in Chapter 17.

The major histocompatibility complex (MHC)

Molecules within this complex were originally defined by their ability to provoke vigorous rejection of grafts exchanged between different members of a species (Milestone 4.2). We have already referred to the necessity for antigens to be associated with class I or class II MHC molecules in order that they may be recognized by T-lymphocytes (Figure 4.8). How antigenic peptides are processed and selected for presentation within MHC molecules and how the TCR sees this complex are discussed in detail in Chapter 5, but let us run through the major points briefly here so that reader will appreciate why these molecules are of huge importance within the immune system.

MHC molecules assemble within the cell where they associate with short peptide fragments derived either from proteins being made by the cell (MHC class I molecules bind to peptides derived from proteins being synthesized within the cell) or proteins that have been internalized by the cell through phagocytosis or pinocytosis (MHC class II molecules bind to peptides derived from proteins made external to the cell). There are some exceptions to these general rules, which we deal with in Chapter 5. We have already made the analogy that this process represents a type of "quality control" checking system

📍 Milestone 4.2—The Major Histocompatibility Complex

Peter Gorer raised rabbit antiserums to erythrocytes from pure strain mice (resulting from >20 brother–sister matings) and, by careful cross-absorption with red cells from different strains, he identified the strain-specific antigen II, now known as H-2 (Table M4.2.1).

He next showed that the rejection of an albino (A) tumor by black (C57) mice was closely linked to the presence of the antigen II (Table M4.2.2) and that tumor rejection was associated with the development of antibodies to this antigen.

Subsequently, George Snell introduced the term **histocompatibility (H)** antigen to describe antigens provoking graft rejection and demonstrated that, of all the potential H antigens, differences at the H-2 (i.e. antigen II) locus provoked the strongest graft rejection seen between various mouse strains. *Poco a poco*, the painstaking studies gradually uncovered a remarkably complicated situation. Far from representing a single gene locus, H-2 proved to be a large complex of multiple genes, many of which were highly

polymorphic, hence the term **major histocompatibility complex (MHC)**. The major components of the current genetic maps of the human HLA and mouse H-2 MHC are drawn in Figure M4.2.1 to give the reader an overall grasp of the complex make-up of this important region (to immunologists we mean!—presumably all highly transcribed regions are important to the host in some way).

Table M4.2.1. Identification of H-2 (antigen II).

Rabbit antiserum to:	Antigens detected on Albino red cells		
	I	II	III
Albino (A)	+++	+++	++
Black (C57)	++	–	++

Table M4.2.2. Relationship of antigen II to tumor rejection.

Antigen II phenotype of recipient strain	Rejection of tumor inoculum (A strain) by:			
	*Pure strain		**(A × C57) F1 backcross to C57	
	–	+	–	+
Ag II + ve (A)	39	0	17 (19.3)	17 (19.5)
Ag II – ve (C57)	0	45	0	44 (39)

*A tumor inoculum derived from an A strain mouse and bearing antigen II is rejected by the C57 host (+ = rejection; – = acceptance).
**Offspring of A × C57 mating were backcrossed to the C57 parent and the resulting progeny tested for antigen II (Ag II) and their ability to reject the tumor. The figures in brackets = number expected if tumor growth is influenced by two dominant genes, one of which determines the presence of antigen II.

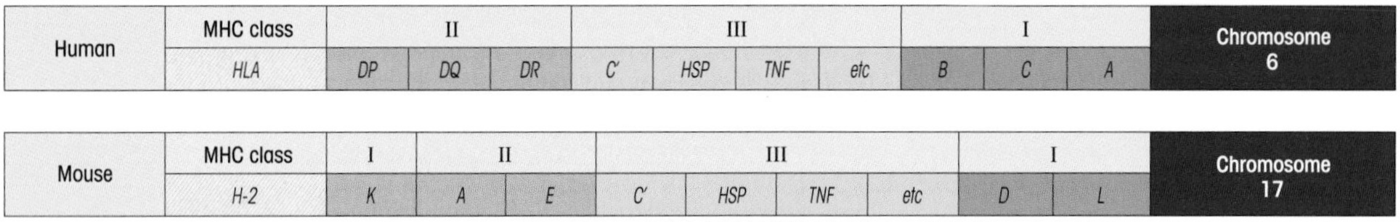

Human	MHC class		II			III				I			Chromosome 6
	HLA	DP	DQ	DR	C'	HSP	TNF	etc	B	C	A		

Mouse	MHC class	I		II			III			I			Chromosome 17
	H-2	K	A	E	C'	HSP	TNF	etc	D	L			

Figure M4.2.1. Main genetic regions of the major histocompatibility complex (MHC).

where a fraction of proteins present in the cell at any given moment are presented to T-cells for inspection to ensure that none of these is derived from nonself. Of course, if a cell happens to harbor a nonself peptide, we want the immune system to know about this as quickly as possible, so that the appropriate course of action can be taken. Thus, MHC class I molecules display peptides that are either self, or that are being made by an intracellular virus or bacterium. MHC class II molecules display peptides that are either extracellular self proteins or proteins being made by extracellular microorganisms. The whole point is to enable a T-cell to inspect what is going on, antigenically speaking, within the cell.

As we shall see, MHC class I molecules serve an important role presenting peptides for inspection by CD8 T-cells that are mainly preoccupied with finding virally infected or "abnormal" cells to kill. Should a TCR-bearing CD8 T-cell recognize a class I MHC-peptide combination that is a good "fit" for its TCR, it will attack and kill that cell. MHC class II molecules, on the other hand, are not expressed on the general cell population but are restricted to cells of the immune system, such as DCs, that have an antigen-presenting function as we already outlined in Chapter 1. Upon recognition of an appropriate MHC class II-peptide combination by a CD4 T-cell, this will result in activation of the latter and maturation to an effector T-cell that can give help to B-cells to make antibody for example. While this is an oversimplification, as we will learn in later chapters, please keep in mind the general idea that MHC class I and II molecules present peptides to CD8- and CD4-retricted T-cells, respectively, for the purposes of allowing these cells to determine whether they should become "activated" and differentiate to effector cells. Let us now look at these molecules in greater detail.

Class I and class II molecules are membrane-bound heterodimers

MHC class I

Class I molecules consist of a heavy polypeptide chain of 44 kDa noncovalently linked to a smaller 12 kDa polypeptide called β_2-**microglobulin**. The largest part of the heavy chain is organized into three globular domains (α_1, α_2 and α_3; Figure 4.17) that protrude from the cell surface; a hydrophobic section anchors the molecule in the membrane and a short hydrophilic sequence carries the C-terminus into the cytoplasm.

The solution of the crystal structure of a human class I molecule provided an exciting leap forwards in our understanding of MHC function. Both β_2-microglobulin and the α_3 region resemble classic Ig domains in their folding pattern (cf. Figure 4.17c). However, the α_1 and α_2 domains, which are most distal to the membrane, form two extended α-helices above a floor created by strands held together in a β-pleated sheet, the whole forming an undeniable **groove** (Figure 4.17b,c). The appearance of these domains is so striking, we doubt whether the reader needs the help of gastronomic analogies such as "two sausages on a barbecue" to prevent any class I structural amnesia. Another curious feature emerged. The groove was occupied by a linear molecule, now known to be a peptide, which had cocrystallized with the class I protein (Figure 4.18).

MHC class II

Class II MHC molecules are also transmembrane glycoproteins, in this case consisting of α and β polypeptide chains of molecular weight 34 kDa and 29 kDa, respectively.

There is considerable sequence homology with class I and structural studies have shown that the α_2 and β_2 domains, the ones nearest to the cell membrane, assume the characteristic Ig fold, while the α_1 and β_1 domains mimic the class I α_1 and α_2 in forming a groove bounded by two α-helices and a β-pleated sheet floor (Figures 4.17a and 4.18).

The organization of the genes encoding the α chain of the human class II molecule HLA-DR and the main regulatory sequences that control their transcription are shown in Figure 4.19.

MHC class I and class II molecules are polygenic

Several different flavors of MHC class I and class II proteins are expressed by most cells. There are three different class I

α-chain genes, referred to as *HLA-A*, *HLA-B* and *HLA-C* in man and *H-2K*, *H-2D* and *H-2L* in the mouse, which can result in the expression of at least three different class I proteins in every cell. This number is doubled if an individual is **heterozygous** for the class I alleles expressed at each locus; indeed, this is often the case due to the **polymorphic** nature of class I genes as we shall discuss later in this chapter.

There are also three different types of MHC class II α- and β-chain genes expressed in humans, *HLA-DQ*, *HLA-DP*, and *HLA-DR*, and two pairs in mice, *H2-A* (I-A) and *H2-E* (I-E). Thus, humans can express a minimum of three different class II molecules, with this number increasing significantly when polymorphisms are considered; this is because different α and β chain combinations can be generated when an individual is heterozygous for a particular class II gene.

The different types of class I and class II molecules all exhibit the same basic structure as depicted in Figure 4.17a and all participate in presenting peptides to T-cells but, because of significant differences in their peptide-binding grooves, **each presents a different range of peptides** to the immune system. This has the highly desirable effect of reducing the probability that peptides derived from pathogen proteins will fail to be presented.

Class I and class II MHC molecules probably evolved from a single ancestral gene that underwent serial gene duplications, followed by diversification due to selective pressure, to generate the different class I and class II genes that we see today (Figure 4.20). Genes that failed to confer any selective advantage or that suffered deleterious mutations were either deleted from the genome or are still present as pseudogenes (genes that fail to express a functional protein); indeed many pseudogenes are present within the MHC region. This type of gene evolution pattern has been termed the **birth and death model** or the accordion model due to the way in which this gene region expanded and contracted during evolution.

Several immune response-related genes contribute to the remaining class III region of the MHC

A variety of other genes that congregate within the MHC chromosome region are grouped under the heading of class III. Broadly, one could say that many are directly or indirectly related to immune defense functions. A notable cluster involves four genes coding for complement components, two of which are for the C4 isotypes C4A and C4B and the other two for C2 and factor B. The cytokines tumor necrosis factor (TNF, sometimes referred to as TNFα) and lymphotoxin (LTα and LTβ) are encoded under the class III umbrella, as are three members of the human 70 kDa heat-shock proteins. As ever, things don't quite fit into the nice little boxes we would like to put them in. Even if it were crystal clear where one region of the MHC ends and another begins (and it isn't), some genes located in the middle of the "classical" (cf. Figure 4.21) class I or II regions should more correctly be classified as part of the

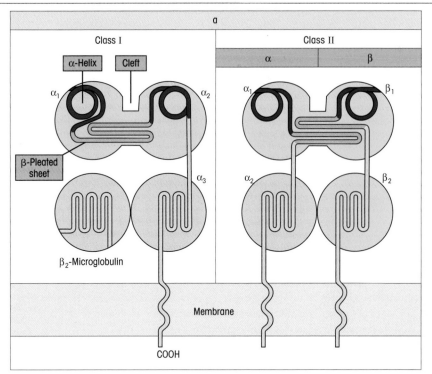

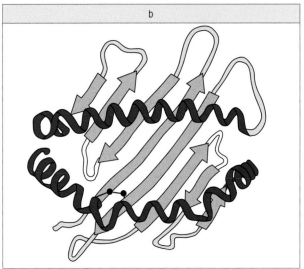

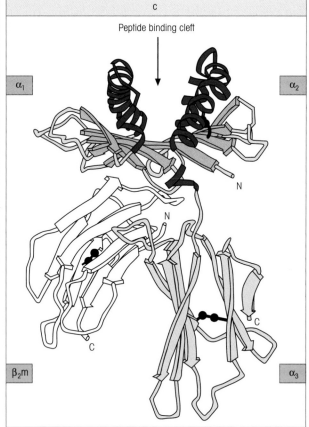

Figure 4.17. Class I and class II MHC molecules.

(a) Diagram showing domains and transmembrane segments; the α-helices and β-sheets are viewed end on. (b) Schematic bird's eye representation of the top surface of human class I molecule (HLA-A2) based on the X-ray crystallographic structure. The strands making the β-pleated sheet are shown as thick gray arrows in the amino to carboxy direction; α-helices are represented as dark red helical ribbons. The inside-facing surfaces of the two helices and the upper surface of the β-sheet form a cleft. The two black spheres represent an intrachain disulfide bond. (c) Side view of the same molecule clearly showing the anatomy of the cleft and the typical Ig-type folding of the α₃- and β₂-microglobulin (β₂m) domains (four antiparallel β-strands on one face and three on the other). (Reproduced from Bjorkman P.J. *et al.* (1987) *Nature* **329**, 506, with permission.)

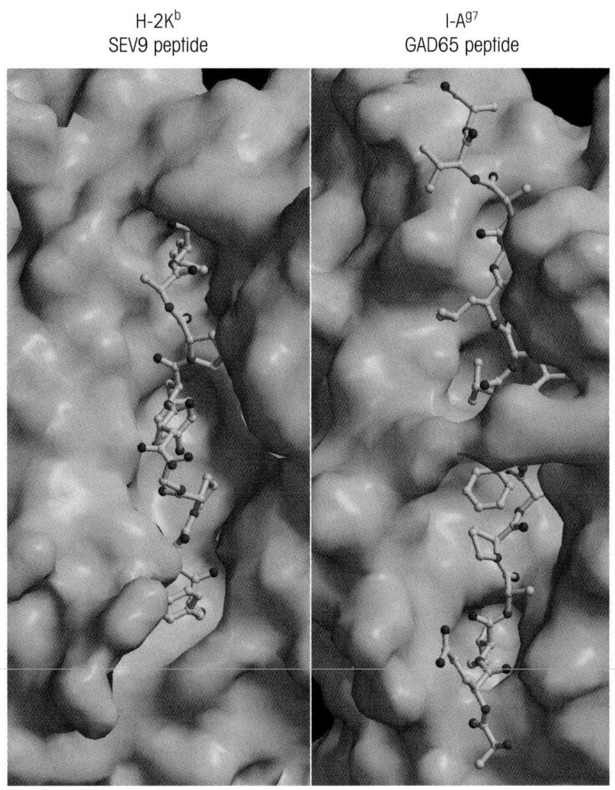

H-2K^b
SEV9 peptide

I-A^g7
GAD65 peptide

Figure 4.18. Surface view of mouse class I and class II MHC molecules in complex with peptide.

Surface solvent-accessible areas of the mouse class I molecule (H-2K^b) in complex with a virus-derived peptide and the mouse class II molecule I-A^g7 in complex with an endogenous peptide. The views shown here are similar to that schematically depicted in Figure 4.17b and look down upon the surface of the MHC molecules. Note that the peptide-binding cleft of class I molecules is more restricted than that of class II molecules with the result that class I-binding peptides are typically shorter than those that bind to class II molecules. (Kindly provided by Dr. Robyn Stanfield and Dr. Ian Wilson, Department of Molecular Biology, The Scripps Research Institute, La Jolla, California, USA.)

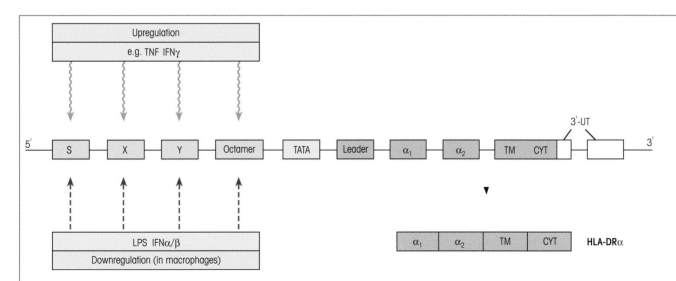

Figure 4.19. Genes encoding human HLA-DRα chain (darker blue) and their controlling elements (regulatory sequences in light blue and TATA box promoter in yellow).

α_1/α_2 encode the two extracellular domains; TM and CYT encode the transmembrane and cytoplasmic segments, respectively. 3′-UT represents the 3′-untranslated sequence. Octamer motifs are also found in virtually all heavy and light chain immunoglobulin *V* gene promoters (cf. Figure 3.21) and in the promoters of other B-cell-specific genes such as *B29* and *CD20*.

Figure 4.20. Birth and death model of MHC evolution.

Different major histocompatibility complex (MHC) genes most likely arose though duplication events that resulted in diversification of the duplicated genes as a result of selective pressure. Genes that confer no selective advantage can suffer deleterious mutations resulting in pseudogenes or may be deleted from the genome altogether. Different environments impose distinct selective pressures, due to different pathogens for example, resulting in a high degree of polymorphism within this gene family. MHC polymorphism is seen primarily within the peptide-binding regions of MHC class I and class II molecules.

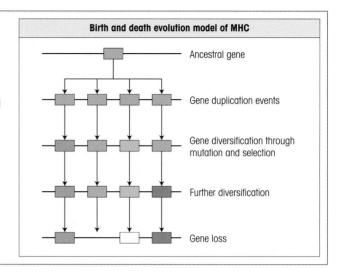

Human	HLA gene	MICB	MICA	B	C	E	A	G	F
	Gene product	MICB	MICA	HLA-B	HLA-C	HLA-E	HLA-A	HLA-G	HLA-F

Mouse	H-2 gene	TAPASIN	K	D	L	Q	T	M	
	Gene product	TAPASIN	H-2K	H-2D	H-2L	Q	T	H-2M	

Figure 4.21. MHC class I gene map.

The "classical" polymorphic class I genes, *HLA-A*, *-B*, *-C* in humans and *H-2K*, *-D*, *-L* in mice, are highlighted with orange shading and encode peptide chains that, together with β₂-microglobulin, form the complete class I molecules originally identified in earlier studies as antigens by the antibodies they evoked on grafting into another member of the same species. Note that only some strains of mice possess an *H-2L* gene. The genes expressed most abundantly are *HLA-A* and *-B* in the human and *H-2K* and *-D* in the mouse. The other class I genes ("class Ib") are termed "nonclassical" or "class I chain-related."

They are oligo- rather than polymorphic or sometimes invariant, and many are silent or pseudogenes. In the mouse there are approximately 15 *Q* (also referred to as *Qa*) genes, 25 *T* (also referred to as *TL* or *Tla*) genes and 10 *M* genes. MICA and MICB are ligands for NK cell receptors. Tapasin is involved in peptide transport (cf. p. 126). The gene encoding this molecule is at the centromeric end of the MHC region and therefore is shown in this gene map with respect to the mouse, but in Figure 4.22, the class II gene map with respect to the human—look at Figure M4.2.1 to see why.

class III cohort. For example, the *LMP* and *TAP* genes concerned with the intracellular processing and transport of T-cell epitope peptides are found in the class II region (see below), but do not have the classical class II structure nor are they expressed on the cell surface.

Gene map of the MHC

The complete sequence of a human MHC was published at the very end of the last millennium after a gargantuan collaborative effort involving groups in England, France, Japan and the USA. The entire sequence, which represents a composite of several MHC haplotypes, comprises 224 gene loci. Of the 128 of these genes that are predicted to be expressed, it is estimated that about 40% of them have functions related to the immune system. It is not clear why so many immune

response-related genes are clustered within this relatively small region, although this phenomenon has also been observed with housekeeping genes that share related functions. Because the location of a gene within chromatin can profoundly influence its transcriptional activity, perhaps it has something to do with ensuring that the genes within this region are expressed at similar levels. Genes found within condensed regions of chromatin are often expressed at relatively low levels and in some cases may not be expressed at all. The region between class II and class I in the human contains 60 or so class III genes. An overall view of the main clusters of class I, II and III genes in the MHC of the mouse and human may be gained from Figure M4.2.1 in Milestone 4.2. More detailed maps of each region are provided in Figures 4.21, 4.22 and 4.23. A number of pseudogenes have been omitted from these gene maps in the interest of simplicity.

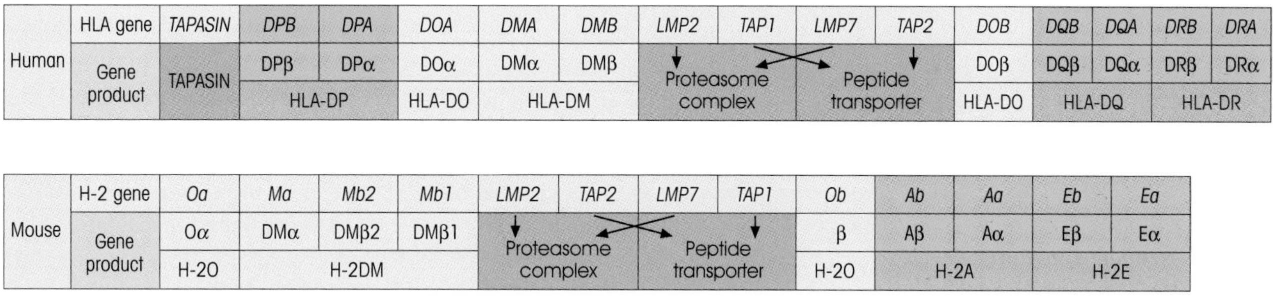

Human	HLA gene	TAPASIN	DPB	DPA	DOA	DMA	DMB	LMP2	TAP1	LMP7	TAP2	DOB	DQB	DQA	DRB	DRA
	Gene product	TAPASIN	DPβ	DPα	DOα	DMα	DMβ	Proteasome complex		Peptide transporter		DOβ	DQβ	DQα	DRβ	DRα
			HLA-DP		HLA-DO	HLA-DM						HLA-DO	HLA-DQ		HLA-DR	

Mouse	H-2 gene	Oa	Ma	Mb2	Mb1	LMP2	TAP2	LMP7	TAP1	Ob	Ab	Aa	Eb	Ea
	Gene product	Oα	DMα	DMβ2	DMβ1	Proteasome complex		Peptide transporter		β	Aβ	Aα	Eβ	Eα
		H-2O	H-2DM							H-2O	H-2A		H-2E	

Figure 4.22. MHC class II gene map.

With "classical" *HLA-DP, -DQ, -DR* in the human and *H-2A (I-A)* and *H-2E (I-E)* in mice more heavily shaded. Both α and β chains of the class II heterodimer are transcribed from closely located genes. There are usually two expressed *DRB* genes, *DRB1* and one of either *DRB3, DRB4* or *DRB5*. A similar situation of a single α chain pairing with different β chains is found in the mouse I-E molecule. The *LMP2* and *LMP7* genes encode part of the proteasome complex that cleaves cytosolic proteins into small peptides that are transported by the *TAP* gene products into the endoplasmic reticulum. *HLA-DMA* and *-DMB* (mouse *H-2DMa, -DMb1* and *-DMb2*) encode the DM αβ heterodimer that removes class II-associated invariant chain peptide (CLIP) from classical class II molecules to permit the binding of high affinity peptides. The mouse H-2DM molecules are often referred to as H-2M1 and H-2M2, although this is a horribly confusing designation because the term *H-2M* is also used for a completely different set of genes that lie distal to the *H-2T* region and encode members of the class Ib family (cf. Figure 4.21). The *HLA-DOA* (alternatively called *HLA-DNA*) and *-DOB* genes (*H-2Oa* and *-Ob* in the mouse) also encode an αβ heterodimer that may play a role in peptide selection or exchange with classical class II molecules. (Reproduced with permission from Horton R. *et al.* (2004) *Nature Reviews Genetics* **5**, 889–899.)

Human	CYP21B	C4B	CYP21A	C4A	BF	C2	HSPA1B	HSPA1A	HSPA1L	LTB	TNF	LTA
Mouse	CYP21A1	C4	CYP21A2	Slp	BF	C2	HSP70-1	HSP70-3	Hsc70t	LTB	TNF	LTA

Figure 4.23. MHC class III gene map.

This region is something of a "rag bag." Aside from immunologically "respectable" products like C2, C4, factor B (encoded by the *BF* gene), tumor necrosis factor (*TNF*), lymphotoxin-α and lymphotoxin-β (encoded by *LTA* and *LTB*, respectively) and three 70kDa heat-shock proteins (the *HSPA1A, HSPA1B* and *HSPA1L* genes in humans, *HSP70-1, HSP70-3* and *Hsc70t* genes in mice), genes not shown in this Figure but nonetheless present in this locus include those encoding valyl tRNA synthetase (*G7a*), NOTCH4, which has a number of regulatory activities, and tenascin, an extracellular matrix protein. Of course many genes may have drifted to this location during the long passage of evolutionary time without necessarily having to act in concert with their neighbors to subserve some integrated defensive function. The 21-hydroxylases (21OHA and B, encoded by *CYP21A* and *CYP21B*, respectively) are concerned with the hydroxylation of steroids such as cortisone. *Slp* (sex-limited protein) encodes a murine allele of C4, expressed under the influence of testosterone.

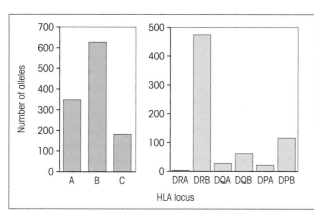

Figure 4.24. Polymorphism within human HLA (human leukocyte antigen) class I and class II genes.

Number of distinct human HLA class I (A, B, C) and class II (DRA, DRB, DQA, DQB, DPA,DPB) alleles at each locus as of January 2005. (Based upon data gathered by the WHO Nomenclature Committee for Factors of the HLA system and published within Marsh S.G. *et al.* (2005) *Tissue Antigens* **65**, 301.)

The cell surface class I molecule, based on a transmembrane chain with three extracellular domains associated with β_2-microglobulin, has clearly proved to be a highly useful structure judging by the number of variants on this theme that have arisen during evolution. It is helpful to subdivide them, first into the **classical class I molecules** (sometimes referred to as class Ia), HLA-A, -B and -C in the human and H-2K, -D and -L in the mouse. These were defined serologically by the antibodies arising in grafted individuals using methods developed from Gorer's pioneering studies (Milestone 4.2). Other molecules, sometimes referred to as class Ib, have related structures and are either encoded within the MHC locus itself ("**nonclassical**" MHC molecules, for example the human HLA-E, -F and -G, HFE, MICA and MICB, the murine H-2T, -Q and -M), or elsewhere in the genome ("**class I chain-related**," including the CD1 family and FcRn). Nonclassical MHC genes are far less polymorphic than the classical MHC, are often invariant, and many are pseudogenes. Many of these nonclassical MHC class I molecules form structures that are very similar to class I molecules and have also been found to either present nonpeptide antigens or canonical (i.e. invariant) peptides that serve roles in monitoring overall cell stress levels. We will discuss these nonclassical MHC molecules in more detail towards the end of this chapter.

The genes of the MHC display remarkable polymorphism

Unlike the immunoglobulin system where, as we have seen, variability is achieved in each individual by a **multigenic** system, the MHC has evolved in terms of variability between individuals with a highly **polymorphic** (literally "many shaped") system based on **multiple alleles** (i.e. alternative genes at each locus). This has likely arisen through **pathogen-driven selection** to form new alleles that may offer increased "fitness" for the individual; in this context, fitness could mean increased protection from an infectious organism. The class I and class II genes are the most polymorphic genes in the human genome; for some of these genes over 600 allelic variants have been identified (Figure 4.24). This implies that there has been intense selective pressure on the MHC gene region and that genes within this region are mutating at rates much faster than at other gene loci.

As is amply illustrated in Figure 4.24, class I HLA-A, -B and -C molecules are highly polymorphic and so are the class II β chains (HLA-DRβ most, -DPβ next and -DQβ third) and, albeit to a lesser extent than the β chains, the α chains of -DP and -DQ. HLA-DRα and β_2-microglobulin are invariant in structure. The amino acid changes responsible for this polymorphism are restricted to the α_1 and α_2 domains of class I and to the α_1 and β_1 domains of class II. It is of enormous significance that they occur essentially in the β-sheet floor and on the inner surfaces of the α-helices that line the central cavity (Figure 4.17a) and also on the upper surfaces of the helices; these are the very surfaces that make contact with the peptides

that these MHC molecules offer up for inspection by TCRs (Figure 4.18). The nonrandom location at which MHC alleles diverge from one another is as a result of positive selection over the course of animal evolution due to host-pathogen interactions. As a consequence of the polymorphic nature of MHC molecules, the spectrum of peptides bound by these molecules is highly variable. In Chapter 5 we will explore in greater detail how peptide interacts with the β-pleated sheet floor of MHC molecules, as these interactions dramatically influence the type of peptides that can be presented by particular molecules. The ongoing drive towards creating new MHC molecules, with slightly altered peptide-binding grooves, is akin to a genetic arms race where the immune system is constantly trying to keep one step ahead of its foe. This genetic one-upmanship has been termed **pathogen-driven balancing selection** because heterozygotes typically have a selective advantage over homozygotes at a given locus.

The MHC region represents an outstanding hotspot with mutation rates two orders of magnitude higher than non-MHC loci. These multiple allelic forms can be generated by a variety of mechanisms: point mutations, recombination, homologous but unequal crossing over and **gene conversion**.

The degree of sequence homology and an increased occurrence of the dinucleotide motif 5′-cytosine–guanine-3′ (to produce what are referred to as CpG islands) seem to be important for gene conversion, and it has been suggested that this might involve a DNA-nicking activity that targets CpG-rich DNA sequences. MHC genes that lack these sequences, for example H-2Ea^d and HLA-DRA, do not appear to undergo gene conversion, whereas those that possess CpG islands act as either donors (e.g. H-2Eb^b, H-2Q2^k, H-2Q10^b), acceptors (e.g. H-2A^b) or both (e.g. H-2K^k, HLA-DQB1). The large number of pseudogenes within the MHC may represent a stockpile of genetic information for the generation of polymorphic diversity in the "working" class I and class II molecules.

Nomenclature

As much of the experimental work relating to the MHC is based on experiments in our little laboratory friend, the mouse, it may be helpful to explain the nomenclature used to describe the allelic genes and their products. If someone says to you in an obscure language "we are having free elections," you fail to understand, not because the idea is complicated but because you do not comprehend the language. It is much the same with the shorthand used to describe the H-2 system that looks unnecessarily frightening to the uninitiated. In order to identify and compare allelic genes within the H-2 complex in different strains, it is usual to start with certain pure homozygous inbred strains, obtained by successive brother–sister matings, to provide the prototypes. The collection of genes in the H-2 complex is called the **haplotype** and the haplotype of each prototypic inbred strain will be allotted a given superscript. For example, the DBA strain haplotype is designated *H-2^d* and the

Strain	Haplotype	MHC designation	I	II				III		I	
C57BL	**b**	*H-2*^{b}	K^b	Ab^b	Aa^b	Eb^b	Ea^b	$C4^b$	etc	D^b	etc.
CBA	**k**	*H-2*^{k}	K^k	Ab^k	Aa^k	Eb^k	Ea^k	$C4^k$	etc	D^k	etc.

Figure 4.25. How the definition of *H-2* haplotype works.

Pure strain mice homozygous for the whole *H-2* region through prolonged brother–sister mating for at least 20 generations are each arbitrarily assigned a **haplotype** designated by a superscript. Thus the particular set of alleles that happens to occur in the strain named C57BL is assigned the haplotype *H-2*^{b} and the particular nucleotide sequence of each allele in its MHC

is labeled as **gene**^{b}, e.g. ***H-2K***^{b}, etc. It is obviously more convenient to describe a given allele by the haplotype than to trot out its whole nucleotide sequence, and it is easier to follow the reactions of cells of known *H-2* make-up by using the haplotype terminology—see, for example, the interpretation of the experiment in Figure 4.26.

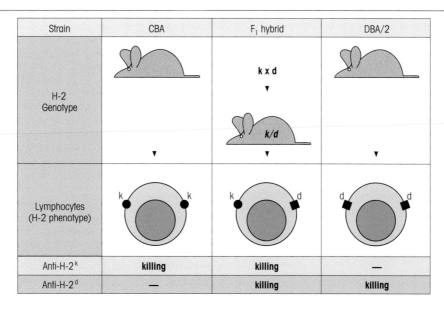

Figure 4.26. Inheritance and codominant expression of MHC genes.

Each homozygous (pure) parental strain animal has two identical chromosomes bearing the *H-2* haplotype, one paternal and the other maternal. Thus in the present example we designate a strain that is *H-2*^{k} as *k/k*. The first familial generation (F1) obtained by crossing the pure parental strains CBA (*H-2*^{k}) and DBA/2 (*H-2*^{d}) has the *H-2* genotype *k/d*. As 100% of F1

lymphocytes are killed in the presence of complement by antibodies to H-2^k or to H-2^d (raised by injecting H-2^k lymphocytes into an H-2^d animal and vice versa), the MHC molecules encoded by both parental genes must be expressed on every lymphocyte. The same holds true for other tissues in the body.

genes constituting the complex are therefore *H-2K*^{d}, *H-2Aa*^{d}, *H-2Ab*^{d}, *H-2D*^{d} and so on; their products will be H-2K^d, H-2A^d and H-2D^d and so forth (Figure 4.25). When new strains are derived from these by genetic recombination during breeding, they are assigned new haplotypes, but the individual genes are designated by the haplotype of the prototype strain from which they were derived. Thus the A/J strain produced by genetic cross-over during interbreeding between (*H-2*^{k} × *H-2*^{d}) F1 mice (Figure 4.26) is arbitrarily assigned the haplotype *H-2*^{a}, but Table 4.4 shows that individual genes in the complex are identified by the haplotype symbol of the original parents.

Inheritance of the MHC

Pure strain mice derived by prolonged brother–sister mating are homozygous for each pair of homologous chromosomes. Thus, in the present context, the haplotype of the MHC derived from the mother will be identical to that from the father; animals of the C57BL strain, for example, will each bear two chromosomes with the *H-2*^{b} haplotype (cf. Table 4.4).

Let us see how the MHC behaves when we cross two pure strains of haplotypes *H-2*^{k} and *H-2*^{d}, respectively. We find that the lymphocytes of the offspring (the F1 generation) all display *both* H-2^k and H-2^d molecules on their surface, i.e. there is

Table 4.4. The haplotypes of the *H-2* complex of some commonly used mouse strains and recombinants derived from them. A/J was derived by interbreeding (k × d) F1 mice, recombination occurring between E (class II) and S (class III) regions*.

		ORIGIN OF INDIVIDUAL REGIONS				
STRAIN	HAPLOTYPE	K	A	E	S	D
C57BL	b	b	b	b	b	b
CBA	k	k	k	k	k	k
DBA/2	d	d	d	d	d	d
A/J	a	k	k	k*	d	d
B.10A(4R)	h4	k	k	b	b	b

codominant expression (Figure 4.26). If we go further and breed F1s together, the progeny have the genotypes *k*, *k/d* and *d* in the proportions to be expected if the **haplotype segregates as a single mendelian trait**. This happens because the H-2 complex spans 0.5 centimorgans, equivalent to a recombination frequency between the *K* and *D* ends of 0.5%, and the haplotype tends to be inherited *en bloc*. Only the relatively infrequent recombinations caused by meiotic cross-over events, as described for the A/J strain above, reveal the complexity of the system.

The tissue distribution of MHC molecules

Essentially, all nucleated cells carry classical class I molecules. These are abundantly expressed on both lymphoid and myeloid cells, less so on liver, lung and kidney and only sparsely on brain and skeletal muscle. In the human, the surface of the placental extravillous cytotrophoblast lacks HLA-A and -B, although there is now some evidence that it may express HLA-C. What is well established is that the extravillous cytotrophoblast and other placental tissues bear HLA-G, a molecule that generally lacks allodeterminants and that does not appear on most other body cells, except for medullary and subcapsular epithelium in the thymus, and on blood monocytes following activation with γ-interferon. The role of HLA-G in the placenta is not fully resolved, but it appears to function as a replacement for classical class I molecules serving to inhibit immune responses against paternal MHC alleles carried by the foetus. Class II molecules, on the other hand, are highly restricted in their expression, being present only on B-cells, dendritic cells, macrophages and thymic epithelium. However, when activated by agents such as γ-interferon, capillary endothelia and many epithelial cells in tissues other than the thymus express surface class II and increased levels of class I.

The nonclassical MHC and class I chain-related molecules

These molecules include the **CD1** family that utilize β$_2$-microglobulin and have a similar overall structure to the classical class I molecules (Figure 4.27). They are, however, encoded by a set of genes on a different chromosome to the MHC, namely on chromosome 1 in humans and chromosome 3 in the mouse. Like its true MHC counterparts, CD1 is involved in the presentation of antigens to T-cells, but the antigen-binding groove is to some extent covered over, contains mainly hydrophobic amino acids, and is accessible only through a narrow entrance. Instead of binding peptide antigens, the CD1 molecules generally present lipids or glycolipids. At least four different CD1 molecules are found expressed on human cells; CD1a, b and c are present on cortical thymocytes, dendritic cells and a subset of B-cells, whilst CD1d is expressed on intestinal epithelium, hepatocytes and all lymphoid and myeloid cells. Mice appear to only express two different CD1 molecules that are both similar to the human CD1d in structure and tissue distribution and are referred to as CD1d1 and CD1d2 (or CD1.1 and CD1.2).

Genes in the MHC itself that encode nonclassical MHC molecules include the H-2T, -Q and -M loci in mice, each of which encodes a number of different molecules. The T22 and T10 molecules, for example, are induced by cellular activation and are recognized directly by γδ TCR without a requirement for antigen, possibly suggesting that they are involved in triggering immunoregulatory γδ T-cells. Other nonclassical class I molecules do bind peptides, such as H-2M3 that presents *N*-formylated peptides produced either in mitochondria or by bacteria.

In the human, **HLA-E** binds a nine-amino acid peptide derived from the signal sequence of HLA-A, -B, -C and -G molecules, and is recognized by the CD94/NKG2 receptors on NK cells and cytotoxic T-cells, as well as by the αβ TCR on some cytotoxic T-cells. HLA-E is upregulated when other HLA alleles provide the appropriate leader peptides, thereby allowing NK cells to monitor the expression of polymorphic class I molecules using a single receptor. The murine homolog, Qa-1, has a similar function.

The stress-inducible MICA and MICB (*M*HC class *I c*hain-related molecules) have the same domain structure as classical class I and display a relatively high level of polymorphism. They are present on epithelial cells, mainly in the gastrointestinal tract and in the thymic cortex, and are recognized by the NKG2D-activating molecule. One possible role for this interaction is in the promotion of NK- and T-cell antitumor responses.

The function of **HLA-F** is unclear, although its expression in placental trophoblasts has led some to suggest that it may play a role in protecting the developing foetus from attack by the maternal immune system. A more definitive role for **HLA-G** in this context has been found. This HLA molecule is also

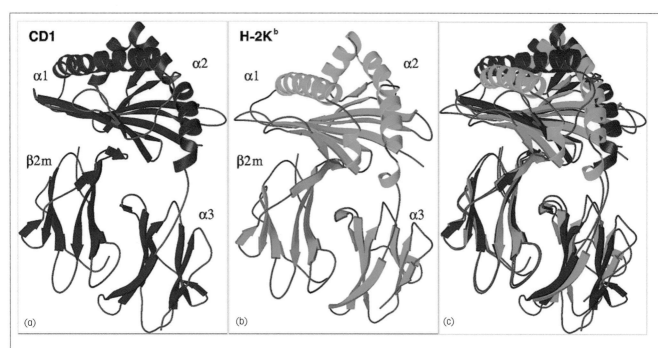

Figure 4.27. Comparison of the crystal structures of CD1 and MHC class I.

(a) Backbone ribbon diagram of mouse CD1d1 (red, α-helices; blue, β-strands). (b) Ribbon diagram of the mouse MHC class I molecule H-2K^b (cyan, α-helices; green, β-strands). (c) Superposition using alignment of β$_2$-microglobulin highlights some of the differences between CD1d1 and H-2K^b. Note in particular the shifting of the α-helices. This produces a deeper and more voluminous groove in CD1d1, which is narrower at its entrance compared with H-2K^b. (Reprinted with permission from Porcelli S.A. *et al.* (1998) *Immunology Today* **19**, 362.)

preferentially expressed on placental trophoblast cells where it plays a role in shielding the foetus from the unwanted attentions of the maternal NK cells and cytotoxic T-cells. It has long been a puzzle why mothers tolerate their genetically non-identical foetuses, as one would normally expect a strong immune response to foreign (i.e. paternal) HLA molecules. While this is partially solved through downregulation of the expression of MHC class I A, B and C molecules on placenta, this would normally attract the attentions of NK cells on the prowl for cells with such missing-self characteristics, as we discussed earlier when dealing with NK receptors. HLA-G expression on the placental-maternal trophoblast interface appears to be a solution to this. The interaction between the immunoglobulin-like transcript-2 (ILT2) molecule on NK cells, which is an inhibitory NK receptor, with HLA-G expressed on placental trophoblasts confers protection against NK-cell-mediated cytolysis.

HFE, previously referred to as HLA-H, possesses an extremely narrow groove that is unable to bind peptides, and it may serve no role in immune defense. However, it binds to the transferrin receptor and appears to be involved in iron uptake. A point mutation (C282Y) in HFE is found in 70–90% of patients with hereditary hemochromatosis.

Nonclassical MHC molecules may be the precursors to classical MHC molecules

Analysis of vertebrate genomes suggests that invariant nonclassical MHC molecules are probably the primordial forerunner to modern polymorphic MHC class I and class II molecules and rather than playing a role in antigen presentation, these molecules were most likely used as primitive "danger signals" that were involved in conveying stress signals to innate immune cells. Thus, expression of these molecules on the cell surface signified a stressed or potentially transformed cell that should be eliminated in the interests of overall organismal fitness. During the course of evolution, such molecules then most likely evolved the ability to bind self peptides, which were initially relatively invariant, followed by the ability to bind highly variable peptides as we now see with classical MHC class I and class II gene products. The appearance of polymorphic MHC molecules, as a consequence of gene duplication events followed by divergence, would have enabled much greater diversity in the range of peptides bound by these molecules. Thus, invariant MHC-like molecules (such as HLA-E, -F, -G and MICA, MICB) tend not to have antigen presenting functions, but perform homeostatic or regulatory roles, permitting cells of the innate immune system to monitor cell health in a relatively antigen nonspecific way.

A good example, that was discussed in the context of NK receptors but is worth going over again, is the HLA-E molecule that binds a nine-amino acid peptide derived from the signal sequence of HLA-A, -B, and -C molecules. Should HLA-E-peptide complexes be absent from cells, this suggests that an infectious agent may be present or that cells are stressed in some way. This results in activation of NK cells via the activating CD94/NKG2 receptors, with consequent NK-mediated killing of such cells. In the absence of class I leader peptides, HLA-E can be stabilized on the surface of stressed cells by heat shock treatment because the HSP-60 signal peptide can also bind in place of HLA class I peptides. However, such HLA-E/HSP-60 leader peptide complexes fail to be recognized by the CD94/NKG2 receptor, once again precipitating attack by the NK cell. Thus, cell stress can override the presentation of class I-derived peptides through competition for HSP-60-derived peptides that would not normally be present at levels high enough to compete effectively in unstressed cells. If this isn't a clever molecular security system, we don't know what is.

The B-cell surface receptor for antigen
- The B-cell inserts its Ig gene product containing a transmembrane segment into its surface where it acts as a specific receptor for antigen.
- Specific antigen induces the formation of B-cell receptor (BCR) microclusters made up of between 50–500 receptors that appear to represent the active form of the BCR.
- The surface Ig is complexed with the membrane proteins Ig-α and Ig-β that become phosphorylated on cell activation and transduce signals received through the Ig antigen receptor.
- The cytoplasmic tails of the Ig-α and Ig-β *immunoreceptor tyrosine-based activation motifs* (ITAMs) that, upon phosphorylation, can recruit phosphotyrosine-binding proteins that play important roles in signal transduction from the BCR.
- The B-cell co-receptor synergises with the BCR to productively activate B-cells.

The T-cell surface receptor for antigen
- The receptor for antigen is a transmembrane dimer, each chain consisting of two Ig-like domains.
- The outer domains are variable in structure, the inner ones constant, rather like a membrane-bound Fab.
- Both chains are required for antigen recognition.
- Most TCRs can only recognize antigen when presented within the context of MHC molecules.
- CD4 and CD8 act as co-receptors, along with the TCR, for MHC molecules. CD4 acts as a co-receptor for MHC class II molecules and CD8 recognizes MHC class I molecules.
- Most T-cells express a receptor (TCR) with α and β chains (TCR2). A separate lineage (TCR1) bearing γδ receptors is transcribed strongly in early thymic ontogeny but is associated mainly with epithelial tissues in the adult.

- The encoding of the TCR is similar to that of immunoglobulins. The variable region coding sequence in the differentiating T-cell is formed by random translocation from clusters of *V*, *D* (for β and δ chains) and *J* segments to give a single recombinant *V(D)J* sequence for each chain.
- Like the Ig chains, each variable region has three hypervariable sequences that function in antigen recognition.
- The CD3 complex, composed of γ, δ, ε and either ζ, ζη or η, covalently linked dimers, forms an intimate part of the receptor and has a signal transducing role following ligand binding by the TCR.

The generation of antibody diversity for antigen recognition
- Ig heavy and light chains and TCR α and β chains generally are represented in the germline by between 33 and 75 variable region genes, between 2 and 27 *D* segment minigenes (Ig heavy and TCR β and δ only) and 3–60 short *J* segments.
- TCR γ and δ chains are encoded by far fewer genes.
- Random recombination of any single *V*, *D* and *J* from each gene cluster generates approximately 6.5×10^3 Ig heavy chain *VDJ* sequences, 350 light chains, 4.5×10^3 TCR α, 1×10^3 TCR β, but only 60 TCR γ and 72 TCR δ.
- Random interchain combination produces roughly 2.4×10^6 Ig, 4.5×10^6 TCR αβ and 4.3×10^3 TCR γδ receptors.
- Further diversity is introduced at the junctions between *V*, *D* and *J* segments by variable combination as they are spliced together by recombinase enzymes and by the N-region insertion of random nontemplated nucleotide sequences. These mechanisms may be particularly important in augmenting the number of specificities that can be squeezed out of the relatively small γδ pool.
- Useless or self-reactive receptors can be replaced by receptor editing.

■ In addition, after a primary response, B-cells but not T-cells undergo high rate somatic mutation affecting the *V* regions.

NK receptors

■ NK cells bear a number of receptors with Ig-type domains and other receptors with C-type lectin domains. Members of both types of receptor family can function as inhibitory or activating receptors to determine whether the target cell should be killed.

■ NK receptors are "hard-wired" (i.e. germline encoded) and achieve diversity through their sheer number rather than through somatic recombination.

■ Loss of MHC class I molecules can provoke attack by NK cells.

■ NK cells can also recognize ligands, typically nonclassical MHC-like molecules, which are upregulated by cells that suffer stress or DNA damage.

MHC

■ MHC molecules act as receptors for antigen and present antigen-derived peptides to T-cells.

■ Each vertebrate species has an MHC identified originally through its ability to evoke very powerful transplantation rejection.

■ Each contains three classes of genes. Class I encodes 44 kDa transmembrane polypeptides associated at the cell surface with β_2-microglobulin. Class II molecules are transmembrane heterodimers. Class III products are heterogeneous but include complement components linked to the formation of C3 convertases, heat-shock proteins and tumor necrosis factors.

■ MHC class I molecules present endogenous peptides synthesized by the cell, while MHC class II molecules present exogenous peptides that have been internalized by the cell.

■ Several different types of MHC class I and class II molecules are expressed by all cells. MHC genes also display remarkable polymorphism. A given MHC gene cluster is referred to as a "haplotype" and is usually inherited *en bloc* as a single mendelian trait, although its constituent genes have been revealed by cross-over recombination events.

■ The highly polymorphic state of MHC class I and class II molecules has most likely arisen as a consequence of pathogen-driven selection and maximizes the number of pathogen-derived peptides that can be presented to the immune system.

■ Classical class I molecules are present on virtually all cells in the body and present peptides to CD8$^+$ cytotoxic T-cells.

■ Class II molecules are particularly associated with B-cells, dendritic cells and macrophages but can be induced on capillary endothelial cells and epithelial cells by γ-interferon. Class II molecules present peptides to CD4$^+$ T-helpers for B-cells and macrophages.

■ The two domains distal to the cell membrane form a peptide binding cavity bounded by two parallel α-helices sitting on a floor of β-sheet strands; the walls and floor of the cavity and the upper surface of the helices are the sites of maximum polymorphic amino acid substitutions.

■ Silent class I genes may increase polymorphism by gene conversion mechanisms.

■ Nonclassical MHC molecules and MHC-like molecules have a number of functions, and include CD1 that presents lipid and glycolipid antigens to T-cells, and HLA-E that presents signal sequence peptides from classical class I molecules to the CD94/NKG2 receptor of NK cells.

■ Nonclassical invariant MHC-like molecules probably represent the primordial forerunners to modern highly polymorphic MHC class I and II molecules.

FURTHER READING

Biassoni R. (2009) Human natural killer receptors, co-receptors, and their ligands. Current Protocols in Immunology. Chapter 14 Unit 14.10. John Wiley & Sons.

Braud V.M., Allan D.S.J. & McMichael A.J. (1999) Functions of nonclassical MHC and non-MHC-encoded class I molecules. *Current Opinion in Immunology* **11**, 100–108.

Call M.E. & Wucherpfennig K.W. (2005) The T cell receptor: critical role of the membrane environment in receptor assembly and function. *Annual Review of Immunology* **23**, 101–125.

Carding S.R. & Egan P.J. (2002) γδ T cells: functional plasticity and heterogeneity. *Nature Reviews Immunology* **2**, 336–345.

Clark D.A. (1999) Human leukocyte antigen-G: new roles for old? *American Journal of Reproductive Immunology* **41**, 117–120.

Flajnik M.F. & Kasahara M. (2010) Origin and evolution of the adaptive immune system: genetic events and selective pressures. *Nature Reviews Genetics* **11**, 47–59.

Garcia K.C. & Adams E.J. (2005) How the T cell receptor sees antigen—a structural view. *Cell* **122**, 333–336.

Gleimer M. & Parham P. (2003) Stress management: MHC class I and class II molecules as receptors of cellular stress. *Immunity* **19**, 469–477.

Godfrey D.I., Rossjohn J. & McCluskey J. (2008) The fidelity, occasional promiscuity, and versatility of T cell receptor recognition. *Immunity* **28**, 304–314.

Grawunder U. & Harfst E. (2001) How to make ends meet in V(D)J recombination. *Current Opinion in Immunology* **13**, 186–194.

Horton R. *et al.* (2004) Gene map of the extended human MHC. *Nature Reviews Genetics* **5**, 889–899.

Hunt JS. (2006) Stranger in a strange land. (Review on HLA-G and pregnancy) *Immunological Reviews* **213**, 36–47.

Kelsoe G. (1999) V(D)J hypermutation and receptor revision: coloring outside the lines. *Current Opinion in Immunology* **11**, 70–75.

Krangel M.S. (2009) Mechanics of T cell receptor gene rearrangement. *Current Opinion in Immunology* **21**, 133–139.

Kumanovics A. *et al.* (2003) Genomic organization of the mammalian MHC. *Annual Review of Immunology* **21**, 629–657.

Kumar V. & McNerney M.E. (2005) A new self: MHC class I-independent natural-killer cell self-tolerance. *Nature Reviews Immunology* **5**, 363–374.

Longerich S., Basu U., Alt F. & Storb U. (2006) AID in somatic hypermutation and class switch recombination. *Current Opinion in Immunology* **18**, 164–174

Mak T.W. (1998) T-cell receptor, αβ. In: Delves P.J. & Roitt I.M. (eds.) Encyclopedia of Immunology, 2nd edn, pp. 2264–2268. Academic Press, London. (See also article by Hayday A. & Pao W. on the γδ TCR; *ibid.*, pp. 2268–2278.)

Matsuda F. *et al.* (1998) The complete nucleotide sequence of the human immunoglobulin heavy chain variable region locus. *Journal of Experimental Medicine* **188**, 2151–2162.

Matthews A.G. & Oettinger M.A. (2009) RAG: a recombinase diversified. *Nature Immunology* **10**, 817–821.

MHC Sequencing Consortium (1999) Complete sequence and gene map of a human major histocompatibility complex. *Nature* **401**, 921–923.

Moody D.B., Zajonc D.M. & Wilson I.A. (2005) Anatomy of CD1–lipid antigen complexes. *Nature Reviews Immunology* **5**, 387–399.

Nemazee D. (2000) Receptor editing in B cells. *Advances in Immunology* **74**, 89–126.

Parham P. (2008) The genetic and evolutionary balances in human NK cell receptor diversity. *Seminars in Immunology* **20**, 311–316.

Prugnolle F. *et al.* (2005) Pathogen-driven selection and worldwide HLA class I diversity. *Current Biology* **15**, 1022–1027.

Raulet D.H. (2004) Interplay of natural killer cells and their receptors with the adaptive immune response. *Nature Immunology* **5**, 996–1002.

Salio M., Silk J.D. & Cerundolo V. (2010) Recent advances in processing and presentation of CD1 bound lipid antigens. *Current Opinion in Immunology* **22**, 81–88.

Sasaki Y. & Kurosaki T. (2010) Immobile BCRs: the safety on the signal trigger. *Immunity* **32**, 143–144.

de Wildt R.M.T. *et al.* (1999) Somatic insertions and deletions shape the human antibody repertoire. *Journal of Molecular Biology* **294**, 701–710.

Now visit **www.roitt.com** to test yourself on this chapter.

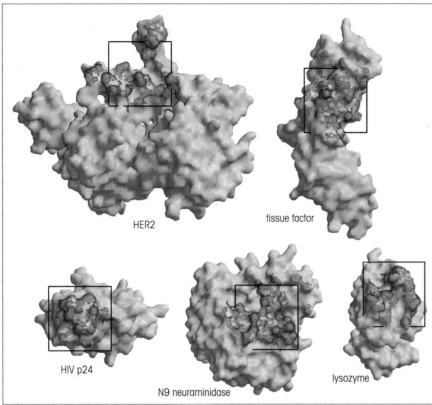

Figure 5.2. Antibody footprints (red) on a range of antigens.

These footprints are determined from crystal structures of the antigens with antibody bound. The footprints are irregular but can be very roughly represented as a square of dimensions 2.5 × 2.5 nm as shown. (Courtesy of Robyn Stanfield.)

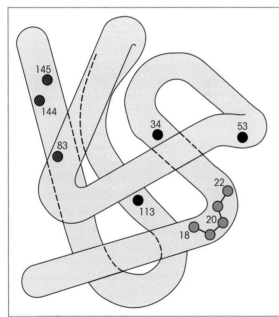

Figure 5.3. Residues contributing to epitopes on the folded peptide chain of myoglobin.

Amino acid residues 34, 53 and 113 (black) contribute to the binding of a monoclonal antibody (mAb) and residues 83, 144 and 145 to the binding of another mAb (red). Both epitopes are clearly discontinuous. By contrast, a third mAb binds to residues 18–22 (green). The mAb binds to isolated peptides containing the sequence corresponding to residues 18–22. The epitope is described as continuous. Much of the myoglobin structure is in a-helical conformation. (Based on Benjamin D.C. *et al.* (1986) *Annual Review of Immunology* **2**, 67.)

however, that an antibody that recognizes a continuous epitope does not bind a random or disordered structure. Rather it recognizes a defined structure that is found in the complete protein but can readily be adopted by the shorter peptide. The structure of an antibody that recognizes a linear epitope in complex with a peptide that contains the epitope is shown in Figure 5.4; note that the structure of the peptide is largely helical in this example.

The antibody complementarity determining regions (CDRs) contact the epitope

The antibody combining site can vary greatly in shape and character depending upon the length and characteristics of the CDRs. Generally most or all of the CDRs contribute to antigen binding but their relative contributions vary. The heavy

Figure 5.4. The structure of an antibody bound to a peptide corresponding to a linear epitope.

The antibody 4E10 neutralizes HIV by binding to a linear epitope on the glycoprotein gp41 on the surface of the virus. The antibody binds to peptides containing the amino acid sequence NWFDIT and peptides containing this sequence can inhibit the binding of 4E10 to gp41. The structure of the Fab fragment of 4E10 bound to a peptide (gold) containing the NWFDIT sequence shows the peptide adopts a helical conformation. It is likely that the antibody recognizes its epitope in a helical conformation on the virus. (Courtesy of Rosa Cardoso.)

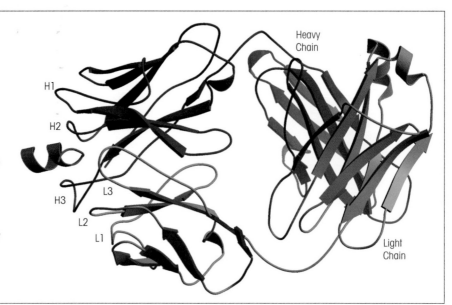

Figure 5.5. Conformational change in an antibody combining site.

(a) An anti-progesterone antibody has a very hydrophobic pocket that is filled by a tryptophan residue (colored red) in the free antibody. (b) To bind progesterone (dark blue), the tryptophan residue swings out of the pocket and the antigen gains access. (Courtesy of Robyn Stanfield.)

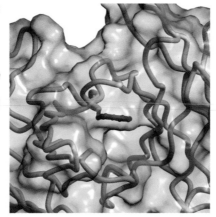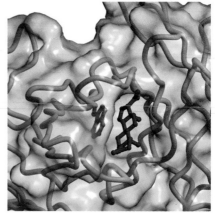

chain CDRs, and particularly CDR H3, tend to contribute disproportionately more to antigen binding. The CDR H3 in human antibodies can be quite long and has a finger-like appearance that could be used to bind into cavities on the antigen. The combining site of antibodies against smaller molecules such as carbohydrates and organic groups (haptens) are often more obviously grooves or pockets rather than the extended surfaces typically found in anti-protein antibodies.

Structural changes and conformational rearrangements can occur in antibodies or antigens on interaction. In other words, on some occasions, the relationship between antibody and antigen will be like a "lock and key" but on other occasions the lock or key or both can be deformed to make a good fit. For the antibody, possible conformational changes include side chain rearrangements, segmental movements of CDRs or of the main-chain backbone, and rotation of the V_L–V_H domain upon antigen binding. Large changes in the conformation of the CDR H3 have been documented in crystal structures of Fab complexes. As shown in Figure 5.5, an antibody to progesterone has

a very hydrophobic combining pocket, which is normally filled with a tryptophan from the CDR H3. Antigen binding involves this residue moving out of the pocket, the antigen molecule moving in and the trytophan stabilizing the antigen binding.

As more and more structures have been solved it has become clear that antibody–antigen interactions come in all shapes and sizes with few general rules. It is important to bear in mind that high-affinity antibodies evolve in each individual following rounds of mutation and selection. There are multiple ways in which high-affinity recognition of an antigen can be achieved, and indeed no two antibody–antigen interactions are exactly the same.

Antigens vs immunogens

An epitope on an antigen may bind very tightly to a given antibody but it may elicit such antibodies infrequently when the antigen is used to immunize an animal. In other words, there may be a perfectly good site on a pathogen for antibody binding but the antibody response to that site is so poor it cannot contribute to antibody protection against the pathogen. We say that the site has low immunogenicity and the consequences can clearly be great.

An extreme example of the distinction between the ability to be recognized by an antibody (which we will term antigenicity) and the ability to elicit antibodies when used to immunize an animal (which we will term immunogenicity) is provided by experiments using small molecules known as haptens such as *m*-aminobenzene sulfonate. Immunization with free hapten produces no antibodies to the hapten (Figure 5.6). However immunization with hapten groups linked to a protein carrier generates antibodies that react with high affinity to hapten alone or linked to a molecule other than the carrier. It is logical to refer to the hapten as the antigen and the hapten–protein complex as the immunogen, although strictly the word "antigen" is derived from "*anti*body *gen*erating" substance.

Identifying B-cell epitopes on a protein

How many epitopes are there on a single protein? This depends upon how one defines an epitope. For the small protein lysozyme (molecular weight ~14 300 daltons), the structures of three noncompeting monoclonal antibodies in complex with the protein antigen have been determined. They have minimally overlapping footprints that cover just under half of the surface of the protein (Figure 5.7). One could extrapolate that a small protein such as this could have of the order of between three and six nonoverlapping epitopes recognized by noncompeting antibodies. The specificity of a given antibody could then be defined by its ability to compete with the three to six "prototype" antibodies. In practice, this is often done; an antibody is said to be directed against a given epitope if it competes with a prototype antibody of known specificity. This is, of course, a rather simplistic view as many antibodies will compete with more than one prototype antibody allowing a more sophisticated B-cell epitope map to be constructed. An even more sophisticated map can be constructed by scanning mutagenesis of the antigen. In the latter case, single positions in the antigen can be substituted by differing amino acids (usually alanine—hence the term "alanine scanning mutagenesis") and the effects on antibody binding measured (see Figure 5.10). At this greater level of precision, it is likely that no two antibodies

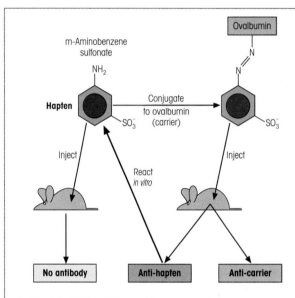

Figure 5.6. Antigenicity and immunogenicity.

A free small molecule hapten will not induce antibodies if injected in to an animal. However, high affinity antibodies specific for the free hapten can be obtained by injecting the hapten conjugated to a protein carrier molecule such as ovalbumin.

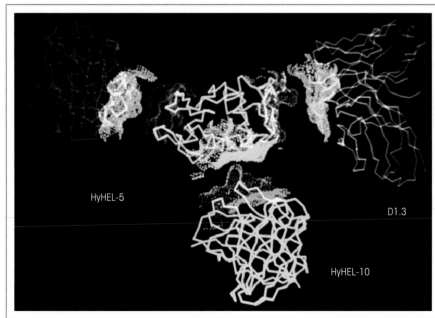

Figure 5.7. Three epitopes on the small protein lysozyme.

The crystal structures of lysozyme bound to three antibodies (HyHEL-5, HyHEL-10 and D1.3) have been determined. In the figure, the Fv fragment of each antibody is shown separated from lysozyme to reveal the footprint of interaction in each case. The three epitopes are nearly nonoverlapping with only a small overlap between HyHEL-10 and D1.3. (After Davies D.R. *et al.* (1990) *Annual Review of Biochemistry* **59**, 439.)

will give exactly the same footprint, and therefore no two antibodies recognize exactly the same epitope.

What determines the strength of the antibody response to a given epitope on a protein? There appear to be a number of factors involved. Perhaps the most important is the accessibility of the epitope on the protein surface. Loops that protrude from the surface of the folded protein tend to elicit particularly good antibody responses. The sites on the hemagglutinin (HA) protein from the surface of influenza virus that elicit important antibody responses are indicated in Figure 5.8. Antibodies to these regions, perhaps elicited by vaccination, neutralize the virus and protect against infection. Mutations in these regions allow the virus to "escape" from neutralizing antibodies and infect human hosts who were protected against the original form of the virus. Influenza epidemics thus directly reflect antibody targeting to certain preferred epitopes. Note that the epitopes are all located towards the part of HA that is distant from the membrane of the influenza virus and more accessible to antibody. Note also that three of the epitopes involve prominent loops on the HA structure. The combination of the ability of loops to accommodate changes in amino acid sequence more readily than more compact structural features and their favored status in eliciting antibody responses is responsible for the frequent association of loops with neutralization escape.

HIV is another virus that exploits the tendency of the antibody system to respond to highly exposed variable loops on the viral surface protein to evade immune control. Following primary infection, it takes some time (weeks) for neutralizing antibodies to reach a level where they begin to inhibit virus replication. These antibodies are typically elicited to exposed loops on the virus. While these antibodies are being elicited, the virus has diversified, i.e. it has become a swarm of related viruses through the errors associated with RNA to DNA transcription of this retrovirus. Among this swarm is a virus that has sequence changes in the epitopes targeted by the neutralizing antibody response that allow it to escape from the response. This new virus becomes predominant. Eventually a response is mounted to this virus and a second new virus emerges and so on. The antibody response chases the virus over many years but never gains control.

One point worthy of note is that accessible loops on protein structures tend to be flexible. Therefore epitope dominance has also been associated with flexible regions of a protein antigen.

Thermodynamics of antibody–antigen interactions

The interaction of antibody and antigen is reversible and can be described by the laws of thermodynamics. In particular, the reaction

$$Ab + Ag \rightleftharpoons Ab\text{–}Ag \text{ complex}$$

can be studied and the position of the equilibrium established under varying conditions. In other words, the amount

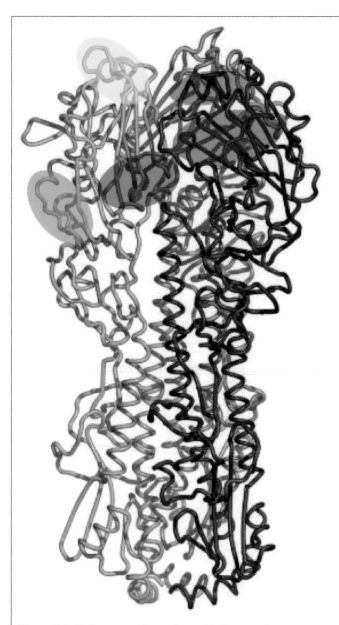

Figure 5.8. Epitopes on the surface of influenza virus hemagglutinin (HA).

The structure of HA from the 1918 flu virus responsible for a pandemic that killed up to 50 million people is shown. The molecule is a homotrimer with monomers shown in cyan, gray and brown. The homotrimers form "spikes" on the surface of the virus. The spikes are anchored to the virus membrane (bottom of the figure). Sialic acid residues on the target cells bind to sites at the top of the spikes resulting in attachment of virus to target cell in the first step of infection. Five principal epitopes on HA are represented as colored ovals located towards the tip of the molecule. Three of the epitopes (yellow, green and purple) involve prominent loop structures. (Courtesy of James Stevens.)

of antibody bound to antigen under different conditions can be estimated. This is crucial information. If antibody coats a virus then it is likely that the virus will be prevented from entering target cells and infection will be avoided. If antibody can become attached to a bacterial cell in a high enough density then complement may be triggered and the cell killed.

The position of equilibrium is described by the association or binding constant, K_a:

$$K_a = [\text{Ab–Ag complex}]/([\text{Ab}] \times [\text{Ag}])$$

where square brackets indicate molar concentrations. The units of K_a are thus mols per liter, (M) or 1/M. If K_a is a large number then the equilibrium is far to the right and Ab–Ag complex formation is favored. Typically high-affinity antibodies have K_a values of the order of 10^8–10^{10} M. Some researchers prefer to think of binding in terms of a dissociation constant, K_d, simply defined as $1/K_a$ and having the units of M. High-affinity antibodies then have K_d values of the order of 10^{-8}–10^{-10} M. As a $K_d = 10^{-9}$ M corresponds to 1 nM, high-affinity antibodies are sometimes referred to as "nM binders." Moderate affinity antibodies such as IgMs are often referred to as μM binders ($K_d = 1$ μM).

Another way to look at the binding equation is that if half the available antigen sites are occupied by antibody then [Ag] = [Ab–Ag complex] and $K_a = 1/[\text{Ab}]$ or $K_d = [\text{Ab}]$. In other words, K_d is equal to the antibody concentration at which half of the antibody is bound. Thus for example a nM binding antibody will begin to complex antigen when its concentration is in the nanomolar range. The antibody will bind very little if it is only in the picomolar (10^{-12}) range of concentrations but will bind very effectively in the μM range. Similarly a μM antibody will be effective in the μM range of concentration but not the nM. For IgG, nM is roughly 0.15 μg/ml and mM is 150 μg/ml. The average concentration of IgG in serum is about 12 mg/ml. Clearly then, if we require that antibodies be present in serum at concentrations where they are going to be effective in binding antigen, many many more specificities can be covered by a set of nM binding (high affinity) antibodies than a set of μM binding antibodies. Indeed, this seems to be largely how Nature operates outside of extreme immunization protocols in animal models. Thus we are mostly protected, at least against re-infection following a primary infection or vaccination, by high affinity antibodies at relatively moderate concentrations.

In the above discussion, we implicitly assume that antibody–antigen interactions are monovalent, involving just one Fab arm of the antibody molecule. In fact they may well be multivalent, which complicates the issues somewhat, but the major points remain intact. We return to multivalency below.

Binding constants for antibody–antigen interactions are often estimated from ELISA measurements but now can be determined with some precision by techniques such as surface plasmon resonance and isothermal calorimetry. For binding of antibodies to antigens on the cell surface, flow cytometry can give a good estimate of binding affinities.

The binding constant for a reaction is directly related to the energy accompanying the reaction by the equation:

$$\Delta G = -RT \ln K_a$$

where ΔG is called the free energy of the reaction, R is the gas constant and T is the temperature in K. ln is natural log = 2.303 × $\log_{10}$. ΔG is then another way of describing how far a reaction will be driven to the left or right at equilibrium under certain conditions. If $K_a = 10^9$ M^{-1}, ΔG approx. −12 kcal/mol; if $K_a = 10^6$ M^{-1}, ΔG approx. −8 kcal/mol. The advantage of considering the ΔG is that it can help in beginning to understand the molecular forces that lead to antibody–antigen interaction. Thus the free energy of a reaction (ΔG) is the net effect of contributions from enthalpy (ΔH) and entropy (ΔS):

$$\Delta G = \Delta H - T \Delta S$$

The enthalpy is the heat of the reaction; the more heat is given out by the reaction (negative ΔH) the more it will be favored (negative ΔG). If heat has to be supplied to the reaction it is disfavored. The more entropy (or disorder) results from the reaction (positive ΔS), the more it is favored. For example, an antibody–antigen interaction would be favored by the formation of a H bond between the two molecules to the tune of approximately 1–3 kcal/mol. A salt bridge would provide a similar or slightly greater amount of energy. The reaction would also be favored by hydrophobic surfaces on the antibody and the antigen coming together because then water that was ordered around the hydrophobic faces would be released to increase entropy. It is estimated that burying 1 nm^2 of hydrophobic surface generates about 2.5 kcal/mol of binding energy. Some of the forces driving protein–protein interactions are summarized in Figure 5.9.

An epitope is often thought of in terms of the region of the antigen contacted by antibody, a picture provided from crystal structure studies of antibody–antigen complexes. However, it should be borne in mind that looking at contacts between antibody and antigen in a crystal structure does not tell us the contributions of individual interactions to the overall binding energy. This can be done by measuring the effects of scanning mutagenesis (see above) on antibody binding measured. The available data then suggest that only a few productive interactions ("hot spots") dominate the energetics of binding; many interactions are neutral or detrimental to binding even in a high affinity antibody–antigen pairing. In the interaction of an antibody with lysozyme, only about a third of the antibody contact residues actually contribute significantly to net binding (Figure 5.10).

A substitution in only one residue of antigen or antibody can be decisive in net binding of antibody to antigen. This can be readily appreciated intuitively. If a bulky residue replaces a small one in the epitope recognized, then the whole antibody–antigen interface may be disrupted. Pathogens typically evade antibodies by mutations in a small number of critical residues.

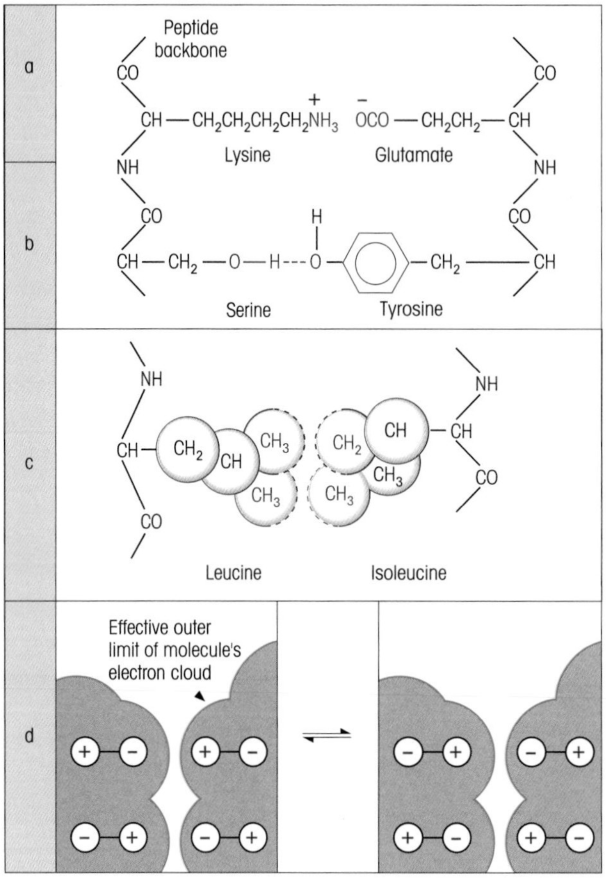

Figure 5.9. Protein–protein interactions.

(a) Coulombic attraction between oppositely charged ionic groups on the two protein side-chains as illustrated by an ionized amino group (NH_3^+) on a lysine of one protein and an ionized carboxyl group ($-COO^-$) of glutamate on the other. The force of attraction is inversely proportional to the square of the distance between the charges. Thus, as the charges come closer together, the attractive force increases considerably: if we halve the distance apart, we quadruple the attraction. Furthermore, as the dielectric constant of water is extremely high, the exclusion of water molecules through the proximity of the interacting residues would greatly increase the force of attraction. Dipoles on antigen and antibody can also attract each other. In addition, electrostatic forces may be generated by charge transfer reactions between antibody and antigen; for example, an electron-donating protein residue such as tryptophan could part with an electron to a group such as dinitrophenyl (DNP) that is electron accepting, thereby creating an effective +1 charge on the antibody and −1 on the antigen. (b) Hydrogen bonding between two proteins involving the formation of reversible hydrogen bridges between hydrophilic groups, such as OH, NH_2 and COOH, depends very much upon the close approach of the two molecules carrying these groups. Although H bonds are relatively weak, because they are essentially electrostatic in nature, exclusion of water between the reacting side-chains would greatly enhance the binding energy through the gross reduction in dielectric constant. (c) Nonpolar, hydrophobic groups such as the side-chains of valine, leucine and isoleucine tend to associate in an aqueous environment. The driving force for this hydrophobic interaction derives from the fact that water in contact with hydrophobic molecules with which it cannot H bond will associate with other water molecules, but the number of configurations that allow H bonds to form will not be as great as that occurring when they are surrounded completely by other water molecules, i.e. the entropy is lower. The greater the area of contact between water and hydrophobic surfaces, the lower the entropy and the higher the energy state. Thus, if hydrophobic groups on two proteins come together so as to exclude water molecules, between them the net surface in contact with water is reduced and the proteins take up a lower energy state than when they are separated (in other words, there is a force of attraction between them). (d) van der Waals force: the interaction between the electrons in the external orbitals of two different macromolecules may be envisaged (for simplicity!) as the attraction between induced oscillating dipoles in the two electron clouds. The nature of this interaction is difficult to describe in nonmathematical terms, but it has been likened to a temporary perturbation of electrons in one molecule effectively forming a dipole, which induces a dipolar perturbation in the other molecule, the two dipoles then having a force of attraction between them; as the displaced electrons swing back through the equilibrium position and beyond, the dipoles oscillate. The force of attraction is inversely proportional to the seventh power of the distance and, as a result, this rises very rapidly as the interacting molecules come closer together.

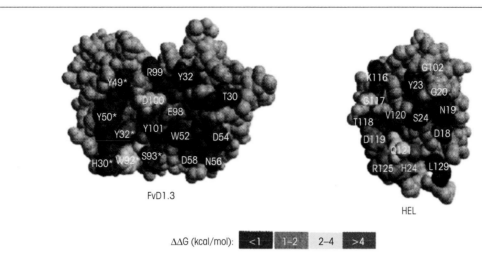

FvD1.3

HEL

ΔΔG (kcal/mol): <1   1–2   2–4   >4

Figure 5.10. Energetic map of an antibody–antigen interface.

The antibody D1.3 (single chain Fv (sFv) shown here) binds with high affinity to hen egg-white lysozyme (HEL) and the crystal structure of the complex has been solved (see Figure 5.7). The energetic contribution of contact residues for both antibody and antigen can be estimated by substituting the residue with the relatively "neutral" residue alanine. The effect can be expressed in terms of the loss of free energy of binding for the interaction on alanine substitution (ΔΔG). A large positive value for ΔΔG shows that the alanine substitution has had a strong detrimental effect on binding and implies that the residue substituted forms a crucial contact in the interface between antibody and antigen. Clearly, most contact residues, particularly on the antibody, contribute little to the overall binding energy. There are clear "hot spots" on both antibody and antigen and the hot spot residues on the antibody side of the interaction correspond to those on the antigen side. (After Sundberg E.J. & Mariuzza R.A. (2002) *Advances in Protein Chemistry* **61**, 119.)

Multivalency in antibody–antigen interactions

The binding of a monovalent Fab fragment to a monovalent antigen can be analyzed in a straightforward way as described above. This should also be true for the corresponding divalent IgG molecule interacting with the monovalent antigen. However, once we consider a divalent IgG (or multivalent antibody of any class) interacting with a multivalent antigen, the analysis of binding becomes more complex.

Consider IgG binding to an antigen that is expressed as multiple copies on a cell surface. If the antigen molecules are appropriately spaced and in an appropriate orientation, IgG may be able to bind divalently (Figure 5.11). This will lead to a higher affinity (often referred to as the avidity or functional affinity) of the IgG for the cell surface than the corresponding Fab. The "bonus effect" of divalent binding can be understood intuitively in terms of the tendency of the divalent IgG to stick better to the cell surface than the corresponding Fab. For the Fab to "fall off" the cell, a series of interactions between a single antibody combining site and the antigen must be broken. For the IgG to fall off, the interactions in two antibody combining sites must be broken simultaneously; a lower probability event. The bonus effect can be thought of in terms of ΔG. Divalent binding will produce a more favorable ΔH because of the use of two antibody combining sites. However, an entropy price will be paid in constraining the Fab arms of the IgG molecule. The net effect in ΔG usually corresponds to an enhanced affinity of the order of 1–100-fold as the bonus effect. It should also be borne in mind that IgG may bind monovalently even

to a multivalent antigen if the antigen molecules are inappropriately spaced or oriented. IgM is decavalent for antigen, which in theory could produce a huge bonus effect in functional affinity. In practice IgMs tend to be rather moderate affinity binders, suggesting limited use of multivalency and/or a high entropy price paid for multivalent binding.

One of the most dramatic effects of multivalent antibody interaction can be seen in the neutralization of toxins. Botulinum neurotoxins cause the paralytic human disease botulism and are considered a major potential bioterrorist threat. Monoclonal antibodies have been generated from phage libraries against the toxin. No single mAb protected mice against lethal challenge with toxin. However, a combination of three mAbs protected mice against a huge challenge with toxin. The difference could be attributed in part to a multivalency bonus effect (cooperative binding of the antibodies with more than one molecule of the toxin) that increased the functional affinities of the antibodies in to the pM range from the nM range in the individual mAbs. The origins of this effect are illustrated for a two-mAb combination in Figure 5.12.

Specificity and cross-reactivity of antibodies

Specificity is a commonly discussed concept in the context of antibodies. It can have different meanings. Sometimes, it is used simply to indicate that the antibody has high affinity for antigen. Generally this means that the antibody has a combining site

(a)

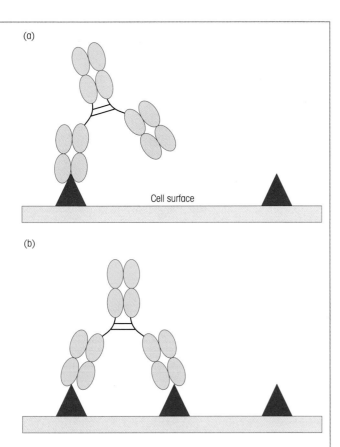

Cell surface

(b)

Figure 5.11. Divalent antibody binding to a cell surface.

The affinity of an antibody that can bind divalently to a multivalent antigen (b), such as may be found on a cell surface, is enhanced relative to an antibody that can only bind monovalently (a).

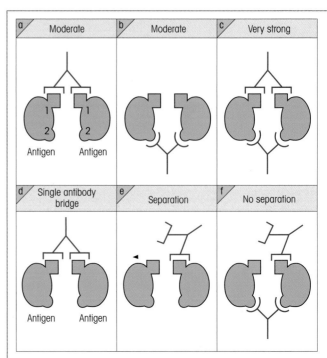

Figure 5.12. The bonus effect of multivalent binding in antibody neutralization of a soluble molecule such as a toxin.

(a–c) It is found that two antibodies binding to nonoverlapping epitopes on a soluble antigen may show considerably enhanced affinity as compared to the antibodies used separately (cooperative binding). (d,e) If only one antibody is present, dissociation of the complex requires only that the interaction between one antibody combining site and its epitope be disrupted. (f) If two antibodies are bound to antigen and one antibody-combining site–epitope interaction is lost as shown, the complex stays together and the released Fab arm is in a position to re-complex. In effect, the k_{off} values for the two antibodies are decreased in the complex and, if an Fab arm is dislodged, the k_{on} value is increased relative to a single bound antibody situation.

that fits very well to an epitope on the antigen and is much less likely to fit other shapes very well. Therefore it is specific for the antigen. However, there may be other shapes that can be accommodated, especially if they are related to the antigenic epitope in composition or character. Most likely is that other molecules will be recognized with lower affinity. It is important to remember from the discussion above that antibodies will be functional at concentrations around their K_d values. So if an antibody has a nM affinity for a given antigen and is present at nM concentrations *in vivo*, cross-reactivities with other antigens in the sub-μM range are unlikely to be functionally significant unless those antigens are at high concentrations.

A second meaning that is attached to "specificity" is the ability to discriminate between molecules. This clearly overlaps with the discussion above but could also be applied to lower affinity antibodies. Thus in genomic studies there has been a demand for antibodies that can distinguish target proteins from many other proteins and identify the target proteins in a variety of assays. This has not necessarily required high affinity but has required good discrimination. Moderate affinity antibodies selected from phage libraries have been used successfully in this arena.

What the T-cell sees

We have on several occasions alluded to the fact that the αβ T-cell receptor sees peptide antigen on the surface of cells associated with an MHC class I or II molecule. Now is the time for us to go into the nuts and bolts of this relationship.

Haplotype restriction reveals the need for MHC participation

It has been established in "tablets of stone" that T-cells bearing αβ receptors, with some exceptions (cf. p. 133), only respond when the antigen-presenting cells express the same MHC haplotype as the host from which the T-cells were derived (Milestone 5.1). This **haplotype restriction** on T-cell recognition tells us unequivocally that MHC molecules are intimately and necessarily involved in the interaction of the

⦿ Milestone 5.1—MHC Restriction of T-cell Reactivity

The realization that the MHC, which had figured for so long as a dominant controlling element in tissue graft rejection, should come to occupy the center stage in T-cell reactions has been a source of fascination and great pleasure to immunologists—almost as though a great universal plan had been slowly unfolding.

One of the seminal observations that helped to elevate the MHC to this lordly position was the dramatic Nobel prize-winning revelation by Doherty and Zinkernagel that cytotoxic T-cells taken from an individual recovering from a viral infection will only kill virally infected cells that share an MHC haplotype with the host. They found that cytotoxic T-cells from mice of the H-2^d haplotype infected with lymphocytic choriomeningitis virus could kill virally infected cells derived from any H-2^d strain but not cells of H-2^k or other H-2 haplotypes. The reciprocal experiment with H-2^k mice shows that this is not just a special property associated with H-2^d (Figure M5.1.1a). Studies with recombinant strains (cf. Table 4.4) pin-pointed class I MHC as the restricting element and this was confirmed by showing that antibodies to class I MHC block the killing reaction.

The same phenomenon has been repeatedly observed in the human. HLA-A2 individuals recovering from influenza have cytotoxic T-cells that kill HLA-A2 target cells infected with influenza virus, but not cells of a different HLA-A tissue-type specificity (Figure M5.1.1b). Note how cytotoxicity could be inhibited by antiserum specific for the donor HLA-A type, but not by antisera to the allelic form HLA-A1 or the HLA-DR class II framework. Of striking significance is the inability of antibodies to the nucleoprotein to block T-cell recognition even though the T-cell specificity in these studies was known to be directed towards this antigen. As the antibodies react with nucleoprotein in its native form, the conformation of the antigen as presented to the T-cell must be quite different.

In parallel, an entirely comparable series of experiments has established the role of MHC class II molecules in antigen presentation to helper T-cells. Initially, it was shown by Shevach and Rosenthal that lymphocyte proliferation to antigen *in vitro* could be blocked by antisera raised between two strains of guinea-pig that would have included antibodies to the MHC of the responding lymphocytes. More stringent evidence comes from the type of experiment in which a T-cell clone proliferating in response to ovalbumin on antigen-presenting cells with the H-2A^b phenotype fails to respond if antigen is presented in the context of H-2A^k. However, if the H-2A^k antigen-presenting cells are transfected with the genes encoding H-2A^b, they now communicate effectively with the T-cells (Figure M5.1.2).

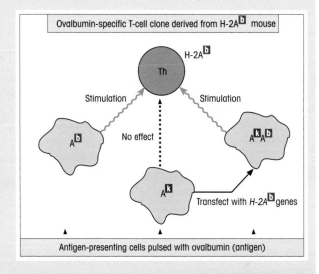

Figure M5.1.2. The T-cell clone only responds by proliferation in vitro when the antigen-presenting cells (e.g. macrophages) pulsed with ovalbumin express the same class II MHC.

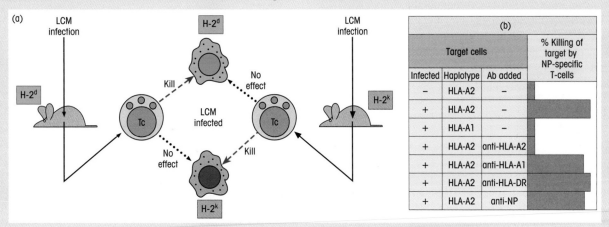

Figure M5.1.1. T-cell killing is restricted by the MHC haplotype of the virus-infected target cells.

(a) Haplotype-restricted killing of lymphocytic choriomeningitis (LCM) virus-infected target cells by cytotoxic T-cells. Killer cells from H-2^d hosts only killed H-2^d-infected targets, not those of H-2^k haplotype and vice versa. (b) Killing of influenza-infected target cells by influenza nucleoprotein (NP)-specific T-cells from an HLA-A2 donor (cf. p. 101 for human MHC nomenclature). Killing was restricted to HLA-A2 targets and only inhibited by antibodies to A2, not to A1, nor to the class II HLA-DR framework or native NP antigen.

antigen-bearing cell with its corresponding antigen-specific T-lymphocyte. We also learn that, generally, cytotoxic T-cells recognize antigen in the context of class I MHC, and helper T-cells interact when the antigen is associated with class II molecules. Accepting then the participation of MHC in T-cell recognition, what of the antigen?

T-cells recognize a linear peptide sequence from the antigen

In Milestone 5.1, we commented on experiments involving influenza nucleoprotein-specific T-cells that could kill cells infected with influenza virus. Killing occurs after the cytotoxic T-cell adheres strongly to its target through recognition of specific surface molecules. It is curious then that the nucleoprotein, which lacks a signal sequence or transmembrane region and so cannot be expressed on the cell surface, can nonetheless function as a target for cytotoxic T-cells, particularly as we have already noted that antibodies to native nucleoprotein have no influence on the killing reaction (see Figure M5.1.1b). Furthermore, **uninfected** cells do not become targets for the cytotoxic T-cells when whole nucleoprotein is added to the culture system. However, if, instead, we add a series of short peptides with sequences derived from the primary structure of the nucleoprotein, the uninfected cells now become susceptible to cytotoxic T-cell attack (Figure 5.13).

Thus was the mystery of T-cell recognition of antigen revealed. T-cells recognize linear peptides derived from protein antigens, and that is why antibodies raised against nucleoprotein in its native three-dimensional conformation do not inhibit killing. Note that only certain nucleoprotein peptides were recognized by the polyclonal T-cells in the donor population and these are to be regarded as T-cell epitopes. When clones are derived from these T-cells, each clone reacts with only one of the peptides; in other words, like B-cell clones, each clone is specific for one corresponding epitope.

Entirely analogous results are obtained when **T-helper** clones are stimulated by antigen-presenting cells to which certain peptides derived from the original antigen have been added. Again, by synthesizing a series of such peptides, the T-cell epitope can be mapped with some precision.

The conclusion is that the **T-cell recognizes both MHC and peptide** and we now know that the peptide, which acts as a T-cell epitope, lies along the groove formed by the α-helices and the β-sheet floor of the class I and class II outermost domains (see Figure 4.17). Just how does it get there?

Processing of intracellular antigen for presentation by class I MHC

Within the cytosol lurk proteolytic structures, the proteasomes, involved in the routine turnover and cellular degradation of proteins (Figure 5.14). Cytosolic proteins destined for antigen presentation, including viral proteins, are degraded to peptides via a pathway involving these structures, and further trimmed by cytosolic proteases including leucine- and aspartyl-

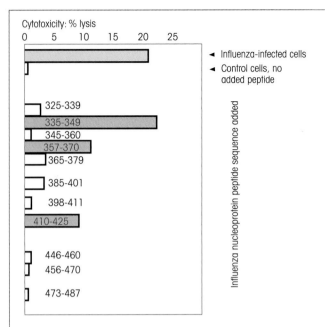

Figure 5.13. Cytotoxic T-cells, from a human donor, kill uninfected target cells in the presence of short influenza nucleoprotein peptides.

The peptides indicated were added to ^{51}Cr-labeled syngeneic (i.e. same as T-cell donor) mitogen-activated lymphoblasts and cytotoxicity was assessed by ^{51}Cr release with a killer to target ratio of 50:1. The three peptides indicated in red induced good killing. (Reproduced from Townsend A.R.M. *et al.* (1986) *Cell* **44**, 959–968, with permission. Copyright ©1986 by Cell Press.)

aminopeptidases. In addition to proteins that are already present in the cytosol, a proportion of membrane-bound and secretory proteins are transported from the ER back into the cytosol. This process may be mediated by the Sec61 multimolecular channel. Proteins that have undergone retrotranslocation from the ER into the cytosol can then be processed for class I presentation, as can proteins derived from mitochondria. Prior to processing, polypeptide antigens are covalently linked to several molecules of the 7.5 kDa protein ubiquitin in an ATP-dependent process. The polyubiquitination targets the polypeptides to the proteasome (Figure 5.14).

Only about 10% of the peptides produced by proteasomes are the optimal length (8–10 amino acids) to fit into the MHC class I groove; about 70% are likely to be too small to function in antigen presentation, and the remaining 20% would either bulge out of the groove (which apparently does happen in some cases) or require further trimming. This additional processing can occur either prior to transport into the ER, by for example cytosolic aminopeptidases, or following transport in which case the *e*ndoplasmic *r*eticulum resident *a*minopeptidases (ERAP)-1 and -2 can be employed. The cytokine IFNγ increases the production of three specialized catalytic proteosomal subunits, β_1i, β_2i and β_5i, which replace the homologous catalytic

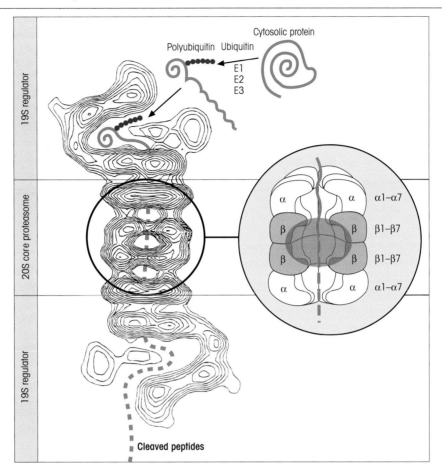

Figure 5.14. Cleavage of cytosolic proteins by the proteasome.

Cytosolic proteins become polyubiquitinated in an ATP-dependent reaction in which the enzyme E1 forms a thiolester with the C-terminus of ubiquitin and then transfers the ubiquitin to one of a number of E2 ubiquitin-carrier proteins. The C-terminus of the ubiquitin is then conjugated to a lysine residue on the polypeptide by one of several E3 ubiquitin-protein ligase enzymes. There is specificity in these processes in that the individual E2 and E3 enzymes have preferences for different proteins. The ubiquitinated cytosolic protein binds to the ATPase-containing 19S regulator where ATP drives the unfolded protein chain into the cylindrical structure of the 20S core proteasome that is made up of 28 subunits arranged in four stacked rings. The two outer rings comprise seven different α-subunits (α_1–α_7) whereas the two rings of the central hydrolytic chamber are each made up of seven different β-subunits (β_1–β_7). Within the hydrolytic chamber the protein is exposed to proteolytic activity (red shading). A novel catalytic mechanism is involved in which the nucleophilic residue that attacks the peptide bonds is the hydroxyl group on the N-terminal threonine residue of the β-subunits. There are three catalytically active subunits, β_1, β_2 and β_5, and they can act on a broad range of polypeptides. However, broadly speaking, the β_1 subunit has "caspase-like "activity and hydrolyses polypeptides after acidic residues, β_2 is "trypsin-like" and cleaves after basic residues, and β_5 is "chymotrypsin-like" in that it hydrolyses peptides after large hydrophobic residues. The β_1i, β_2i and β_5i molecules associated with the IFNγ-induced immunoproteasome show similar specificities but generally produce longer peptides, have reduced post-acidic cleavage and enhanced trypsin and chymotrypsin activity compared to their counterparts in the housekeeping proteasome. (Based on Peters J.-M. *et al.* (1993) *Journal of Molecular Biology* **234**, 932–937 and Rubin D.M. & Finley D. (1995) *Current Biology* **5**, 854–858.)

subunits in the housekeeping proteasome to produce what has been termed the **immunoproteasome**, a process that modifies the cleavage specificity in order to tailor peptide production for class I binding.

Both proteasome- and immunoproteasome-generated peptides are translocated into the ER by two members of the ATP-binding cassette (ABC) transporter family; the *t*ransporters associated with *a*ntigen *p*rocessing (TAP1 and TAP2) (Figure 5.15). It has been proposed that TAP1 and TAP2 bind ATP and ADP, respectively, and that prior to peptide entry into the peptide-binding cavity the TAP pore is only open at the cytosolic surface. Upon peptide entry the cytosolic nucleotide-binding domains close and the luminal end opens to allow the peptide to access the ER.

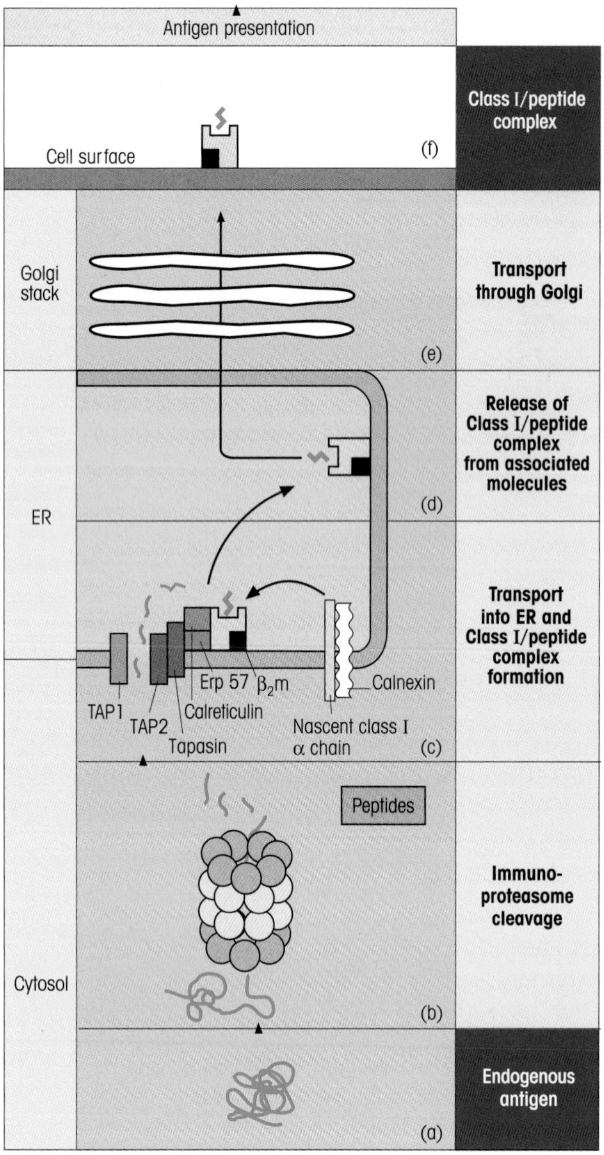

Figure 5.15. Processing of endogenous antigen and presentation by class I MHC.

Cytosolic proteins (a) are degraded by the proteasome complex (b) into peptides that are transported into the endoplasmic reticulum (ER) by the transporters associated with antigen processing (TAP)1 and TAP2 members of the ABC family of ATP-dependent transport proteins (c). Under the influence of the peptide loading complex (PLC; which comprises TAP1/2 together with calreticulin, tapasin and ERp57) the peptides are loaded into the groove of the membrane-bound class I MHC. ERp57 isomerizes disulfide bonds to ensure the correct conformation of the class I molecule. Tapasin forms a bridge between TAP1/2 and the other PLC components and is covalently linked to ERp57, which in turn is noncovalently bound to the calreticulin. Following peptide loading the peptide–MHC complex is released from the PLC (d), traverses the Golgi system (e), and appears on the cell surface (f) ready for presentation to the T-cell receptor. Mutant cells deficient in TAP1/2 do not deliver peptides to class I and cannot function as cytotoxic T-cell targets.

The newly synthesized class I heavy chain is retained in the ER by the lectin-like chaperone calnexin, which binds to the monoglucosylated N-linked glycan of the nascent heavy chain. Calnexin assists in protein folding and promotes assembly with β2-microglobulin. The calnexin is then replaced with calreticulin, which has similar lectin-like properties and, together with TAP1/2, tapasin and ERp57 (57 kDa ER thiol oxidoreductase), constitutes the peptide loading complex (PLC). The tapasin bridge ensures that the empty class I molecule sits adjacent to the TAP pores in the ER, thereby facilitating the loading of peptides. Upon peptide loading, the class I molecule dissociates from the PLC, and the now stable peptide–class I heavy chain–β2-microglobulin trimer traverses the Golgi stack and reaches the surface where it is a sitting target for the cytotoxic T-cell.

Processing of extracellular antigen for class II MHC presentation follows a different pathway

Class II MHC complexes with antigenic peptide are generated by a fundamentally different intracellular mechanism, as the antigen-presenting cells that interact with T-helper cells need to sample the antigen from the *extra*cellular compartment. In essence, a trans-Golgi vesicle containing MHC class II has to meet up with a late endosome containing exogenous protein antigen taken into the cell by an endocytic mechanism.

Regarding the class II molecules themselves, these are assembled from α and β chains in the ER in association with the transmembrane **invariant chain (Ii)** (Figure 5.16) that trimerizes to recruit three MHC class II molecules into a nonameric complex. Ii has several functions. First, it acts as a dedicated chaperone to ensure correct folding of the nascent class II molecule. Second, an internal sequence of the luminal portion of Ii sits in the MHC groove to inhibit the precocious binding of peptides in the ER before the class II molecule reaches the endocytic compartment containing antigen. Additionally, combination of Ii with the αβ class II heterodimer inactivates a retention signal and allows transport to the Golgi. Finally, targeting motifs in the N-terminal cytoplasmic region of Ii ensure delivery of the class II-containing vesicle to the endocytic pathway.

Meanwhile, exogenous protein is taken up by endocytosis. The enzyme GILT (interferon-γ-induced lysosomal thiol reductase) is present in the endosomes and will break any disulfide bonds that are present in the engulfed proteins. As the early endosome undergoes progressive acidification, the proteins are processed into peptides by a range of proteolytic enzymes (see Figure 5.16 legend). The late endosomes characteristically acquire *l*ysosomal-*a*ssociated *m*embrane *p*roteins (LAMPs), which are implicated in enzyme targeting, autophagy (see below) and lysosomal biogenesis. These late endosomes fuse with the vacuole containing the class II–Ii complex. Under the acidic conditions within these *M*HC class *II*-enriched *c*ompartments (MIICs), AEP and cathepsins S and L degrade

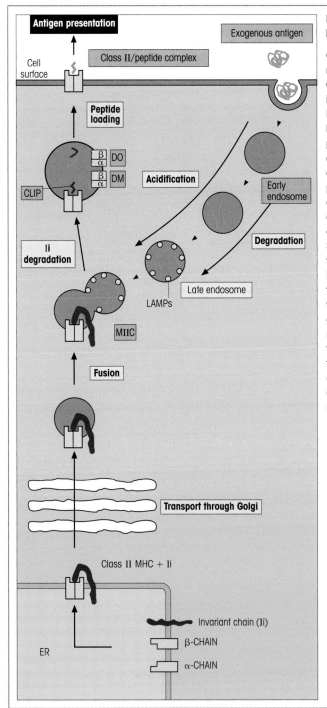

Figure 5.16. Processing of exogenous antigen and presentation by class II MHC.

Class II molecules with Ii are assembled in the endoplasmic reticulum (ER) and transported through the Golgi to the trans-Golgi reticulum (actually as a nonamer consisting of three invariant, three α and three β chains—not shown). There the class II-containing vacuole fuses with a late endosome which has lysosomal characteristics and contains peptides generated by partial degradation of proteins derived from the endocytic uptake of exogenous antigen. This fusion generates a so-called MHC class II-enriched compartment, MIIC. Particularly implicated in the processing of exogenous antigen in the endosomes are the cysteine proteases cathepsin S and L, both of which have endopeptidase activity, as do both cathepsin D and asparagine endopeptidase (AEP) which might also partake in this process. Subsequently, the exopeptidases cathepsin B and X are thought to trim the C-terminus, and cathepsins C and H to trim the N-terminus of the peptides either prior to or after their binding into the MHC class II groove. Degradation of the invariant chain leaves the CLIP (*cl*ass II-associated *i*nvariant chain *p*eptide) lying in the groove but, under the influence of the DM molecule, this is replaced by the peptides derived from exogenous antigen, and the complexes are transported to the cell surface for presentation to T-helper cells. This version of events is supported by the finding of high concentrations of invariant chain CLIP associated with class II in the MIIC vacuoles of DM-deficient mutant mice that are poor presenters of antigen to T-cells.

Ii except for the part sitting in the MHC groove that, for the time being, remains there as a peptide referred to as CLIP (*cl*ass II-associated *i*nvariant chain *p*eptide). An MHC-related dimeric molecule, DM, then catalyzes the removal of CLIP and keeps the groove open so that peptides generated in the endosome can be inserted (Figure 5.17). Initial peptide binding is determined by the concentration of the peptide and its on-rate, but DM may subsequently assist in the removal of lower affinity peptides to allow their replacement by high affinity peptides, i.e. act as a peptide editor permitting the incorporation of peptides with the most stable binding characteristics, namely those with a slow off-rate. Particularly in B-cells an additional MHC-related molecule, DO, associates with DM bound to class II and modifies its function in a pH-dependent fashion. Its effect may be to favor the presentation of antigens internalized via the BCR over those taken up by

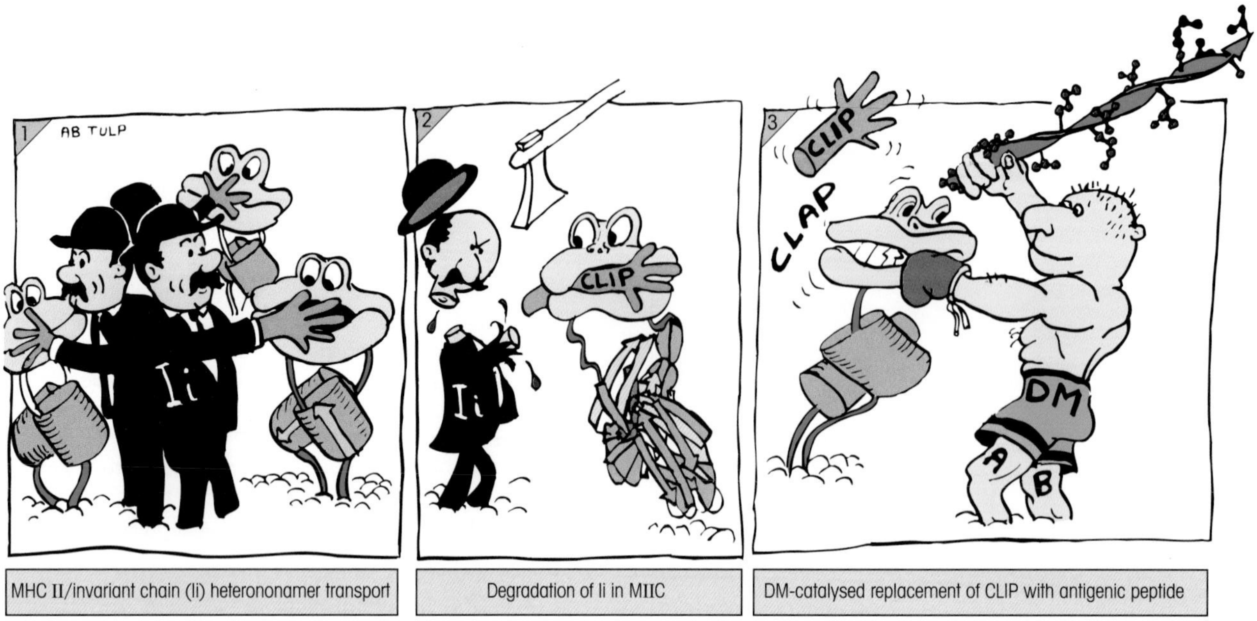

| MHC II/invariant chain (Ii) heterononamer transport | Degradation of Ii in MIIC | DM-catalysed replacement of CLIP with antigenic peptide |

Figure 5.17. MHC class II transport and peptide loading illustrated by Tulp's gently vulgar cartoon. (Reproduced from Benham A. *et al.* (1995) *Immunology Today* **16**, 359–362, with permission of the authors and Elsevier Science Ltd.)

fluid phase endocytosis. The class II–peptide complexes are eventually transported to the membrane for presentation to T-helper cells.

Cross-presentation of antigens

We have just seen how MHC class I presents endogenous antigen whilst MHC class II presents exogenous antigen. However, approximately 25% of class I molecules present antigen of exogenous origin and up to 20% of MHC class II molecules present peptides derived from either cytoplasmic or nuclear antigens. Indeed, naive cytotoxic T-cells require dendritic cells for their activation but most viruses are not tropic for dendritic cells and therefore not naturally present in the cytosol of the professional APCs. Given the two separate pathways (endogenous/class I, exogenous/class II) outlined in the previous sections, how can this be achieved? The answer to this conundrum lies in the phenomenon of "cross-presentation." Phagocytosed or endocytosed antigens can sneak out of the vacuole into which they have been engulfed and gain entry to the cytosol (Figure 5.18a). The escape route may involve the Sec61 multimolecular channel. Once they enter the cytosol they are fair game for ubiquitination and subsequent degradation by the proteasome, followed by TAP-mediated transfer into the ER, and presentation by MHC class I. It is also possible that some endocytosed antigens can be loaded directly into recycling MHC class I molecules within the endosome without the need to be first processed in the cytosol. In addi-

tion to dendritic cells, macrophages also seem to be able to play the cross-presentation game, albeit less efficiently.

Conversely, proteasome-derived peptides within the cytosol, such as those derived from viral capsids, are potential clients for the class II groove and could make the journey to the MIIC. This can occur by a process known as autophagy in which portions of cytoplasm, which will potentially contain peptides generated from the proteasome, are engulfed internally by structures referred to as autophagosomes (Figure 5.18b). Autophagy has been shown to happen constitutively in professional antigen-presenting cells. The peptide-containing autophagosome can then fuse with the MHC class II-containing MIIC, where proteolytic cleavage of any intact proteins may also take place. From then on events parallel those described for the presentation of exogenous antigens, with the peptides exchanging with CLIP, and transfer of peptide–MHC to the cell surface. During periods of cell stress a second pathway, chaperone-mediated autophagy, can be employed involving members of the heat-shock protein 70 family that bind to the protein to be processed. The protein complex is then recognized by lysosome-associated membrane protein 2a (LAMP-2a) and dragged into the lumen of the lysosome for subsequent processing.

The nature of the "groovy" peptide

The MHC grooves impose some well-defined restrictions on the nature and length of the peptides they accommodate

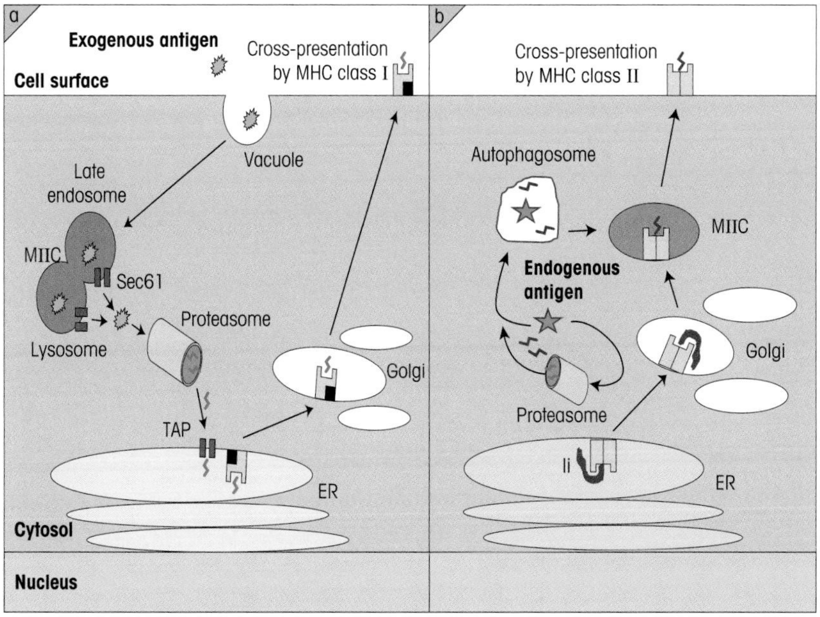

Figure 5.18. Cross-presentation of antigen.

(a) Engulfed exogenous antigens are able to access the class I processing pathway by entering the cytosol from the MHC class II compartments (MIIC), perhaps through Sec61 channels. Other routes for the presentation of peptides derived from exogenous antigens on MHC class I may include peptide exchange with MHC class I molecules recycling from the cell membrane. (b) Cross-presentation can also work the "other way round" with cytosolic peptides generated from the proteasome (and also intact endogenous antigens) undergoing autophagy to gain entry into the class II processing and presentation pathway. ER, endoplasmic reticulum.

Table 5.1. Natural MHC class I peptide ligands contain two allele-specific anchor residues. (Based on Rammensee H.G., Friede T. & Stevanovic S. (1995) *Immunogenetics* **41**, 178.) Letters represent the Dayhoff code for amino acids; where more than one residue predominates at a given position, the alternative(s) is given; • = any residue.

Class I allele	Amino acid position								
	1	2	3	4	5	6	7	8	9
H-2K^d	•	Y	•	•	•	•	•	•	I/L
H-2K^b	•	•	•	•	Y/F	•	•	L/M	
H-2D^b	•	•	•	•	N	•	•	•	L/M/I
HLA-A*0201	•	L/M/I	•	•	•	•	•	•	L/V/I/M
HLA-B*2705	•	R	•	•	•	•	•	•	R/K/L/F

and the pattern varies with different MHC alleles. However, at the majority of positions in the peptide ligand, a surprising degree of redundancy is permitted and this relates in part to residues interacting with the T-cell receptor rather than the MHC.

Binding to MHC class I

X-ray analysis reveals the peptides to be tightly mounted along the length of the groove in an extended configuration with no breathing space for α-helical structures (Figure 5.19). The forces involved in peptide binding to MHC and in TCR binding to peptide–MHC are similar to those seen between antibody and antigen, i.e. noncovalent. The N-terminus of the bound peptide is tightly hydrogen-bonded independently of the MHC allele to conserved residues at one end of the groove, whilst the C-terminus engages in hydrogen bonding and ionic interactions at the other end of the groove.

The naturally occurring peptides can be extracted from purified MHC class I and sequenced. They are predominantly 8–10 residues long; longer peptides bulge upwards out of the cleft. Analysis of the peptide pool sequences indicates amino acids with defined characteristics at certain key positions (Table 5.1). These are called **anchor positions** and represent the amino acid side-chains required to fit into allele-specific pockets in the MHC groove (Figure 5.20a). There are usually two, sometimes three, such major anchor positions for class I-binding peptides, one at the C-terminal end and the other frequently at peptide position 2 (P2), but sometimes at other

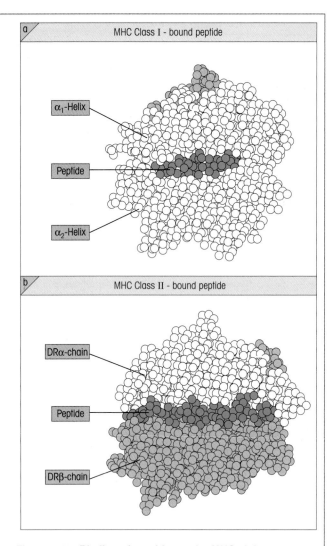

Figure 5.19. Binding of peptides to the MHC cleft.

T-cell receptor (TCR) "view" looking down on the α-helices lining the cleft (cf. Figure 4.17b) represented in space-filling models. (a) Peptide 309–317 from HIV-1 reverse transcriptase bound tightly within the class I HLA-A2 cleft. In general, one to four of the peptide side-chains points towards the TCR, giving a solvent accessibility of 17–27%. (b) Influenza hemagglutinin 306–318 lying in the class II HLA-DR1 cleft. In contrast with class I, the peptide extends out of both ends of the binding groove and from four to six out of an average of 13 side-chains point towards the TCR, increasing solvent accessibility to 35%. (Based on Vignali D.A.A. & Strominger J.L. (1994) *The Immunologist* **2**, 112, with permission of the authors and publisher.)

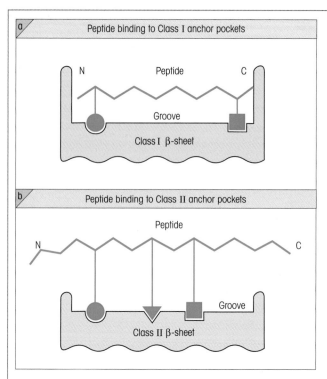

Figure 5.20. Allele-specific pockets in the MHC-binding grooves bind the major anchor residue motifs of the peptide ligands.

Cross-section through the longitudinal axis of the MHC groove. The two α-helices forming the lateral walls of the groove lie horizontally above and below the plane of the paper. (a) The class I groove is closed at both ends. The anchor at the carboxy terminus is invariant but the second anchor very often at P2 may also be at other positions depending on the MHC allele (cf. Table 5.1). (b) By contrast, the class II groove is open at both ends and does not constrain the length of the peptide. There are usually three or four major anchor pockets with, for example, P1 dominant for HLA-DR1 and P4 dominant for HLA-DR3.

positions. For example, the highly prevalent HLA-A*0201 has pockets for leucine, methionine or isoleucine at peptide position P2 and for leucine, valine, isoleucine or methionine at P9. Sometimes, a major anchor pocket may be replaced by two or three more weakly binding secondary pockets. Even with the constraints of two or three anchor motifs, each MHC class I allele can accommodate a considerable number of different peptides. Thus, so long as the criteria for the anchor positions are met, the other amino acids in the sequence can vary.

Except in the case of viral infection, the natural class I ligands will be self peptides derived from proteins endogenously synthesized by the cell, histones, heat-shock proteins, enzymes, leader signal sequences, and so on. It turns out that 75% or so of these peptides originate in the cytosol and most of them will be in low abundance, say 100–400 copies per cell. Thus proteins expressed with unusual abundance, such as oncofetal proteins in tumors and viral antigens in infected cells, should be readily detected by resting T-cells.

Binding to MHC class II

Unlike class I, where the allele-independent hydrogen-bonding to the peptide is focused at the N- and C-termini, the class

II groove residues hydrogen-bond and use other noncovalent interactions along the entire length of the peptide with links to the atoms forming the main chain. With respect to class II allele-specific binding pockets for peptide side-chains, motifs based on three or four major anchor residues seem to be the order of the day (Figure 5.20b). Secondary binding pockets with less strict preference for individual side-chains can still modify the affinity of the peptide–MHC complex, while "nonpockets" may also influence preferences for particular peptide sequences, especially if steric hindrance becomes a factor. Unfortunately, we cannot establish these preferences for the individual residues within a given peptide. This is because although the length of the class II groove is similar to that of class I, the open nature of the groove in class II places no constraint on the length of the ligand. The peptide is therefore able to dangle nonchalantly from each end of the groove, quite unlike the strait-jacket of the class I ligand site (Figures 5.19 and 5.20). Thus, as noted earlier, each class II molecule binds a collection of peptides with a spectrum of lengths ranging from eight to 30 amino acid residues, and analysis of such a naturally occurring pool isolated from the MHC would not establish which amino acid side-chains were binding preferentially to the nine available sites within the groove. One approach to get around this problem is to study the binding of soluble class II molecules to very large libraries of random-sequence nonapeptides expressed on the surface of bacteriophages (cf. the combinatorial phage libraries, p. 146). The idea is emerging that each amino acid in a peptide contributes independently of the others to the total binding strength, and it should be possible to compute each contribution quantitatively from these random binding data, so that ultimately we could predict which sequences in a given protein antigen would bind to a given class II allele.

Because of the accessible nature of the groove as the native molecule is unfolded and reduced, but before any degradation need occur, the high affinity epitopes could immediately bury themselves in the class II-binding groove where they are protected from internal proteolysis. At least for the HLA-DR1 molecule it has been shown that peptide binding leads to a transition from a more open conformation to one with a more compact structure extending throughout the peptide-binding groove. Trimming of the N- and C-terminal ends of the peptide can then take place after the peptides have bound to the MHC. Several factors will influence the relative concentration of peptide–MHC complex formed: the affinity for the groove as determined by the fit of the anchors, enhancement or hindrance by internal residues (sequences outside the binding residues have little or no effect on peptide-binding specificity), sensitivity to proteases and disulfide reduction, and downstream competition from determinants of higher affinity.

The range of concentration of the different peptide complexes that result will engender a hierarchy of epitopes with respect to their ability to interact with T-cells; the most effec-

tive will be **dominant**, the less so **subdominant**. Dominant, and presumably subdominant, **self** epitopes will generally induce tolerance during T-cell ontogeny in the thymus (see p. 288). Complexes with some self peptides that are of relatively low abundance will not tolerize their T-cell counterparts and these autoreactive T-cells constantly pose an underlying threat of potential autoimmunity. These are **cryptic** epitopes, and we will discuss their possible relationship to autoimmune disease in Chapter 18.

The αβ T-cell receptor forms a ternary complex with MHC and antigenic peptide

When soluble TCR preparations produced using recombinant DNA technology are immobilized on a sensor chip, they can bind MHC–peptide complex specifically with rather low affinities (K_a) in the 10^4 to $10^7 M^{-1}$ range. This low affinity and the relatively small number of atomic contacts formed between the TCRs and their MHC–peptide ligands when T-cells contact their target cell make the contribution of TCR recognition to the binding energy of this cellular interaction fairly trivial. The brunt of the attraction rests on the antigen-independent major adhesion molecule pairs, such as LFA-1–ICAM-1 and CD2–LFA-3 that are recruited into the immunological synapse (cf. Figure 8.12), but any subsequent triggering of the T-cell by MHC–peptide antigen must involve signaling through the T-cell receptor.

Topology of the ternary complex

Of the three complementarity determining regions present in each TCR chain, CDR1 and CDR2 are much less variable than CDR3 that, like its immunoglobulin counterpart, has (D)J sequences that result from a multiplicity of combinatorial and nucleotide insertion mechanisms (cf. p. 88). As the MHC elements in a given individual are fixed, but great variability is expected in the antigenic peptide, a logical model would have CDR1 and CDR2 of each TCR chain contacting the α-helices of the MHC, and the CDR3 concerned in binding to the peptide. In accord with this view, several studies have shown that T-cells that recognize small variations in a peptide in the context of a given MHC restriction element differ only in their CDR3 hypervariable regions.

The combining sites of the TCRs that have been crystallized to date are relatively flat (Figure 5.21), which would be expected given the need for complementarity to the gently undulating surface of the peptide–MHC combination (Figure 5.22a). In most of the structures so far solved, recognition involves the TCR lying either diagonally or orthogonally (Figure 5.22b,c) across the peptide–MHC with the TCR Vα CDR1 and CDR2 overlying the MHC class II β₁-helix or class I α₂-helix, and the Vβ CDR1 and CDR2 overlying

Figure 5.21. T-cell receptor antigen combining site.

Although the surface is relatively flat, there is a cleft between the CDR3α and CDR3β that can accommodate a central upfacing side-chain of the peptide bound into the groove of an MHC molecule. The surface and loop traces of the Vα CDR1 and CDR2 are colored magenta, Vβ CDR1 and CDR2 blue, Vα CDR3 and Vβ CDR3 yellow, and the Vβ fourth hypervariable region, which makes contact with some superantigens, orange. (Reproduced from Garcia K.C. *et al.* (1996) *Science* **274**, 209–219, with permission.)

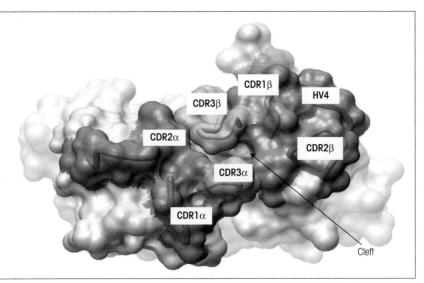

Figure 5.22. Complementarity between MHC–peptide and T-cell receptor.

(a) Backbone structure of a T-cell receptor (TCR) recognizing a peptide presented by the MHC class I molecule H-2Kᵇ. The TCR is in the top half of the picture, with the α chain in pink and its CDR1 colored magenta, CDR2 purple and CDR3 yellow. The β chain is colored light blue with its CDR1 cyan, CDR2 navy blue, CDR3 green and the fourth hypervariable loop orange. Below the TCR is the MHC α chain in green and β₂-microglobulin in dark green. The peptide with side-chains at positions P1, P4 and P8 is colored yellow. (Reproduced from Garcia K.C. *et al.* (1998) *Science* **279**, 1166–1172, with permission.) (b) The same complex looking down onto a molecular surface representation of the H-2Kᵇ in yellow, with the diagonal docking mode of the TCR in a backbone worm representation colored pink. The dEV8 peptide is drawn in a ball and stick format. (c) By contrast, here we see the orthogonal docking mode of a TCR recognizing a peptide presented by MHC class II. The TCR (scD10) backbone worm representation shows the Vα in green and Vβ in blue, and the I-Aᵏ class II molecular surface representation has the α chain in light green and the β chain in orange, holding its conalbumin-derived peptide. (Reproduced from Reinherz E.L. *et al.* (1999) *Science* **286**, 1913–1921, with permission.)

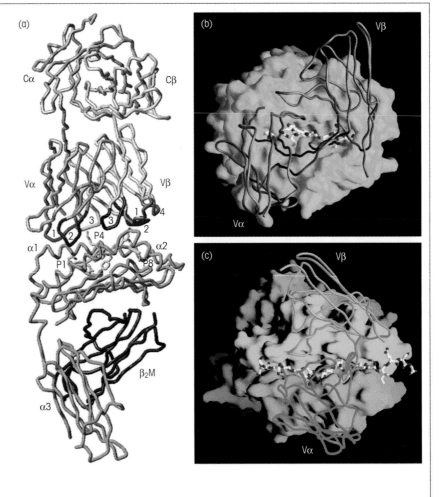

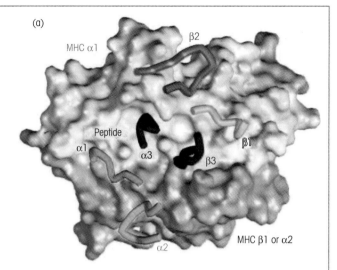

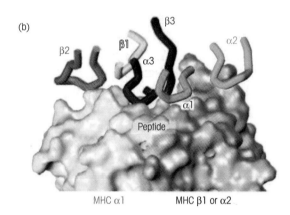

Figure 5.23. TCR CDR3 recognition of peptide presented by MHC.

(a) Contacts between the CDR1–3 loops of the α and β chains of a T-cell receptor (TCR) and a space-filling surface of MHC and peptide. The example shown here is a mouse TCR bound to the H2 I-A^b presenting a 13-mer peptide. The α1 region of MHC is colored cyan, the β1 or α2 region of MHC magenta and the peptide yellow. The CDR loops of the TCR α and β chains are indicated (α1 is CDR1 of the α chain, and so on). (b) Elevation perspective of the interactions (Reproduced from Marrack P. et al. (2008) *Annual Review of Immunology* **26**, 171–203, with permission).

the α₁-helix of MHC class I or class II (Figure 5.23) The more variable CDR3 regions make contact with the peptide, particularly focusing in on the middle residues (P4 to P6). There is evidence to suggest that the TCR initially binds to the MHC in a fairly peptide-independent fashion, followed by conformational changes particularly in the peptide-recognising CDR3 loops of the TCR to permit optimal contact with the peptide. Activation through the TCR-CD3 complex can operate if these adjustments permit more stable and multimeric binding.

T-cells with a different outlook

Nonclassical class I molecules can also present antigen

MHC class I-like molecules

In addition to the highly polymorphic classical MHC class I molecules (HLA-A, -B and -C in the human and H-2K, -D and -L in the mouse), there are other loci encoding MHC molecules containing β₂-microglobulin with relatively non-polymorphic heavy chains. These are **H-2M**, **-Q** and **-T** in mice, and **HLA-E**, **-F** and **-G** in *Homo sapiens.*

The **H-2M3** molecule encoded by the H-2M locus is unusual in that its peptide-binding groove has many nonpolar amino acids designed to facilitate the binding of the hydrophobic *N*-formyl methionine residue of peptides derived from bacterial proteins, which can then be presented to T-cells. Expression of H-2M3 is limited by the availability of these peptides so that high levels are only seen during prokaryotic infections. The demonstration of H-2M3-restricted CD8⁺ αβ T-cells specific for *Listeria monocytogenes* encourages the view that this class I-like molecule could underwrite a physiological function in infection. Discussion of the role of HLA-G expression in the human extravillous cytotrophoblast will arise in Chapter 16 (see p. 441).

The family of CD1 non-MHC but class I-like molecules presents lipid antigens

After MHC class I and class II, the CD1 family (see p. 108) represents a third lineage of antigen-presenting molecules recognized by T-lymphocytes. Just like MHC class I heavy chain, the CD1 polypeptide chain associates with β₂-microglobulin, and the overall structure is indeed similar to that of classical class I molecules, although the topology of the binding groove is altered (see Figure 4.27).

CD1 molecules can present a broad range of **lipid, glycolipid** and **lipopeptide** antigens, and even certain small organic molecules, to clonally diverse αβ and γδ T-cells and, for CD1d, to NKT cells (see below). A common structural motif facilitates CD1-mediated antigen presentation and comprises a hydrophobic region of a branched or dual acyl chain and a hydrophilic portion formed by the polar or charged groups of the lipid and/or its associated carbohydrate or peptide. The hydrophobic regions are buried in the deep binding groove of CD1, whilst the hydrophilic regions, such as the carbohydrate structures, are recognized by the TCR (Figure 5.24). In this solved crystal structure, the αβ TCR recognizes CD1d plus α-galactosylceramide by docking in parallel to the complex (Figure 5.25). This is rather different to the diagonal or orthogonal binding usually seen with αβ TCR recognition of peptide–MHC (Figure 5.26).

Ligands for CD1a include the sulphatide sphingolipid and mycopeptides such as didehydroxymycobactin from *Mycobacterium tuberculosis;* for CD1b are mycolic acid and carbohydrate structures such as the mycobacterial cell wall

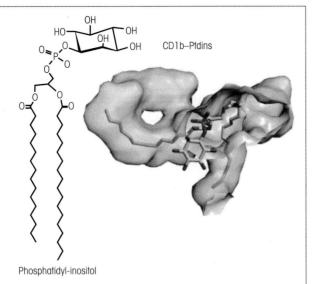

Figure 5.24. Antigen presentation by CD1.

In this example the binding of phosphatidylinositol (Ptdins) to CD1b is shown with the binding pocket represented from a top view, looking directly into the groove. Aliphatic backbones are in green, phosphor atom in blue and oxygen atoms in red. (Reproduced with permission from Hava D.L. *et al.* (2005) *Current Opinion in Immunology* **17**, 88–94.)

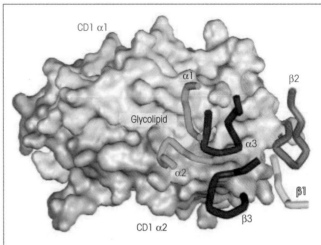

Figure 5.25. T-cell receptor (TCR) recognition of CD1d-presented antigen.

αβ TCR recognition of α-galactosylceramide presented by CD1d. The α1 (colored cyan) and α2 (magenta) regions of CD1d and the glycolipid (*yellow*) are shown, together with the CDR loops of the TCR α and β chains. Note the TCR binding is towards one end of the CDld molecule. Because the lipid component of the antigen is buried within the CD1d molecule, recognition of α-galactosylceramide by the TCR involves only the protruding glycosyl head. The TCR α chain CDR1 (α1) interacts only with the antigen whereas the α chain CDR3 (α3) interacts with both the antigen and CD1d. Recognition of the antigen does not involve the TCR β chain, whose CDR2 (β2) and CDR3 (β3) bind to CD1d. The α chain CDR2 (α2) and β chain CDR1 (β1) are not involved in binding to the CD1d-antigen complex in this solved crystal structure. (Reproduced from Marrack P. *et al.* (2008) *Annual Review of Immunology* **26**, 171–203, with permission).

Figure 5.26. Comparison of TCR recognition of CD1d–lipid and MHC–peptide.

(a) T-cell receptor (TCR) α-chain (yellow) and β-chain (blue) binding to α-galactosylceramide (magenta) presented by CD1d (green). (b) TCR α -chain (purple) and β-chain (cyan) binding to MHC (grey) and peptide (magenta). (c) Parallel docking mode seen with TCR (CDR1α, yellow; CDR2α, green; CDR3α, cyan; CDR1β, magenta; CDR2β, orange; CDR3β, blue) recognition of α-galactosylceramide (magenta) presented by CD1d (α-helices, pale green). (d) Diagonal docking mode of a typical TCR (CDR loops colored as in (c)) with peptide–MHC. In (c) and (d) the center of mass between the Vα and Vβ domain is indicated by the black line. (Reproduced from Borg N.A. *et al.* (2007) *Nature* **448**, 44–49, with permission).

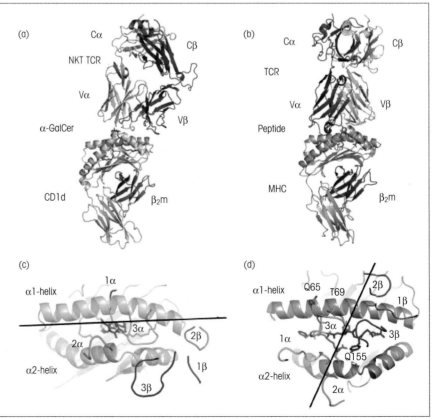

component lipoarabinomannan; and for CD1c include myco-bacterial mannosyl-1-phosphodolichol. Possible microbial ligands for CD1d are still under investigation, but α-galactosylceramide from marine sponges is known to be a very potent stimulator of invariant NKT (iNKT, see below) cells when presented by this molecule. The fifth member of the family, CD1e, appears to be involved in the processing of glycolipids prior to their presentation by other CD1 family members. Both endogenous and exogenous lipids can be presented by CD1 and, like MHC class I, the CD1 heavy chain complexes initially with calnexin in the endoplasmic reticulum and is then subsequently replaced with calreticulin. The protein Erp57 is then recruited into the complex. Subsequent dissociation of the complex permits the binding of β$_2$-microglobulin and, in a step involving the microsomal triglyceride-transfer protein (MTP), the insertion of endogenous lipid antigens into the CD1 antigen-binding region. Just like their proteinaceous colleagues, exogenously derived lipid and glycolipid antigens are delivered to the acidic endosomal compartment. Localization of CD1b, c and d molecules to the endocytic pathway is mediated by a tyrosine-based cytosolic targeting sequence in the cytoplasmic tail. CD1a, which lacks this targeting motif, traffics through early recycling endosomes. Both humans and mice deficient in prosaposin, a precursor molecule of the sphingolipid activator proteins (SAPs) saposin A–D, are defective in the presentation of lipid antigens to T-cells. Various lines of enquiry indicate that these molecules are involved in the transfer of lipid antigens to CD1 in the endosomes.

Some T-cells have NK markers

NKT-cells possess the NK1.1 marker, characteristic of NK cells, together with a T-cell receptor. There are two populations, one with diverse TCRs and the other referred to as invariant NKT-cells (iNKT cells). In the latter population the TCR bears an invariant α chain (Vα24Jα18 in humans, Vα14Jα18 in mice) with no N-region modifications and an extremely limited β chain repertoire based upon Vβ11 in the human and Vβ8.2, Vβ7 and Vβ2 in the mouse. They recognize lipid antigens such as α-galactosylceramide and isoglobosides presented by CD1d and constitute a major component of the T-cell compartment, accounting for 20–30% of T-cells in bone marrow and liver in mice, and up to 1% of spleen cells. Upon activation, NKT-cells rapidly secrete IL-4 and IFNγ and thereby can be involved in the stimulation of many cell types including dendritic cells, NK cells and B-cells.

γδ TCRs have some features of antibody

Unlike αβ T-cells, γδ T-cells recognize antigens directly without a requirement for antigen processing. In the mouse, γδ T-cells have been isolated that directly recognize the MHC class I molecule I-E^k and the nonclassical MHC molecules T10 and T22. Neither the polymorphic residues associated with peptide binding to classical MHC molecules nor the peptide itself is involved. T10 and T22 are expressed by αβ T-cells following

their activation, and it has therefore been suggested that γδ T-cells specific for these nonclassical MHC molecules may exert a regulatory function. Stressed or damaged cells appear to be powerful activators of γδ cells, and certain heat-shock proteins (e.g. hsp60) can act as stimulators of these cells. Low molecular weight **phosphate-containing nonproteinaceous** antigens, such as isopentenyl pyrophosphate and ethyl phosphate, which occur in a range of microbial and mammalian cells, have also been identified as potent stimulators.

Evidence for direct recognition of antigen by γδ T-cells came from experiments such as those involving a γδ T-cell clone specific for the herpes simplex virus glycoprotein-1. This clone could be stimulated by the native protein bound to plastic, suggesting that the cells are triggered by cross-linking of their receptors by antigen that they recognize in the intact native state just as antibodies do. There are structural arguments to give weight to this view. The CDR3 loops, which are critical for foreign antigen recognition by T-cells and antibodies, are comparable in length and relatively constrained with respect to size in the α and β chains of the αβ TCR, reflecting a relative constancy in the size of the MHC–peptide complexes to which they bind. CDR3 regions in the immunoglobulin light chains are short and similarly constrained in length, but in the heavy chains they are longer on average and more variable in length, related perhaps to their need to recognize a wide range of epitopes. Quite strikingly, the γδ TCRs resemble antibodies in that the γ chain CDR3 loops are short with a narrow length distribution, while in the δ chain they are long with a broad length distribution. Therefore, in this respect, the **γδ TCR resembles antibody** more than the αβ TCR. The X-ray crystallographic structure of a γδ TCR bound to its ligand, the nonclassical MHC molecule T22 mentioned above, has been solved. In this example the extended CDR3 loop of the δ chain, particularly the Dδ2 segment encoded by a non-mutated (germline) sequence, mediates most of the binding with a minor contribution also made by the CDR3 of the γ chain. Whilst structural determinations of additional γδ TCR–antigen complexes will reveal whether this type of interaction is representative of other γδ TCRs, the broad length distribution of the different CDR3 Vδ loops suggests that γδ TCRs will generally have topographically more adventurous binding sites than the TCRs of αβ T-cells, thereby facilitating the ability of γδ T-cells to interact with intact rather than processed antigen.

A particular subset of γδ cells, which possess a diverse range of TCRs utilizing different *D* and *J* gene segments but always using the same *V* gene segments, V*γ*9 and V*δ*2, can expand *in vivo* to comprise a large proportion (up to 50%) of all peripheral blood T-cells during a diverse range of infections. These Vγ9Vδ2 T-cells recognize alkylamines and organophosphates. Indeed, individual Vγ9Vδ2 T-cells can recognize **both** positively charged alkylamines **and** negatively charged molecules such as ethyl phosphate. However, this should be fairly straightforward for the receptor given the small hapten-like size of these antigens. A number of alkylamine antigens are produced by human pathogens, including *Salmonella typhimurium*, *Listeria monocytogenes*, *Yersinia enterocolitica* and *Escherichia coli*.

The above characteristics provide the γδ cells with a distinctive role complementary to that of the αβ population and enable them to function in the direct recognition of microbial pathogens and of damaged or stressed host cells. Very interestingly, activated γδ T-cells can express classical MHC class II and the CD80/CD86 co-stimulatory molecules and thereby act as professional antigen-presenting cells for the activation of αβ T-cells. Additionally they are able to indirectly facilitate antigen presentation because their secretion of TNFα induces expression of class II and CD80/CD86 in resting dendritic cells.

Superantigens stimulate whole families of lymphocyte receptors

Bacterial toxins represent one major group of T-cell superantigens

Whereas an individual peptide complexed to MHC will react with antigen-specific T-cells that represent a relatively small percentage of the T-cell pool because of the requirement for specific binding to particular CDR3 regions, a special class of molecule has been identified that stimulates the 5–20% of the total T-cell population expressing the same TCR Vβ family structure. These molecules do this irrespective of the antigen specificity of the receptor. They are referred to as **superantigens** and do not need to be processed by the antigen-presenting cell, instead cross-linking the class II and Vβ independently of direct interaction between MHC and TCR molecules (Figure 5.27).

The pyogenic toxin superantigen family can cause food poisoning, vomiting and diarrhea and includes *Staphylococcus aureus* enterotoxins (SEA, SEB and several others), staphylococcal toxic shock syndrome toxin-1 (TSST-1), streptococcal superantigen (SSA) and several streptococcal pyogenic exotoxins (SPEs). Although these molecules all have a similar structure, they stimulate T-cells bearing different Vβ sequences. They are strongly mitogenic for these T-cells in the presence of MHC class II expressing cells. SEA is one of the most potent T-cell mitogens known, causing marked proliferation in the concentration range 10^{-13} to 10^{-16} M. Like the other superantigens it can cause a "cytokine storm" involving the release of copious amounts of IL-2, IFNγ, TNFα, TNFβ (lymphotoxin) and other cytokines, and of mast cell leukotrienes, which form the basis for its ability to produce toxic shock syndrome. Other superantigens, not belonging to the pyogenic toxin superantigen family, include staphylococcal exfoliative toxins (ETs), *Mycoplasma arthritidis* mitogen (MAM) and *Yersinia pseudotuberculosis* mitogen (YPM).

Endogenous retroviruses can act as superantigens

Very many years ago, Festenstein made the curious observation that B-cells from certain mouse strains produce powerful pro-

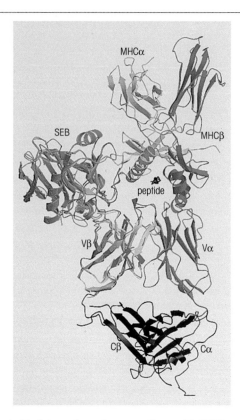

Figure 5.27. Interaction of superantigen with MHC and TCR.

In this composite model, the interaction with the superantigen staphylococcal enterotoxin B (SEB) involves SEB wedging itself between the T-cell receptor (TCR) Vβ chain and the MHC, effectively preventing interaction between the TCR and the peptide in the groove, and between the TCR β chain and the MHC. Thus direct contact between the TCR and the MHC is limited to Vα amino acid residues. (Reproduced from Li H. *et al.* (1999) *Annual Review of Immunology* **17**, 435–466, with permission.) Other superantigens disrupt direct TCR interactions with peptide–MHC to varying extents, and in some cases (e.g. *Mycoplasma arthritidis* mitogen) there is no direct contact at all between the TCR and peptide/MHC.

liferative responses in roughly 20% of unprimed T-cells from another strain of identical MHC. The Mls gene product responsible for inciting this proliferation is encoded by the open reading frame (ORF) located in the 3′ long terminal repeat of mouse mammary tumor viruses (MMTV). These are retroviruses that are transmitted as infectious agents in milk and are specific for B-cells. They associate with class II MHC in the B-cell membrane and act as superantigens through their affinity for certain TCR Vβ families in a similar fashion to the bacterial toxins.

In humans, EBV infection of B-cells transactivates the HERV-K18 *env* gene of an endogenous retroviral superantigen. Polyclonal activation of T-cells can also occur in response to antigens from viruses other than retroviruses, for example rabies virus nucleocapsid protein.

Microbes can also provide B-cell superantigens

Staphylococcal protein A reacts not only with the Fcγ region of IgG but also with 15–50% of polyclonal IgM, IgA and IgG F(ab′)$_2$, all of which belong to the V$_H$3 family. This superantigen is mitogenic for B-cells through its recognition by a discontinuous binding sequence composed of amino acid residues from FR1, CDR2 and FR3 of the V$_H$ domain. The human immunodeficiency virus (HIV) glycoprotein gp120 also reacts with immunoglobulins that utilize V$_H$3 family members. The binding site partially overlaps with that for protein A and utilizes amino acid residues from FR1, CDR1, CDR2 and FR3.

The recognition of different forms of antigen by B- and T-cells is advantageous to the host

It is our conviction that this section deals with a subject of the utmost importance, which is at the epicenter of immunology.

Antibodies combat microbes and their products in the extracellular body fluids where they exist essentially in their native form (Figure 5.28a). Clearly it is to the host's advantage for the B-cell receptor to recognize epitopes on the **native molecules**.

αβ T-cells have quite a different job. In the case of cytotoxic T-cells, and the T-cells that activate infected macrophages, they have to seek out and bind to the infected cells and carry out their effector function face to face with the target. First, with respect to proteins produced by intracellular infectious agents, the MHC molecules act as markers to tell the effector T-lymphocyte that it is encountering a cell. Second, the T-cell does not want to attack an uninfected cell on whose surface a native microbial molecule happens to be sitting purely by chance, nor would it wish to have its antigenic target on the appropriate cell surface blocked by an excess of circulating antibody. Thus it is of benefit for the infected cell to express the microbial antigen on its surface in a form distinct from that of the native molecule. As will now be more than abundantly clear, the evolutionary solution was to make the T-cell recognize a processed peptide derived from the intracellular antigen and to hold it as a complex with the surface MHC molecules. The single T-cell receptor then recognizes both the **MHC cell marker** and the **peptide infection marker** in one operation (Figure 5.28b). Given that virtually all nucleated cells can

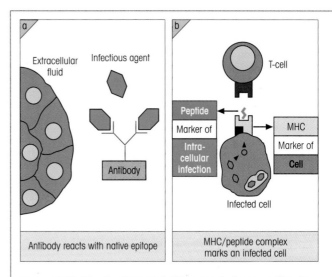

Figure 5.28. The fundamental difference between antibody and αβ T-cell receptor (TCR) recognition of antigen.

(a) Antibodies are formed against the native, not denatured, form of infectious agents that are attacked in the extracellular fluids. (b) Effector T-cells recognize infected cells by two surface markers: the MHC is a signal for the cell, and the foreign peptide is present in the MHC groove as it is derived from the proteins of an intracellular infectious agent. Further microbial cell surface signals can be provided by undegraded antigens and low molecular weight phosphate-containing antigens (seen by γδ T-cells), and lipids and glycolipids presented by CD1 molecules.

become infected with some virus or other, it is necessary for the MHC class I cell marker to be expressed by all nucleated cells in the body because cytotoxic killing requires intimate cell contact between the effector cytotoxic CD8$^+$ αβ T-cell and the class-I-expressing target (infected) cell. In contrast, the job of activating most helper and regulatory T-cells (which because they usually act by secreting cytokines do not need to directly contact the cells they influence) can be handed over to designated professional antigen-presenting cells that, in addition to expressing MHC class I, also express the MHC class II which is required for presentation of peptides to these CD4$^+$ αβ T-cells.

A comparable situation arises when CD1 molecules substitute for MHC in antigen presentation to T-cells, in this case associating with processed microbial lipids and glycolipids. The physiological role of the γδ cells has yet to be fully unraveled.

Antibody recognition
- Antibodies recognize molecular shapes (epitopes) on antigens.
- Most protein epitopes are discontinuous involving key residues from different parts of the linear sequence of the protein, although some are continuous and can be mimicked by linear peptides.
- The antibody-combining site forms a complementary surface to the epitope on the antigen and largely involves the CDRs of the antibody.
- Antibody-combining sites come in many shapes and sizes; anti-protein antibodies tend to have more extended recognition surfaces than antibodies to carbohydrates or peptides that are more likely to involve grooves or pockets.

- Both antibody and antigen can sometimes undergo local changes in conformation to permit interaction.

Eliciting antibodies

- Antigenicity (the ability of an antigen to be recognized by antibodies) can be distinguished from immunogenicity (the ability of an antigen (immunogen) to elicit antibodies when used to immunize an animal).
- Small molecule haptens only elicit antibodies when linked to a protein carrier molecule.
- Certain epitopes, usually those with the greatest accessibility on the surface of the protein, e.g. loops, elicit far stronger antibody responses than others.
- Many viruses, such as influenza and HIV, use the tendency of the antibody response to focus on immunodominant epitopes to "escape" antibody control.

Thermodynamics of antibody–antigen interaction

- Antibody–antigen interaction is reversible and subject to the laws of thermodynamics.
- The tendency of antibody and antigen to interact is reflected in a binding constant (K_a) and a free energy for the interaction (δG).
- Physiologically active antibodies mostly have binding constants of the order of 10^9/M ("nM binders").
- The energetics of antibody–antigen interaction is dominated by a few "hot spots."
- Multivalency can greatly enhance functional antibody affinity with significant physiological consequences, e.g. in toxin inactivation.
- High affinity physiologically active antibodies generally have much lower affinities for antigens other than the target antigen, i.e. they have low cross-reactivity.

T-cell recognition

- $\alpha\beta$ T-cells see antigen in association with MHC molecules.
- The T-cells are restricted to the haplotype of the cell to which they were initially primed.
- Protein antigens are processed by antigen-presenting cells to form small linear peptides that associate with the MHC molecules, binding to the central groove formed by the α-helices and the β-sheet floor.

Processing of antigen for presentation by class I MHC

- Endogenous cytosolic antigens such as viral proteins are cleaved by **immunoproteasomes** and the peptides so formed are **transported** to the ER by the TAP1/2 system.
- The peptide then dissociates from TAP1/2 and forms a stable heterotrimer with newly synthesized class I MHC heavy chain and β_2-microglobulin.
- This **peptide–MHC complex** is then transported to the surface for presentation to cytotoxic T-cells.

Processing of antigen for presentation by class II MHC

- The α and β chains of the **class II molecule** are synthesized in the ER and complex with membrane-bound **invariant chain (Ii)**.
- This facilitates transport of the vesicles containing class II across the Golgi and directs them to an acidified late endosome containing exogenous protein taken into the cell by endocytosis or phagocytosis.
- Proteolytic degradation of Ii in the class II enriched compartments (MIIC) leaves a peptide referred to as CLIP, which protects the MHC groove.
- Processing by endosomal proteases degrades the antigen to peptides, which replace the CLIP.
- The **class II–peptide** complex now appears on the cell surface for presentation to T-helper cells.

Cross-presentation

- Exogenous antigens can also be presented by MHC class I in dendritic cells through a post-endocytic pathway involving transfer into the cytosol by channels created by the Sec61 multimolecular complex followed by conventional proteasomal processing.
- By contrast, autophagy can transfer cytosolic peptides and proteins to the MIIC for subsequent presentation by class II.

The nature of the peptide

- Class I peptides are held in extended conformation within the MHC groove.
- They are usually 8–10 residues in length and have two or three key **anchors**, relatively invariant residues that bind to allele-specific pockets in the MHC.
- Class II peptides are between eight and 30 residues long, extend beyond the groove and usually have three or four anchor residues.
- The other amino acid residues in the peptide are greatly variable and are recognized by the T-cell receptor.

Complex between TCR, MHC and peptide

- The first and second hypervariable regions (CDR1 and CDR2) of each TCR chain mostly contact the MHC α-helices, while the CDR3s, having the greatest variability, interact with the antigenic peptide.

Some T-cells are independent of classical MHC molecules

■ MHC class I-like molecules, such as murine H-2M, are relatively nonpolymorphic and can present antigens such as bacterial *N*-formylmethionine peptides.

■ The CD1 family of non-MHC class I-like molecules can present antigens such as lipid and glycolipid mycobacterial antigens.

■ γδ T-cells resemble antibodies in recognizing whole unprocessed molecules such as low-molecular-weight, phosphate-containing, nonproteinaceous molecules.

Superantigens

■ These are potent mitogens that stimulate whole lymphocyte subpopulations sharing the same TCR Vβ or immunoglobulin V_H family independently of antigen specificity.

■ *Staphylococcus aureus* enterotoxins are powerful human superantigens that cause food poisoning and toxic shock syndrome.

■ T-cell superantigens are not processed but cross-link MHC class II and TCR Vβ independently of their direct interaction.

■ Mouse mammary tumor viruses are B-cell retroviruses that are superantigens in the mouse.

Recognition of different forms of antigen by B- and T-cells is an advantage

■ B-cells recognize epitopes on the native antigen; this is important because antibodies react with native antigen in the extracellular fluid.

■ Cytotoxic T-cells must contact infected cells and, to avoid confusion between the two systems, the infected cell signals itself to the T-cell by the combination of MHC class I and degraded antigen.

■ Helper and regulatory T-cells also recognize antigen that has been broken down into peptides, but in this case the MHC involved is the class II molecule found only on professional antigen-presenting cells.

FURTHER READING

Amigorena S. & Savina A. (2010) Intracellular mechanisms of antigen cross presentation in dendritic cells. *Current Opinion in Immunology* **22**, 109–117.

Boes M., Stoppelenburg A.J. & Sillé F.C.M. (2009) Endosomal processing for antigen presentation by CD1 and class I major histocompatibility complex: roads to display or destruction. *Immunology* **127**, 163–170.

Burton D.R., Stanfield R.L. & Wilson I.A. (2005) Antibody versus HIV in a clash of evolutionary titans. *Proceedings of the National Academy of Sciences USA* **102**, 14943–14948.

Chapman H.A. (2006) Endosomal proteases in antigen presentation. *Current Opinion in Immunology* **18**, 78–84.

Crotzer V.L. & Blum J.S. (2009) Autophagy and its role on MHC-mediated antigen presentation. *Journal of Immunology* **182**, 3335–3341.

Davies D.R. & Padlan E.A. (1990) Antibody–antigen complexes. *Annual Reviews of Biochemistry* **59**, 439–473.

Davis S.J. et al. (2003) The nature of molecular recognition by T-cells. *Nature Immunology* **4**, 217–224.

Finley D. (2009) Recognition and processing of ubiquitin-protein conjugates by the proteasome. *Annual Review of Biochemistry* **78**, 477–513.

Fraser J.D. & Proft T. (2008) The bacterial superantigen and superantigen-like proteins. *Immunological Reviews* **255**, 226–243.

Godfrey D.I., Rossjohn J. & McCluskey J. (2008) The fidelity, occasional promiscuity, and versatility of T cell receptor recognition. *Immunity* **28**, 304–314.

Heath W.R. et al. (2004) Cross-presentation, dendritic cell subsets, and the generation of immunity to cellular antigens. *Immunological Reviews* **199**, 9–26.

Marrack P. et al. (2008) Evolutionarily conserved amino acids in TCR V regions and MHC control their interaction. *Annual Review of Immunology* **26**, 171–203.

Moody D.B., Zajonc D.M. & Wilson I.A. (2005) Anatomy of CD1–lipid antigen complexes. *Nature Reviews Immunology* **5**, 387–399.

Nowakowski A. et al. (2002) Potent neutralization of botulinum neurotoxin by recombinant oligoclonal antibody. *Proceedings of the National Academy of Sciences USA* **99**, 11346–11350.

Padlan E.A. (1994) Anatomy of the antibody molecule. *Molecular Immunology* **31**, 169–217.

Procko E. et al. (2009) The mechanism of ABC transporters: general lessons from structural and functional studies of an antigenic peptide transporter. *The FASEB Journal* **23**, 1287–1302.

Raghavan M., Cid N.D., Rizvi S.M. & Peters L.R. (2008) MHC class I assembly: out and about. *Trends in Immunology* **29**, 436–443.

Rudd P.M. *et al.* (2001) Glycosylation and the immune system. *Science* **291**, 2370–2376.

Speak A.O., Cerundolo V. & Platt F.M. (2008) CD1d presentation of glycolipids. *Immunology and Cell Biology* **86**, 588–597.

Sundberg E.J. & Mariuzza R.A. (2002) Molecular recognition in antibody–antigen complexes. *Advances in Protein Chemistry* **61**, 119–160.

Trombetta E.S. & Mellman I. (2005) Cell biology of antigen processing *in vitro* and *in vivo*. *Annual Review of Immunology* **23**, 975–1028.

van den Eynde B.J. & Morel S. (2001) Differential processing of class I-restricted epitopes by the standard proteasome and the immunoproteasome. *Current Opinion in Immunology* **13**, 147–153.

Wearsch P.A. & Cresswell P. (2008) The quality control of MHC class I peptide loading. *Current Opinion in Cell Biology* **20**, 624–631.

Now visit **www.roitt.com** to test yourself on this chapter.

CHAPTER 6
Immunological methods and applications

Key Topics

Just to Recap ...

Now that the reader is familiar with all of the major elements of the innate and adaptive immune systems, it is instructive to consider how these elements can be manipulated *in vitro* and *in vivo*, either in the quest for further knowledge of immunity, or for the development of reagents (primarily antibody-based) that can be used for a huge number of applications. It is also very useful to know how immunologists go about the task of discovering the knowledge we have gamely tried to summarize within these pages. The methods and applications described in this chapter will hopefully explain how, in practical terms, one would go about measuring cytokine production by individual T-cell subsets, or antibody production by B-cells, or apoptosis induced by NK cells, and so on.

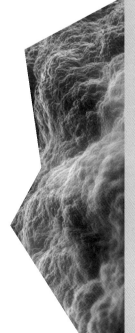

Roitt's Essential Immunology, Twelfth Edition. Peter J. Delves, Seamus J. Martin, Dennis R. Burton, Ivan M. Roitt.
© 2011 Peter J. Delves, Seamus J. Martin, Dennis R. Burton, Ivan M. Roitt. Published 2011 by Blackwell Publishing Ltd.

Introduction

This chapter is structured such that we will progress from molecular- to cell-based techniques, and then on to whole animal-based approaches. We will initially consider how antibodies can be generated and purified, how they can in turn be used to purify their specific antigen from complex mixtures of antigen, how they can be used to functionally mimic natural ligands for the purposes of stimulating cell function, or conversely, inhibiting specific functions, as well as many other applications. We will then take a look at a series of variations on the theme of using antibody to detect antigen in cells, in tissues, in fluids as well as solid supports (such as protein arrays) and we will also explore how the discrete regions within an antigen that are recognized by antibodies, or T-cell receptors (i.e. their specific epitopes), can be mapped. The second half of the chapter is devoted to cell-based methods that are used to assess the functionality and interactions between cells of the immune system. We will discuss how cells of the immune system can be isolated, phenotyped, functionally assessed, and genetically manipulated both *in vitro* as well as *in vivo*. We will then look at some of the animal models that are commonly used by immunologists and how genetically engineered animals can be produced.

Many of the procedures we discuss in this chapter have been painstakingly developed and refined by several generations of immunologists and range from the straightforward to the highly complex. It is sobering to be reminded that, when we make statements such as *"an antibody was generated,"* the work involved typically takes many months, if not years. Similarly, while *"gene X was knocked out in the mouse"* rolls off the tongue in a mere two seconds, you can take it from us that the procedure itself occupied someone for a couple of years.

Making antibodies to order

In addition to being quite handy for protecting our bodies from harmful infectious agents, antibodies are also incredibly useful and exquisitely specific reagents for detecting and quantitating other proteins, as well as many other substances. Antibodies have, quite literally, numerous practical applications; ranging from the purification of proteins using antibody-based affinity columns, the detection of circulating hormones in blood or urine samples for clinical diagnosis, the exploration of expression and subcellular localization of proteins, as immunotherapeutics in cancer therapy and as antidotes for snake and spider bites. Indeed, to the research scientist, a world without antibodies is very hard to contemplate as these molecules are used daily as highly specific and reliable probes for virtually every protein under the sun, in a multitude of contexts. We shall now take a look, in practical terms, at how these wonderfully adaptable proteins can be produced in the laboratory.

Generation of polyclonal antibodies

Although antibodies can be raised against practically any organic substance, some molecules elicit antibody responses much more readily than others. Proteins usually make excellent immunogens (i.e. substances that can elicit an immune response), although the immune response will typically be concentrated against small regions within the protein (called epitopes or antigenic determinants) spanning approximately five to eight amino acids. As we discussed earlier (see Chapter 5), an epitope represents the minimal structure required for recognition by antibody and a relatively large molecule, such as a protein, will usually contain multiple epitopes. Thus, injection of the average antigen into an animal will almost always

elicit the production of a mixture of antibodies that are directed against different epitopes within the antigen. It is also quite possible that some of the antibodies within this mixture may be directed towards epitopes that are also found in other antigens. Such antibodies are said to be cross-reactive against the other antigen to which they also bind. Small organic molecules are typically poor immunogens when injected on their own; the immune system appears unable to recognize these structures efficiently. Notwithstanding this, immunologists have found that such molecules can be made visible to the immune system by covalent coupling to a carrier protein, such as bovine serum albumin (BSA), which is intrinsically immunogenic. Such small molecules are called haptens (see Figure 5.6).

To generate an antibody against a protein of interest, the standard approach is to inject small samples of the protein (in the microgram range) into an animal such as a rabbit. However, administration of antigen alone is rarely sufficient to provoke a robust immune response, even if the antigen is composed of a high proportion of nonself determinants; co-administration of an **adjuvant** is required (Figure 6.1). While it is not entirely clear exactly how adjuvants work, one important role they peform is to **activate dendritics cells (DCs) and other antigen-presenting cells (APCs)** at the site of antigen delivery (see p. 30). Recall from Chapter 1 that activation of APCs dramatically enhances their ability to provide the co-stimulatory signals that are required for efficient T- and B-cell activation upon encounter with antigen. The reader will recall that pathogen-associated molecular patterns (PAMPs) are typically required to trigger maturation of dendritic cells and trigger their movement to secondary lymphoid tissues for the purposes of presenting nonself antigens to T-cells, which in turn provides T-cell-dependent help to B-cells for class switching, affinity maturation and optimum antibody production.

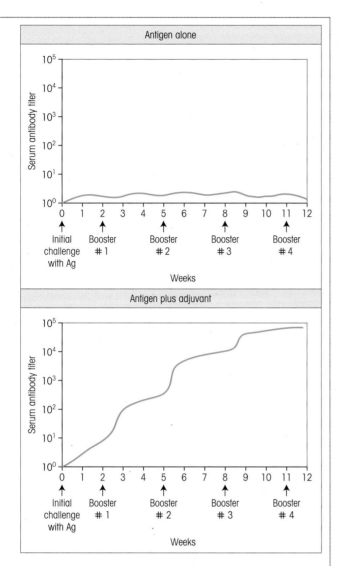

Figure 6.1. Production of polyclonal antibodies.

Repeated immunization with antigen (Ag) plus adjuvant is required to generate efficient antibody responses as immunization with antigen alone is usually ineffective. Polyclonal antisera are generated by immunizing, with a combination of antigen plus adjuvant, several times over a 12-week period. Serum antibody titre (i.e. the highest dilution giving a positive test) frequently increases after each successive boost with antigen.

Potent adjuvants are usually crude preparations of bacterial extracts that contain mixtures of Toll-like receptor (TLR) ligands such as LPS or peptidoglycan. In essence, most adjuvants are mixtures of PAMPs, which activate DCs and other cells of the innate immune system through their pattern recognition receptors (PRRs). Because DCs are incapable of providing essential co-stimulatory signals to T-cells unless activated through their PRRs, antigens that lack intrinsic PRR-binding activity will fail to activate DCs and therefore fail to elicit potent immune responses on their own.

As we outlined in Chapter 2, because a single dose of antigen usually elicits a relatively modest response (see Figure 2.13), the antigen is therefore injected several times over a period of 12 weeks or so. During this time, the concentration of antibodies (what is usually referred to as **antibody titer**) directed against the immunogen will increase (Figure 6.1). All going well, we will now have an antiserum that is *enriched* with antibodies against our protein of interest and this can be used as a probe in many different contexts; to localize an antigen within a cell, to quantify it within a mixture of other antigens, to neutralize its biological activity, and many other applications (these are elaborated upon later in this chapter).

It is important to remind ourselves here that antisera generated in this way will also contain considerable amounts of other antibodies (directed against a variety of determinants) that the animal happens to have made in the recent past. These antibodies will usually be of a significantly lower titer than those directed against the antigen we have repeatedly used for immunization, but they can cause problems and may need to be removed from our antiserum for several applications. Fortunately, this can be achieved by **affinity purification** where specific antigen is immobilized on a solid support and used to "fish" out its specific antibody from a crude mixture of antibodies (see Figure 6.6).

Because many antigens contain several distinct epitopes, antisera generated by injection of antigen will typically contain a mixture of antibodies directed against different antigenic determinants on the molecule. Some of these antibodies will bind to the antigen with high avidity, some will not, some will only recognize the native form of the antigen, while others will still recognize the antigen following denaturation to eliminate tertiary structure. Such antisera are said to be **polyclonal** as they contain a mixture of antibodies that are predominantly, although not exclusively, directed against the immunogen to which they were raised.

The monoclonal antibody revolution

First in rodents

A fantastic technological breakthrough was achieved by Georges Köhler and César Milstein who devised a technique for the production of "immortal" clones of cells making single antibody specificities by fusing normal antibody-forming cells with an appropriate B-cell tumor line. Normal untransformed B-cells cannot be grown in culture for long periods of time and quickly die off unless immortalized. This truly paradigm-shifting method enables individual B-cell clones to be grown in tissue culture and expanded to a point where enormous quantities of antigen-specific antibody can be produced. These so-called **"hybridomas"** are selected out in a tissue culture medium that fails to support growth of the parental cell types and, by successive dilutions or by plating out, single clones can be established (Figure 6.2). These clones can be grown up in the ascitic form in mice when quite prodigious titers of **monoclonal antibody** can be attained, but bearing in mind the imperative to avoid using animals wherever feasible, propagation in large-scale culture is to be preferred. Remember that, even in a good antiserum, over 90% of the Ig molecules have

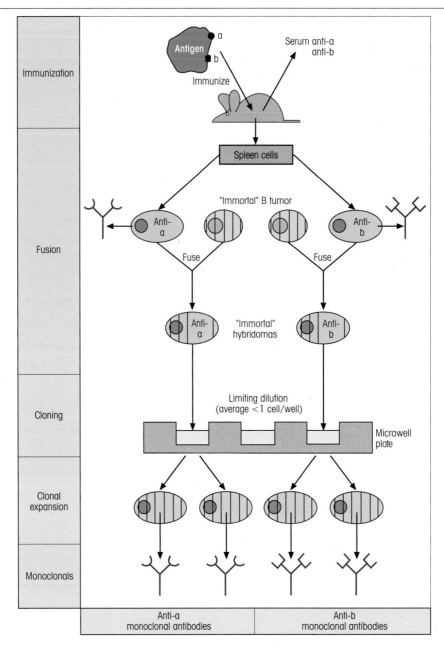

Figure 6.2. Production of monoclonal antibodies.

Mice immunized with an antigen bearing (shall we say) two epitopes, a and b, develop spleen cells making anti-a and anti-b and which appear as antibodies in the serum. The spleen is removed and the individual cells are fused in polyethylene glycol with constantly dividing (i.e. "immortal") B-tumor cells selected for a purine enzyme deficiency and usually for their inability to secrete Ig. The resulting cells are distributed into micro-well plates in HAT (hypoxanthine, aminopterin, and thymidine) medium that kills off the fusion partners. They are seeded at such a dilution that on average each well will contain less than one hybridoma cell. Each hybridoma—the fusion product of a single antibody-forming cell and a tumor cell—will have the ability of the former to secrete a single species of antibody and the immortality of the latter enabling it to proliferate continuously. Thus, clonal progeny can provide an unending supply of antibody with a single specificity—the monoclonal antibody. In this example, we considered the production of hybridomas with specificity for just two epitopes, but the same technique enables monoclonal antibodies to be raised against complex mixtures of multiepitopic antigens. Fusions using rat cells instead of mouse may have

certain advantages in giving a higher proportion of stable hybridomas, and monoclonals that are better at fixing human complement, a useful attribute in the context of therapeutic applications to humans involving cell depletion.

Naturally, for use in the human, the ideal solution is the production of purely human monoclonals. Human myeloma fusion partners have not found wide acceptance as they tend to have low fusion efficiencies, poor growth and secretion of the myeloma Ig which dilutes the desired monoclonal. A nonsecreting heterohybridoma (to avoid the formation of mixed antibody specificities) obtained by fusing a mouse myeloma with human B-cells can be used as a productive fusion partner for antibody-producing human B-cells. Other groups have turned to the well-characterized murine fusion partners, and the heterohybridomas so formed grow well, clone easily and are productive. There is some instability from chromosome loss and it appears that antibody production is maintained by translocation of human *Ig* genes to mouse chromosomes. Fusion frequency is even better if Epstein–Barr virus (EBV)-transformed lines are used instead of B-cells.

little or no avidity for the antigen, and the "specific antibodies" themselves represent a whole spectrum of molecules with different avidities directed against different determinants on the antigen. What a contrast is provided by monoclonal antibodies, where all the molecules produced by a given hybridoma are identical: they have the same Ig class and allotype, the same variable region, structure, idiotype, affinity and specificity for a given epitope.

The large amount of nonspecific, relative to antigen-specific, Ig in a polyclonal antiserum means that background binding to antigen in any given immunological test may be uncomfortably high. This problem is greatly reduced with a monoclonal antibody preparation, as all the antibody is antigen-specific, thus giving a much superior "signal : noise" ratio. By being directed towards single epitopes on the antigen, monoclonal antibodies frequently show high specificity in terms of their low cross-reactivity with other antigens.

An outstanding advantage of the monoclonal antibody as a reagent is that it provides a single standard material for all laboratories throughout the world to use in an unending supply if the immortality and purity of the cell line are nurtured; antisera raised in different animals, on the other hand, may be as different from each other as chalk and cheese. The monoclonal approach again shows a clean pair of heels relative to conventional strategies in the production of antibodies specific for individual components in a complex mixture of antigens. The uses of monoclonal antibodies are truly legion and include: immunoassay, diagnosis of malignancies, tissue typing, serotyping of microorganisms, the separation of individual cell types with specific surface markers (e.g. lymphocyte subpopulations), therapeutic neutralization of inflammatory cytokines and "magic bullet" therapy with cytotoxic agents coupled to antitumor-specific antibody—these and many other areas have been transformed by hybridoma technology.

Catalytic antibodies

An especially interesting development with tremendous potential is the recognition that a monoclonal antibody to a stable analog of the transition state of a given reaction can act as an enzyme ("abzyme") in catalyzing that reaction. The possibility of generating enzymes to order promises a very attractive future, and some exceedingly adroit chemical maneuvers have already extended the range of reactions that can be catalyzed in this way. A recent demonstration of sequence-specific peptide cleavage with an antibody that incorporates a metal complex cofactor has raised the pulse rate of the *cognoscenti*, as this is an energetically difficult reaction that has an enormous range of applications. Another innovative approach is to immunize with an antigen that is so highly reactive that a chemical reaction occurs in the antibody combining site. This recruits antibodies that are not only complementary to the active chemical, but are also likely to have some enzymic power over the immunogen–substrate complex. Thus, using this strategy, an antibody with exceptionally broad substrate specificity for efficient catalysis

of aldol and retro-aldol reactions was obtained. A key feature of this antibody is a reactive lysine buried within a hydrophobic pocket in the binding site. The antibody remains catalytically active for several weeks following i.v. injection into mice and has therapeutic potential for a version of antibody-directed enzyme prodrug therapy (see p. 471), here with the enzyme component being a catalytic antibody.

Large combinatorial antibody libraries created by random association between pools of heavy and light chains and expressed on bacteriophages (see below) can be screened for catalytic antibodies by using the substrate in a solid-phase state. Cleavage by the catalytic antibody leaves a solid-phase product that can now be identified by a double antibody system using antibodies specific for the product as distinct from the substrate.

An area of great interest is the presence of catalytic auto-antibodies in certain groups of patients, with hydrolytic antibodies against vasoactive intestinal peptide, DNA and thyroglobulin having been described. Catalytic antibodies capable of factor VIII hydrolysis have also recently been discovered in hemophiliacs given this clotting factor, the antibodies preventing the coagulation function of the factor VIII.

Human monoclonals can be made

While scientists were quick to realize that monoclonal antibodies would make powerful and highly specific therapeutic agents, particularly for the treatment of cancer, this proved to be rather more difficult than originally anticipated. Mouse monoclonals injected into human subjects for therapeutic purposes are frightfully immunogenic and the human anti-mouse antibodies (HAMA in the trade) so formed are a wretched nuisance, accelerating clearance of the monoclonal from the blood and possibly causing hypersensitivity reactions; they also prevent the mouse antibody from reaching its target and, in some cases, block its binding to antigen. In some circumstances it is conceivable that a mouse monoclonal taken up by a tumor cell could be processed and become the MHC-linked target of cytotoxic T-cells or help to boost the response to a weakly immunogenic antigen on the tumor cell surface. In general, however, logic points to removal of the xenogeneic (foreign) portions of the monoclonal antibody and their replacement by human Ig structures using recombinant DNA technology. Chimeric constructs, in which the V_H and V_L mouse domains are spliced onto human C_H and C_L genes (Figure 6.3a), are far less immunogenic in humans.

A more refined approach is to graft the six complementarity determining regions (CDRs) of a high affinity rodent monoclonal onto a completely human Ig framework without loss of specific reactivity (Figure 6.3b). This is not a trivial exercise, however, and the objective of fusing human B-cells to make hybridomas is still appealing, taking into account not only the gross reduction in immunogenicity, but also the fact that, within a species, antibodies can be made to subtle differences such as major histocompatibility complex (MHC)

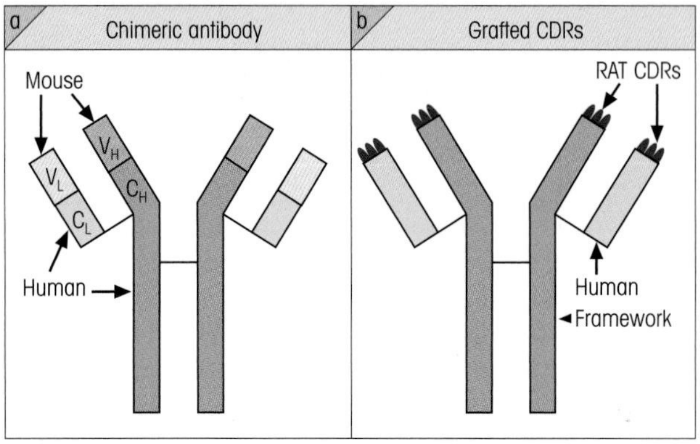

Figure 6.3. Genetically engineering rodent antibody specificities into the human.

(a) Chimeric antibody with mouse variable regions fused to human Ig constant regions. (b) "Humanized" rat monoclonal in which gene segments coding for all six complementarity determining regions (CDRs) are grafted on to a human Ig framework.

polymorphic molecules and tumor-associated antigens on other individuals. In contrast, xenogeneic responses are more directed to immunodominant structures common to most subjects, making the production of variant-specific antibodies more difficult. Notwithstanding the difficulties in finding good fusion partners, large numbers of human monoclonals have been established. A further restriction arises because the peripheral blood B-cells, which are the only B-cells readily available in the human, are not normally regarded as a good source of antibody-forming cells.

Immortalized Epstein–Barr virus-transformed B-cell lines have also been used as a source of human monoclonal antibodies. Although these often produce relatively low affinity IgM antibodies, some useful higher-affinity IgG antibodies can occasionally be obtained. The cell lines frequently lose their ability to secrete antibody if cultured for long periods of time, although they can sometimes be rescued by fusion with a myeloma cell line to produce hybridomas, or the genes can be isolated and used to produce a recombinant antibody.

A radically different approach involves the production of transgenic xenomouse strains in which megabase-sized unrearranged human Ig *H* and *κ* light chain loci have been introduced into mice whose endogenous murine *Ig* genes have been inactivated. Immunization of these mice yields high-affinity (10^{-10}–10^{-11} M) human antibodies that can then be isolated using hybridoma or recombinant approaches. Potent anti-inflammatory (anti-IL-8) and anti-tumor (anti-epidermal growth factor receptor) therapeutic agents have already been obtained using such mice.

There is still a snag in that even human antibodies can provoke anti-idiotype responses; these may have to be circumvented by using engineered antibodies bearing different idiotypes for subsequent injections. Even more desirable would be if the prospective recipients could be first made tolerant to the

idiotype, perhaps by coadministering the therapeutic antibody together with a nondepleting anti-CD4.

Despite the difficulties involved, a battery of humanized monoclonals has now been approved for therapeutic use. These include: anti-IL-2 (kidney transplant rejection), anti-VEGF (colorectal cancer), anti-TNFα (rheumatoid arthritis), anti-CD11a (psoriasis), anti-CD52 (B-cell chronic lymphocytic leukaemia), anti-CD33 (acute myelogenous leukaemia), anti-HER2 (a subset of metastatic breast cancers) and several others (cf. Table 17.2). Many more are currently in the clinical trial pipeline and are likely to become routinely used in clinical practice in the coming years.

Engineering antibodies

There are other ways around the problems associated with the production of human monoclonals that exploit the wiles of modern molecular biology. Reference has already been made to the "humanizing" of rodent antibodies (Figure 6.3), but an important new strategy based upon **bacteriophage expression** and **selection** has achieved a prominent position. In essence, mRNA from primed human B-cells is converted to cDNA (complementary DNA) and the antibody genes, or fragments therefrom, expanded by the polymerase chain reaction (PCR). Single constructs are then made in which the light and heavy chain genes are allowed to combine randomly in tandem with the gene encoding bacteriophage coat protein III (pIII) (Figure 6.4). This **combinatorial library** containing most random pairings of heavy and light chain genes encodes a huge repertoire of antibodies (or their fragments) expressed as fusion proteins with pIII on the bacteriophage surface. The extremely high number of phages produced by *E. coli* infection can now be panned on solid-phase antigen to select those bearing the highest affinity antibodies attached to their surface (Figure 6.4). Because the genes that encode these highest affinity antibodies are already present within the selected phage, they can readily be cloned and the antibody expressed in bulk. It should be recognized that this **selection** procedure has an enormous advantage over techniques that employ **screening** because the number of phages that can be examined is several logs higher.

Combinatorial libraries have also been established using mRNA from **unimmunized** human donors. V_H, V_k and V_l genes are expanded by PCR and randomly recombined to form single-chain Fv (scFv) constructs (Figure 6.5a) fused to phage pIII. Soluble fragments binding to a variety of antigens have been obtained. Of special interest are those that are autoantibodies to molecules with therapeutic potential such as CD4 and tumor necrosis factor-α (TNFα); lymphocytes expressing such autoantibodies could not be obtained by normal immunization as they would probably be tolerized, but the random recombination of V_H and V_L can produce entirely new specificities under conditions *in vitro* where tolerance mechanisms do not operate.

Although a "test-tube" operation, this approach to the generation of specific antibodies does resemble the affinity maturation of the immune response *in vivo* (see p. 254) in the sense

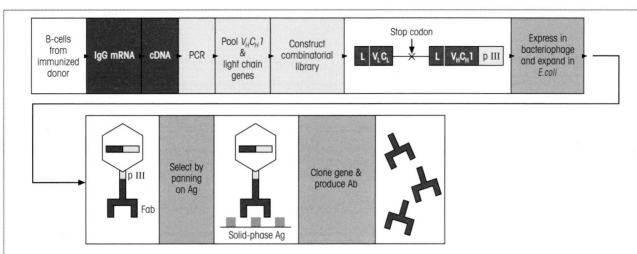

Figure 6.4. Selection of antibody genes from a combinatorial library.

B-cells from an immunized donor (in one important experiment, human memory peripheral blood cells were boosted with tetanus toxoid antigen after transfer to SCID mice; Duchosal M.A. *et al.* (1992) *Nature* **355**, 258) are used for the extraction of IgG mRNA and the light chain (V_LC_L) and V_HC_H1 genes (encoding Fab) randomly combined in constructs fused to the bacteriophage pIII coat protein gene as shown. These were incorporated into phagemids such as pHEN1 and expanded in *E. coli*. After infection with helper phage, the recombinant phages bearing the highest affinity were selected by rounds of panning on solid-phase antigen so that the genes encoding the Fab fragments could be cloned. Ab, antibody; Ag, antigen; L, bacterial leader sequence.

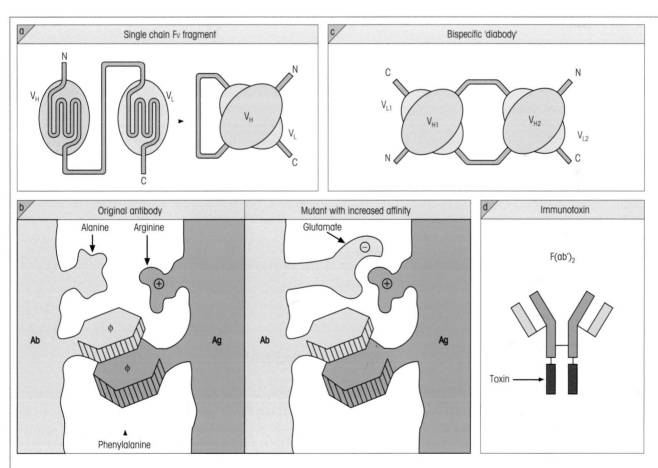

Figure 6.5. Other engineered antibodies.

(a) A single gene encoding V_H and V_L joined by a sequence of suitable length gives rise to a single-chain Fv (scFv) antigen-binding fragment. (b) By site-specific mutagenesis of residues in or adjacent to the complementarity determining region (CDR), it is possible to increase the affinity of the antibody. (c) Two scFv constructs expressed simultaneously will associate to form a "diabody" with two specificities. These bispecific antibodies have a number of uses. Note that such a bispecific antibody (Ab) directed to two different epitopes on the same antigen (Ag) will have a much higher affinity due to the "bonus effect" of cooperation between the two binding sites (cf. p. 122). (d) Potential "magic bullets" can be constructed by fusing the gene for a toxin (e.g. ricin) to the Fab.

that antigen is the determining factor in selecting out the highest affinity responders.

In order to increase the affinities of antibodies produced by these techniques, antigen can be used to select higher affinity mutants produced by random mutagenesis or even more effectively by site-directed replacements at mutational hotspots (Figure 6.5b), again mimicking the natural immune response that involves random mutation and antigen selection (see pp. 248–250). Affinity has also been improved by gene "shuffling" in which a V_H gene encoding a reasonable affinity antibody is randomly combined with a pool of V_L genes and subjected to antigen selection. The process can be further extended by mixing the V_L from this combination with a pool of V_H genes. It has also proved possible to shuffle individual CDRs between variable regions of moderate affinity antibodies obtained by panning on antigen, thereby creating antibodies of high affinity from relatively small libraries. The isolation of high-affinity, llama, heavy-chain antibody V_{HH} fragments from immunized animals represents yet another approach.

Other novel antibodies have been created. In one construct, two scFv fragments associate to form an antibody with two different specificities (Figure 6.5c). Another consists of a single heavy chain variable region domain (DAB) whose affinity can be surprisingly high—of the order of 20 nM. If it were possible to overcome the "stickiness" of these miniantibodies, their small size could be exploited for tissue penetration. The design of potential "magic bullets" for immunotherapy can be based on fusion of a toxin (e.g. ricin) to an antibody Fab (Figure 6.5d).

Fields of antibodies

Not only can the genes for a monoclonal antibody be expressed in bulk in the milk of lactating animals but plants can also be exploited for this purpose. So-called "**plantibodies**" have been expressed in bananas, potatoes and tobacco plants. One can imagine a high-tech farmer drawing the attention of a bemused visitor to one field growing anti-tetanus toxoid, another anti-meningococcal polysaccharide, and so on. Multifunctional plants might be quite profitable with, say, the root being harvested as a food crop and the leaves expressing some desirable gene product. At this rate there may not be much left for science fiction authors to write about!

Drugs can be based on the CDRs of minibodies

Millions of **minibodies** composed of a segment of the V_H region containing three β-strands and the H1 and H2 hypervariable loops were generated by randomization of the CDRs and expressed on the bacteriophage pIII coat protein. By panning the library on functionally important ligand-binding sites, such as hormone receptors, useful lead candidates for drug design programs can be identified and their affinity improved by loop optimization, loop shuffling and further selection.

Purification of antigens and antibodies by affinity chromatography

The principle is simple and *very* widely applied. Antigen or antibody is bound through its free amino groups to cyanogen bromide-activated Sepharose particles or some other solid support. Immobilized antibody, for example, can be used to extract the corresponding antigen out of solution, in which it is present as one component of a complex mixture, by absorption to its surface. The uninteresting garbage is washed away and the required ligand released from the affinity absorbent by disruption of the antigen–antibody bonds by changing the pH or adding chaotropic ions such as thiocyanate (Figure 6.6). This technique can be used to identify the antigen to which an antibody binds where this is not known; in the case of an autoantibody for example. A very similar approach can also be used to identify **binding partners** for an antigen; such molecules will usually stay attached to the antigen if the immunopurification procedure is carried out under gentle conditions. Many of the proteins that participate in T-cell receptor (TCR) signal transduction, for instance, were initially identified by using antibodies directed against known TCR signalling components to pull out these components from complex protein mixtures, along with their binding-partners. Isolated llama heavy chain (V_{HH}) fragments are proving to be valuable for repeated cycles of antigen purification because of their resistance to denaturation by repeated cycles of exposure to low pH.

In a similar manner, an antigen immunosorbent can be used to absorb out an antibody from a mixture whence it can be purified by elution (Figure 6.6). This is especially useful where an antiserum displays high levels of nonspecific reactivity against other antigens rendering it unusable. Affinity-purification of such an antiserum, by means of the antigen that was used to generate it, can often dramatically improve its specificity.

Modulation of biological activity by antibodies

To detect antibody

A number of biological reactions can be inhibited by addition of specific antibody. Thus the agglutination of red cells by interaction of influenza virus with receptors on the erythrocyte surface can be blocked by antiviral antibodies and this forms the basis for their serological detection. A test for antibodies to salmonella H antigen present on the flagella depends upon their ability to inhibit the motility of the bacteria *in vitro*. Likewise, mycoplasma antibodies can be demonstrated by their inhibitory effect on the metabolism of the organisms in culture.

Using antibody as an inhibitor

The successful treatment of cases of drug overdose with the Fab fragment of specific antibodies has been described and may

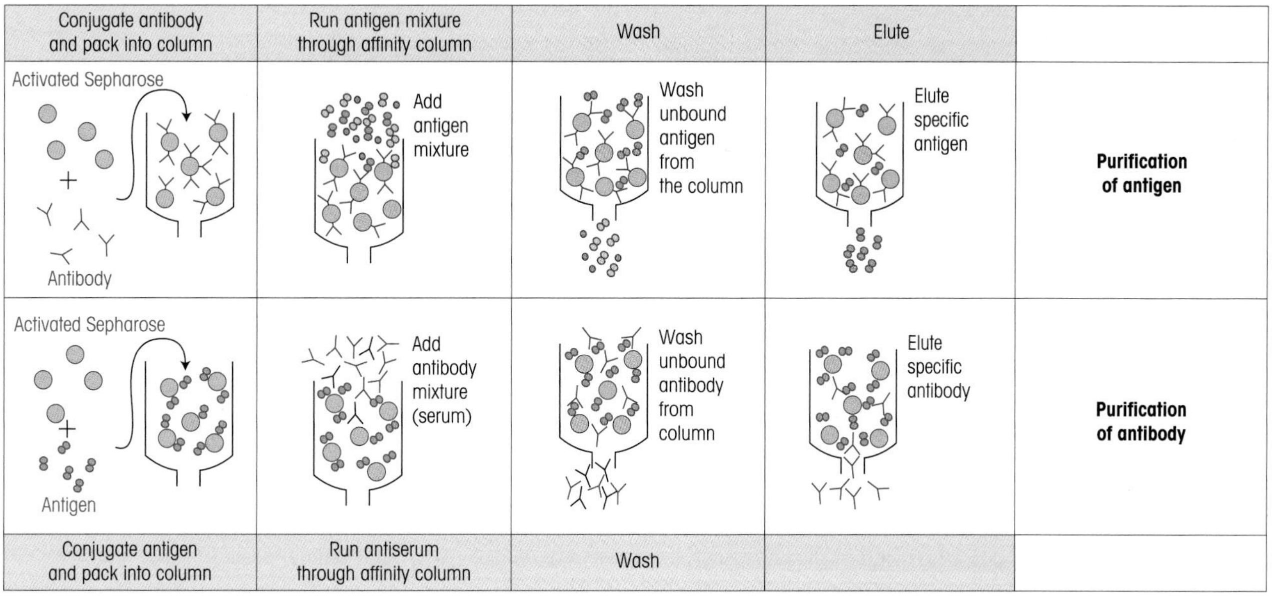

Figure 6.6. Affinity purification of antigen and antibody.

Antibody can be immobilized on activated sepharose and used to affinity-purify antigen. Depending on the conditions used to carry out the assay, antigen-associated proteins may also be captured by this procedure. For the purification of specific antibody from a polyclonal antiserum, antigen is immobilized on Sepharose beads and nonspecific unbound antibodies fail to be captured and can be washed away. After capture, specific antibody can be eluted by transiently lowering the pH or increasing the salt concentration of the buffer.

become a practical proposition if a range of hybridomas can be assembled. Conjugates of cocaine with keyhole limpet hemocyanin (the latter is used as a carrier to elicit efficient Ab production to cocaine) can provoke neutralizing antibodies. Antibodies to hormones such as insulin and thyroid-stimulating hormone (TSH), or to cytokines, can be used to probe the specificity of biological reactions *in vitro*. For example, the specificity of the insulin-like activity of a serum sample on rat epididymal fat pad can be checked by the neutralizing effect of an antiserum. Such antibodies can be effective *in vivo*, and anti-TNF treatment of patients with rheumatoid arthritis has confirmed the role of this cytokine in the disease process. Likewise, as part of the worldwide effort to prevent disastrous overpopulation, attempts are in progress to immunize against chorionic gonadotropin using fragments of the β chain coupled to appropriate carriers, as this hormone is needed to sustain the implanted ovum.

In a totally different context, antibodies raised against myelin-associated neurite growth inhibitory proteins revealed their importance in preventing nerve repair, in that treatment with these antibodies permitted the regeneration of corticospinal axons after a spinal cord lesion had been induced in adult rats. This quite remarkable finding significantly advances our understanding of the processes involved in regeneration and gives ground for cautious optimism concerning the develop-

ment of treatment for spinal cord damage, although for various reasons this may not ultimately be based on antibody therapy.

Using antibody as an activator

Antibodies can also be used to substitute for natural biological ligands, either because the ligand is unknown, is difficult to purify, or would require a small mortgage to be able to afford it! For example, antibodies can be used instead of ligand to stimulate cell-surface receptors that propagate signals into the cell upon cross-linking. Normally, the natural ligand for the receptor would promote receptor cross-linking but antibodies can be used to mimic this very efficiently. Such an approach has been used to great effect to study intracellular events that take place upon stimulation of T- or B-cell receptor complexes by antibodies directed against these receptors or associated proteins (such as the CD3 complex). In a similar vein, antibodies directed against the Fas (CD95) cell surface receptor can substitute for the natural ligand (FasL/CD95L) in order to stimulate the receptor and study the consequences of this. In the latter case, stimulation of Fas by anti-Fas antibodies induces rapid programmed cell death (apoptosis) in cells bearing this receptor (Figure 6.7). Another good example is the induction of histamine release from mast cells by divalent F(ab′)$_2$ anti-FcεRI but not by the univalent fragment. Antibody-induced

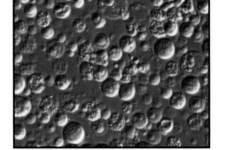

Untreated   anti-Fas

Figure 6.7. Antibody-induced receptor activation.

Transformed Jurkat T-cells were either left untreated, or were treated with anti-Fas IgM antibody for 4 hours. Cross-linking of the Fas (CD95) receptor with antibody activates the receptor and results in a signal transduction cascade that culminates in activation of a series of cysteine proteases, called caspases, that provoke apoptosis in the stimulated cell. Apoptotic cells exhibit plasma membrane blebbing and collapse of the cell into small fragments or vesicles termed "apoptotic bodies." Similar effects are also seen when the natural ligand, FasL, is used instead of anti-Fas antibody. (Kindly provided by Dr. Colin Adrain, Dept. of Genetics, Trinity College, Dublin, Ireland.)

Figure 6.8. The basis of fluorescence antibody tests for identification of tissue antigens or their antibodies.

⬤ = fluorescein labeled.

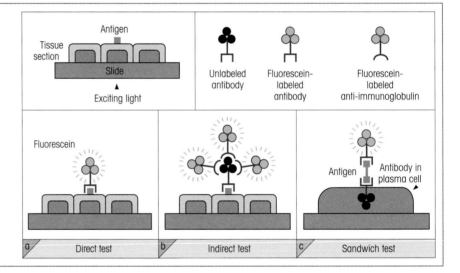

activation can be used to study the signal transduction cascade downstream of receptor engagement by ligand, even where the ligand has not yet been identified.

Immunodetection of antigen in cells and tissues

Immunofluorescence microscopy

Antibodies can be used as highly sensitive probes to explore the subcellular localization of a protein (or other antigenic determinant) within a cell or a tissue. Because fluorescent dyes such as fluorescein and rhodamine can be coupled to antibodies without destroying their specificity, the conjugates can combine with antigen present in a tissue section and be visualized using a microscope equipped with an appropriate light source (typically UV light). Looked at another way, the method can also be used for the detection of antibodies directed against antigens already known to be present in a given tissue section or cell preparation. Before applying the antibody to the cell or tissue preparation, samples require fixation and permeabilization in order to preserve cellular structures and to permit free passage of antibody across the plasma membrane. There are two general ways in which the test is carried out.

Direct test with labeled antibody

The antibody to the tissue antigen is directly conjugated with the fluorochrome and applied to the sample (Figure 6.8a). Binding of the antibody to the antigen is betrayed by that part of the cell becoming fluorescent when illuminated using UV light. For example, suppose we wished to show the distribution

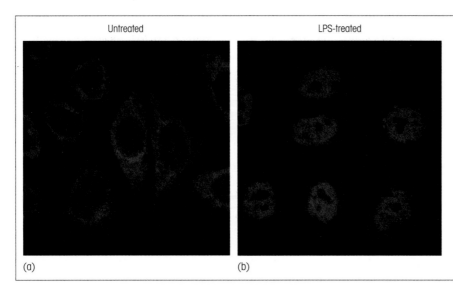

Untreated   LPS-treated

(a)   (b)

Figure 6.9. Immunolocalization of a transcription factor upon receptor stimulation.

Transformed human monocytes (THP-1 cells) were either left untreated (a), or were stimulated with bacterial lipopolysaccharide (LPS) for 2 hours (b). Cells were then fixed and immunostained with an anti-NFκB antibody. Note that in unstimulated cells NFκB is abundantly present in the cell cytoplasm but is excluded from the nucleus, whereas the reverse is true in LPS-stimulated cells. (Courtesy of Dr. Lisa Bouchier-Hayes, St. Jude's Hospital, Memphis, USA.)

of a thyroid autoantigen reacting with the autoantibodies present in the serum of a patient with Hashimoto's disease, a type of thyroid autoimmunity. We would isolate IgG from the patient's serum, conjugate it with fluorescein, and apply it to a section of human thyroid on a slide. When viewed in the fluorescence microscope we would see that the cytoplasm of the follicular epithelial cells was brightly stained (cf. Figure 18.1a).

Let's consider another example to illustrate the versatility of this technique. We have just generated a monoclonal antibody to a transcription factor (NFκB for example) that is known to be important for LPS-induced macrophage activation and IL-1β production. We could compare resting versus LPS-treated macrophages to determine whether the transcription factor does anything "interesting" upon exposure of macrophages to LPS. Recall from Chapter 1 (see Figure 1.9) that NFκB is normally tethered in the cytoplasm and prevented from gaining access to the nucleus as a result of interaction with its inhibitor, IκB. Upon stimulation of the TLR4 receptor with LPS, a chain of signal transduction events is set in motion that culminates in the degradation of IκB freeing up NFκB to translocate to the nucleus and initiate gene transcription (see Figure 1.9). Thus, using an antibody against NFκB we would observe that, whereas resting macrophages contain lots of NFκB, it all appears to be in the cytoplasm. However, we would also certainly note that within minutes of exposure to LPS, practically all of the NFκB had moved to the nucleus (Figure 6.9).

By using two (or even three) antisera conjugated to dyes that emit fluorescence at different wavelengths (Figure 6.10), several different antigens can be identified simultaneously in the same preparation. In Figure 2.7e, direct staining of fixed plasma cells with a mixture of rhodamine-labeled anti-IgG and fluorescein-conjugated anti-IgM craftily demonstrates that these two classes of antibody are produced by different cells. The technique of coupling biotin to the antiserum and then finally staining with fluorescent avidin is often employed.

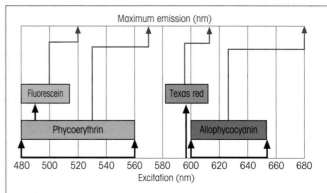

Maximum emission (nm)

Fluorescein   Texas red

Phycoerythrin   Allophycocyanin

480   500   520   540   560   580   600   620   640   660   680

Excitation (nm)

Figure 6.10. Fluorescent labels used in immunofluorescence microscopy and flow cytometry.

The fluorescein longer wave emission overlaps with that of Texas red and is corrected for in the software. The phycobiliproteins of red algae and cyanobacteria effect energy transfer of blue light to chlorophyll for photosynthesis; each molecule has many fluorescent groups giving a broad excitation range, but fluorescence is emitted within a narrow wavelength band with such high quantum efficiency as to obviate the need for a second amplifying antibody.

Indirect test with labeled secondary antibody

In this double-layer technique, which is the most commonly adopted approach, the unlabeled antibody (the primary antibody) is applied directly to the tissue and visualized by treatment with a fluorochrome-conjugated anti-immunoglobulin serum (the secondary antibody; Figure 6.8b). Anti-immunoglobulin antisera are widely available conjugated to different fluorochromes.

This technique has several advantages. In the first place the fluorescence is brighter than with the direct test as several fluorescent anti-immunoglobulins bind on to each of the antibody molecules present in the first layer (Figure 6.8b). Second, even when many sera have to be screened for specific antibodies it is only necessary to prepare (or, more usually the case, purchase) a single secondary antibody. Furthermore, the method has great flexibility. For example, by using a mixture of primary antibodies directed against different target antigens, it is possible to compare the relative positions and/or expression of two different antigens within the same cell. Note, however, that in the latter scenario the primary antibodies must not have been generated in the same species or the secondary reagent will not be able to discriminate between them. For example, to simultaneously label cytochrome *c* and tubulin in the same cell, one would need to use anti-tubulin antibody that has been raised in the mouse, in combination with anti-cytochrome *c* antibody that has been raised in rabbit, or vice versa. By using species-specific secondary detection reagents (i.e. anti-mouse and anti-rabbit Ig) that are labeled with different fluorochromes, it is a simple matter to detect both proteins within the same cell (Figure 6.11).

Further applications of the indirect test may be seen in Chapter 18.

Confocal microscopy

Fluorescence images at high magnification are usually difficult to resolve because of the flare from slightly out of focus planes above and below the object. The resulting blurred images are usually of little help in exploring the finer points of cellular

architecture. All that is now a thing of the past, with the advent of **scanning confocal microscopy** that focuses the laser light source on a narrow plane within the cell and collects the fluorescence emission in a photomultiplier tube (PMT) with a confocal aperture. Fluorescence from planes above and below the object plane fails to reach the PMT and so the sharpness of the image is dramatically enhanced over conventional immunofluorescence microscopy (Figure 6.11). An X–Y scanning unit enables the whole of the specimen plane to be interrogated *quantitatively* and, with suitable optics, three or four different fluorochromes can be used simultaneously. The instrument software can compute three-dimensional fluorescence images from an automatic series of such X–Y scans accumulated in the Z axis (Figure 6.12) and rotate them at the whim of the operator. Such Z-stacks can be used to reconstruct a three-dimensional view of a cell, tissue or organelle, and offer unparalleled insights into cell and molecular structure. Timelapse experiments can also be carried out using the confocal microscope and this often transforms our understanding of events previously only viewed as snapshots in time. Often, seeing really is believing!

Flow cytometry

When a cell population is immunostained for a particular marker (CD4 for example) a subset of the population may express this marker at high levels, a different subset may express

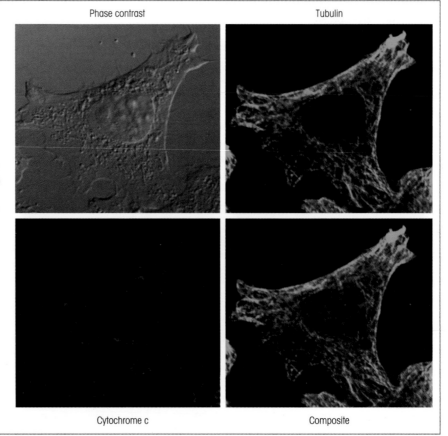

Figure 6.11. Confocal immunofluorescence microscopy.

Human HeLa cell immunostained with mouse anti-b-tubulin antibody detected with FITC-labeled anti-mouse Ig (green) and rabbit anti-cytochrome *c* antibody detected with Texas red-labeled anti-rabbit Ig (red). Cells were also stained with the DNA-binding dye, DAPI (blue). A phase contrast image of the same cell is also shown for comparison. Images were acquired on an Olympus Fluoroview 1000 confocal microscope. (Courtesy of Dr. Petrina Delivani, Dept. of Genetics, Trinity College Dublin, Ireland.)

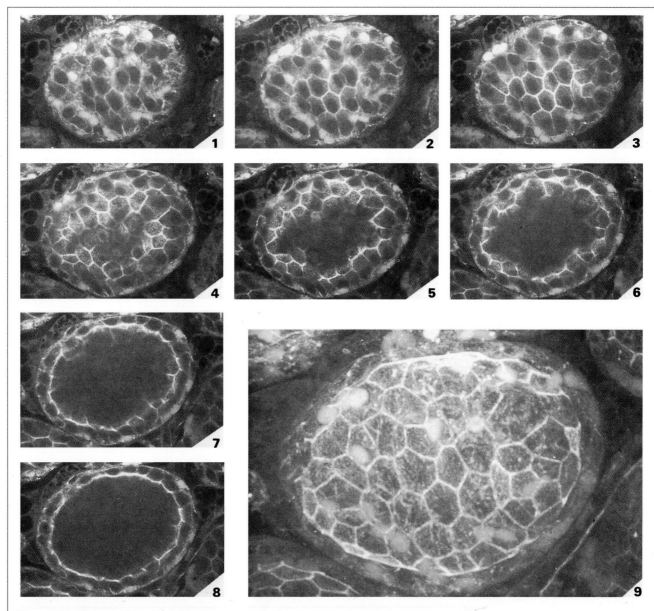

Figure 6.12. Construction of a three-dimensional fluorescence image with the confocal microscope.

A spherical thyroid follicle in a thick razor-blade section of rat thyroid fixed in formalin was stained with a rhodamine–phalloidin conjugate that binds F-actin (similar results obtained with antibody conjugates). Although the sample was very thick, the microscope was focused on successive planes at 1-mm intervals from the top of the follicle (image no. 1) to halfway through (image no. 8), the total of the images representing a hemisphere. Note how the fluorescence in one plane does not interfere with that in another and that the composite photograph (image no. 9) of images 1–8 shows all the fluorescence staining in focus throughout the depth of the hemisphere. Clearly the antibody is staining hexagonal structures close to the apical (inner) surface of the follicular epithelial cells. Erythrocytes are visible near the top of the follicle. (Negatives kindly supplied by Dr. Anna Smallcombe were taken by Bio-Rad staff on a Bio-Rad MRC-600 confocal imaging system using material provided by Professor V. Herzog and Fr. Brix of Bonn University, Germany.)

the same marker at low levels and the remainder of the population may be negative. To add further complexity, one may wish to examine simultaneously the expression of a different marker (CD8 for example) to determine whether expression of these proteins is mutually exclusive. Assessment of the percentage of cells in a population expressing either CD4 or CD8, or both, would be quite a chore using fluorescence microscopy or confocal microscopy, as this would involve manual counting of several hundred cells to obtain reliable figures. Quite apart from the labor involved, such analyses would also be quite subjective and results may vary depending on the skill of the operator. Fortunately, the **flow cytometer** makes such determinations rather trivial as this instrument can analyze the fluorescence levels associated with thousands of cells per minute in a highly reproducible and quantitative way (Figure 6.13).

In its most basic form, the flow cytometer is an instrument equipped with a fluid-handling system capable of moving thousands of cells in **single file** through a narrow chamber illuminated by a laser. The passage of an immunolabeled cell through the chamber (called a **flow cell**) results in excitation of the fluorochrome attached to the cell by the laser. The resulting emission from the fluorochrome is detected by a sensitive photomultiplier-based detector that permits precise quantitation of the fluorescence associated with the cell. Thus it is possible to rapidly discriminate between cells that are negative, slightly positive or highly positive for a given marker or antigen. Most modern flow cytometers are equipped with three or four lasers of different wavelengths (along with associated detectors) and each laser-detector combination can gather signals from different fluorochromes (Figure 6.14). As a result, it is possible to immunostain a cell population for four different markers (with a different fluorochrome-labeled antibody used for each one) and to gather data relating to the expression of all four markers as the cell passes through the flow cytometer.

The good news doesn't end there; the flow cytometer is also capable of providing information relating to **cell size** and **granularity** (organelle density) due to the way in which the laser light is scattered or reflected as it passes through the cell. The latter information (called forward and side scatter) is also very useful as this alone is often enough to permit discrimination between distinct cell types (Figure 6.15a).

Thus, the flow cytometer records quantitative data relating to the antigen content and physical nature of each individual cell, with multiple parameters being assessed per cell to give a phenotypic analysis on a single cell rather than a population average. With the impressive number of monoclonal antibodies and of fluorochromes to hand, highly detailed analyses are now feasible, with a notable contribution to the diagnosis of leukemia.

We can also probe the cell *interior* in several ways. Permeabilization to allow penetration by fluorescent antibodies (preferably with small Fab or even single-chain Fv fragments) gives readout of cytokines and other intracellular proteins. Cell cycle analysis can be achieved with DNA-binding dyes such as propidium iodide to measure DNA content (Figure 6.15b) and antibody detection of BrdU incorporation to visualize DNA synthesis. In addition, fluorescent probes for intracellular pH, thiol concentration, Ca^{2+}, Mg^{2+} and Na^+ have been developed.

Other labeled antibody methods

A problem with fluorescent conjugates is that the signals emitted by these probes fade within a relatively short time; photobleaching of the fluorescent label upon exposure to an

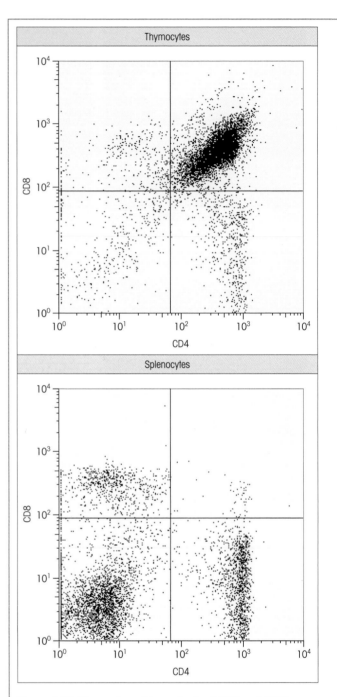

Figure 6.13. Flow cytometric analysis of CD4 and CD8 expression in thymocytes and splenocytes.

Mouse thymocytes and splenocytes were stained using FITC-conjugated anti-CD4 and rhodamine-conjugated anti-CD8 antibodies. Note that the majority of thymocytes are positive for both CD4 and CD8 and are therefore present in the upper right quadrant; thymocytes single-positive for CD4 (bottom right) or CD8 (top left) are also detected, as are double-negative cells (bottom left). In the spleen, few double-positive cells are found, with the majority of cells (most likely B-cells) negative for CD4 or CD8 along with cells that are single-positive for either marker. (Data kindly provided by Professor Thomas Brunner and Daniela Kassahn.)

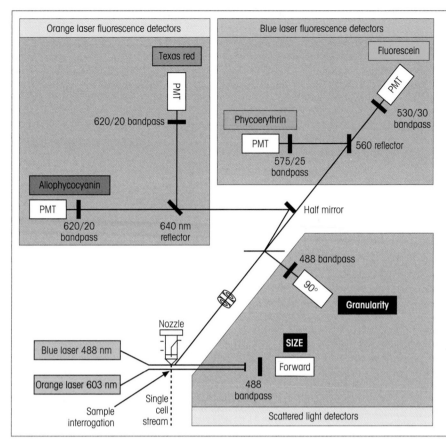

Figure 6.14. Six-parameter flow cytometry optical system for multicolor immunofluorescence analysis.

Cell fluorescence excited by the blue laser is divided into green (fluorescein) and orange (phycoerythrin) signals, while fluorescence excited by the orange laser is reflected by a mirror and divided into near red (Texas red) and far red (allophycocyanin) signals. Blue light scattered at small forward angles and at 90° is also measured in this system, providing information on cell size and internal granularity respectively. PMT, photomultiplier tube. (Based closely on Hardy R.R. (1998) In: Delves P.J. & Roitt I.M. (eds.) *Encyclopedia of Immunology*, 2nd edn, p. 946. Academic Press, London.) The recent use of three lasers and nine different fluorochromes pushes the system even further, providing 11 parameters!

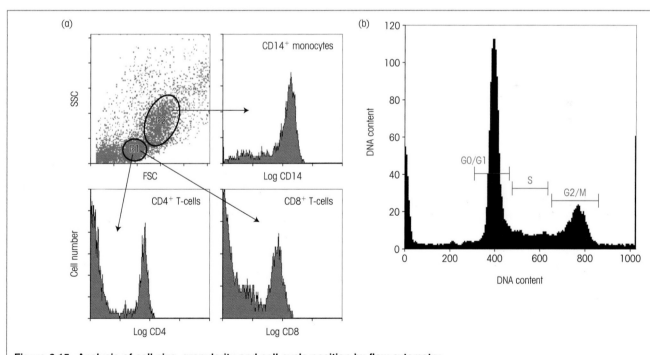

Figure 6.15. Analysis of cell size, granularity and cell cycle position by flow cytometry.

(a) Staining of peripheral blood with anti-CD4, anti-CD8, and anti-CD14 antibodies followed by analysis of cells by forward-scatter (FSC) and side-scatter (SSC) characteristics (top left). Cells with low forward- and side-scatter characteristics (lymphocytes, R1) were analyzed for CD4 or CD8 expression, as indicated. Cells with high forward- and side-scatter characteristics (monocytes, R2) were analyzed for CD14 expression. (Data kindly provided by Professor Thomas Brunner.) (b) Cell cycle analysis of transformed Jurkat T-cells by propidium iodide staining. The fluorescent DNA-binding dye, propidium iodide, stains cells in proportion to their DNA content; cells with normal diploid (2N) DNA content appear in the G0/G1 phase of the cell cycle, cells actively synthesizing DNA have greater than 2N DNA content and are therefore assigned to S-phase, whereas cells with 4N (diploid) DNA content are in G2 or mitosis (G2/M). (Courtesy of Dr. Colin Adrain, Trinity College Dublin, Ireland.)

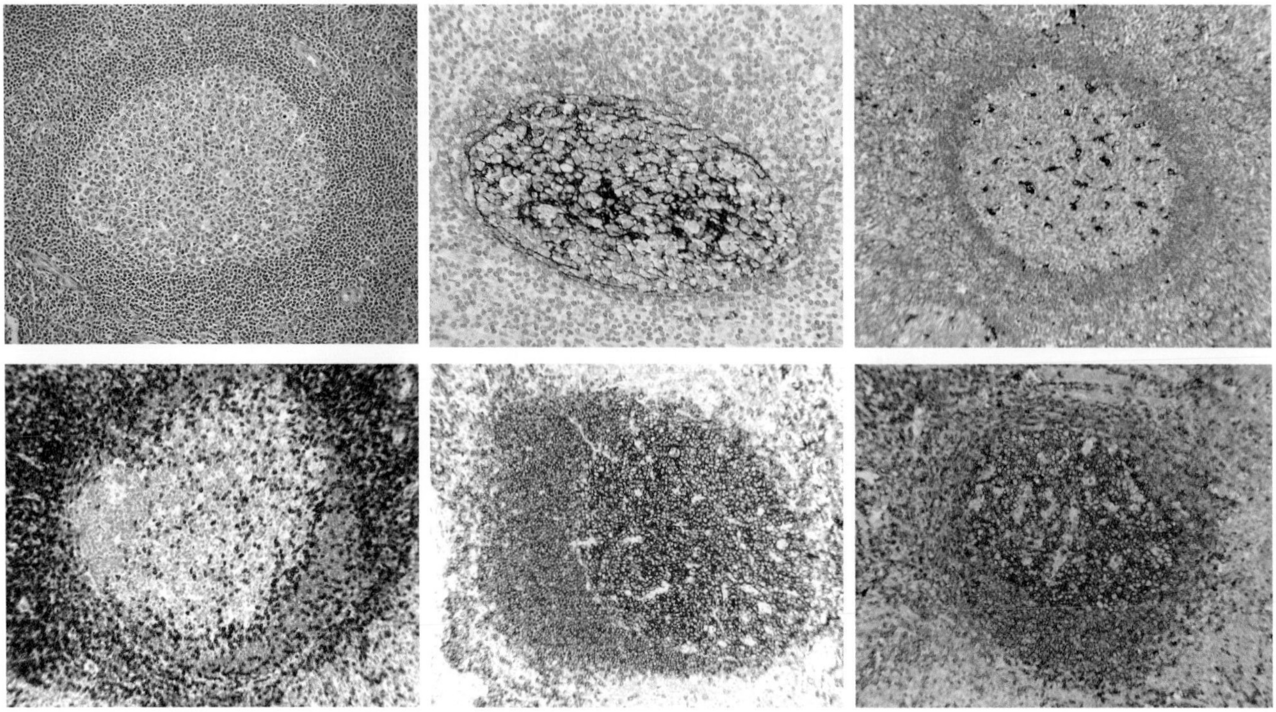

H & E	Anti-CD21	Anti-CD68
Anti-CD3	Anti-CD20	Anti-CD3 (brown) Anti-CD20 (red)

Figure 6.16. Immunohistochemical analysis of human tonsil follicle centers.

Human tonsil preparations were stained either with the histochemical stain hematoxylin and eosin (H&E), or were immunostained with antibodies against CD21 (complement receptor 2, expressed on follicular dendritic cells and B-cells), CD68 (expressed on macrophages), CD3 (T-cells), CD20 (B-cells), or a combination of anti-CD3 and anti-CD20, as shown. (Images kindly provided by Dr. Andreas Kappeler, University of Bern, Switzerland.)

excitation source (such as UV light) can also occur. In practice, this is not a problem so long as the labeled sample is analyzed in a timely fashion. However, enzymes such as alkaline phosphatase (cf. Figure 1.10d) or horseradish peroxidase can be coupled to antibodies and then visualized by conventional histochemical methods under the light microscope (Figure 6.16). Such stains are relatively stable and are particularly useful for staining tissue sections as opposed to cell suspensions.

Colloidal gold bound to antibody is being widely used as an electron-dense immunolabel by electron microscopists. At least three different antibodies can be applied to the same section by labeling them with gold particles of different size (cf. Figure 8.16). A new ultra-small probe consisting of Fab′ fragments linked to undecagold clusters allows more accurate spatial localization of antigens and its small size enables it to mark sites that are inaccessible to the larger immunolabels. However, clear visualization requires a high-resolution scanning transmission electron microscope.

Detection and quantitation of antigen by antibody

Immunoassay of antigen by ELISA

The ability to establish the concentration of an analyte (i.e. a substance to be measured) through fractional occupancy of its specific binding reagent is a feature of any ligand-binding system (see Milestone 6.1), but because antibodies can be raised to virtually any structure, its application is most versatile in immunoassay.

Large analytes, such as protein hormones, are usually estimated by a noncompetitive two-site assay in which the original ligand binder and the labeled detection reagent are both antibodies (see Figure M6.1.1). By using monoclonal antibodies directed to two different epitopes on the same analyte, the system has greater power to discriminate between two related analytes; if the fractional cross-reactivity of the first antibody

The appreciation that a ligand could be measured by the fractional occupancy (*F*) of its specific binding agent heralded a new order of sensitive wide-ranging assays. Ligand-binding assays were first introduced for the measurement of thyroid hormone by thyroxine-binding protein (Ekins) and for the estimation of hormones by antibody (Berson & Yalow). These findings spawned the technology of radioimmunoassay, so called because the antigen had to be trace-labeled in some way and the most convenient candidates for this were radioisotopes.

The relationship between fractional occupancy and analyte concentration [An] is given by the equation:

$$F = 1 - (1/1 + K[An])$$

where *K* is the association constant of the ligand-binding reaction. *F* can be measured by noncompetitive or competitive

assays (Figure M6.1.1) and related to a calibration curve constructed with standard amounts of analyte.

For competitive assays, the maximum theoretical sensitivity is given by the term *e/K* where *e* is the experimental error (coefficient of variation). Suppose the error is 1% and *K* is 10^{11} M^{-1}, the maximum sensitivity will be 0.01×10^{-11} M $= 10^{-13}$ M or 6×10^{7} molecules/ml. For noncompetitive assays, labels of very high specific activity could give sensitivities down to 10^{2}–10^{3} molecules/ml under ideal conditions. In practice, however, as the sensitivity represents the lowest analyte concentration that can be measured against a background containing zero analyte, the error of the measurement of background poses an ultimate constraint on sensitivity.

Figure M6.1.1. The principle of ligand-binding assays.

The ligand-binding agent may be in the soluble phase or bound to a solid support as shown here, the advantage of the latter being the ease of separation of bound from free analyte. After exposure to analyte, the fractional occupancy of the ligand-binding sites can be determined by competitive or noncompetitive assays using labeled reagents (in orange) as shown. Ab, antibody.

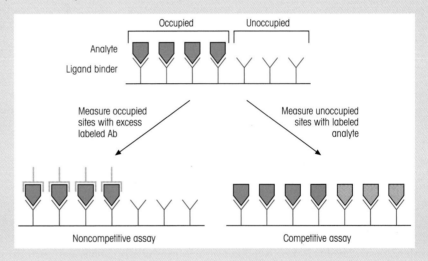

for a related analyte is 0.1 and of the second also 0.1, the final readout for cross-reactivity will be as low as 0.1 × 0.1, i.e. 1%. Using chemiluminescent and time-resolved fluorescent probes, highly sensitive assays are available for an astonishing range of analytes. For small molecules like drugs or steroid hormones, where two-site binding is impractical, competitive assays (see Figure M6.1.1) are appropriate.

The **ELISA (enzyme-linked immunosorbent assay)** is one of the most commonly used techniques for measuring antigens, such as cytokines, from serum or cell culture fluid. The technique is quite straightforward and involves immobilizing antibody to the protein of interest within the plastic wells of a microtiter plate. Unbound protein-binding sites within the plate are then blocked by incubation with an irrelevant protein such as albumin. Samples containing the antigen of interest are then added to the antibody-coated wells and incubated for a couple of hours to allow *capture* of the antigen by antibody. Following washing to remove nonbinding material, the bound antigen is then *detected* by adding a second antibody

that is directed against a different binding-site on the antigen to the one recognized by the capture antibody. The antigen is now sandwiched between the two antibodies giving rise to the terms **"sandwich ELISA"** or **antigen-capture assay**. The detection antibody is conjugated to an enzyme such as horseradish peroxidase or alkaline phosphatase that, upon addition of the enzyme substrate, produces a colored or chemiluminescence reaction product. Comparison between a range of standards of known concentration enables the concentration of antigen in the test samples to be calculated.

The nephelometric assay for antigen

If antigen is added to a solution of excess antibody, the amount of complex that can be assessed by forward light scatter in a nephelometer (cf. p. 164) is linearly related to the concentration of antigen. With the ready availability of a wide range of monoclonal antibodies that facilitate the standardization of the method, nephelometry is frequently used for the estimation of

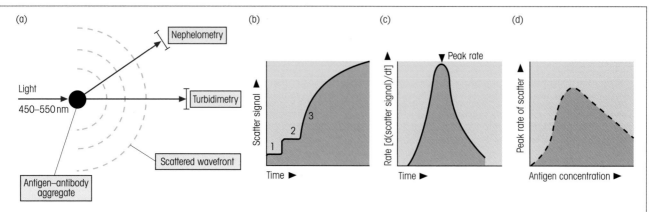

Figure 6.17. Rate nephelometry.

(a) On addition of antiserum, small antigen–antibody aggregates form (cf. Figure 6.24) that scatter incident light filtered to give a wavelength band of 450–550 nm. For nephelometry, the light scattered at a forward angle of 70° or so is measured. (b) After addition of the sample (1) and then the antibody (2), the rate at which the aggregates form (3) is determined from the scatter signal. (c) The software in the instrument then computes the maximum rate of light scatter, which is related to the antigen concentration as shown in (d). (Copied from the operating manual for the "Array" rate reaction automated immunonephelometer with permission from Beckman Coulter Ltd.)

immunoglobulins, C3, C4, haptoglobin, ceruloplasmin and C-reactive protein in those favored laboratories that can sport the appropriate equipment. Very small samples down in the range 1–10 µl can be analyzed. Turbidity of the sample can be a problem; blanks lacking antibody can be deducted but a more satisfactory solution is to follow the **rate of formation** of complexes that is proportional to antigen concentration as this obviates the need for a separate blank (Figure 6.17). Because soluble complexes begin to be formed in antigen excess, it is important to ensure that the value for antigen was obtained in antibody excess by running a further control in which additional antigen is included.

Immunoblotting (western blotting)

This widely adopted technique can be used to determine the **relative molecular mass** of a protein and to explore its behavior within a complex mixture of other proteins. Issues relating to whether the protein of interest is upregulated, downregulated, cleaved, phosphorylated, glycosylated or ubiquitinated in response to a particular stimulus can be addressed by immuno-blot analysis. This involves first running a mixture of proteins through a gel matrix that is formed by polymerization of acry-lamide and bisacrylamide between a pair of glass plates. **Polyacrylamide gel electrophoresis (PAGE)** of proteins is typically carried out using protein mixtures that have been denatured by heating in the presence of a detergent, sodium dodecylsulfate (SDS). SDS is a negatively charged molecule that becomes covalently coupled to proteins along their length upon exposure to heat; apart from denaturing the protein, this also imparts a negative charge in proportion to its length. Upon introduction of the protein sample to the gel and the application of a vertical electric field from the top of the gel to the bottom, proteins are repelled from the negative pole (the cathode) and

migrate towards the positive pole (the anode). Due to the molecular sieving effect of the gel matrix, proteins within the mixture become resolved into discrete zones (bands) with the smallest proteins moving furthest through the gel (Figure 6.18).

In order to probe the electrophoretically separated protein mixture with antibody to identify the protein of interest, it is necessary to allow the antibody access to the proteins within the gel. Because antibodies are relatively large proteins they cannot readily penetrate the gel matrix; the solution to this problem is to "blot" the gel onto a positively charged mem-brane that traps the charged proteins and immobilizes them on the surface of the membrane (Figure 6.18). This is achieved by again applying an electric field to the gel to drive the pro-teins horizontally out of the gel onto the blotting membrane; polyvinylidene difluoride (PVDF) and nitrocellulose-based membranes are typically used for this purpose. The blot can then be probed with either polyclonal or monoclonal antibod-ies directed against the protein of interest. Binding of antibody is detected using horseradish peroxidase-conjugated anti-Ig secondary antibodies, followed by application of a suitable enzyme substrate (Figure 6.19).

Obviously, such a procedure will not work with antigens that are irreversibly denatured by this detergent, and it is best to use polyclonal antisera for blotting to increase the chance of including antibodies to whichever epitopes do survive the denaturation procedure; a surprising number do.

Immunoprecipitation of antigen complexes

Antibodies immobilized on a solid support, such as agarose beads, can be used to purify an antigen from a complex mixture of other antigens to explore the nature of the antigen and the proteins to which it binds (Figure 6.20). To illustrate this approach, let us imagine that we have generated a monoclonal

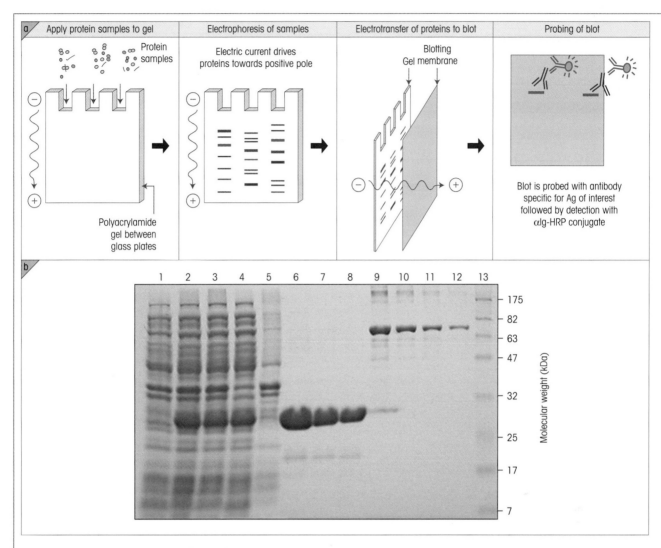

Figure 6.18. Principle of immunoblot analysis.

(a) Denatured protein mixtures can be separated on the basis of their relative mobilities through a gel matrix that is formed by polymerizing acrylamide and bis-acrylamide, to form polyacrylamide, between closely spaced (1.0–1.5 mm) glass plates. Prior to loading on the gel, proteins are first denatured by heating in a sample buffer containing SDS followed by introduction to the sample wells of the gel and application of an electric current for 2–3 hours. Separated proteins are then electrotransferred onto blotting membranes composed of PVDF or nitrocellulose that can then be probed with antibody, followed by detection of bound antibody using anti-Ig conjugated to horseradish peroxidase or similar. (b) SDS-PAGE gel of various cell lysates (lanes 1–5), purified proteins (lanes 6–12) and molecular weight markers (lane 13), stained with Coomassie Blue dye to reveal all proteins ran on the gel. (Data kindly provided by Dr. Sean Cullen, Trinity College Dublin, Ireland.)

antibody against a cell-surface receptor, such as TLR4, that is known to play an important role in the recognition of pathogen components. We would like to **immunoprecipitate (IP)** the receptor in the (possibly vain!) hope that there will be a protein hanging onto the cytoplasmic tail of the receptor that may shed some light upon how the receptor signals deep into the bowels of the cell. To do this, we would immunoprecipitate the receptor using our lovingly prepared anti-TLR4 monoclonal antibody immobilized on agarose beads. We would then wash away unbound material by centrifugation of the beads a couple of times in a suitable wash buffer, followed by applying the immunoprecipitated material onto an SDS-PAGE gel to

see what we have bagged. In the event that only the receptor has been immunoprecipitated, we would, to our obvious dismay, see only a single band on the gel along with bands corresponding to the antibody that we have used to perform the IP. Any unexpected bands are candidate receptor-interacting proteins that we can identify by picking a sample of the protein spot from the gel and subjecting this to mass spectrometry or protein sequencing analysis. The cynics among you will guess that this is often rather simpler in theory than in practice. However, given that the sensitivity of protein identification techniques has increased in leaps and bounds in recent years, such approaches have become increasingly fruitful.

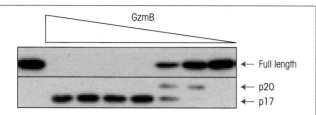

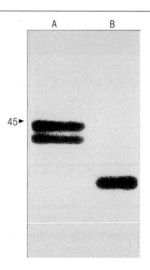

Figure 6.19. Immunoblot analysis.

Analysis of caspase-3 processing by the CTL/NK protease, granzyme B (GzmB). Protein extracts, derived from Jurkat T-cells, were incubated in the presence of decreasing concentrations of granzyme B, a serine protease that is delivered into target cells upon attack by CTLs or NK cells. Cell lysates were then separated on an SDS-PAGE gel followed by transfer to nitrocellulose membrane and immunoblotted with antibodies against caspase-3. Note how caspase-3 becomes processed (cleaved) by the higher concentrations of granzyme B; such processing activates the caspase-3 precursor within the target cells and promotes apoptosis. (Data kindly provided by Dr. Colin Adrain, Trinity College Dublin, Ireland.)

Figure 6.20. Immunoprecipitation of membrane antigen.

Analysis of membrane-bound class I MHC antigens (cf. p. 101). The membranes from human cells pulsed with ^{35}S-labeled methionine were solubilized in a detergent, mixed with a monoclonal antibody to HLA-A and -B molecules and immunoprecipitated with staphylococci. An autoradiograph (a) of the precipitate run in SDS–PAGE shows the HLA-A and B chains as a 43 000 molecular weight doublet (the position of a 45 000 marker is arrowed). If membrane vesicles are first digested with protease K before solubilization, a labeled band of molecular weight 39 000 can be detected (b) consistent with a transmembrane orientation of the HLA chain: the 4000 Da hydrophilic C-terminal fragment extends into the cytoplasm and the major portion, recognized by the monoclonal antibody and by tissue typing reagents, is present on the cell surface (cf. Figure 4.17). (From data and autoradiographs kindly supplied by Dr. M.J. Owen.)

Immunoprecipitation can also be used to test whether protein A binds to protein B by coexpressing these proteins within the same cell, followed by immunoprecipitation of protein A (or protein B) using a suitable antibody and running on an SDS-PAGE gel. Following transfer of the gel to a membrane support by Western blotting, the membrane can now be probed with antibodies directed against protein B to see whether it has co-immunoprecipitated with protein A. The latter technique is undoubtedly the most widely used form of the IP method and has been employed to great effect in the study of protein–protein interactions.

Chromatin immunoprecipitation (ChIP) assays

This interesting modification of the standard immunoprecipitation assay can analyse the repertoire of gene promoter sequences (or other regions within DNA) a transcription factor or other DNA-binding protein is bound to under a particular experimental condition. For example, if we would like to explore the range of gene promoters that NFκB binds to under unstimulated versus stimulated (e.g. LPS-treatment) conditions we could perform a ChIP experiment. Here's how the method works. Cells are incubated for a defined period of time in the presence or absence of a stimulus (LPS in this example), followed by brief treatment with a chemical cross-linking agent (e.g. formaldehyde) to ensure that any transcription factor bound to a promoter will remain bound under the conditions of the assay. After chemical cross-linking of protein–DNA complexes, cells are then lysed and the mixture is sonicated to shear very high molecular weight DNA into smaller more manageable fragments. Then an antibody specific to our transcription factor of interest (i.e. NFκB in this instance) is used to immunoprecipitate the protein from the mixture. The clever bit is that, due to the cross-linking step, our transcription factor will be bound to the regions of DNA (i.e. the promoters to which it was bound) it was actively transcribing when we ended the experiment. We can then carry out a PCR reaction on the immunoprecipitated samples using primers specific for genes we think might be regulated by the transcription factor of interest. If our transcription factor has bound to a promoter region of a gene, then the corresponding DNA fragment will be amplified when we carry out the PCR assay on that sample. We can then compare the amount of DNA amplified under the control versus treated conditions to determine whether the treatment (i.e. LPS in this instance) has enhanced binding of our transcription factor to specific gene promoters.

ChIP on Chip assays

In a further modification of the standard ChIP assay, as described above, a ChIP on Chip (DNA microarray) assay can be carried out. This permits a more global analysis of the DNA fragments immunoprecipitated with a particular transcription factor, where, rather then looking for specific gene sequences by PCR, we can more objectively look at all of the immunoprecipitated DNA fragments through hybridization with a

DNA microarray chip that carries sequences from a huge variety of genes. Such arrays can carry gene fragments, arrayed in specific spot locations on a solid support (called a chip), that represent the whole genome, or can be more restricted and carry gene fragments representative of all cytokines, or chemokines, and so on. This type of assay involves carrying out a standard ChIP experiment, as described above, followed by applying the DNA fragments so captured onto a DNA chip. This allows identification all the DNA sequences bound to the protein of interest under the experimental condition.

Protein and antibody microarrays

With the ready availability of cDNA copies of essentially all human genes, it is now possible to express virtually any human protein "off-the-shelf" and to purify it to homogeneity using simple molecular tricks. This is also true for protein-coding genes from several species of yeast, many bacteria, the fruitfly and other organisms. Using large-scale protein expression approaches, arrays of proteins have been produced that contain thousands of independent proteins, or protein fragments, arranged on glass slides as discrete microdots. On such arrays, each microdot contains a single protein and the identity of this protein is known from its position within the array. Such arrays can be probed with an antiserum, or monoclonal antibody, to determine the spectrum of proteins to which the antibody reacts. Thus, it may be possible in the near future to determine the full spectrum of autoantibodies (and their relative titer) present in a patient sample in a single step. One has only to cross-reference the spots "lighting up" after incubation with antibody with a list that specifies the identity of the protein that has been placed within those particular spots (Figure 6.21). Such arrays are likely to be useful for the identification of novel autoantigens, for the rapid diagnosis and classification of autoimmune conditions, and may also be useful for monitoring disease progression. Additional applications include the rapid determination of proteins that cross-react against monoclonal or polyclonal antibodies. In practice, smaller arrays focused on particular disease states are used for diagnostic purposes.

Similar to protein arrays, antibodies can also be arrayed as discrete spots on glass slides or other solid supports. Such arrays can be used to capture multiple antigens from the same sample simultaneously. Thus, for example, an anti-cytokine antibody array can be used to detect the presence of multiple cytokines within the same sample.

Epitope mapping

T-cell epitopes

Where the primary sequence of the whole protein is known, the identification of T-cell epitopes is comparatively straightforward. As these epitopes are linear in nature, multipin solid-phase synthesis can be employed to generate a series of overlapping peptides, 8–9-mers for cytotoxic T-cells and usually 10–14-mers for T-helpers (Figure 6.22), and their

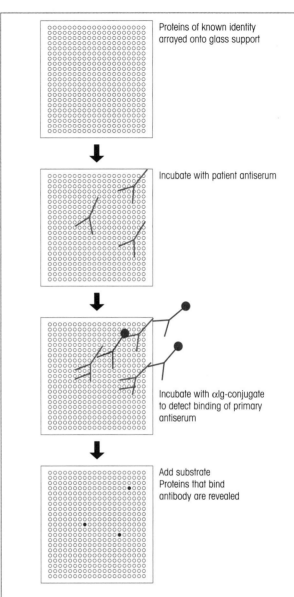

Proteins of known identity arrayed onto glass support

Incubate with patient antiserum

Incubate with αIg-conjugate to detect binding of primary antiserum

Add substrate
Proteins that bind antibody are revealed

Figure 6.21. Serum profiling by protein microarray analysis.

Protein arrays, consisting of thousands of proteins of known identity arrayed in a specific order, can be probed with a sample of a patient's serum to determine the range of proteins to which there are antibodies present. Bound antibodies can be detected with appropriate anti-Ig secondary antibody that leads directly to the identity of the proteins within the positive spots.

ability to react with antigen-specific T-cell lines or clones can be deciphered to characterize the active epitopes.

Dissecting out T-cell epitopes where the antigen has not been characterized is a more daunting task. Randomized peptide libraries can be produced but strategies need to be devised in order to keep these within manageable numbers. Information from the accumulated data deposited in various databanks can be used to identify key anchor residues and libraries constructed that maintain the relevant amino acids at

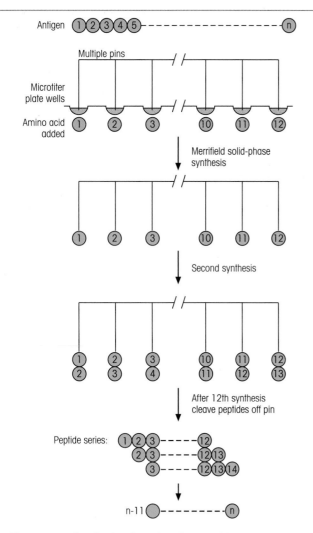

Antigen ①②③④⑤ - - - - - - - - - - - - - - ⓷

Figure 6.22. Synthesis of overlapping peptide sequences for (PEPSCAN) epitope analysis.

A series of pins that sit individually in the wells of a 96-well microtiter plate each provide a site for solid-phase synthesis of peptide. A sequence of such syntheses as shown in the figure provides the required nests of peptides. Incorporation of a readily cleavable linkage allows the soluble peptide to be released as the synthesis is terminated.

these positions. Thus, a positional scanning approach employs a peptide library in which one amino acid at a particular position is kept constant and all the different amino acids are used at the other positions.

B-cell epitopes

If they are **linear** protein epitopes formed directly from the primary amino acid sequence, then binding of antibody to individual overlapping peptides synthesized as described above will identify them. Unfortunately, most epitopes on globular proteins recognized by antibody are **discontinuous** and this makes the job rather demanding, as one cannot predict which residues are likely to be brought together in space to form the epitope. To the extent that small linear sequences may contribute to a discontinuous epitope, the overlapping peptide strategy may provide some clues.

A potentially promising approach to this problem of mimicking the residues that constitute such epitopes (termed **mimotopes** by Mario Geysen) is through the production of libraries of bacteriophages bearing all possible random hexapeptides. These are produced by ligating degenerate oligonucleotide inserts (coding for hexapeptides) to a bacteriophage coat protein in a suitable vector; appropriate expression in *E. coli* can provide up to 10^9 different clones. The beauty of the system is that a bacteriophage expressing a given hexapeptide on its external coat protein also bears the sequence encoding the hexapeptide in its genome (cf. p. 147). Accordingly, sequential rounds of selection, in which the phages react with a biotinylated monoclonal antibody and are then panned on a streptavidin plate, should isolate those bearing the peptides that mimic the epitope recognized by the monoclonal; nucleotide sequencing will then give the peptide structure.

Even nonproteinaceous antigens can occasionally be mimicked using peptide libraries, one example being the use of a D-amino acid hexapeptide library to identify a mimotope for *N*-acetylglucosamine. Others have used a single-chain Fv (scFv) library to isolate an idiotypic mimic of a meningococcal carbohydrate.

Estimation of antibody

As antigens and antibodies are defined by their mutual interactions, they can each be used to quantify each other. Before we get down to details, it is worth posing the question "What does serum 'antibody content' mean?"

If we have a solution of a monoclonal antibody, we can define its affinity and specificity with considerable confidence and, if pure and in its native conformation, we will know that the concentration of antibody is the same as that of the measurable immunoglobulin in ng/ml or whatever. When it comes to measuring the antibody content of an antiserum, the problem is of a different order because the immunoglobulin fraction is composed of an enormous array of molecules of varying abundance and affinity (Figure 6.23a).

An **average** K_a for the whole IgG can be obtained by analyzing the overall interaction with antigen as a mass action equation. But how can the **antibody content** of the IgG be defined in a meaningful way? The answer is of course that one would usually wish to describe antibody in practical functional terms: does a serum protect against a given infectious dose of virus, does it promote effective phagocytosis of bacteria, does it permit complement-mediated bacteriolysis, does it neutralize toxins, and so on? For such purposes, very low affinity molecules would be useless because they form such inadequate amounts of complex with the antigen.

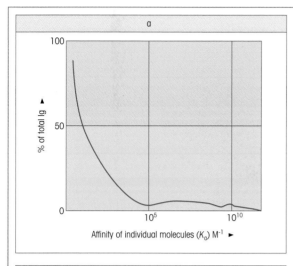

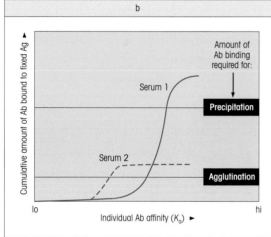

Figure 6.23. Distribution of affinity and abundance of IgG molecules in an individual serum.

(a) Distribution of affinities of IgG molecules for a given antigen in the serum of a hypothetical individual. There is a great deal of low-affinity antibody that would be incapable of binding to antigen effectively, and much lower amounts of high-affinity antibody whose skewed distribution is assumed to arise from exposure to infection. (b) Relationship of affinity distribution to positivity in tests for antigen binding. Rearranging the mass action equation, for all molecules of the same affinity K_x and concentration of unbound antibody $[Ab_x]$: the amount of complex formed $[AgAb] \propto K_x[Abx]$ for fixed $[Ag]$.

Starting with the lowest affinity molecules in the serum, we have charted the cumulative total of antibody bound for each antibody species up to and including the one being plotted. As might be expected, the very low affinity antibodies make no contribution to the tests. Serum 2 has more low affinity antibody and virtually no high affinity, but it can produce just enough complex to react in the sensitive agglutination test although, unlike serum 1, it forms insufficient to give a positive precipitin. Because of its relatively high "content" of antibody, serum 1 can be diluted to a much greater extent than serum 2 and yet still give positive agglutination, i.e. it has a higher titer. The precipitin test is less sensitive, requiring more complex formation, and serum 1 cannot be diluted much before this test becomes negative, i.e. the precipitin titer will be far lower than the agglutination titer for the same serum.

At the practical level in a diagnostic laboratory, the functional tests are labor intensive and therefore expensive, and a compromise is usually sought by using immunochemical assays that measure a composite of medium to high affinity antibodies and their abundance. The majority of such tests usually measure the total amount of antibody binding to a given amount of antigen; this could be a modest amount of high affinity antibody or much more antibody of lower affinity, or all combinations in between. Sera are compared for high or low "antibody content" either by seeing how much antibody binds to antigen at a fixed serum dilution, or testing a series of serum dilutions to see at which level a standard amount of antibody just sufficient to give a positive result is bound. This is the so-called **antibody titer**. To take an example, a serum might be diluted, say, 10 000 times and still just give a positive agglutination test (cf. Figure 6.29). This titer of 1:10 000 enables comparison to be made with another much "weaker" serum that has a titer of only, say, 1:100. Note that the titer of a given serum will vary with the sensitivity of the test, as much smaller amounts of antibody are needed to bind to antigen for a highly sensitive test, such as agglutination,

than for a test of low sensitivity, such as precipitation, which requires high concentrations of antibody–antigen product (Figure 6.23b).

To summarize: the "effective antibody contents" of different sera can be compared by seeing how much antibody binds to the fixed amount of test antigen, or the titer can be determined, i.e. how far the serum can be diluted before the test becomes negative. This is a compromise between abundance and affinity and for practical purposes is used as an approximate indicator of biological effectiveness.

Antigen–antibody interactions in solution

The classical precipitin reaction

When an antigen solution is added progressively to a potent antiserum, antigen–antibody precipitates are formed (Figure 6.24a,b). The cross-linking of antigen and antibody gives rise to three-dimensional lattice structures, as suggested by John Marrack, which coalesce, largely through Fc–Fc interaction, to form large precipitating aggregates. As more and more antigen is added, an optimum is reached (Figure 6.24b) after which

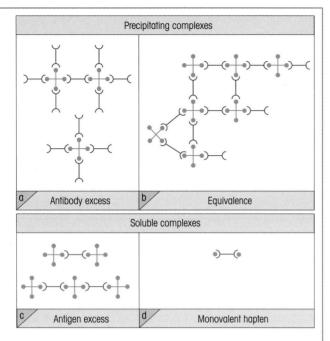

Figure 6.24. Diagrammatic representation of complexes formed between a hypothetical tetravalent antigen (⊹) and bivalent antibody (◯—◯) mixed in different proportions. In practice, the antigen valencies are unlikely to lie in the same plane or to be formed by identical determinants as suggested in the figure. (a) In extreme antibody excess, the antigen valencies are saturated and the molar ratio Ab:Ag approximates to the valency of the antigen. (b) At equivalence, most of the antigen and antibody combines to form large lattices that aggregate to produce typical immune precipitates. (c) In extreme antigen excess, where the two valencies of each antibody molecule become rapidly saturated, the complex Ag$_2$Ab tends to predominate. (d) A monovalent hapten binds but is unable to cross-link antibody molecules.

consistently less precipitate is formed. At this stage the supernatant can be shown to contain soluble complexes of antigen (Ag) and antibody (Ab), many of composition Ag$_4$Ab$_3$, Ag$_3$Ab$_2$ and Ag$_2$Ab (Figure 6.24c). In extreme antigen excess (Figure 6.24c), ultracentrifugal analysis reveals the complexes to be mainly of the form Ag$_2$Ab, a result directly attributable to the two combining sites (divalence) of the IgG antibody molecule (cf. electron microscope study, Figure 3.10).

Serums frequently contain up to 10% of nonprecipitating antibodies that are effectively monovalent because of the asymmetric presence of oligosaccharide on one antigen-binding arm of the antibody molecule that stereochemically blocks the combining site. Also, frank precipitates are only observed when antigen, and particularly antibody, is present in fairly hefty concentrations. Thus, when complexes are formed that do not precipitate spontaneously, more devious methods must be applied to detect and estimate the antibody level.

Nonprecipitating antibodies can be detected by nephelometry

The small aggregates formed when dilute solutions of antigen and antibody are mixed create a cloudiness or turbidity that can be measured by forward angle scattering of an incident light source (nephelometry). Greater sensitivity can be obtained by using monochromatic light from a laser and by adding polyethylene glycol to the solution so that aggregate size is increased. In practice, nephelometry is applied more to the detection of antigen than antibody (cf. Figure 6.17).

Complexes formed by nonprecipitating antibodies can be precipitated

The relative antigen-binding capacity of an antiserum that forms soluble complexes can be estimated using radiolabeled antigen. The complex can be brought out of solution either by changing its solubility or by adding an anti-immunoglobulin reagent as in Figure 6.25.

Measurement of antibody affinity

As discussed in earlier chapters (cf. p. 118), the binding strength of antibody for antigen is measured in terms of the association constant (K_a) or its reciprocal, the dissociation constant (K_d), governing the reversible interaction between them and defined by the mass action equation at equilibrium:

$$K_a = \frac{[\text{AgAb complex}]}{[\text{free Ag}][\text{free Ab}]}$$

With small haptens, equilibrium dialysis can be employed to measure K_a, but usually one is dealing with larger antigens and other techniques must be used. One approach is to add increasing amounts of radiolabeled antigen to a fixed amount of antibody, and then separate the free from bound antibody by precipitating the soluble complex as described above (e.g. by an anti-immunoglobulin). The reciprocal of the bound, i.e. complexed, antibody concentration can be plotted against the reciprocal of the free antigen concentration, so allowing the affinity constant to be calculated (Figure 6.26a). For an antiserum this will give an affinity constant representing an average of the heterogeneous antibody components and a measure of the effective number of antigen-binding sites operative at the highest levels of antigen used.

Various types of ELISA have been developed that provide a measure of antibody affinity. In one system the antibody is allowed to first bind to its antigen, and then a chaotropic agent such as thiocyanate is added in increasing concentration in order to disrupt the antibody binding; the higher the affinity of the antibody, the more agent that is required to reduce the binding. Another type of ELISA for measuring affinity is the indirect competitive system devised by Friguet and associates (Figure 6.26b). A constant amount of antibody is incubated

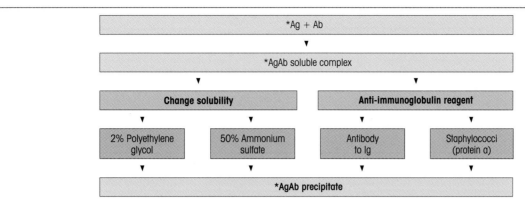

Figure 6.25. Binding capacity of an antiserum for labeled antigen (*Ag) by precipitation of soluble complexes either: (i) by changing the solubility so that the complexes are precipitated while the uncombined Ag and Ab remain in solution, or (ii) by adding a precipitating anti-immunoglobulin antibody or staphylococcal organisms that bind immunoglobulin Fc to the protein A on their surface; the complex can then be spun down. The level of label (e.g. radioactivity) in the precipitate will be a measure of antigen-binding capacity.

with a series of antigen concentrations and the free antibody at equilibrium is assessed by secondary binding to solid-phase antigen. In this way, values for K_a are not affected by any distortion of antigen by labeling. This again stresses the superiority of determining affinity by studying the **primary reaction** with antigen in the **soluble state** rather than conformationally altered through binding to a solid phase.

Increasingly, affinity measurements are obtained using **surface plasmon resonance**. A sensor chip consisting of a monoclonal antibody coupled to dextran overlying a gold film on a glass prism will totally internally reflect light at a given angle (Figure 6.27a). Antigen present in a pulse of fluid will bind to the sensor chip and, by increasing its size, alter the angle of reflection. The system provides data on the kinetics of association and dissociation (and hence K) (Figure 6.27b) and permits comparisons between monoclonal antibodies and also assessment of subtle effects of mutations.

Agglutination of antigen-coated particles

Whereas the cross-linking of multivalent protein antigens by antibody leads to precipitation, cross-linking of cells or large particles by antibody directed against surface antigens leads to agglutination. As most cells are electrically charged, a reasonable number of antibody links between two cells are required before the mutual repulsion is overcome. Thus agglutination of cells bearing only a small number of determinants may be difficult to achieve unless special methods such as further treatment with an antiglobulin reagent are used. Similarly, the higher avidity of multivalent IgM antibody relative to IgG makes the former more effective as an agglutinating agent, molecule for molecule (Figure 6.28).

Agglutination reactions are used to identify bacteria and to type red cells; they have been observed with leukocytes and

platelets, and even with spermatozoa in certain cases of male infertility due to sperm agglutinins. Because of its sensitivity and convenience, the test has been extended to the identification of antibodies to soluble antigens that have been artificially coated on to erythrocytes, latex or gelatin particles. Agglutination of IgG-coated latex is used to detect rheumatoid factors. Similar tests using antigen-coated particles can be carried out in U-bottom microtiter plates in which the settling pattern on the bottom of the well may be observed (Figure 6.29); this provides a more sensitive indicator than macroscopic clumping. Quantification of more subtle degrees of agglutination can be achieved by nephelometry or Coulter counting.

Immunoassay for antibody using solid-phase antigen

The principle

The antibody content of a serum can be assessed by the ability to bind to antigen that has been immobilized by physical adsorption to a plastic tube or microtiter plate with multiple wells; the bound immunoglobulin may then be estimated by addition of a labeled anti-Ig raised in another species (Figure 6.30). Consider, for example, the determination of DNA autoantibodies in SLE (cf. p. 479). When a patient's serum is added to a microwell coated with antigen (in this case DNA), the autoantibodies will bind to the antigen and the remaining serum proteins can be readily washed away. Bound antibody can now be estimated by addition of ^{125}I-labeled purified rabbit anti-human IgG; after rinsing out excess unbound reagent, the radioactivity of the tube will clearly be a measure of the autoantibody content of the patient's serum. The distribution of antibody in different classes can be determined by using

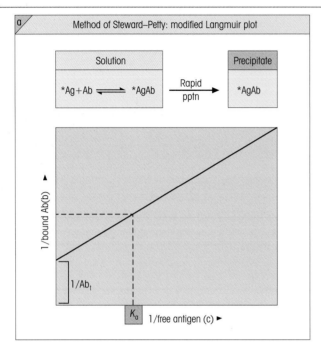

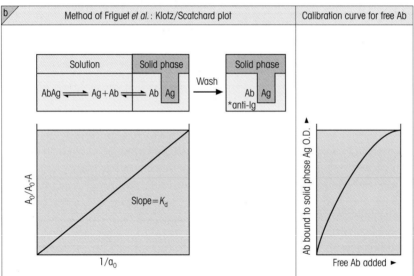

Figure 6.26. Determination of affinity with large antigens.

The equilibria between antibody (Ab) and antigen (Ag) at different concentrations are determined as follows:

(a) For a polyclonal antiserum one can use the Steward–Petty modification of the Langmuir equation:

$$1/b = 1/(Ab_t \cdot c \cdot K_a) + 1/Ab_t$$

where Ab_t = total Ab combining sites, b = bound Ab concentration, c = free Ag concentration and K_a = average affinity constant. At infinite Ag concentration, all Ab sites are bound and $1/b = 1/Ab_t$. When half the Ab sites are bound, $1/c = K_a$.
(b) The method of Friguet et al. for monoclonal antibodies. First, a calibration curve for free antibody is established by estimating the proportion binding to solid-phase antigen, bound antibody being measured by enzyme-labeled anti-Ig (ELISA: see text). Using the calibration curve, the amount of free Ab in equilibrium with Ag in solution is determined by seeing how much of the Ab binds to solid-phase Ag (the amount of solid-phase antigen is insufficient to affect the solution equilibrium materially). Combination of the Klotz and Scatchard equations gives:

$$A_o/A_o - A = 1 + K_d/a_o$$

where A_o = ELISA optical density (OD) for Ab in the absence of Ag, A = OD in the presence of Ag concentration a_o where a_o is approximately 10× concentration of Ab. The slope of the plot gives K_d. (Labeled molecules are marked with an asterisk.)

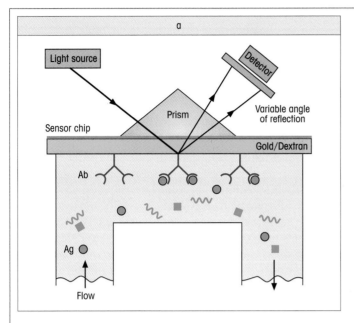

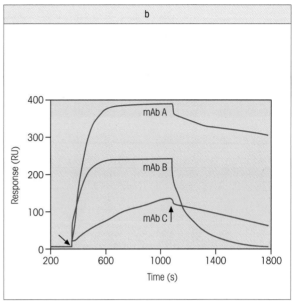

Figure 6.27. Surface plasmon resonance.

(a) The principle: as antigen (Ag) binds to the antibody-coated sensor chip it alters the angle of reflection. (b) This signals the rates of association during the antigen pulse and dissociation. In this example, the same antigen was injected over three immobilized monoclonal antibodies (mAbs). The arrows point to the beginning and end of the antigen injection, which is followed by buffer flow. Note the differences between the antibodies in the association and dissociation rates. (Data kindly provided by Dr. R. Karlsson, Biacore AB, and reproduced from Panayotou G. (1998) Surface plasmon resonance. In: Delves P.J. & Roitt I.M. (eds.) *Encyclopedia of Immunology*, 2nd edn. Academic Press, with permission.) The system can be used with antigen immobilized on the sensor chip and antibody in the fluid phase, or can be applied to any other single ligand-binding assay.

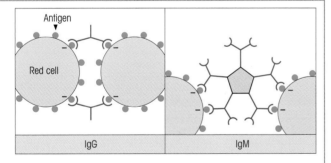

Figure 6.28. Mechanism of agglutination of antigen-coated particles by antibody cross-linking to form large macroscopic aggregates. If red cells are used, several cross-links are needed to overcome the electrical charge at the cell surface. IgM is superior to IgG as an agglutinator because of its multivalent binding and because the charged cells are further apart.

specific antisera. Take the radioallergosorbent test (RAST) for IgE antibodies in allergic patients. The allergen (e.g. pollen extract) is covalently coupled to an immunoabsorbent, in this case a paper disk, which is then treated with patient's serum. The amount of specific IgE bound to the paper can now be estimated by the addition of labeled anti-IgE.

A wide variety of labels available

Whilst providing extremely good sensitivity, radiolabels have a number of disadvantages, including loss of sensitivity during storage due to radioactive decay, the deterioration of the labeled reagent through radiation damage, and the precautions needed to minimize human exposure to radioactivity. Therefore, other types of label are often employed in immunoassays.

ELISA. Enzymes that give a colored soluble reaction product are currently the most commonly used labels, with horseradish peroxidase (HRP) and calf intestine alkaline phosphatase (AP) being by far the most popular. *Aspergillus niger* glucose oxidase, soy bean urease and *Escherichia coli* β-galactosidase provide further alternatives. One clever ploy for amplifying the phosphatase reaction is to use nicotinamide adenine dinucleotide phosphate (NADP) as a substrate to generate NAD that now acts as a coenzyme for a second enzyme system.

Other labels. Enzyme-labeled streptococcal protein G or staphylococcal protein A will bind to IgG. Conjugation with the vitamin biotin is frequently used as this can readily be detected by its reaction with enzyme-linked avidin or streptavidin (the latter gives lower background binding), both of which bind with ferocious specificity and affinity ($K = 10^{15} M^{-1}$).

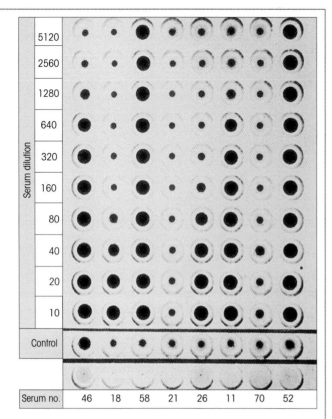

Figure 6.29. Red cell hemagglutination test for thyroglobulin autoantibodies. Thyroglobulin-coated cells were added to dilutions of patients' serums. Uncoated cells were added to a 1 : 10 dilution of serum as a control. In a positive reaction, the cells settle as a carpet over the bottom of the cup. Because of the "V"-shaped cross-section of these cups, in negative reactions the cells fall into the base of the "V," forming a small, easily recognizable button. The reciprocal of the highest serum dilution giving an unequivocally positive reaction is termed the titer. The titers reading from left to right are: 640, 20, >5120, neg, 40, 320, neg, >5120. The control for serum no. 46 was slightly positive and this serum should be tested again after absorption with uncoated cells.

Chemiluminescence systems based on the HRP-catalyzed enhanced luminol reaction, where light from the oxidized luminol substrate is intensified and the signal duration increased by the use of an enhancing reagent, provide increased sensitivity and dynamic range. Special mention should be made of time-resolved fluorescence assays based upon chelates of rare earths such as europium 3+, although these have a more important role in antigen assays.

Detection of immune complex formation

Many techniques for detecting circulating complexes have been described and because of variations in the size, complement-fixing ability and Ig class of different complexes, it is useful to apply more than one method. Two fairly robust methods for general use are:

1 Precipitation of complexed IgG from serum at concentrations of polyethylene glycol that do not bring down significant amounts of IgG monomer, followed by estimation of IgG in the precipitate by single radial immunodiffusion (SRID) or laser nephelometry; and
2 Binding of C3b-containing complexes to beads coated with bovine conglutinin (cf. p. 20) and estimation of the bound Ig with enzyme-labeled anti-Ig.

Other techniques include: (i) estimation of the binding of ^{125}I-C1q to complexes by coprecipitation with polyethylene glycol, (ii) inhibition by complexes of rheumatoid factor-induced aggregation of IgG-coated particles, and (iii) detection with radiolabeled anti-Ig of serum complexes capable of binding to the C3b (and to a lesser extent the Fc) receptors on the Raji cell line. Sera from patients with immune complex disease often form a cryoprecipitate when allowed to stand at 4°C. Measurement of serum C3 and its conversion product C3c is sometimes useful.

Tissue-bound complexes are usually visualized by the immunofluorescence staining of biopsies with conjugated anti-immunoglobulins and anti-C3 (cf. Figure 15.18).

Isolation of leukocyte subpopulations

Because of the complexity of the interactions between cells of the immune system, it is often well-nigh impossible to sort out who is doing what to whom unless one adopts a reductionist approach by purifying specific cell populations to study in isolation. Clearly, this approach also has its pitfalls as purified cell populations often behave differently *in vitro* to the way they do *in vivo*. However, the combination of *in vitro* and *in vivo* approaches has been very powerful and each has its place in the immunologist's armory. A number of techniques are routinely employed to enrich immune cell populations to varying degrees of purity. Most of these rely upon unique characteristics of particular cell populations ranging from their size, ability to adhere to plastic, or expression of a particular cell surface antigen. Antibodies to particular CD markers are especially useful for isolating specific populations of leukocytes when used in conjunction with a range of clever panning methods, as we shall see below.

Bulk techniques

Separation based on physical parameters

Separation of cells on the basis of their differential **sedimentation rate**, which roughly correlates with **cell size**, can be carried out by centrifugation through a density gradient. Cells can be increased in mass by selectively binding particles such as red cells to their surface, the most notable example being the rosettes formed when sheep erythrocytes bind to the CD2 marker present on human T-cells.

Buoyant density is another useful parameter. Centrifugation of whole blood over isotonic Ficoll–Hypaque (sodium metri-

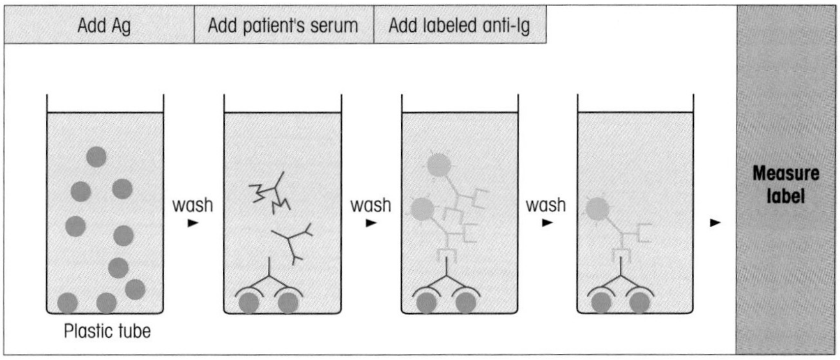

Add Ag	Add patient's serum	Add labeled anti-Ig	

wash ▶   wash ▶   wash ▶   ▶   **Measure label**

Plastic tube

Figure 6.30. Solid-phase immunoassay for antibody.

To reduce nonspecific binding of IgG to the solid phase after adsorption of the first reagent, it is usual to add an irrelevant protein, such as dried skimmed milk powder or bovine serum albumin, to block any free sites on the plastic. Note that the conformation of a protein often alters on binding to plastic, e.g.

a monoclonal antibody that distinguishes between the apo and holo forms of cytochrome *c* in solution combines equally well with both proteins on the solid phase. Covalent coupling to carboxy-derivatized plastic or capture of the antigen (Ag) substrate by solid-phase antibody can sometimes lessen this effect.

zoate) of density 1.077g/ml leaves the mononuclear cells (lymphocytes, monocytes and natural killer (NK) cells) floating in a band at the interface, while the erythrocytes and polymorphonuclear leukocytes, being denser, travel right down to the base of the tube (Figure 6.31). **Adherence** to plastic surfaces largely removes phagocytic cells, while passage down nylon-wool columns greatly enriches lymphocyte populations for T-cells at the expense of B-cells.

Separation exploiting biological parameters

Actively phagocytic cells that take up small iron particles can be manipulated by a magnet deployed externally. Lymphocytes that divide in response to a polyclonal activator (see p. 217), or specific antigen, can be eliminated by allowing them to incorporate 5-bromodeoxyuridine (BrdU); this renders them susceptible to the lethal effect of UV irradiation.

Selection by antibody

Several methods are available for the selection of cells specifically coated with antibody, some of which are illustrated in Figure 6.32. Addition of complement or anti-Ig toxin conjugates will eliminate such populations. Magnetic beads coated with anti-Ig form clusters with antibody-coated cells that can be readily separated from uncoated cells. Another useful bulk selection technique is to pan antibody-coated cells on anti-Ig adsorbed to a surface. One variation on this theme used to isolate bone marrow stem cells with anti-CD34 is to coat the cells with biotinylated antibody and select with an avidin column or avidin magnetic beads. Cocktails of antibodies coated onto beads are used in cell separation columns for the depletion of specific populations leading to, for example, enriched CD4⁺CD45RA⁻ or CD4⁺CD45RO⁻ lymphocytes.

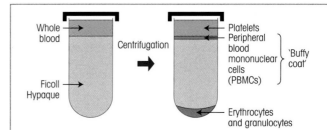

Figure 6.31. Separation of leukocytes by density gradient centrifugation.

Whole blood is carefully layered onto Ficoll–Hypaque or similar medium of known density, followed by centrifugation at 800*g* for 30 min. This results in the sedimentation of erythrocytes and granulocytes to the bottom of the centrifuge tube. A peripheral blood mononuclear cell "buffy coat" consisting mainly of T- and B-lymphocytes, NK cells and monocytes is found at the interface between the two layers.

Cell selection by FACS

Cells coated with fluorescent antibody can be separated by fluorescence-activated cell sorting (FACS) as described in Milestone 6.2 and Figure 6.33 (see more in-depth discussion under "Flow cytometry," p. 152). The technique is relatively simple but the technology required to achieve it is highly sophisticated. Cells are typically stained with antibodies against particular cell surface markers (such as CD4 or CD19) and cells that are positive or negative for this marker are sorted into different collection tubes by the instrument.

Enrichment of antigen-specific populations

Selective expansion of antigen-specific T-cells by repeated stimulation with antigen and presenting cells in culture, usually

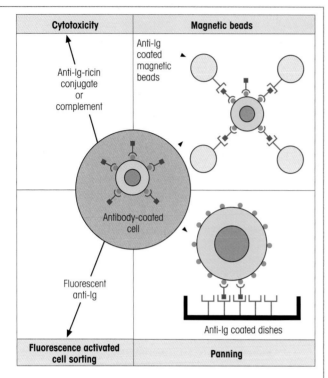

Figure 6.32. Major methods for separating cells coated with a specific antibody.

alternated with interleukin-2 (IL-2) treatment, leads to an enrichment of heterogeneous T-cells specific for different epitopes on the antigen. Such **T-cell lines** can be distributed in microtiter wells at a high enough dilution such that **on average** there is less than one cell per well; pushing the cells to proliferate with antigen or anti-CD3 produces single T-cell clones that can be maintained with much obsessional care and attention, but my goodness they can be a pain! Potentially immortal **T-cell hybridomas**, similar in principle to B-cell hybridomas, can be established by fusing cell lines with a T-tumor line and cloning.

Generation of dendritic cells *in vitro*

Because of the difficulty of isolating large quantities of dendritic cells, many immunologists produce these *in vitro* by inducing their differentiation from freshly isolated bone marrow. The procedure involves extracting bone marrow from the long bones of mice followed by addition of GM-CSF for 11 days. The resulting cells are predominantly MHC class II+, CD11c+, CD8− DCs and are responsive to stimulation with many PAMPs. Similar methods can also be used to produce DCs from splenocyte cultures.

Immortalization of primary B-cells

Because primary B-cells rapidly die off in culture, procedures have been established for the transformation of these cells using Epstein–Barr virus (EBV) that selectively immortalizes B-cells

and allows their indefinite growth *in vitro*. The procedure used to generate EBV-transformed B-cell lines was established over 25 years ago and is still widely used. EBV particles are obtained from an EBV-infected cell line through lysis. Human lymphocyte cultures are then inoculated with the free virus, which enters B-cells via the CD2I (CR2) cell surface molecule (receptor for complement C3 fragments). Propagation of EBV-infected cultures for several weeks then leads to the emergence of immortalized B-cells. However, EBV-specific cytotoxic T-cells (Tc) can emerge in culture, which kill the infected B-cells, leading a failure to produce transformed cells. This can be countered either by removing T-cells using immunodepletion methods (as outlined above), by suppressing T-cell activation by adding cyclosporin A to the cultures, or by addition of T-cell polyclonal activators (such as phytohaemagglutinin [PHA]) that stimulates rapid T-cell proliferation and apoptosis before Tc cells can be generated.

Cellular interactions *in vitro*

It is obvious that the methods outlined above for depletion, enrichment and isolation of individual cell populations enable the investigator to study cellular interactions through judicious combining of various purified populations. These interactions are usually more effective when the cells are operating within some sort of stromal network resembling the set-up of the tissues where their function is optimally expressed. For example, colonization of murine fetal thymus rudiments in culture with T-cell precursors enables one to follow the pattern of proliferation, maturation, TCR rearrangement and positive and negative selection normally seen *in vivo* (cf. pp. 290–291). An even more refined system involves the addition of selected lymphoid populations to disaggregated stromal cells derived from fetal thymic lobes depleted of endogenous lymphoid cells with deoxyguanosine. The cells can be spun into a pellet and co-cultured in hanging drops; on transfer to normal organ culture conditions after a few hours, reaggregation to intact lobes takes place quite magically and the various differentiation and maturation processes then unfold.

Animals populated essentially by a single T-cell specificity can be produced by introducing the T-cell receptor α and β genes from a T-cell clone, as a transgene (see below); as the genes are already rearranged, their presence in every developing T-cell will switch off any other Vβ gene recombinations.

No one has succeeded in cloning primary B-cells as they die rapidly upon introduction to cell culture. It is possible however to culture immortalized B-cell hybridomas or EBV-transformed cell lines, and, as with T-cells, transgenic animals expressing the same antibody in all of their B-cells have been generated.

Gene expression analysis

The analysis of gene expression patterns can tell us a lot about what a cell or cell population is doing, or about to do, at a particular moment in time. To analyze the cohort of genes that

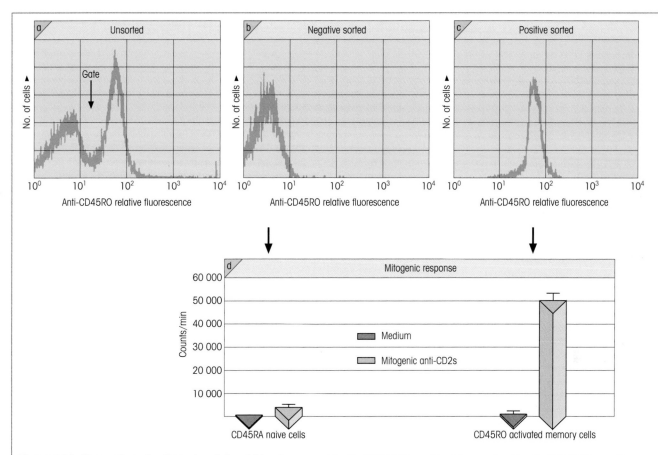

Figure 6.33. Separation of activated peripheral blood memory T-cells (CD45RO positive) from naive T-cells (CD45RO negative; but positive for the CD45RA isoform) in the FACS after staining the surface of the living cells in the cold with a fluorescent monoclonal antibody to the CD45RO (see p. 256). The unsorted cells showed two peaks (a); cells with fluorescence intensity lower than the arbitrary gate were separated from those with higher intensity giving (b) negative (CD45RA) and (c) positive (CD45RO) populations, which were each tested for their proliferative response to a mixture of two anti-CD2 monoclonals (OKT11 and GT2) in the presence of 10% antigen-presenting cells (d). ^{3}H-Thymidine was added after 3 days and the cells counted after 15 h. Clearly the memory cell population proliferated, whereas the naive population did not. (Data kindly provided by D. Wallace and R. Hicks.)

are expressed by a cell population, either at a steady-state level or in response to a particular stimulus, messenger RNA (mRNA) is extracted and is analyzed by a method that enables genes of interest to be detected. mRNA can be analyzed by northern blot, in which a single gene probe is hybridized to the mRNA sample, or by reverse transcriptase (RT)-primed PCR in which genes of interest can be amplified by initially making a cDNA copy using RT followed by gene amplification by means of specific primers that are complementary to the sequence of interest. While northern blotting and RT-PCR can give information concerning more than one transcript, this usually requires significant amounts of mRNA and is relatively slow.

The development of microarray technologies now permits the simultaneous measurement of expression of thousands of genes in a single experiment. Oligonucleotides or cDNA fragments are robotically spotted onto a gene chip and cDNA generated from, for example, T-cell mRNA is labeled and

hybridized to the genes on the microarray. This provides a quantitative comparison of expression for every gene present on the chip. By accumulating such data it is possible to build up a complete picture of which genes are expressed in which cells (Figure 6.34). One area in which this technology is being rapidly deployed is in the analysis of differences in gene expression between a tumor cell and its normal counterpart, thereby illuminating possible targets for therapeutic intervention.

All that glitters is not gold however and it is certainly true to say that DNA microarrays are not a solution to all our problems. Background is a troublesome feature of this type of approach and often threatens to drown out interesting data in a cacophony of experimental noise. Well controlled experimental set-ups are a must for large-scale microarray approaches, otherwise any gene expression differences observed could well be due to slamming the tissue culture incubator door rather than the intended stimulus. The term "garbage in, garbage out" comes to mind in these situations.

⚲ Milestone 6.2—The Fluorescence-activated Cell Sorter (FACS)

The FACS was developed by the Herzenbergs (Leonard and Leonore) and their colleagues to quantify the surface molecules on individual white cells by their reaction with fluorochrome-labeled monoclonal antibodies and to use the signals so generated to separate cells of defined phenotype from a heterogeneous mixture.

In this elegant but complex machine, the fluorescent cells are made to flow obediently in a single stream past a laser beam. Quantitative measurement of the fluorescence signal in a suitably placed photomultiplier tube relays a signal to the cell as it emerges in a single droplet; the cell becomes

charged and can be separated in an electric field (Figure M6.2.1). Extra sophistication can be introduced by using additional lasers and fluorochromes, and both 90° and forward light scatter. This is elaborated upon in the section on flow cytofluorimetry describing how this technique can be used for quantitative multiparameter analysis of single-cell populations (cf. Figure 6.14). Suffice to state that these latest FACS machines permit the isolation of cells with a complex phenotype from a heterogeneous population with a high degree of discrimination.

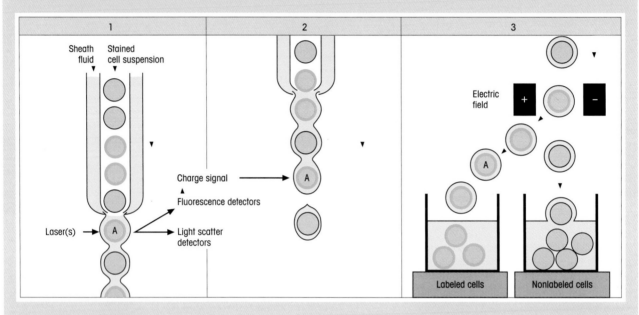

Figure M6.2.1. The principle of the FACS for flow cytofluorimetry of the fluorescence on stained cells (green rimmed circles) and physical separation from unstained cells. The charge signal can be activated to separate cells of high from low fluorescence and, using light scatter, of large from small size and dead from living.

Assessment of functional activity

The activity of phagocytic cells

The major tests employed to assess neutrophil function are summarized in Table 6.1.

Dendritic cell responsiveness

As we discussed in Chapter 1, dendritic cells and other APCs, such as macrophages, typically respond to pathogen-associated molecular patterns (PAMPs) and danger-associated molecular patterns (DAMPs) through secretion of cytokines as well as upregulation of surface B7 family ligands and MHC class II molecules (c.f. Figure 1.27). PAMP stimulation of DCs, as well as macrophages, also typically leads to the production of multiple cytokines such as TNF, IL-1β, IL-6, IL-8, GM-CSF, IFNα, IFNβ and others. Thus, cytokine production is a con-

venient assay of PAMP-mediated activation of DCs and macrophages.

Lymphocyte responsiveness

When lymphocytes are stimulated by antigen or polyclonal activators *in vitro* they usually undergo cell division (cf. Figure 4.1) and release cytokines. Cell division is normally assessed by the incorporation of radiolabeled ^{3}H-thymidine or ^{125}I-labeled UdR (5-iododeoxyuridine) into the DNA of the dividing cells. Cell division can also be measured by incorporation of fluorescent lipophilic dyes, such as CFSE, into the plasma membrane of lymphocytes or other cells. Upon division of cells labeled in this way, the fluorescent dye is equally partitioned to each of the daughter cells such that each daughter has only half the dye content of the parent (Figure 6.35a). The decrease in membrane dye content can be measured accurately using a

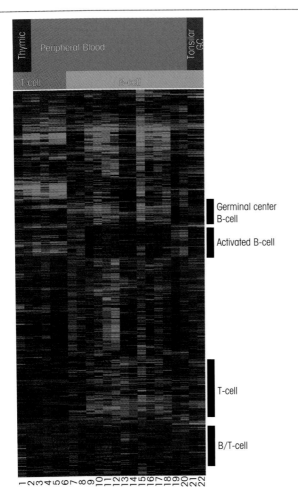

Figure 6.34. Gene expression during lymphocyte development and activation.

The data were generated from over 3.8 million measurements of gene expression made on 13637 genes using 243 microarrays. Each experiment represents a different cell population. For example, experiment 1 utilized polyclonally activated fetal CD4+ thymic cells, whereas experiment 2 shows the same population prior to stimulation. Overexpressed or induced genes are colored red, underexpressed or repressed genes green. Certain gene expression signatures become apparent in the different cell populations, indicated on the right. For example, the T-cell gene expression signature includes CD2, TCR, TCR signaling molecules and many cytokines. (Reproduced with permission of the authors and the publishers from Alizadeh A.A. & Staudt L.M. (2000) *Current Opinion in Immunology* **12**, 219.)

Table 6.1. Evaluation of neutrophil function.

Function	Test
Phagocytosis	Measure the uptake of particles such as latex or bacteria by counting or by chemiluminescence
Respiratory burst	Measure reduction of nitroblue tetrazolium
Intracellular killing	Microbicidal test using viable *Staphylococcus aureus*
Directional migration	Movement through filters up concentration gradient of chemotactic agent such as formyl.Met.Leu.Phe
Surface LFA-1 and CR3 upregulation	Ascertained with monoclonal antibody staining

number of cell divisions the labeled cells subsequently undergo by measuring their dye content.

Cytokines released into the culture medium can be measured by immunoassay or by a bioassay using a cell line dependent on a particular cytokine for its growth and survival. Individual cells synthesizing cytokines can be enumerated in the flow cytometer by permeabilizing and staining intracellularly with labeled antibody (see below); alternatively the ELISPOT technique (see below) can be applied. As usual, molecular biology has a valuable, if more sophisticated, input as T-cells transfected with an IL-2 enhancer–*lacZ* construct will switch on *lacZ* β-galactosidase expression on activation of the IL-2 cytokine response (cf. p. 212) and this can be readily revealed with a fluorescent or chromogenic enzyme substrate.

The ability of cytotoxic T-cells to kill their cell targets extracellularly is usually evaluated by a chromium release assay. Target cells are labeled with ^{51}Cr and the release of radioactive protein into the medium over and above that seen in the controls is the index of cytotoxicity. The test is repeated at different ratios of effector to target cells. A similar technique is used to measure extracellular killing of antibody-coated or uncoated targets by NK cells. Now a word of caution regarding the interpretation of *in vitro* assays. As one can manipulate the culture conditions within wide limits, it is possible to achieve a result that might not be attainable *in vivo*. Let us illustrate this point by reference to cytotoxicity for murine cells infected with lymphocytic choriomeningitis virus (LCMV) or vesicular stomatitis virus (VSV). The most sensitive *in vitro* technique proved to be chromium release from target cells after secondary stimulation of the lymphocytes. However, this needs 5 days, during which time a relatively small number of memory CD8 cytotoxic T-cell precursors can replicate and surpass the threshold required to produce a measurable assay. Nonetheless, a weak cytotoxicity assay under these conditions was not reflected

flow cytometer and this gives information concerning the number of cell divisions a cell has undergone as it was labeled (Figure 6.35b). This method is especially useful when using mixed cell populations where it is important to know which cell type is dividing; by membrane labeling of purified cells, followed by adding these cells into a mixed cell population or even injecting these into an animal, it is possible to track the

Figure 6.35. Analysis of cell proliferation by CFSE-labeling.

Lymphocytes, or other cells with proliferative potential, can be labeled with the fluorescent lipophilic dye, CFSE, and subsequently analyzed for partitioning of fluorescent dye into daughter cells. (a) Schematic depiction of a CFSE-anti-labeling experiment and corresponding flow cytometry plots. (b) Human peripheral T-cells were labeled with CFSE and stimulated with plate-coated anti-CD3 monoclonal antibody for 4 days. Left panel: no stimulation; right panel: anti-CD3 stimulation. Numbers and bars on the top of each histogram refer to respective division peaks with the peak of undivided cells to the extreme right in each histogram. (Courtesy of Dr. Antione Attinger.)

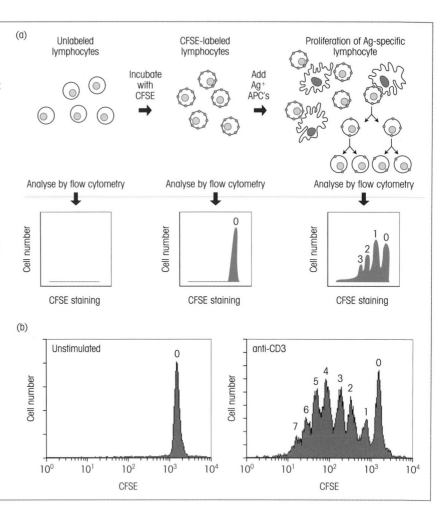

Detection of T-cell subsets through staining for expression of cytokines

Cytokine production by T-cell populations was for many years carried out at the population level, using ELISA assays, for example. This is because cytokines, with some exceptions, are typically rapidly secreted as they are synthesized. However, two approaches now make it possible to directly measure cytokine production at the cellular level. One approach, utilizes inhibitors of cytokine export (e.g. metabolic poisons such as brefeldin A that trap cytokines within the endoplasmic reticulum) to block cytokine secretion such that these molecules can be immunostained once cellular permeabilization has been achieved. Cell populations treated in this way can then be **stained for intracellular cytokines** using specific antibodies, followed by analysis by flow cytometry, as described earlier. The other approach makes use of bispecific antibodies that can simultaneously bind to a T-cell marker (such as CD4) while the other Fab is specific for a cytokine. In this application of the technique, cytokines are captured as they are secreted from

cells but, due to the bispecific nature of the antibody, which is tethered to the cell surface, the cytokine also becomes stably attached to the cell making it. The **captured cytokine** can then be detected by use of a different cytokine specific antibody conjugated to a fluorochrome.

Apoptosis

Programed cell death occurs frequently in the immune system and is particularly important for the resolution of immune responses. Antigen-driven clonal expansion of T- and B-cells is typically followed by death of many of these cells within a relatively short period, with the remaining cells making up the memory cell population; interference with this cell elimination process can result in accumulation of lymphocytes that may break tolerance and result in autoimmunity. The Fas (CD95) receptor plays an important role in peripheral tolerance and homeostatic control of lymphocyte cell populations; inactivation of this membrane receptor protein, or its ligand, in the mouse results in severe enlargement of the spleen and lymph nodes due to accumulation of lymphocytes that would normally have been eliminated through Fas-dependent apoptosis (Figure 6.36). Engagement of the Fas receptor on activated lymphocytes normally results in rapid induction of apoptosis in these cells (Figure 6.7). Cytotoxic T-cells also eliminate target cells by inducing apoptosis through a variety of strategies. Apoptosis is also important in shaping the T- and B-cell repertoires; negative selection of both lymphocyte populations involves triggering apoptosis.

A variety of approaches can be used to measure apoptosis, ranging from morphological assessment (see Figure 6.7) or by exploiting biochemical alterations to the cell that occurs during this process. One of the most widely used assays for apoptosis takes advantage of the fact that phosphatidylserine (PS), a phospholipid that is normally confined to the inner leaflet of the plasma membrane, becomes exposed on the outer leaflet during apoptosis. This can be readily detected using fluorescently labeled annexin V, a PS-binding protein; apoptotic cells display markedly enhanced binding of annexin V relative to healthy cells (Figure 6.37).

Other assays take advantage of the fact that extensive DNA fragmentation is also a common feature of apoptosis and this can be assessed by agarose gel electrophoresis of DNA extracted from apoptotic cells or the TUNEL (*T*dT-mediated d*U*TP (deoxyuridine triphosphate) *n*ick *e*nd *l*abeling) assay; the latter assay utilizes the enzyme terminal deoxynucleotidyl transferase (TdT) to add biotinylated nucleotides to the 3' ends of DNA fragments and this can then be detected using fluorescently labeled streptavidin. Several members of the caspase family of cysteine proteases become activated during apoptosis and this can be assessed by immunoblot analysis (Figure 6.19) or by using labeled synthetic substrate peptides that can be cleaved by active caspases.

Precursor frequency

The magnitude of lymphocyte responses in culture is closely related to the number of antigen-specific lymphocytes capable of responding. Because of the clonality of the responses, it is possible to estimate the frequency of these antigen-specific precursors by **limiting dilution analysis**. In essence, the method depends upon the fact that, if one takes several replicate aliquots of a given cell suspension that would be expected to contain *on average* one precursor per aliquot, then Poisson distribution analysis shows that 37% of the aliquots will contain *no* precursor cells (through the randomness of the sampling). Thus, if aliquots are made from a series of dilutions of a cell suspension and incubated under conditions that allow the precursors to mature and be recognized through some amplification scheme, the dilution at which 37% of the aliquots give negative responses will be known to contain an average of one precursor cell per aliquot, and one can therefore calculate the precursor frequency in the original cell suspension. An example is shown in some detail in Figure 6.38.

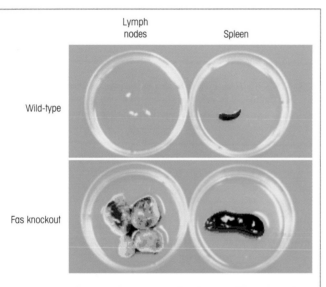

Figure 6.36. Gross enlargement of spleen and lymph nodes from Fas "knockout" mice.

Lymph nodes and spleen from wild type versus Fas knockout mice are compared. Both organs are increased approximately 20-fold in size in the knockout due to accumulation of excess T- and B-cells due to a failure of peripheral deletion in these animals. (Kindly provided by Professor Shigekazu Nagata and adapted from Adachi M. *et al.*, 1995 *Nature Genetics* **11**, 294, with permission.)

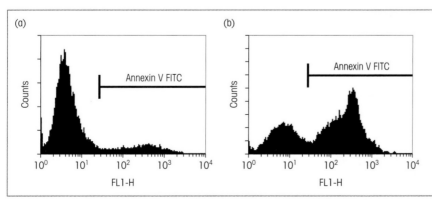

Figure 6.37. Analysis of apoptosis by Annexin V-labeling.

Phosphatidylserine (PS) is externalized on the outer leaflet of the plasma membrane during apoptosis and this can be readily detected using the PS-binding protein, Annexin V. (a) Untreated human T-lymphoblastoid cells; and (b) apoptotic T-lymphoblastoid cells were stained with FITC-conjugated annexin V. (Data kindly provided by Dr. Gabriela Brumatti.)

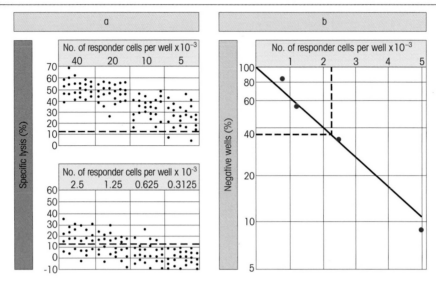

Figure 6.38. Limiting dilution analysis of cytotoxic T-cell precursor frequency in spleen cells from a BALB/c mouse stimulated with irradiated C57BL/6 spleen cells as antigen. BALB/c splenic responder cells were set up in 24 replicates at each concentration tested together with antigen and an excess of T-helper factors. The generation of cytotoxicity in each well was looked for by adding ^{51}Cr-labeled tumor cells (EL-4) of the C57BL/6 haplotype; cytotoxicity was then revealed by measuring the release of soluble ^{51}Cr-labeled intracellular material into the medium. (a) The points show the percentage of specific lysis of individual wells. The dashed line indicates three standard deviations above the medium release control, and each point above that line is counted as positive for cytotoxicity. (b) The data replotted in terms of the percentage of negative wells at each concentration of responder cells over the range in which the data titrated (5×10^{-3}/well to 0.625×10^{-3}/well). The dashed line is drawn at 37% negative wells and this intersects the regression line to give a precursor (T_{cp}) frequency of 1 in 2327 responder cells. The regression line has an r^2 value of 1.00 in this experiment. (Reproduced with permission from Simpson E. & Chandler P. (1986) In: Weir D.M. (ed.) *Handbook of Experimental Immunology*, Figure 68.2. Blackwell Scientific Publications, Oxford.)

It has been argued that limiting dilution analysis often underestimates the true precursor frequency. This is likely because cells generally do not survive very well when cultured in isolation (i.e. as a single cell per well) because most cells, with few exceptions, require signals from other cells to survive. Martin Raff showed that in the absence of such signals cells typically undergo apoptosis. An accurate measure of the percentage of lymphocytes bearing a specific antigen receptor can be obtained by flow cytometry of cells stained with labeled antigen. In the case of B-cells this is fairly straightforward, given that their antigen receptors recognize native antigen. However, it is only recently that technical finesse, in the form of peptide–MHC tetramers, has brought this technique to T-cells (Figure 6.39). This approach overcomes the problem of the relatively weak intrinsic affinity of TCR for peptide–MHC by presenting a tagged peptide–MHC as a multivalent tetramer, thereby exploiting the bonus effect of multivalency (cf. p. 122). Peptide–MHC complexes are produced by permitting recombinant MHC molecules to refold with the appropriate synthetic peptide. The recombinant MHC molecules are biotinylated on a special carboxy-terminal extension, that ensures that the biotin is incorporated at a distance from the site to

which the TCR binds, and mixed with fluorescently labeled streptavidin, which not only binds biotin with a very high affinity but also has a valency of four with respect to the biotin—hence the formation of tetramers.

Numerous adaptations of this technology are appearing. For example, incubation of tetramers bound to their cognate TCR leads to internalization at 37°C; by tagging them with a toxin individual T-lymphocytes of a single specificity can be eliminated. Another approach is to use the FACS to directly sort stained cells into an ELISPOT microtiter plate in which cytokine secretion is measured, providing a functional analysis of the cells.

Enumeration of antibody-forming cells

The immunofluorescence sandwich test

This is a double-layer procedure designed to visualize specific intracellular antibody. If, for example, we wished to see how many cells in a preparation of lymphoid tissue were synthesizing antibody to pneumococcus polysaccharide, we would first fix the cells with ethanol to prevent the antibody being washed away during the test, and then treat with a solution of the

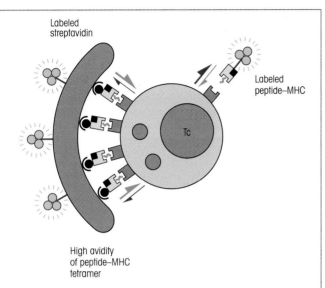

Figure 6.39. Peptide–MHC tetramer.

A single fluorochrome-labeled peptide–MHC complex (top right) has only a low affinity for the TCR and therefore provides a very insensitive probe for its cognate receptor. However, by biotinylating (•) the MHC molecules and then mixing them with streptavidin, which has a valency of four with respect to biotin binding, a tetrameric complex is formed which has a much higher functional affinity (avidity) when used as a probe for the specific TCRs on the T-cell surface.

polysaccharide antigen. After washing, a fluorescein-labeled antibody to the polysaccharide would then be added to locate those cells that had specifically bound the antigen.

The name of the test derives from the fact that antigen is sandwiched between the antibody present in the cell substrate and that added as the second layer (Figure 6.8c).

Plaque techniques

Antibody-secreting cells can be counted by diluting them in an environment in which the antibody formed by each individual cell produces a readily observable effect. In one technique, developed from the original method of Niels Jerne and Albert Nordin, the cells from an animal immunized with sheep erythrocytes are suspended together with an excess of sheep red cells and complement within a shallow chamber formed between two microscope slides. On incubation, the antibody-forming cells release their immunoglobulin that coats the surrounding erythrocytes. The complement will then cause lysis of the coated cells and a **plaque** clear of red cells will be seen around each antibody-forming cell (Figure 6.40). Direct plaques obtained in this way largely reveal IgM producers as this antibody has a high hemolytic efficiency. To demonstrate IgG synthesizing cells it is necessary to increase the complement binding of the erythrocyte–IgG antibody complex by adding a rabbit anti-IgG serum; the "indirect plaques" thus developed can be used to enumerate cells making antibodies in different immunoglobulin subclasses, provided that the appropriate rabbit antisera are available. The method can be extended by coating an antigen such as pneumococcus

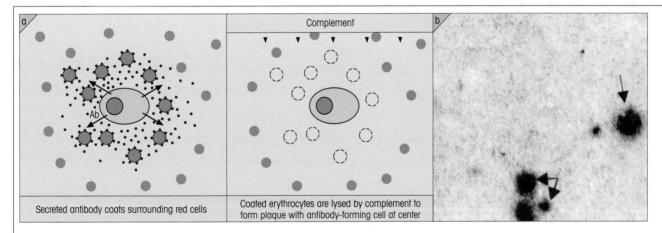

Figure 6.40. Jerne plaque technique for enumerating antibody-forming cells (Cunningham modification).

(a) The *direct* technique for cells synthesizing IgM hemolysin is shown. The *indirect* technique for visualizing cells producing IgG hemolysins requires the addition of anti-IgG to the system. The difference between the plaques obtained by direct and indirect methods gives the number of "IgG" plaques. The *reverse plaque* assay enumerates total Ig-producing cells by capturing secreted Ig on red cells coated with anti-Ig. Multiple plaque assays can be carried out by a modification using microtiter plates. (b) Photograph of plaques that show as circular dark areas (some of which are arrowed) under dark-ground illumination. They vary in size depending upon the antibody affinity and the rate of secretion by the antibody-forming cell. (Courtesy of C. Shapland, P. Hutchings and Professor D. Male.)

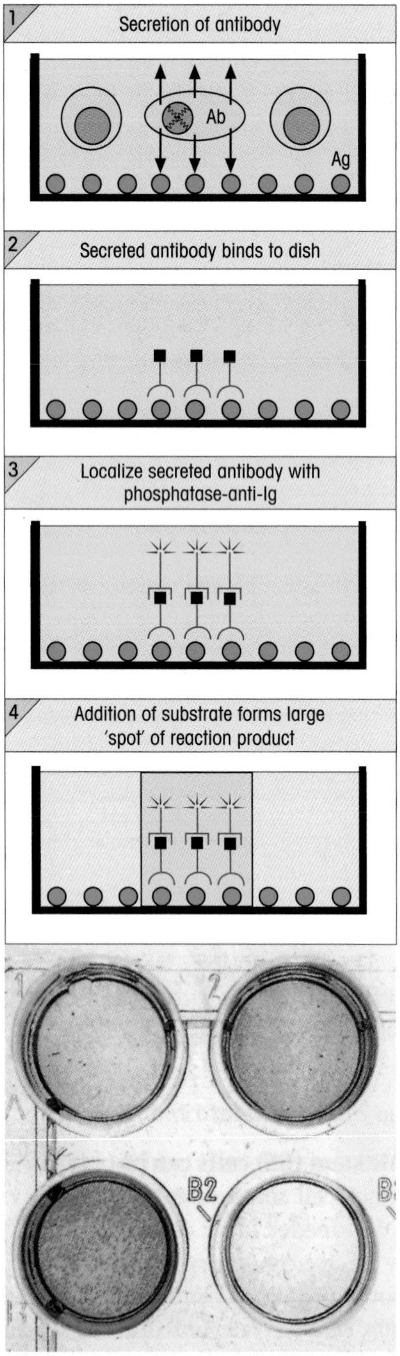

Figure 6.41. ELISPOT (from ELISA spot) system for enumerating antibody-forming cells.

The picture shows spots formed by hybridoma cells making autoantibodies to thyroglobulin revealed by alkaline phosphatase-linked anti-Ig (courtesy of P. Hutchings). Increasing numbers of hybridoma cells were added to the top two and bottom left-hand wells that show corresponding increases in the number of "ELISPOTs." The bottom right-hand well is a control using a hybridoma of irrelevant specificity.

polysaccharide on to the red cell, or by coupling hapten groups to the erythrocyte surface.

In the **ELISPOT** modification, the antibody-forming cell suspension is incubated in microtiter wells containing filters coated with antigen. The secreted antibody is captured locally and is visualized, after removal of the cells, by treatment with enzyme-labeled anti-Ig and development of the color reaction with the substrate. The macroscopic spots can be readily enumerated (Figure 6.41).

Manipulation of the immune system in animal models

The laboratory mouse has proved incredibly informative for our understanding of the vertebrate immune system. There are many cleaver ways in which the murine immune system can be manipulated to tease out the complexities of immune function. What follows is a limited selection of approaches.

Adoptive cell transfer

It is possible to use relatively low doses of X-ray or γ-radiation to eliminate endogenous lymphocytes, while sparing other tissues, followed by transfer of lymphocytes specific for a particular antigen to study in relative isolation *in vivo*. Many other variations on this theme are possible such as transfer of discrete T-cell subsets, e.g. CD4+ T-cells immunodepleted *ex vivo* for CTLA-4-expressing cells can permit the study the role of the latter in negatively regulating T-cell activation.

Generation of bone marrow chimeras

Once again, the starting point is an irradiated mouse. Animals ablated in such a way may be reconstituted by injection of bone marrow hematopoietic stem cells that provide the precursors of all the formed elements of the blood (cf. Figure 11.1). These chimeras of host plus hematopoietic grafted cells can be manipulated in many ways to analyze cellular function, such as the role of the thymus in the maturation of T-lymphocytes from bone marrow stem cells (Figure 6.42).

T-cell depletion *in vivo*

This can be achieved by **thymectomy**, the surgical removal of the thymus at birth, that results in a dramatic depletion of T-cells. Alternatively, thymectomy of an adult mouse, followed by reconstitution with wild type bone marrow results in reconstitution of all hematopoietic cell types except T-cells, due to the essential role of the thymus for T-cell development.

Spontaneous mutant mice lacking T-cells

Homozygous *nude* mice, which carry a spontaneous mutation in the *Foxn1nu* gene, lack a thymus and are consequently devoid of T-cells. Such mice are also hairless, giving rise to their rather

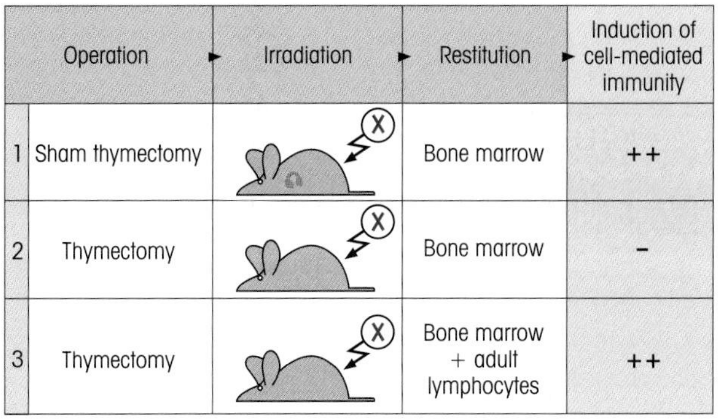

	Operation	Irradiation	Restitution	Induction of cell-mediated immunity
1	Sham thymectomy	(X)	Bone marrow	++
2	Thymectomy	(X)	Bone marrow	–
3	Thymectomy	(X)	Bone marrow + adult lymphocytes	++

Figure 6.42. Maturation of bone marrow stem cells under the influence of the thymus

to become immunocompetent lymphocytes capable of cell-mediated immune reactions. X-irradiation (X) destroys the ability of host lymphocytes to mount a cellular immune response, but the stem cells in injected bone marrow can become immunocompetent and restore the response (1) unless the thymus is removed (2), in which case only already immunocompetent lymphocytes are effective (3). Incidentally, the bone marrow stem cells also restore the levels of other formed elements of the blood (red cells, platelets, neutrophils, monocytes) that otherwise fall dramatically after X-irradiation, and such therapy is crucial in cases where accidental or therapeutic exposure to X-rays or other antimitotic agents seriously damages the hematopoietic cells.

appropriate name. Apart from their role in the study of immunodeficiency and T-cell development, such mice are also commonly used as graft or tumor recipients; such mice readily accept tissue from other mouse strains (allografts) as well as different species (xenografts) due to their almost complete lack of T-cells that are required to mount graft rejections.

Mice with severe combined immunodeficiency (SCID)

Mice with defects in the genes encoding the IL-2 receptor γ chain, the nucleotide salvage pathway enzymes adenosine deaminase or purine nucleoside phosphorylase, or the RAG enzymes, develop SCID due to a failure of B- and T-cells to differentiate. These special animals can be reconstituted with various human lymphoid tissues and their functions and responses analyzed. Coimplantation of contiguous fragments of human fetal liver (hematopoietic stem cells) and thymus allows T-lymphopoiesis, production of B-cells and maintenance of colony-forming units of myeloid and erythroid lineages for 6–12 months. Adult peripheral blood cells injected into the peritoneal cavity of SCID mice treated with growth hormone can sustain the production of human B-cells and antibodies and can be used to generate human hybridomas making defined monoclonal antibodies. Immunotherapeutic antitumor responses can also be played with in these animals.

Genetic engineering of cells and model organisms

Insertion and modification of genes in mammalian cells

Because gene transfer into primary (i.e. untransformed) mammalian cells is inefficient, it is customary to use immortal cell lines for such **transfections** and to include a selectable marker such as neomycin resistance. Genes can be introduced into cells using bacterial plasmid vectors; however, because cells do not readily take up free DNA, methods to improve the rate of uptake have been developed. Increased uptake can be achieved through precipitating plasmid DNA using calcium phosphate or by electroporation where an electric current is used to open transient pores in the plasma membrane. Another approach is to incorporate the plasmid into liposomes, which fuse with the cell membrane. Direct microinjection of DNA is also effective but is labor intensive and requires specialized equipment. Integration of the gene into the genome of a virus such as vaccinia provides an easy ride into the cell, although more stable long-term transfections are obtained with modified retroviral vectors. One of the latest fads is transfection by biolistics, the buzz word for biological ballistics. DNA coated on to gold microparticles is literally fired from a high-pressure helium gun and penetrates the cells; even plant cells with their cellulose coats are easy meat for this technology. Skin and surgically exposed tissues can also be penetrated with ease.

Studying the effect of *adding* a gene, then, does not offer too many technological problems. How does one assess the impact of *removing* a gene? One versatile strategy to delete endogenous gene function is to target the gene's mRNA as distinct from the gene itself. Nucleotide sequences complementary to the mRNA of the target gene are introduced into the cell, usually in a form that allows them to replicate. The **antisense** molecules so produced base pair with the target mRNA and block translation into protein. Although antisense RNA approaches showed early promise, this approach has been largely superseded by a recent innovation called **RNA interference (RNAi)**.

RNAi can be used to "knock down" expression of particular target genes within a cell by introducing a double-stranded (ds) RNA molecule homologous to the target gene. This method takes advantage of a natural antiviral system that selectively targets mRNA when it is detected in double-stranded form in the cell; normally dsRNA spells trouble, as this form of RNA is rarely present in cells unless they are infected by a virus. The cellular machinery that naturally responds to dsRNA selectively degrades only mRNAs that are homologous to the dsRNA molecule that initiated the response. In theory, this can be mimicked by synthesizing a dsRNA copy of the gene to be silenced and introducing this into the cell; in practice there are problems with this approach when using mammalian cells and so an alternative strategy is widely employed (Figure 6.43). Short-interfering RNA (siRNA) molecules of 21–25 nucleotides, homologous to the gene of interest, can be synthesized and these overcome some of the nonspecific effects seen with large dsRNA molecules. Because of the simplicity of the siRNA approach, genome-wide cell-based screens are underway to knockdown essentially every gene in the genome and explore the consequences of this. It is important to note however that gene knockdown approaches are rarely, if ever, 100% effective and there is always the uncertainty that any observed effects could also be due to unintentional silencing of other genes along with the gene of interest.

Introducing new genes into animals

Establishing "designer mice" bearing new genes

Female mice are induced to superovulate and are then mated. The fertilized eggs are microinjected with the gene and surgically implanted in females. Between 5% and 40% of the implanted oocytes develop to term and, of these, 10–25% have copies of the injected gene, stably integrated into their chromosomes, detectable by PCR. These "founder" transgenic animals are mated with nontransgenic mice and pure transgenic lines are eventually established (Figure 6.44).

Expression of the transgene can be directed to particular tissues if the relevant promoter is included in the construct, for example the thyroglobulin promoter will confine expression to the thyroid. A different approach is to switch a gene on and off at will by incorporating an inducible promoter. Thus, the metallothionein promoter will enable expression of its linked gene only if zinc is added to the drinking water given to the mice. One needs to confirm that only the desired expression is obtained as, in some situations, promoters may misbehave leading to "leaky" expression of the associated gene.

Transgenes introduced into embryonic stem cells

Embryonic stem (ES) cells can be obtained by culturing the inner cell mass of mouse blastocysts. After transfection with the appropriate gene, the transfected cells can be selected and reimplanted after injection into a new blastocyst. The resulting mice are chimeric, in that some cells carry the transgene and others do not. The same will be true of germ cells and, by breeding for germ-line transmission of the transgene, pure strains can be derived (Figure 6.45).

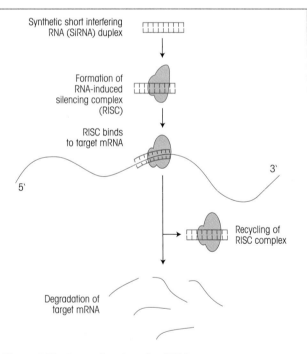

Figure 6.43. Gene silencing via siRNA.

Synthetic short-interfering double-stranded RNA molecules (siRNAs), complementary to a gene of interest, are introduced into cells by transfection and, in complex with proteins within the transfected cell, lead to the formation of an RNA-induced silencing complex (RISC) that binds to mRNA molecules complementary to the introduced siRNA. This results in degradation of the target mRNA and recycling of the RISC to target additional mRNA molecules.

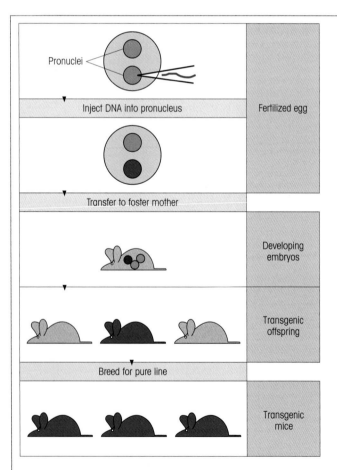

Figure 6.44. Production of pure strain transgenic mice by microinjection of fertilized egg, implantation into a foster mother and subsequent inbreeding.

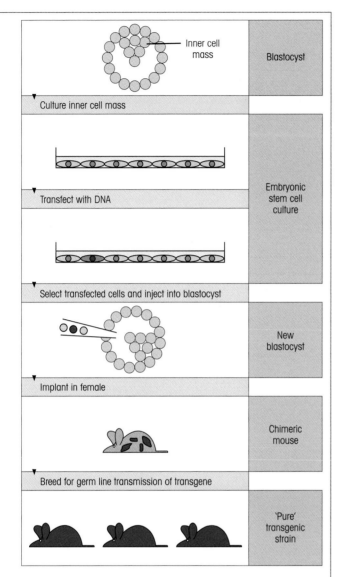

Figure 6.45. Introduction of a transgene through transfection of embryonic stem cells.

The transfected cells can be selected, e.g. for homologous recombinant "knockouts," before reimplantation.

Table 6.2. Some gene "knockouts" and their effects.

Knockout target	Phenotype of knockout mice
CD8 α-chain	Absence of cytotoxic T-cells
p59^{fynT}	Defective signaling in thymocytes but not peripheral T-cells
HOX 11	No spleen
FcεRI α-chain	Resistant to cutaneous and systemic anaphylaxis
IgM μ-chain membrane exon	Absence of B-cells
IL-6	No bone loss when ovariectomized (implications for osteoporosis?)
IL-18	Susceptible to *Leishmania major*; shift from Th1 to Th2 response (decreased IFNγ and increased IL-4 production)
MHC class II Aβ	Decreased CD4 T-cells; inflammatory bowel disease
Perforin	Impaired CTL and NK cell function
TAP1	Lack CD8 cells
TNFR-1	Resistant to endotoxic shock; susceptible to *Listeria*

Modified from Brandon (1995) *Current Biology* **5**, 625.

and center. Just a few examples of knockout mice of interest to immunologists are listed in Table 6.2.

It is not a particularly rare finding to observe that knocking out a gene leads to unexpected developmental defects. Although this in itself can provide important information concerning the role of the gene in developmental processes, it can frustrate the original aim of the experiment. Indeed, a number of knockouts are nonviable due to embryonic lethality. Never fear, ingenuity once again triumphs, in this case by the harnessing of viral or yeast recombinase systems. Instead of using a nonfunctional gene to create the knockout mouse, the targeting construct contains the normal form of the gene but flanked with recognition sequences (*loxP* sites) for a recombinase enzyme called Cre. These mice are mated with transgenic mice containing the bacteriophage P1-derived *Cre* transgene linked to an inducible or tissue-specific promoter. The endogenous gene of interest will be deleted only when and where Cre is expressed thereby creating a **tissue-specific** or **conditional knockout** (Figure 6.47). The Cre/*loxP* system can also be organized in such a way as to turn on expression of a gene by incorporating a stop sequence flanked by *loxP* sites.

Mice in which an endogenous gene is purposefully replaced by a functional gene, be it a modified version of the original gene or an entirely different gene, are referred to as **"knocked in mice."** Hence, in the example above, knocking in a *loxP*

The advantage over microinjection is that the cells can be selected after transfection, and this is especially important if **homologous recombination** is required in order to generate "**knockout mice**" lacking the gene that has been targeted. In this case, a DNA sequence that will disrupt the reading frame of the endogenous gene is inserted into the ES cells. Because homologous recombination is a rare event compared to random integration, selectable markers are incorporated into the construct in order to transfer only those ES cells in which the endogenous gene has been deleted (Figure 6.46). This is a truly powerful technology and the whole biological community has been suffused with boxing fever, knocking out genes right, left

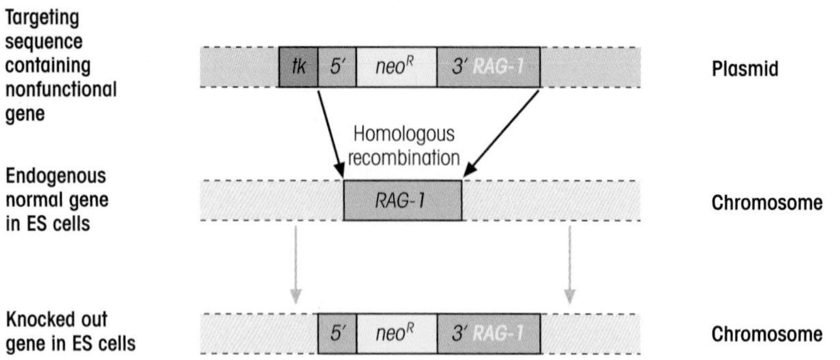

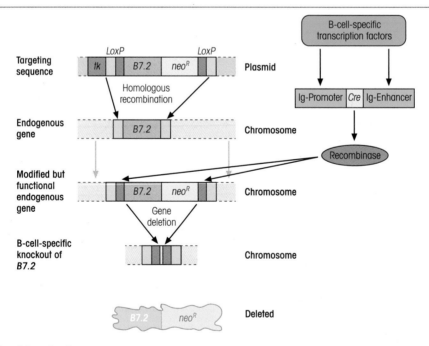

Figure 6.46. Gene disruption by homologous recombination with plasmid DNA containing a copy of the gene of interest (in this example *RAG-1*) into which a sequence specifying neomycin resistance (*neo^R*) has been inserted in such a way as to destroy the *RAG-1* reading frame between the 5′ and 3′ ends of the gene. Embryonic stem (ES) cells in which the targeting sequence has been incorporated into the chromosomal DNA by homologous recombination will be resistant to the neomycin analog G418. Stem cells in which nonhomologous recombination into chromosomal DNA has occurred would additionally incorporate the *thymidine kinase* (*tk*) gene that can be used to destroy such cells by culturing them in the presence of ganciclovir, leaving only ES cells in which homologous recombination has been achieved. These are then used to create a knockout mouse.

Figure 6.47. Conditional knockout.

The endogenous gene that is under study (here *B7.2*) is homologously replaced in ES cells with an identical gene, as in Figure 6.46, but here flanked by *loxP* sequences (brown boxes) and with the *neo^R* gene incorporated in a nondisruptive manner purely for selection purposes. Nonhomologous recombinants will contain the *tk* gene and are eliminated using ganciclovir. Transgenic animals are then generated from ES cells that are resistant to G418. If homozygous *B7.2–loxP*

transgenics are mated with mice that contain a transgene for the Cre recombinase under the control of specific regulatory elements, only those cells in which the promoter is active will produce the Cre enzyme necessary to delete the sequence flanked by *loxP*. The example given would represent an experiment aimed at investigating the effect of specifically knocking out *B7.2* in B-cells whilst maintaining its expression in, for example, dendritic cells.

flanked gene leads eventually to a knocked out gene in a selected cell type.

Gene therapy in humans

We seem to be catching up with science fiction and are in the early stages of being able to correct genetic misfortune by the introduction of "good" genes. For example, one form of severe combined immunodeficiency (SCID) is due to a mutation in the γc gene that encodes a subunit of the cytokine receptors for IL-2, -4, -7, -9, -15 and -21. Correction of this defect in children has been achieved by *in vitro* transfer of the normal gene into CD34$^+$ bone marrow stem cells using a vector derived from a Moloney retrovirus, a convincing proof of principle for human gene therapy.

Major problems yet to be overcome concern both the *efficiency* of delivery of replacement genes as well as *targeting* of the gene-delivery vector to the desired cell population. Where it is possible to remove the target cell population and treat *ex vivo* the risk of mis-targeting to other tissues is diminished but not entirely eliminated. In situations where the target tissue cannot be removed for treatment, the efficiency of gene delivery can be poor. Other risks include insertion of the replacement gene at random chromosomal sites; insertion into a tumor suppressor gene for example would be highly undesirable and may lead to tumor development. Some gene delivery vectors such as adeno-associated virus (AAV) insert at predictable chromosomal locations and seem the way forward in this regard. This still leaves the problem of efficient gene delivery *in vivo*. Viruses represent the most efficient gene delivery vehicles, being perfectly adapted to the task of invading human tissues and inserting their genomes. Thus it is not surprising that the most promising gene delivery vectors are currently assembled around modified forms of adenovirus, AAV, and lentiviruses such as HIV. Ironically, the immune system turns out to be one of the biggest obstacles to efficient gene delivery due to robust immune responses against these viral vectors. However, some viruses (such as AAV) provoke only modest or ineffective immune responses that can be exploited, in this instance at least, to our benefit.

Making antibodies to order

- Polyclonal antisera can be generated by repeated immunization with antigen.
- Polyclonal antibodies recognize a mixture of determinants on the antigen.
- Adjuvants are required for efficient immune responses to antigen.
- Immortal hybridoma cell lines making monoclonal antibodies provide powerful immunological reagents and insights into the immune response. Applications include enumeration of lymphocyte subpopulations, cell depletion, immunoassay, cancer diagnosis and imaging, purification of antigen from complex mixtures, and recently the use of monoclonals as artificial enzymes (catalytic antibodies).
- Genetically engineered human antibody fragments can be derived by expanding the V_H and V_L genes from unimmunized, but preferably immunized, donors and expressing them as completely randomized combinatorial libraries on the surface of bacteriophage. Phages bearing the highest affinity antibodies are selected by panning on antigens and the antibody genes can then be cloned from the isolated viruses.
- Single-chain Fv (scFv) fragments encoded by linked V_H and V_L genes and even single heavy chain domains can be created.
- The human anti-mouse antibody (HAMA) response is a significant obstacle to use of mouse monoclonal antibodies for therapeutic purposes.

- The HAMA response against mouse monoclonal antibodies can be reduced by producing chimeric antibodies with mouse variable regions and human constant regions or, better still, using humanized antibodies in which all the mouse sequences except for the CDRs are replaced by human sequences.
- Humanized antibodies are now in clinical use for the treatment of a variety of conditions such as rheumatoid arthritis and B-cell lymphoma.
- Transgenic mice bearing human *Ig* genes can be immunized. The mice produce high affinity fully human antibodies.
- Recombinant antibodies can be expressed on a large scale in plants.
- Combinatorial libraries of diabodies containing the H1 and H2 V_H CDR may be used to develop new drugs.

Purification of antigen and antibody by affinity chromatography

- Insoluble immunoabsorbents prepared by coupling antibody to Sepharose can be used to affinity-purify antigens from complex mixtures and reciprocally to purify antibodies.
- Affinity chromatography can also be used to co-purify proteins that serve as binding partners of antigens.

Modulation of biological activity

- Antibodies can be detected by inhibition of biological functions such as viral infectivity or bacterial growth.

- Inhibition of biological function by known antibodies helps to define the role of the antigen, be it a hormone or cytokine for example, in complex responses *in vivo* and *in vitro.*
- Activation of biological function by receptor-stimulating or receptor-cross-linking antibodies can substitute for natural ligand and can be used to explore biological function *in vitro* or *in vivo.*

Immunodetection of antigen in cells and tissues

- Antibodies can be used as highly specific probes to detect the presence of antigen in a tissue and to explore the subcellular localization of antigen. Antigens can be localized if stained by fluorescent antibodies and viewed in a fluorescence microscope.
- Fixation and permeabilization of cells permits entry of antibodies and allows intracellular antigens to be detected.
- Confocal microscopy scans a very thin plane at high magnification and provides quantitative data on extremely sharp images of the antigen-containing structures that can also be examined in three dimensions.
- Antibodies can either be labeled directly or visualized by a secondary antibody, a labeled anti-Ig.
- Different fluorescent labels can be conjugated to secondary antibodies enabling simultaneous detection of several different antigens in the same cell.
- Flow cytometry is a highly quantitative means of detecting fluorescence associated with immunolabeled or dye-labeled cells and thousands of cells per minute can be analyzed by such instruments.
- In a flow cytometer single cells in individual droplets are interrogated by one or more lasers and quantitative data using different fluorescent labels can be logged, giving a complex phenotypic analysis of each cell in a heterogeneous mixture. In addition, forward scatter of the laser light defines cell size and 90° scatter, cell granularity.
- Fluorescent antibodies or their fragments can also be used for staining intracellular antigens in permeabilized cells. Intracellular probes for pH, Ca^{2+}, Mg^{2+}, Na^+, thiols and DNA content are also available.
- Antibodies can be enzyme-labeled for histochemical definition of antigens at the light microscope level, or coupled with different-sized colloidal gold particles for ultrastructural visualization in the electron microscope.

Detection and quantitation of antigen by antibody

- Exceedingly low concentrations of antigens can be measured by immunoassay techniques that depend upon the relationship between Ag concentration and fractional occupancy of the binding antibody. Occupied sites are measured with a high specific activity second antibody directed to a different epitope; alternatively, unoccupied sites can be estimated by labeled Ag.
- Antigens can be separated on the basis of molecular mass upon electrophoresis through polyacrylamide gels. Antigens separated in this way can be blotted onto PVDF or nitrocellulose membranes and their presence detected by probing with suitable antibodies.
- Antigens and antigen-associated molecules can be immunoprecipitated using antibodies that recognize the antigen in its native form.
- Higher concentrations of antigens are frequently estimated by nephelometry.
- Protein microarrays, containing thousands of proteins immobilized on a solid support, can be probed with antibody for the simultaneous screening of many antigens. Similarly, antibody microarrays can be used to screen for the presence of multiple antigens in a single sample.

Epitope mapping

- Overlapping nests of peptides derived from the linear sequence of a protein can map T-cell epitopes and the linear elements of B-cell epitopes. Bacteriophages encoding all possible hexapeptides on their surface have provided some limited success in identifying discontinuous B-cell determinants.

Estimation of antibody

- The antibody content of a polyclonal antiserum is defined entirely in operational terms by the nature of the assay employed.
- Nonprecipitating antibodies can be measured by laser nephelometry or by salt or anti-Ig coprecipitation with radioactive antigen.
- Affinity is measured by a variety of methods including surface plasmon resonance, which gives a measure of both the on- and off-rates.
- Antibodies can also be detected by macroscopic agglutination of antigen-coated particles, and by one of the most important methods, ELISA, a two-stage procedure in which antibody bound to solid-phase antigen is detected by an enzyme-linked anti-Ig.

Isolation of leukocyte subpopulations

- Cells can be separated on the basis of physical characteristics such as size, buoyant density and adhesiveness.

■ Phagocytic cells can be separated by a magnet after taking up iron particles, and cells that divide in response to a specific stimulus, e.g. antigen, can be eliminated by ultraviolet light after incorporation of 5-bromodeoxyuridine.

■ Antibody-coated cells can be eliminated by complement-mediated cytotoxicity or anti-Ig–ricin conjugates; they can be isolated by panning on solid-phase anti-Ig or by cluster formation with magnetic beads bearing anti-Ig on their surface.

■ Smaller numbers of cells can be fractionated by coating with a fluorescent monoclonal antibody and separating them from nonfluorescent cells in the FACS.

■ Antigen-specific T-cells can be enriched as lines or clones by driving them with antigen; fusion to appropriate T-cell tumor lines yields immortal antigen-specific T-cell hybridomas.

Gene expression analysis

■ mRNA expression can be analyzed by northern blotting or RT-PCR.

■ A complete picture of cellular gene expression is now attainable by hybridization to microarray chips.

Assessment of functional activity

■ Lymphocyte responses to antigen are monitored by proliferation and/or cytokine release. Proliferation can be measured by uptake of ^{3}H-labeled thymidine or by CFSE-labeling.

■ Individual cells secreting cytokines can be identified by the ELISPOT technique in which the secreted product is captured by a solid-phase antibody and then stained with a second labeled antibody.

■ Extracellular killing by cytotoxic T-cells, and NK cells, can be measured by the release of radioactive ^{51}Cr from prelabeled target cells.

■ Apoptosis can be measured by assessment of annexin V binding, which detects the externalization of phosphatidylserine on the outer leaflet of the plasma membrane of dying cells.

■ The precursor frequency of effector T-cells can be measured by staining the cells with peptide–MHC tetramers or by limiting dilution analysis.

■ Antibody-forming cells can be enumerated, either by an immunofluorescence sandwich test or by plaque techniques in which the antibody secreted by the cells causes complement-mediated lysis of adjacent red cells, or is captured by solid-phase antigen in an ELISPOT assay.

■ Functional activity can be assessed by cellular reconstitution experiments in which leukocyte sets and selected lymphoid tissue can be transplanted into unresponsive hosts such as X-irradiated recipients or SCID mice. Defined cell populations can also be separated and selectively recombined *in vitro*.

■ Antibodies can be used to probe cellular function by cross-linking cell surface components or by selective destruction of particular intracellular sites by laser irradiation of chromophore-conjugated specific antibodies that localize to the target area by penetrating permeabilized cells.

Genetic engineering of cells

■ Genes can be inserted into mammalian cells by transfection using calcium phosphate precipitates, electroporation, liposomes and microinjection.

■ Genes can also be taken into a cell after incorporation into vaccinia or retroviruses.

■ Endogenous gene function can be inhibited by antisense RNA, RNA interference, short-interfering RNA or by homologous recombination with a disrupted gene.

■ Transgenic mice bearing an entirely new gene introduced into the fertilized egg by microinjection of DNA can be established as inbred lines.

■ Genes can be introduced into embryonic stem cells; these modified stem cells are injected back into a blastocyst and can develop into founder mice from which pure transgenic animals can be bred. One very important application of this technique involves the disruption of a targeted gene in the embryonic stem cell by homologous recombination, producing "knockout" mice lacking a specific gene. Conditional knockouts employ recombinase systems such as Cre/*loxP* in order to control the deletion either temporally or in a tissue-specific manner.

■ "Knock in" mice have a specified endogenous gene homologously replaced with either a variant of that gene or an entirely different gene.

■ Human gene therapy promises an exciting future but has to overcome major obstacles concerning safe and effective delivery of therapeutic genes. Delivery of genes by vectors based on retroviruses or adeno-related virus is under intensive investigation.

■ Robust immune responses to many viral vectors reduce their utility as gene delivery vehicles.

FURTHER READING

Alkan S.S. (2004) Monoclonal antibodies: the story of a discovery that revolutionized science and medicine. *Nature Reviews Immunology* **4**, 153–156.

Altman J.D. & Davis M.M. (2003) MHC–peptide tetramers to visualize antigen-specific T cells. *Current Protocols in Immunology* Chapter 17, Unit 17.3, John Wiley & Sons.

Ausubel F.M., Brent R., Kingston R.E., Moore D.D., Seidman J.G., Smith J.A. & Struhl K. (eds.) (2010) *Current Protocols in Molecular Biology.* John Wiley, New York.

Bonifacino J.S., Dasso M., Harford J.B., Lippincott-Schwartz J. & Yamada K.M. (eds.) (2010) *Current Protocols in Cell Biology.* John Wiley, New York.

Brandtzaeg P. (1998) The increasing power of immunohistochemistry and immunocytochemistry. *Journal of Immunological Methods* **216**, 49–67.

Brannigan J.A. & Wilkinson A.J. (2002) Protein engineering 20 years on. *Nature Reviews Molecular and Cell Biology* **3**, 964–970.

Carter L.L. & Swain S.L. (1997) Single cytokine analysis of cytokine production. *Current Opinion in Immunology* **9**, 177–182.

Cavazzana-Calvo S. *et al.* (2000) Gene therapy of human severe combined immunodeficiency (SCID)-XI disease. *Science* **288**, 669–672.

Chatenoud L. (2003) CD3-specific antibody-induced active tolerance: from bench to bedside. *Nature Reviews Immunology* **3**, 123–132.

Chowdhury P.S. & Pastan I. (1999) Improving antibody affinity by mimicking somatic hypermutation *in vitro*. *Nature Biotechnology* **17**, 568–572.

Coligan J.E., Bierer B.E., Margulies D.H., Shevach E.M. & Strober W. (eds.) (2010) *Current Protocols in Immunology.* John Wiley, New York.

Collas P. (2009) The state-of-the-art of chromatin immunoprecipitation. *Methods Mol Biol.* **567**, 1–25.

Delves P.J. (1997) *Antibody Production.* J. Wiley & Sons, Chichester.

Fishwild D.M. *et al.* (1996) High-avidity human IgGk monoclonal antibodies from a novel strain of minilocus transgenic mice. *Nature Biotechnology* **14**, 845–851.

Friguet B., Chafotte A.F., Djavadi-Ohaniance L. & Goldberg M.E.J. (1985) Measurements of the true affinity constant in solution of antigen–antibody complexes by enzyme-linked immunosorbent assay. *Journal of Immunological Methods* **77**, 305–319.

George A.J., Lee L. & Pitzalis C. (2003) Isolating ligands specific for human vasculature using *in vivo* phage selection. *Trends in Biotechnology* **5**, 199–203.

Green L.L. (1999) Antibody engineering via genetic engineering of the mouse: xenomouse strains are a vehicle for the facile generation of therapeutic human monoclonal antibodies. *Journal of Immunological Methods* **231**, 11–23.

Huppi K., Martin S.E. & Caplen N.J. (2005) Defining and assaying RNAi in mammalian cells. *Molecular Cell* **17**, 1–10.

Lacroix-Desmazes S. *et al.* (1999) Catalytic activity of antibodies against factor VIII in patients with hemophilia A. *Nature Medicine* **5**, 1044–1047.

Lefkovits I. & Waldmann H. (1999) *Limiting Dilution Analysis of Cells of the Immune System*, 2nd edn. Oxford University Press, Oxford.

Letsch A. & Scheibenbogen C. (2003) Quantification and characterization of specific T-cells by antigen-specific cytokine production using ELISPOT assay or intracellular cytokine staining. *Methods* **31**, 143–149.

Liu M. *et al.* (2004) Gene-based vaccines and immunotherapeutics. *Proceedings of the National Academy of Sciences USA* **101**, Suppl. 2, 14567–14571.

Martin S.J. Ed. (2008) Apoptosis. *Methods* **44**, 197–285.

Malik V.S. & Lillehoj E.P. (1994) *Antibody Techniques.* Academic Press, London. [Laboratory manual of pertinent techniques for production and use of monoclonal antibodies for the nonimmunologist.]

McGuinness B.T. *et al.* (1996) Phage diabody repertoires for selection of large numbers of bispecific antibody fragments. *Nature Biotechnology* **14**, 1149–1154.

Monroe R.J. *et al.* (1999) RAG2:GFP knockin mice reveal novel aspects of RAG2 expression in primary and peripheral lymphoid tissues. *Immunity* **11**, 201–212.

Mosier D.E. (ed.) (1996) Humanizing the mouse. *Seminars in Immunology* **8**, 185–268.

Ogg G.S. & McMichael A.J. (1998) HLA–peptide tetrameric complexes. *Current Opinion in Immunology* **10**, 393–396.

Pinilla C. *et al.* (1999) Exploring immunological specificity using synthetic peptide combinatorial libraries. *Current Opinion in Immunology* **11**, 193–202.

Robinson J.P. & Babcock G.F. (eds.) (1998) *Phagocyte Function: A Guide for Research and Clinical Evaluation.* Wiley-Liss, New York.

Sambrook J. & Russell D.W. (2001) *Molecular Cloning: A Laboratory Manual*, 3rd edn. Cold Spring Harbor Laboratory Press, New York.

Shabat D., Rader C., List B., Lerner R.A. & Barbas C.F., III (1999) Multiple event activation of a generic prodrug trigger by antibody catalysis. *Proceedings of the National Academy of Sciences USA* **96**, 6925–6930.

Storch W.B. (2000) *Immunofluorescence in Clinical Immunology: A Primer and Atlas*. Birkhäuser Verlag AG, Basel.

Vaughan T.J. *et al.* (1996) Human antibodies with subnanomolar affinities isolated from a large nonimmunized phage display library. *Nature Biotechnology* **14**, 309–314.

Weir D.M. *et al.* (eds.) (1996) *Handbook of Experimental Immunology*, 5th edn. Blackwell Scientific Publications, Oxford.

Zola H. (1999) *Monoclonal Antibodies*. Bios Scientific Publishers, Oxford.

Now visit **www.roitt.com** to test yourself on this chapter.

CHAPTER 7

The anatomy of the immune response

Key Topics

Just to Recap ...

Acquired immune responses are mediated by antigen-specific lymphocytes. The population frequency of each specificity is low, and therefore the relevant clones of lymphocytes are selected by antigen to be expanded up in number by extensive proliferation. Cytotoxic T-cells and most B-cells, both of which are antigen specific, require assistance from antigen-specific helper T-cells. Furthermore, the CD4$^+$ helper T-cells require antigen to be presented to them by MHC class II$^+$ professional antigen-presenting cells. These stringent cellular interactions dictate that, unlike innate responses, the acquired immune responses need to be initiated in a highly structured environment.

Introduction

For an effective acquired immune response, an intricate series of cellular events must occur. Antigen must be detected and then processed by antigen-presenting cells, which subsequently make contact with and activate helper T-cells to stimulate B-cells and cytotoxic T-cell precursors. Additionally, various factors such as cytokines are required to support lymphocyte proliferation and

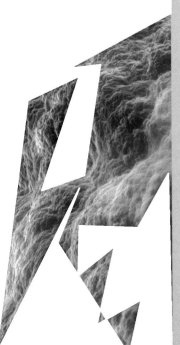

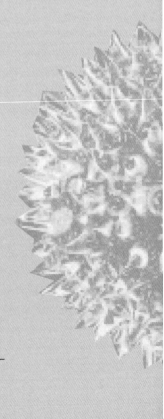

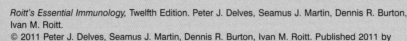

Roitt's Essential Immunology, Twelfth Edition. Peter J. Delves, Seamus J. Martin, Dennis R. Burton, Ivan M. Roitt.

Introduction *(Continued)*

then bring about cellular differentiation. Furthermore, memory cells for secondary responses must be formed and the whole response coordinated so that it is adequate but not excessive and is appropriate to the type of infection being dealt with. The integration of the complex cellular interactions that form the basis of the immune response takes place within the organized architecture of secondary lymphoid tissue, which includes the lymph nodes, spleen and unencapsulated tissue lining the respiratory, gastrointestinal and genitourinary tracts.

Organized lymphoid tissue

Lymphocytes are derived from bone marrow hematopoietic stem cells; although B-cells become fully mature in the **bone marrow** itself, the precursors of T-cells must exit the bone marrow and travel via the blood to the **thymus**, where they develop into mature T-cells (Figure 7.1). As these are the locations in which the lymphocytes are produced they are referred to as the **primary lymphoid organs**. The role of the bone marrow in hematopoiesis and of the thymus in T-cell development will be discussed in Chapter 11, whereas the function of the bone marrow as a major site of antibody production is discussed later in the current chapter (p. 200).

The **secondary lymphoid organs** and tissues are the locations in which acquired immune responses are generated. These tissues, the **lymph nodes**, **spleen** and mucosa-associated lymphoid tissue (**MALT**) become populated by macrophages, dendritic cells and lymphocytes. In essence, the lymph nodes receive antigen either draining directly from the tissues or carried by MHC class II⁺ dendritic cells, the spleen monitors the blood and the unencapsulated lymphoid tissue of the MALT is strategically integrated into mucosal surfaces of the body as a forward defensive system based on IgA secretion.

The anatomical disposition of these lymphoid tissues is illustrated in Figure 7.2. The lymphatics and associated lymph nodes form an impressive network, draining the fluid (lymph) from the body tissues and returning it to the blood by way of the thoracic duct (Figure 7.3).

Communication between these tissues and the rest of the body is maintained by a pool of recirculating lymphocytes that passes from the blood into the lymph nodes, spleen and other tissues and back to the blood by the major lymphatic channels such as the thoracic duct (Figure 7.4 and see 7.12).

Lymphocytes traffic between lymphoid tissues

This traffic of lymphocytes between the tissues, the bloodstream and the lymph nodes enables these antigen-specific cells

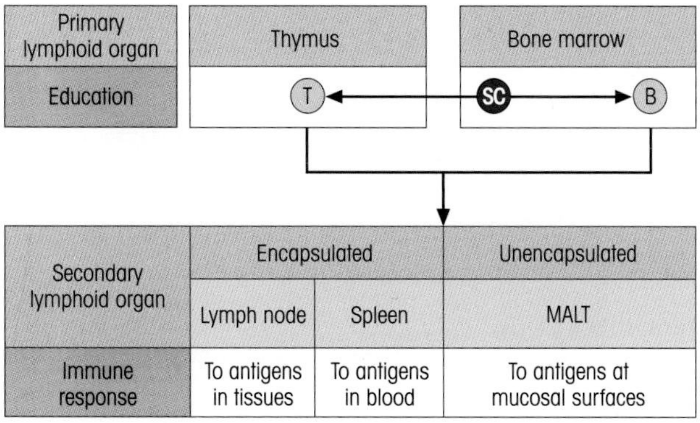

Primary lymphoid organ	Thymus		Bone marrow	
Education		T ◄──── SC ────► B		

Secondary lymphoid organ	Encapsulated		Unencapsulated
	Lymph node	Spleen	MALT
Immune response	To antigens in tissues	To antigens in blood	To antigens at mucosal surfaces

Figure 7.1. The functional organization of lymphoid tissue.

Hematopoietic stem cells (SC) arising in the bone marrow differentiate into immunocompetent T- and B-cells in the primary lymphoid organs and then colonize the secondary lymphoid tissues where immune responses are organized. The mucosa-associated lymphoid tissue (MALT) together with diffuse collections of cells in the lamina propria and the lungs produces antibodies for mucosal secretions.

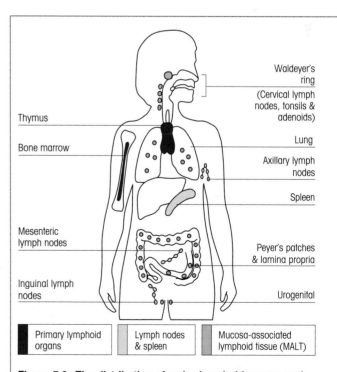

Figure 7.2. The distribution of major lymphoid organs and tissues throughout the body.

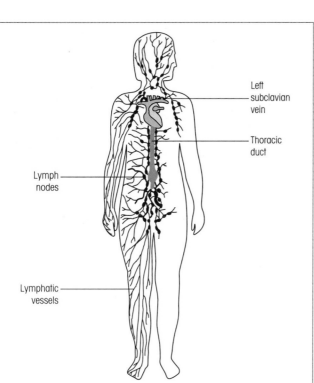

Figure 7.3. The network of lymph nodes and lymphatics.

Lymph nodes occur at junctions of the draining lymphatics. The lymph finally collects in the thoracic duct and thence returns to the bloodstream via the left subclavian vein.

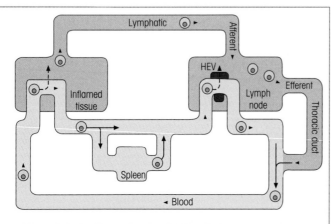

Figure 7.4. Traffic and recirculation of lymphocytes through encapsulated lymphoid tissue and sites of inflammation.

Blood-borne lymphocytes enter inflamed tissues when they recognize upregulated adhesion molecules on the blood vessel endothelium and enter lymph nodes by passing through the high-walled endothelium of the postcapillary venules (HEV). They leave via the draining lymphatics. The efferent lymphatics join to form the thoracic duct, which returns the lymphocytes to the bloodstream. In the spleen, which lacks HEVs, lymphocytes enter the lymphoid area (white pulp) from the arterioles, pass to the sinusoids of the erythroid area (red pulp) and leave by the splenic vein (see Figure 7.9b). Traffic through the mucosal immune system is elaborated in Figure 7.12.

to seek "their" antigen and to be recruited to sites at which a response is occurring, while the dissemination of memory cells and their progeny enables a more widespread response to be organized throughout the lymphoid system. Thus, antigen-reactive cells are depleted from the circulating pool of lymphocytes within 24 hours of antigen first localizing in the lymph nodes or spleen; several days later, after proliferation at the site of antigen localization, a peak of activated cells appears in the thoracic duct. When antigen reaches a lymph node in a primed animal, there is a dramatic fall in the output of cells in the efferent lymphatics, a phenomenon described variously as "cell shutdown" or "lymphocyte trapping." This process involves a reduced responsiveness of lymphocytes to sphingosine 1-phosphate (S1P), a molecule that signals lymphocytes to exit the lymph node. The shutdown phase is followed by an output of activated cells that peaks at around 80 hours.

Naive lymphocytes home to lymph nodes

Naive lymphocytes can enter a lymph node either through the afferent lymphatics or by guided passage across the specialized **high-walled endothelium of the postcapillary venules (HEVs)** (Figure 7.5). If arriving via the HEV their entry is determined by a series of **homing receptors** on the lymphocyte that include the **integrin** superfamily member LFA-1 ($\alpha_L\beta_2$, Table 7.1), the selectin family member L-selectin and the chemokine receptor CCR7. Their ligands on the endothelium act as **vascular addressins**. Thus, L-selectin recognises the highly glycosylated and sulfated sialomucins GlyCAM-1 and

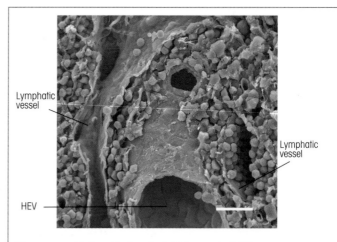

Figure 7.5. High-walled endothelial venule (HEV).

Scanning electronic micrograph of rat mesenteric lymph node showing loosely packed lymphocytes around an HEV (blue) and lymphatic vessels (yellow). (The black hole at the top of the HEV is an artifact where a tributary of the HEV was lost during preparation.) The lymph node was sliced with a vibratome that removes many of the free lymphocytes from the lumen of the HEV and the lymphatic vessels. Scale bar = 20 μm. Micrograph kindly supplied by O. Ohtani.

Table 7.1. The integrin superfamily. In general, the integrins are concerned with intercellular adhesion and adhesion to extracellular matrix components. Various members are involved in embryogenesis, cell growth, differentiation, motility, programmed cell death and tissue maintenance. Many of them are also involved in cell signal transduction. They are $\alpha\beta$ heterodimers selected from 18 α chains and 8 β chains, which pair to form 24 different combinations. A structure called the I (inserted) domain is present in many integrin subunits and contains the metal ion-dependent adhesion site (MIDAS) that, in the presence of Mg^{2+}, is involved in binding the Arg.Gly.Asp (RGD) motif on many of the ligands essential for cell adhesion. The $\alpha_v\beta_3$ and $\alpha_v\beta_5$ integrin ligand MFG-E8 is expressed by a variety of cell types, including IDC and macrophages in secondary lymphoid tissues where it plays a role in phagocytosis of apoptotic B-cells. LAP binds to, and thereby inhibits, the activity of TGFβ.BSP, bone sialoprotein; CO, collagen; CR3, complement receptor 3; DEL-1, developmental endothelial locus-1; FG, fibrinogen; FN, fibronectin; FX, factor X; GPIIb/IIIa, integrin glycoproteins IIb and IIIa; ICAM, intercellular adhesion molecule; IDC, interdigitating dendritic cell; IEL, intraepithelial lymphocyte; JAM-1, junctional adhesion molecule-1; LAP-TGFβ, latency associated peptide–transforming growth factor-β complex; LFA, leukocyte function-associated molecule; LM, laminin; LPAM, lymphocyte Peyer's patch adhesion molecule; Mφ, macrophage; MAdCAM, mucosal addressin cell adhesion molecule; MFG-E8, milk fat globule epidermal growth factor-8; MMP, matrix metalloproteinase; Mo, monocyte; N, neutrophil; NK, natural killer cell; NN, nephronectin; OP, osteopontin; THR, thrombospondin; TN, tenascin; VCAM, vascular cell adhesion molecule; VLA, very late antigen (although they are not all expressed late!); VN, vitronectin; VWF, von Willebrand factor. *CD markers are explained on p. 284. –, no CD designation yet assigned.

Integrin	CD designation	Expression	Ligand
$\alpha_1\beta_1$ (VLA-1)	CD49a/CD29	Widespread	CO, LM
$\alpha_2\beta_1$ (VLA-2)	CD49b/CD29	Widespread	CO, LM, THR
$\alpha_3\beta_1$ (VLA-3)	CD49c/CD29	Widespread	LM, THR
$\alpha_4\beta_1$ (VLA-4)	CD49d/CD29	Widespread	CD14, FN, MADCAM-1, OP, THR, VCAM-1
$\alpha_5\beta_1$ (VLA-5)	CD49e/CD29	Widespread	FN, OP
$\alpha_6\beta_1$ (VLA-6)	CD49f/CD29	Widespread	LM
$\alpha_7\beta_1$	–/CD29	Widespread	LM
$\alpha_8\beta_1$	–/CD29	Widespread	FN, OP, TN, VN
$\alpha_9\beta_1$	–/CD29	Widespread	OP, TN, VECAM-1
$\alpha_{10}\beta_1$	–/CD29	Widespread	CO, LM
$\alpha_{11}\beta_1$	–/CD29	Musculoskeletal	CO
$\alpha_v\beta_1$	CD51/CD29	Most leukocytes	FN, LAP-TGFβ, OP
$\alpha_L\beta_2$ (LFA-1)	CD11a/CD18	Most leukocytes	ICAM-1,-2,-3, -4, JAM-1
$\alpha_M\beta_2$ (CR3 [Mac-1])	CD11b/CD18	N, Mo, Mø	C3bi, FG, FX, ICAM-1, -4
$\alpha_X\beta_2$ (p150, 95)	CD11c/CD18	IDC, IEL, NK, Mo, Mø	C3bi, CO, FG, ICAM-1,-2, -4 VCAM-1
$\alpha_D\beta_2$	CD11d/CD18	Mø	ICAM-3, VECAM-1
$\alpha_{IIb}\beta_3$ (GPIIb/IIIa)	CD41/CD61	Megakaryocytes, platelets	FG, FN, THR, VN, VWF
$\alpha_v\beta_3$	CD51/CD61	Widespread	BSP, DEL-1, FG, FIBRILLIN, FN, LAP-TGFβ, MFG-E8, OP, PECAM-1, THR, TN, VN, VWF
$\alpha_6\beta_4$	CD49f/CD104	Epithelium, endothelium, Schwann cells, T-cells	LM
$\alpha_v\beta_5$	CD51/–	Widespread	BSP, DEL-1, MFG-E8, OP, VN
$\alpha_v\beta_6$	CD51/–	Epithelium	FN, LAP-TGFβ, OP
$\alpha_4\beta_7$ (LPAM-1)	CD49d/–	T-cells, B-cells	FN, MAdCAM-1, OP, VCAM-1
$\alpha_E\beta_7$	–/–	IEL	E-cadherin
$\alpha_v\beta_8$	CD51/–	Neurons	LAP-TGFβ

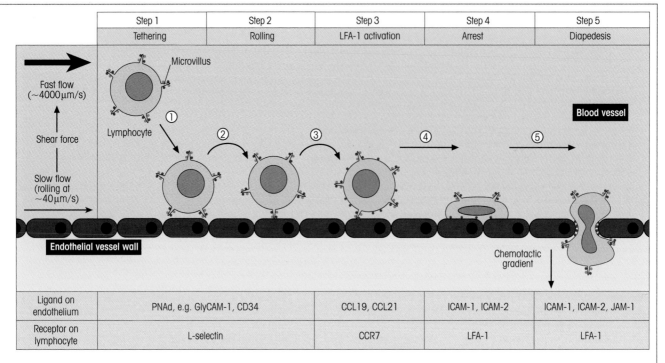

	Step 1	Step 2	Step 3	Step 4	Step 5
	Tethering	Rolling	LFA-1 activation	Arrest	Diapedesis
Ligand on endothelium	PNAd, e.g. GlyCAM-1, CD34		CCL19, CCL21	ICAM-1, ICAM-2	ICAM-1, ICAM-2, JAM-1
Receptor on lymphocyte	L-selectin		CCR7	LFA-1	LFA-1

Figure 7.6. Homing and transmigration of lymphocytes into peripheral lymph nodes.

Fast-moving lymphocytes are tethered (Step 1) to the vessel walls of the tissue they are being guided to enter through an interaction between specific homing receptors, such as L-selectin (•) located on the microvilli of the lymphocyte, and its peripheral node addressin (PNAd) ligands on the vessel wall. PNAd comprises several molecules, including CD34 and GlyCAM-1, which possess fucosylated, sulfated and sialylated Lewis^x structures. Various chemokine receptors (•) are also present on these T- and B-cells. After rolling along the surface of the endothelial cells (Step 2), activation of the lymphocyte LFA-1 integrin (•) (cf. Table 7.1) occurs (Step 3) in response to stimulation by chemokines. For T-cells this step is mainly regulated by CCL19 and CCL21 binding to CCR7 as shown, whereas for B-cells CXCL13 binding to CXCR5 provides additional signals. Note that, because LFA-1 is absent from the microvilli, firm binding occurs by the body of the lymphocyte to its ligands, ICAM-1/2, on the endothelium. This process results in cell arrest and flattening (Step 4) followed by migration of the lymphocyte between adjacent endothelial cells, a process referred to as diapedesis, which involves LFA-1 binding not only to ICAM-1/2 but additionally to the junctional adhesion molecule-1 (JAM-1), which is present between the endothelial cells (Step 5).

CD34 present on the HEVs of peripheral lymph nodes (Figure 7.6). Chemokines (a family of molecules with chemotactic and other functions) presented by vascular endothelium play a key role in triggering lymphocyte arrest, the chemokine receptors on the lymphocyte being involved both in binding to their ligand and in the functional activation of integrins. Thus, naive lymphocytes, and also dendritic cells, express the CCR7 chemokine receptor and are therefore directed into peripheral lymph nodes by virtue of the fact that the HEVs in the nodes display the chemokines CCL19 and CCL21 (cf. Table 9.2) on their luminal surface. Whilst CCL21 is produced by the endothelial cells themselves, CCL19 is secreted by the network of fibroblastic reticular cells (FRCs) within the lymph node and subsequently transferred to the HEV. The *plt/plt* mouse, which lacks expression of both of these chemokines, not unsurprisingly exhibits defective T-cell migration into peripheral lymph nodes. Chemokine activation of integrins occurs as a result of the chemokine signals facilitating their lateral mobility in the cell membrane and also by inducing structural changes in the integrins that results in a state of increased affinity.

Transmigration into the lymph node occurs in three stages

Steps 1 and 2: Tethering and rolling

In order for the lymphocyte to become attached to the HEVs, it has to overcome the shear forces created by the blood flow. This is effected by a force of attraction between the homing receptors and their ligands on the vessel wall that operates through microvilli on the leukocyte surface (Figure 7.6). After this tethering process, the lymphocyte rolls along the endothelial cell, with L-selectin and other adhesion molecules on the lymphocyte binding to their ligands on the endothelium. The selectins generally terminate in a lectin domain (hence "selectin"), as might be expected given the oligosaccharide nature of the ligands.

Steps 3 and 4: LFA-1 activation resulting in firm adhesion

This process leads to activation and recruitment of LFA-1 to the nonvillous surface of the lymphocyte. This integrin binds very strongly to ICAM-1 and -2 on the endothelial cell, the intimate contact causing the lymphocyte rolling to be arrested and a flattening of the lymphocyte.

Step 5: Diapedesis

The flattened lymphocyte now uses the LFA-1 to bind to the ICAMs and junctional adhesion molecule-1 (JAM-1) on the endothelial cells to elbow its way between the endothelial cells and into the tissue in response to chemotactic signals.

Lymphocyte homing to other tissues

Homing of activated and memory lymphocytes to other tissues involves a similar process but with different receptors and ligands involved (Figure 7.7). Dendritic cells from the appropriate tissue appear to play an important role in selectively imprinting the correct address code during their activation of naive T-cells. Cells concerned in mucosal immunity are imprinted to enter Peyer's patches by binding to HEVs in this location. In other cases involving migration into normal and inflamed tissues, the lymphocytes bind to and cross nonspecialized flatter endothelia.

It is essential that once activated in secondary lymphoid tissues the lymphocytes of appropriate antigen-specificity can rapidly be deployed to the site of the infection. The upregulated expression of the VLA-4 and LFA-1 integrins on these activated antigen-specific cells permits them to detect, respectively, the VCAM-1 and ICAM-1 cell adhesion molecules that

become expressed on vascular endothelium in response to IL-1 production in inflamed tissues.

Lymph nodes

The encapsulated tissue of the lymph nodes acts as a filter for lymph draining the body tissues (Figure 7.8a). The lymph, which will contain any foreign antigens present in the tissues, enters the subcapsular sinus by the afferent lymphatic vessels. The subcapsular sinus surrounds the entire lymph node and, together with the trabecular sinuses, allow larger antigens to either be engulfed by the resident macrophages lining the subcapsular and medullary sinuses, or to pass unimpeded to the efferent lymphatics (Figures 7.4 and 7.8b). The resident macrophages, together with dendritic cells that have taken up antigen in the tissues and arrive via the afferent lymphatics, can both act as antigen-presenting cells for T-cells in the lymph node.

Naive B-cells, irrespective of their antigen specificity, are able to use their complement receptors to transport immune complexes from the subcapsular sinus to specialized **follicular dendritic cells** (FDCs) for subsequent presentation to antigen-specific B-cells. The developmental origin of FDCs is still debated but they are nonhematopoietic cells, clearly distinct from interdigitating dendritic cells, and probably derived from mesenchymal stem cells. They are nonphagocytic and lack lysosomes but have very elongated processes that make intimate contact with B-lymphocytes.

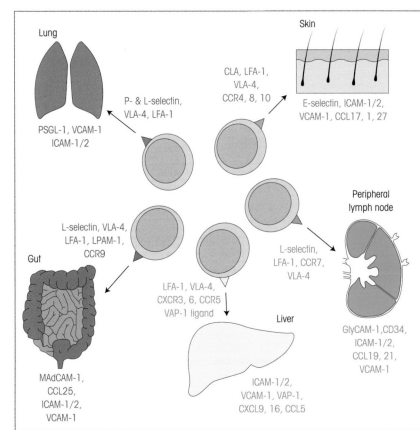

Figure 7.7. Access to tissues require the correct address code.

T-cells (and also dendritic cells) destined for various locations carry a combination code of cell surface molecules that recognize their respective ligands on the vascular endothelium at their destination. Some ligand–ligand pairs are the same irrespective of the destination tissue, such as LFA-1 binding to ICAM-1 and -2, and VLA-4 ($\alpha_4\beta_1$) integrin binding to VCAM-1. Other interactions utilize adhesion molecules that bind to ligands expressed at specific locations. Those for gut and skin are fairly well established, whilst those mediating homing to lung and liver remain somewhat speculative. L-selectin recognizes GlyCAM-1 and CD34 on peripheral lymph node endothelium but recognises MAdCAM-1 (mucosal vascular addressin cell adhesion molecule-1) on gut endothelium. Both L- and P-selectin bind PSGL-1 (P-selectin glycoprotein ligand-1) on lung endothelium. The recognition of E-selectin by CLA (cutaneous lymphocyte antigen) directs skin bound lymphocytes to the correct location. In addition, chemokine receptors (cf. Table 9.2) recognize tissues displaying particular chemokines.

Figure 7.8. Lymph node.

(a) Human lymph node, low-power view. GC, germinal center; LM, lymphocyte mantle; MC, medullary cords; MS, medullary sinus; PA, paracortex; SF, secondary follicles; SS, subcapsular sinus. (b) Diagrammatic representation of section through a whole node. Each lymph node is served by several afferent lymphatic vessels but usually has only one efferent lymphatic vessel. (c) The conduit networks that permeate the lymph node parenchyma are composed of collagen bundles enclosed by fibroblastic reticular cells. The networks are filled with lymph and act to transport small antigens and chemokines to different areas of the lymph node. (d) Secondary lymphoid follicle showing germinal center surrounded by a mantle of small B-lymphocytes stained by anti-human IgD labeled with horseradish peroxidase (brown color). There are few IgD-positive cells in the center but both areas contain IgM-positive B-lymphocytes. (e) The differentiation of B-cells during passage through different regions of an active germinal center. Macrophages engulf apoptotic B-cells in the basal light zone. Plasma cell precursors leave the germinal center before reaching full maturity, whereas memory B-cells can either leave the germinal center or enter the mantle zone. FDC, follicular dendritic cell; Mø, macrophage. ((a) Photographed by P.M. Lydyard; (d) by K.A. MacLennan.)

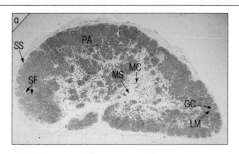

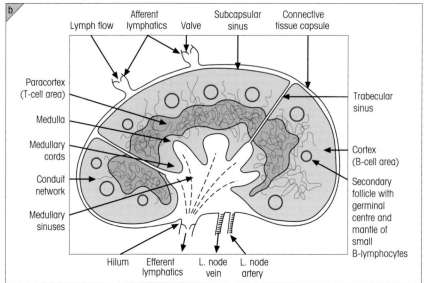

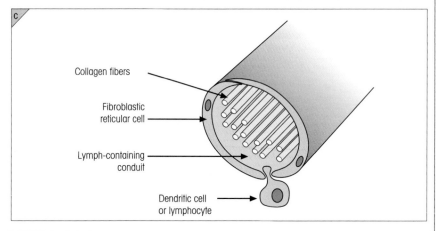

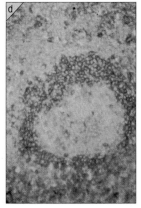

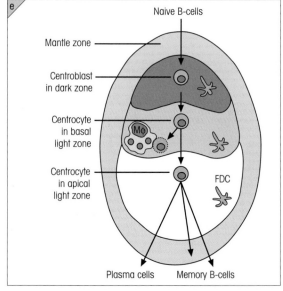

Within the lymph node parenchyma there are very extensive conduit networks composed of collagen fibers ensheathed by **fibroblastic reticular cells** (FRCs) to form 200 nm–3 μm diameter channels (Figure 7.8c). Lymph containing small antigens (below approximately 70 kDa), chemokines, and other low molecular weight substances passes through the channels of the conduit system to permeate the lymph node. Because the FRCs do not form a complete seal around the channels both dendritic cells and lymphocytes are able to extend protuberances into the conduits thereby both accessing the antigen-containing lymph and receiving chemokine signals. What is so striking about the organization of the lymph node is that the T- and B-lymphocytes are very largely separated into different anatomical compartments, a process directed to a large extent by these chemokines. Lymph node stromal cells (and to a lesser extent IDCs) secrete CCL19 and CCL21 in the paracortex that is deposited locally on the surface of the HEVs and FRCs, thereby attracting CCR7-bearing T-cells. In contrast, CXCL13 produced by stromal cells in the cortex attracts CXCR5-positive B-cells.

B-cell areas

The follicular aggregations of B-lymphocytes are a prominent feature of the outer cortex. In the unstimulated node they are present as spherical collections of cells termed **primary follicles**, but after antigenic challenge they form **secondary follicles** that consist of a corona or mantle of concentrically packed, resting, small B-lymphocytes possessing both IgM and IgD on their surface surrounding a pale-staining **germinal center** (Figure 7.8d,e). This center contains large, usually proliferating, B-blasts, a minority of T-cells, scattered conventional reticular macrophages containing "tingible bodies" of phagocytosed lymphocytes, and a tight network of FDCs. The B-cell-activating factor (BAFF), a TNF family member, is produced by FDCs and promotes B-cell survival in the germinal center by inhibiting apoptosis of proliferating B-cells. Germinal centers are greatly enlarged in secondary antibody responses during which they constitute sites of B-cell maturation and the generation of B-cell memory.

In the absence of antigen drive, the primary follicles are composed of a mesh of FDCs whose spaces are filled with recirculating, but resting, small B-lymphocytes. On priming with a T-dependent antigen (i.e. antigen for which the B-cells require cooperation from T-helper cells; cf. p. 217) the primary follicles develop into secondary follicles containing germinal centers in which the FDC network becomes colonized by specific B-cells undergoing exponential growth. These proliferating cells form what is referred to as the dark zone due to the dense packing of the lymphocytes with the production of around 10^4 so-called centroblasts. Recruitment of B-cells to the dark zone of the germinal center is dependent on the local production of the CXCL12 chemokine detected by CXCR4 on the B-cells. The centroblasts displace the original resting B-cells that now form the follicular mantle. These highly mitotic centroblasts, with no surface IgD (sIgD) and very little sIgM, then differentiate into centrocytes within a less densely packed area of the germinal centre called the basal light zone. The centrocytes are noncycling and begin to upregulate their expression of sIg. At this stage there is very extensive apoptotic cell death of B-cells with inappropriate specificity and/or affinity, giving rise to DNA fragments that are visible as "tingible bodies" within the macrophages, the disposal system for the dead cells. The survivors undergo their final differentiation in the apical light zone. A proportion of those that are shunted down the **memory** cell pathway take up residence in the mantle zone population, the remainder joining the recirculating B-cell pool. Other germinal centre B-cells in the apical light zone differentiate into plasmablasts with a well-defined endoplasmic reticulum, prominent Golgi apparatus and cytoplasmic Ig; these migrate to become plasma cells in the medullary cords, which project between the medullary sinuses (Figure 7.8b). This maturation of antibody-forming cells at a site distant from that at which antigen triggering has occurred is also seen in the spleen, where plasma cells are found predominantly in the marginal zone. It is thought that this movement of cells acts to prevent the generation of high local concentrations of antibody within the germinal center, so avoiding neutralization of the antigen and premature shutting off of the immune response.

The remainder of the outer cortex is also essentially a B-cell area with scattered T-cells.

T-cell areas

T-cells are mainly confined to a region referred to as the paracortex, or thymus-dependent area (Figure 7.8a,b). In nodes taken from children with selective T-cell deficiency, or from neonatally thymectomized mice, the paracortical region is seen to be virtually devoid of lymphocytes. Techniques such as intravital multiphoton scanning laser microscopy allow observation of lymphocyte behavior within lymphoid tissue. T-cells are seen to move rapidly and randomly within the paracortex, desperately trying to find an IDC bearing "their" antigen. Should the TCR on the T-cell recognize the cognate MHC–peptide, a stable binding occurs that is largely cemented by LFA-1 on the T-cell binding to ICAM-1 on the IDC. An immunological synapse is generated and contact maintained for 8–24 hours in order to fully activate the T-cell.

Spleen

The spleen is divided into the white pulp, which functions as a secondary lymphoid tissue, and the macrophage-rich red pulp, which is responsible for the removal by phagocytosis of aging erythrocytes, platelets and some blood-borne pathogens. The lymphoid tissue forming the white pulp is seen as circular or elongated areas (Figure 7.9a) within the erythrocyte-containing red pulp, which possesses blood-filled venous sinusoids lined with macrophages. As in the lymph node, the T- and B-cell areas of the white pulp are segregated (Figure 7.9b). In

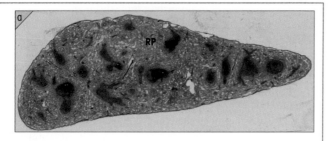

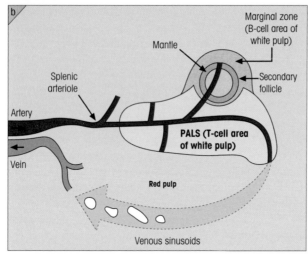

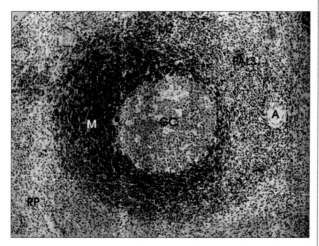

Figure 7.9. Spleen.

(a) Low-power view of human spleen showing red pulp (RP) and lymphoid white pulp (WP). Mallory's triple stain. Kindly provided by G. Campbell. (b) Diagrammatic representation of an area of white pulp surrounded by red pulp. (c) High-power view of germinal center (GC) and lymphocyte mantle (M) surrounded by marginal zone (MZ) and red pulp (RP). Adjacent to the follicle, an arteriole (A) is surrounded by the periarteriolar lymphoid sheath (PALS) predominantly consisting of T-cells. Note that the marginal zone is present only above the secondary follicle. (Photographed by I.C.M. MacLennan.)

addition to acting as a very effective blood filter removing effete cells, the spleen is also important in generating immune responses against blood-borne antigens, especially if they are particulate. Plasmablasts and mature plasma cells are present in the marginal zone extending into the red pulp (Figure 7.9c).

The skin immune system

Pathogens will first be encountered at body surfaces, either the skin or the mucosae (see below). The surfaces of the body are endowed with a variety of external barriers against infection (cf. Figure 1.6), and only if these are breached will the cells of the immune system come into play. In a normal, noninflamed, state the epidermis is provided with resident Langerhans cells and T-cells whilst the underlying dermis contains dendritic cells, T-cells, macrophages and mast cells. There is a continuous migration of leukocytes into the skin from the blood vessels, with these cells looking out for signs of infection and then returning to the circulation via the lymphatic system and lymph nodes. Should a pathogen provoke an inflammatory reaction in the skin then other cells of the immune system will fairly rapidly appear on the scene, including neutrophils, monocytes, eosinophils and plasma cells. In diseases such as atopic eczema the number of leukocytes in the skin substantially increases. Cutaneous inflammation is directed by several adhesion molecules amongst which LFA-1 and VLA-4 integrins and cutaneous leukocyte antigen (CLA) have key roles (Figure 7.7). The CCR4 chemokine receptor is expressed by most CLA+ T-cells, with its ligand CCL17 being presented on blood vessel walls in the skin. Another chemokine, CCL27 is expressed by keratinocytes and its receptor, CCR10, on a subpopulation of CLA+ T-cells. Some of the CLA+ T-cells present in the skin are CD4+ Foxp3+ regulatory cells.

Mucosal immunity

Many pathogens infect mucosal surfaces, for example following ingestion, inhalation or sexual transmission. The gastrointestinal, respiratory and genitourinary tracts are guarded immunologically by subepithelial accumulations of cells and by lymphoid tissues that are not constrained by a connective tissue capsule (Figure 7.10). These may occur as diffuse collections of lymphocytes, plasma cells and phagocytes throughout the lung and the lamina propria (connective tissue) of the intestinal wall (Figure 7.10c), or as organized mucosa-associated lymphoid tissue (MALT) with well-formed follicles. In humans, the latter includes the lingual, palatine and pharyngeal tonsils, the Peyer's patches of the small intestine (Figure 7.10a) and the appendix. Gut-associated lymphoid tissue is separated from the lumen by columnar epithelium with tight junctions and a mucous layer. This epithelium is interspersed with microfold (M)-cells (Figures 7.10b and 7.11); specialized antigen-transporting cells with short, irregular microvillae on their apical surface that endocytose antigens.

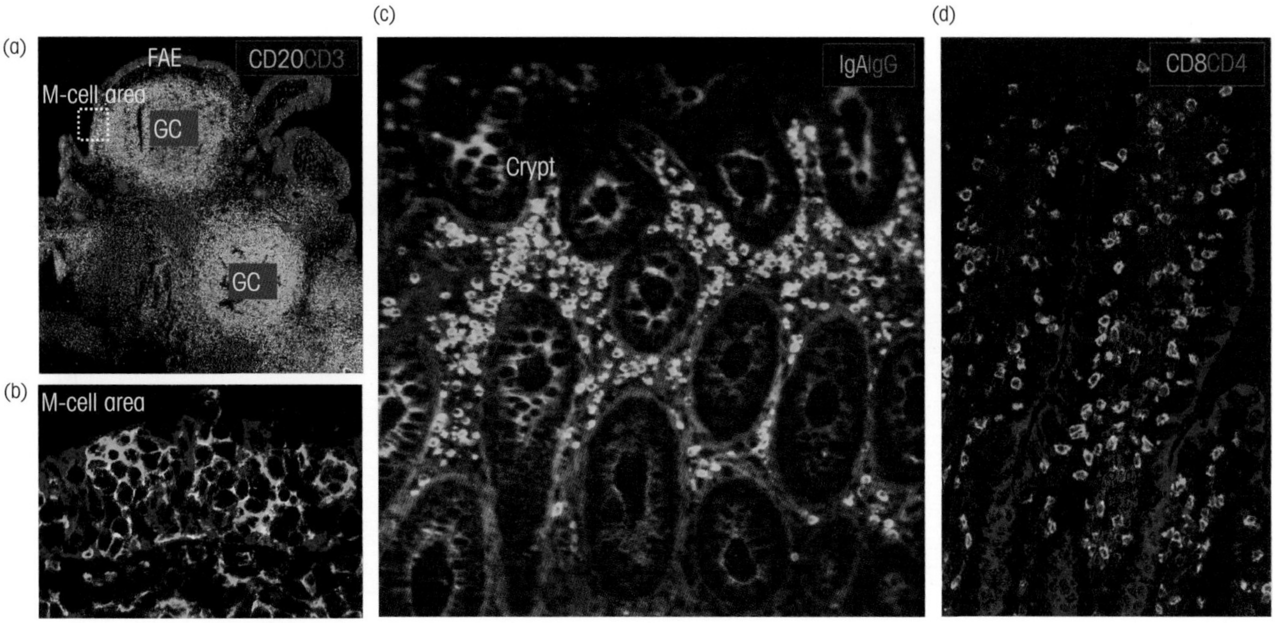

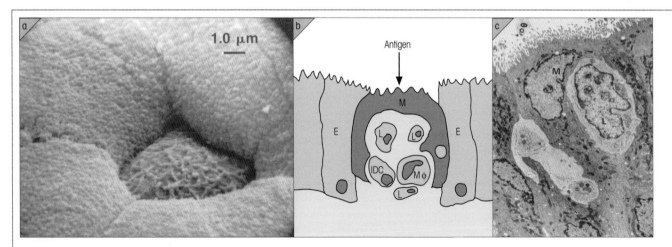

Figure 7.10. Gut-associated immunity.

(a) Immunofluorescence staining indicating the B-cells (with anti-CD20, green), T-cells (with anti-CD3, red) and the follicle-associated epithelium (FAE) (with anti-cytokeratin, blue) in Peyer's patch of human small intestine. GC, germinal center; M-cell, microfold cell. (b) Details from the antigen-sampling microfold-cell (M-cell) area. (c) Staining for IgA (green) and IgG (red) in a section of human large bowel mucosa. Crypt epithelium shows selective transport of IgA. Only a few scattered IgG-producing cells are seen in the lamina propria, together with numerous IgA plasma cells (staining bright green). (d) Staining for CD4 (red) and CD8 (green) T-cells in human duodenal mucosa. The epithelium of the villi is blue (cytokeratin). The weak CD4 expression seen in the background is either macrophages or dendritic cells. (Reproduced from Brandtzaeg P. & Pabst R. (2004) *Trends in Immunology* **25**, 570–577 with permission from the publishers.)

Figure 7.11. M-cell within Peyer's patch epithelium.

(a) Scanning electron micrograph of the surface of the Peyer's patch epithelium. The antigen-sampling M-cell in the center is surrounded by absorptive enterocytes covered by closely packed, regular microvilli. Note the irregular and short microfolds of the M-cell. (Reproduced with permission of the authors and publishers from Kato T. & Owen R.L. (1999) In Ogra R. *et al.* (eds) *Mucosal Immunology,* 2nd edn. Academic Press, San Diego.) (b) After uptake and transcellular transport by the M-cell (M), antigen is processed by macrophages and dendritic cells, which present antigen to T-cells in Peyer's patches and mesenteric lymph nodes. E, enterocyte; IDC, interdigitating dendritic cell; L, lymphocyte; Mφ, macrophage. (c) Electron photomicrograph of an M-cell (M in nucleus) with adjacent lymphocyte (L in nucleus). Note the flanking epithelial cells are both absorptive enterocytes with a typical brush border. (Lead citrate and uranyl acetate, ×1600.) ((b) Based on Sminia T. & Kraal G. (1998) In Delves P.J. & Roitt I.M. (eds) *Encyclopedia of Immunology,* 2nd edn, p. 188. Academic Press, London.)

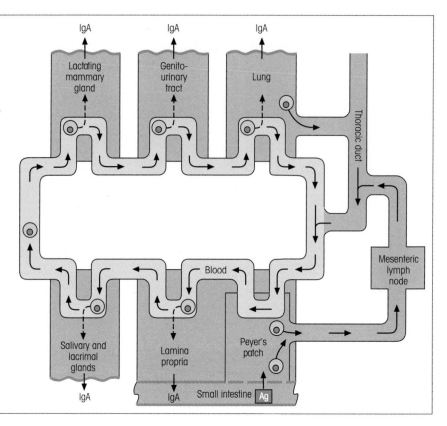

Figure 7.12. Circulation of lymphocytes within the mucosa-associated lymphoid system.

Antigen-stimulated cells move from Peyer's patches to colonize the lamina propria and the other mucosal surfaces (〰〰〰), forming what has been described as a common mucosal immune system.

The endocytic vesicles carry the antigen to be exocytosed at the basal surface for the attention of intraepithelial lymphocytes, dendritic cells and macrophages (Figure 7.11b,c).

Collectively the cells and tissues involved in mucosal immunity form an interconnected secretory system within which B-cells committed to IgA (or IgE) synthesis may circulate (Figure 7.12). It is however noteworthy that, unlike other mucosal tissues, in both the female and male reproductive tract the dominant isotype is often plasma-derived IgG.

Peyer's patches form the site for induction of immune responses in the gut

Foreign material, including bacteria, is taken up by M-cells and passed on to the underlying Peyer's patch antigen-presenting cells, which then activate the appropriate lymphocytes. Thus, the **Peyer's patches** constitute the **inductive site** for immune responses in the gut. After their activation is induced the lymphocytes travel via the lymph to the mesenteric lymph nodes where additional activation and proliferation may occur. A special feature of antigen-presenting cells from Peyer's patches, mesenteric lymph nodes and the lamina propria is that they contain a population of CD103+ dendritic cells that express retinal dehydrogenase enzymes that convert vitamin A to retinoic acid. Why is this relevant? Well, because it turns out that stimulation through lymphocyte retinoic acid receptors (RARs) induces T-cells to upregulate both the LPAM-1 ($\alpha_4\beta_7$) integrin and the CCR9 gut homing receptors, as well as enhancing the differentiation of Foxp3+ regulatory T-cells and favoring the production of IgA producing B-cells.

The "imprinted" T-lymphocytes then move via the thoracic duct into the bloodstream and finally on to the **lamina propria** (Figure 7.12). In this **responsive site** they assist the IgA-forming B-cells that, because they are now broadly distributed, protect a wide area of the bowel with protective antibody. T- and B-cells also appear in the lymphoid tissue of the lung and in other mucosal sites guided by the interactions of specific homing receptors with appropriate HEV addressins as discussed earlier. It is noteworthy that intranasal immunization is particularly effective at generating antibody production in the genitourinary tract.

Intestinal lymphocytes

The LPAM-1 integrin ligand, MAdCAM-1, is present on the intestinal lamina propria postcapillary venules (Figure 7.13) and thus facilitates the arrival of the intestinal T-cells. These cells bear a phenotype roughly comparable to that of peripheral blood lymphocytes: namely >95% T-cell receptor (TCR) $\alpha\beta$ and a CD4:CD8 ratio of 7:3, and seem to mainly be activated or memory cells. Unwarranted immune responses in the gut may be dampened down following the secretion of IL-10 and transforming growth factor-β (TGFβ) by inducible regulatory T-cells. Within the lamina propria there is also a generous sprinkling of activated B-cells and plasma cells secreting IgA for transport by the poly-Ig receptor to the intestinal lumen (cf. p. 68).

Intestinal **intraepithelial lymphocytes** (IELs) are quite a different "kettle of fish." Both they, and intraepithelial dendritic cells, express high levels of the $\alpha_E\beta_7$ integrin, which binds

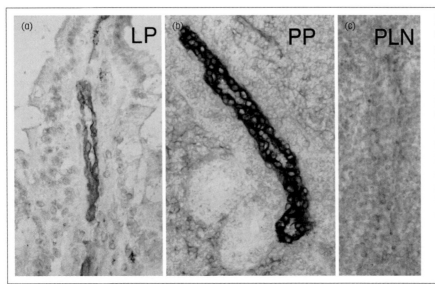

Figure 7.13. Selective expression of the mucosal vascular addressin MAdCAM-1 on endothelium involved in lymphocyte homing to gastrointestinal sites.

Immunohistologic staining reveals the presence of MAdCAM-1 (a) on postcapillary venules in the small intestinal lamina propria (LP) and (b) on high-walled endothelium of the postcapillary venules (HEVs) in Peyer's patches (PP), but its absence from (c) HEV in peripheral lymph nodes (PLN). (Reproduced with permission from Butcher E.C. *et al.* (1999) *Advances in Immunology* **72**, 209.)

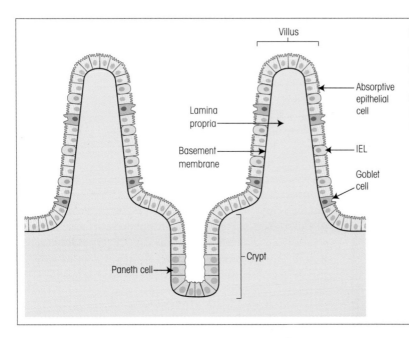

Figure 7.14. Intraepithelial lymphocytes (IELs).

IELs are seen interspersed among the epithelial cells of the villi in the intestine. The absorptive cells with prominent microvilli digest and absorb nutrients, the goblet cells secrete mucus, and the Paneth cells in the crypts secrete lysozyme and defensins.

E-cadherin on the intestinal epithelial cells thereby localizing the IELs between the epithelial cells (Figure 7.14). They are mostly T-cells, about 10% of which in humans bear a γδ TCR. In other species γδ T-cells may represent up to 40% of the IEL T-cells. Of those bearing an αβ TCR, most are CD8+ positive and in mice can be divided into two populations. One-third of them possess the conventional form of CD8, which is a heterodimer composed of a CD8 α chain and a CD8 β chain. However, two-thirds of them instead express a CD8 αα homodimer, which is almost exclusively found only on IELs. Although CD8 αα TCR γδ T-cells exist in both human and mice, the existence of CD8 αα TCR αβ T-cells IELs in humans is controversial.

Those IELs that are conventional T-cells with an αβ TCR and a CD8 αβ heterodimer recognize peptide–MHC. However, αβ TCR IELs that express CD8 αα are efficiently generated in both class I and CD1 knockout mice and therefore do not recognize antigen presented by either of these molecules. Whether these IELs are restricted by nonclassical MHC molecules (cf. p. 108) such as TL and Qa1 remains unclear, but it has been postulated that they act as a relatively primitive first line of defense at the outer surfaces of the body. The MHC class I chain-related (MIC) family members MICA and MICB (cf. p. 108) seem to be involved in the activation of human γδ TCR IELs.

Reflect for a moment on the fact that roughly 10^{14} bacteria reside in the intestinal lumen of the normal adult human. During an infection many of these will be pathogens rather than friendly commensals. Combined with the barrier of mucins produced by goblet cells and the protective zone of secreted IgA antibodies, these collections of intestinal lymphocytes represent a crucial line of defense. Indeed, the number of IEL in the small intestine of the mouse accounts for nearly 50% of the total number of T-cells in all lymphoid organs.

Bone marrow is a major site of antibody synthesis

Although B-cells mature in the bone marrow from hematopoietic stem cells, upon maturation most naive B-cells leave for the secondary lymphoid organs and tissues where they can encounter antigen. This release from the bone marrow may be regulated by sphingosine 1-phosphate, which is known to control the exit of lymphocytes from the thymus and lymph nodes. Activated B-cells can recirculate back to the bone marrow and cluster around vascular sinusoids. In this location they are able to partake in the generation of antibody responses to blood-borne pathogens and their survival is maintained by bone marrow dendritic cells secreting the cytokine MIF (macrophage migration inhibitory factor). The bone marrow is known to be the major residence of long lived plasma cells (Figure 7.15), the precursors of which are generated in the germinal centers of secondary lymphoid tissues. Thus, the bone marrow is a major source of serum Ig. Both B and T memory cells are also present.

The liver contains a variety of immune system cells

The liver is supplied with both venous blood from the intestine and arterial blood, and therefore is well placed to monitor

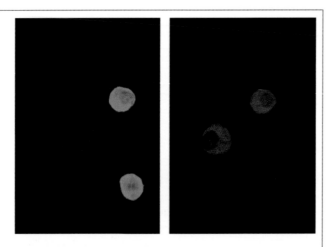

Figure 7.15. Plasma cells in human bone marrow.

Cytospin preparation stained with rhodamine (orange) for IgA heavy chain and fluorescein (green) for lambda light chain. Both images are of the same field, one showing the green fluoresence, the other the orange fluorescence. Thus, one cell is IgA.λ, another IgA.non-λ and the third is non-IgA.λ positive. (Photograph kindly supplied by R. Benner, W. Hijmans and J.J. Haaijman.)

circulating antigens. It plays an important role in innate responses, including the production of acute phase proteins (see p. 24). Together with the spleen, it is the main location to which immune complexes are transported for their subsequent destruction. In the case of the liver this is carried out by Kupffer cells—the resident macrophages of this organ. A relatively high proportion of NK and NKT cells is present, and it is known that CD1d on dendritic cells is able to present microbial glycolipids to liver NKT cells (cf. p. 135). The human liver also contains large numbers of conventional T-cells that can be activated locally by a variety of antigen-presenting cells including interdigitating dendritic cells, Kupffer cells and liver sinusoidal endothelial cells. Nonetheless, the liver tends to be a rather tolerogenic environment due to the presence of high levels of IL-10 and PD-L1 (programed death-1 ligand-1) and therefore the threshold for T-cell activation is set rather high.

The enjoyment of privileged sites

Certain locations in the body, for example brain, anterior chamber of the eye and testis, are referred to as **immunologically privileged sites** because antigens located within them do not provoke reactions against themselves. It has long been known, for example, that foreign corneal grafts can take up long-term residence, and a number of viruses have been expanded by repeated passage through animal brain.

Generally, privileged sites are protected by rather strong blood–tissue barriers and low permeability to hydrophilic compounds and carrier-mediated transport systems. Functionally insignificant levels of complement reduce the threat of acute inflammatory reactions and unusually high concentrations of immunosuppressive cytokines, such as IL-10 and TGFβ (cf. p. 243), quash any unruly Th1-lymphocyte activity. Immune privilege can also be maintained by Fas (CD95)-induced apoptosis of autoaggressive cells. Lesley Brent put it rather well: "It may be supposed that it is beneficial to the organism not to turn the anterior chamber or the cornea of the eye, or the brain, into an inflammatory battlefield, for the immunological response is sometimes more damaging than the antigen insult that provoked it."

The handling of antigen

Where does antigen go when it enters the body? If it penetrates the tissues, it will be carried by the lymph to the draining lymph nodes. Antigens that are encountered in the upper respiratory tract, intestine or reproductive tract are trapped by local MALT, whereas antigens in the blood provoke a reaction in the spleen.

Macrophages are general antigen-presenting cells

"Classically," it has always been recognized that antigens draining into lymphoid tissue are taken up by macrophages. The antigens are then partially, if not completely, broken down in the phagolysosomes; some may escape from the cell in a soluble form to be taken up by other antigen-presenting cells such as dendritic cells, and a fraction may reappear at the surface as a processed peptide associated with class II major histocompatibility molecules. Although resting resident macrophages express very little if any MHC class II, antigens are usually encountered in the context of a microbial infectious agent that can activate the macrophage to express class II following engagement of pattern recognition receptors such as TLR4 by bacterial lipopolysaccharide (LPS). Macrophages are also induced to express MHC class II following exposure to IFNγ or engagement of CD35 (complement receptor 1).

Interdigitating dendritic cells present antigen to naive T-lymphocytes

Notwithstanding the impressive ability of the mighty macrophage to present antigen, there is one function where it is deficient, namely the priming of naive T-lymphocytes. Animals that have been depleted of macrophages, by selective uptake of liposomes containing the drug dichloromethylene diphosphonate, are as good as their controls with intact macrophages in responding to T-dependent antigens. We must conclude that cells other than macrophages prime T-helper cells, and it is now generally accepted that these are the interdigitating dendritic cells (IDCs). These cells, which are of bone marrow origin, have the awesome capacity to process four times their own volume of extracellular fluid in 1 hour, thereby facilitating antigen capture and processing in their abundant intracellular MHC class II-rich compartments (MIIC; cf. p. 126).

The IDCs are therefore the *crème de la crème* of the antigen-presenting cells and, if pulsed with antigen before injection into animals, usually produce stunning immune responses. In this connection, it is relevant to note that large numbers of these dendritic cells can be generated from peripheral blood by culture with granulocyte–macrophage colony-stimulating factor (GM-CSF) (cf. p. 231) to promote proliferation and IL-4 to suppress macrophage overgrowth. Their use in immunotherapy is beginning to be explored, e.g. by pulsing autologous dendritic cells with the patient's tumor antigens and then reinjecting them to evoke an immune response.

Precursor dendritic cells in the blood that are destined to become skin Langerhans' cells express cutaneous leukocyte antigen (CLA), directing their homing to skin via interaction with E-selectin on the relevant vascular endothelial cells just as occurs for cutaneous T-cells. The Langerhans' cells, and dendritic cells in other tissues, act as antigen sampling agents. They are only moderately phagocytic but display extremely active receptor-mediated endocytosis and pinocytosis. Receptors involved in antigen capture, including the mannose receptor, various TLRs, and Fc receptors for both IgG and IgE, are present on dendritic cells. The expression of cell surface MHC class II, and of adhesion and co-stimulatory molecules, is low at this early stage of the dendritic cells' life.

However, as they differentiate into fully fledged antigen-presenting cells, they decrease their phagocytic and endocytic activity, show reduced levels of molecules involved in antigen capture, but dramatically increase their MHC class II. Co-stimulatory molecules such as CD40, CD80 (B7.1) and CD86 (B7.2) are also upregulated at this stage, as is the ICAM-1 adhesion molecule that contributes to both the migratory and antigen-presenting properties of these cells. Their expression of a number of chemokine receptors including CCR5 and CXCR4 (cf. Table 9.2) means that they are attracted to and migrate into T-cell areas in lymphoid tissue and, incidentally, because they also express CD4 they become susceptible to infection by HIV (see p. 386).

Two separate developmental pathways for IDCs have been described, the myeloid pathway, which generates CD11c⁺ interstitial **myeloid dendritic cells** and skin Langerhans' cells, and the lymphoid pathway, which produces **plasmacytoid dendritic cells** that lack or express only very low levels of CD11 and can produce large amounts of interferon-α and -β. There appears to be a number of subpopulations of myeloid dendritic cells, although this area is still somewhat shaky.

In the absence of activation, dendritic cells lack expression of co-stimulatory molecules such as CD80 and CD86. Antigen presented by these "tolerogenic" dendritic cells will cause T-cell anergy or deletion, or induce regulatory T-cells to secrete immunosuppressive cytokines such as IL-10 and TGFβ. In some circumstances dendritic cells can also exhibit a regulatory phenotype by secreting indoleamine 2,3-dioxygenase (IDO), which catalyzes the depletion of trytophan, in the absence of which T-cells undergo apoptosis.

To summarize, the scenario for T-cell priming appears to be as follows. Peripheral dendritic cells such as the Langerhans' cells (cf. Figure 2.7f), which bind to skin keratinocytes through surface expression of E-cadherin, can pick up and process antigen. As differentiation proceeds, they lose their E-cadherin and produce collagenase, presumably to facilitate their crossing of the basement membrane. They then travel as "veiled" cells in the lymph (Figure 7.16a) before settling down as IDCs in the paracortical T-cell zone of the draining lymph node (Figure 7.16b). There the IDC delivers the antigen with co-stimulatory signals (Figure 7.17) for potent stimulation of naive and subsequently of activated, specific T-cells, which take advantage of the large surface area to bind to the MHC–peptide complexes on the IDC membrane.

We will meet IDCs again in Chapter 11 when we discuss their central role within the thymus where they present self-peptides to developing autoreactive T-cells and trigger their apoptotic execution (known more gently as "clonal deletion"; cf. p. 295).

Follicular dendritic cells bind immune complexes and stimulate B-cells

The FcγRIIB, FcεRII and CR1 (CD35) and CR2 (CD21) complement receptors (cf. p. 321) on the surface of the

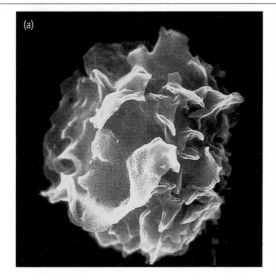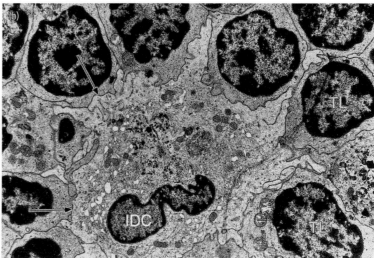

Figure 7.16. Interdigitating dendritic cells (IDCs).

(a) Scanning electron micrograph of a veiled cell, the morphological form adopted by IDCs as they travel in the afferent lymph. (b) IDC in the thymus-dependent area of the rat lymph node. Intimate contacts are made with the surface membranes (arrows) of the surrounding T-lymphocytes (TL) (×2000). In contrast to these interdigitating dendritic cells that present processed antigen to T-cells, the follicular dendritic cells in germinal centers present intact antigen to B-cells. ((a) Courtesy of G.G. MacPherson. (b) Reproduced with permission of the authors and publishers from Kamperdijk E.W.A., Hoefsmit E.Ch.H., Drexhage H.A. & Balfour B.H. (1980) In: Van Furth R. (ed.) *Mononuclear Phagocytes,* 3rd edn. Rijhoff Publishers, The Hague.)

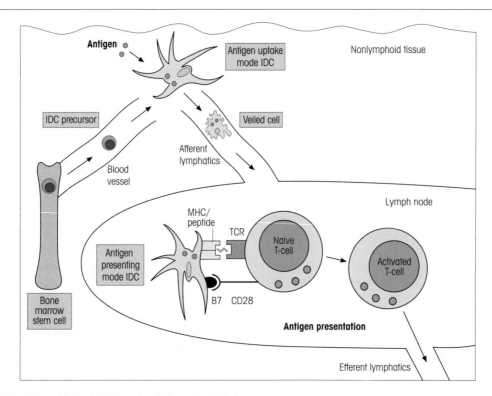

Figure 7.17. Migration of interdigitating dendritic cells (IDCs).

The precursors of the IDCs are derived from bone marrow stem cells. They travel via the blood to nonlymphoid tissues. At this stage in their life these IDCs, e.g. Langerhans' cells in skin, are specialized for antigen uptake. Subsequently they travel via the afferent lymphatics as veiled cells (cf. Figure 7.16a) to take up residence within secondary lymphoid tissues (cf. Figure 7.16b) where they express high levels of MHC class II and co-stimulatory molecules such as B7 (CD80 and CD86). These cells are highly specialized for the activation of naive T-cells. The activated T-cell may carry out its function in the lymph node or, after imprinting with relevant homing molecules, recirculate to the appropriate tissue.

nonphagocytic MHC class II-negative **follicular dendritic cells** (FDC) enables these cells to trap complexed antigen very efficiently and hold it in its native form on their surface for extended periods. Memory B-cells can then be stimulated by recognition of the retained antigen and co-stimulated through the B-cell CD21 (cf. p. 221) recognizing complement fragments held on the surface of the FDC. There is evidence to suggest that intact antigens can be retained by FDCs for many months or possibly even longer.

Classically, a secondary response would be initiated at the T-helper cell level by antigen, alone or as an immune complex, being taken up by IDCs and macrophages, processed, and then presented to the TCR as peptide-MHC. However, the capture of immune complexes on the surface of FDCs opens up an alternative pathway. One to three days after secondary challenge, the filamentous dendrites on the follicular cells, to which the immune complexes are bound, form into beads that break off as structures called "iccosomes" (immune complex-coated bodies). These bind to germinal center B-cells that then endocytose and process the antigen for presentation by the B-cell MHC class II, and subsequent stimulation of T-helper cells to kick off the secondary response.

Organized lymphoid tissue
- The complexity of acquired immune responses is catered for by a sophisticated structure.
- Lymph nodes filter and screen lymph flowing from the body tissues while spleen filters the blood.
- B- and T-cell areas are separated under the direction of chemokines.
- B-cell structures appear in the lymph node cortex as primary follicles that become secondary follicles with germinal centers after antigen stimulation.
- Germinal centers with their meshwork of follicular dendritic cells expand B-cell blasts produced by secondary antigen challenge and direct their differentiation into memory cells and antibody-forming plasma cells.

Mucosal immunity
- Specialized antigen-transporting M-cells provide the gateway for antigens to the mucosal lymphoid tissue.
- Lymphoid tissue guarding the gastrointestinal tract is unencapsulated but has an ordered structure (tonsils, Peyer's patches, appendix). There are also diffuse cellular collections in the lamina propria. Intraepithelial lymphocytes are mostly T-cells and include some novel subsets, e.g. CD8 αα-bearing cells that recognize antigens presented by nonclassical MHC molecules.
- Together with the subepithelial accumulations of cells lining the mucosal surfaces of the respiratory and genitourinary tracts, these cells and lymphoid tissues form the "secretory immune system," which bathes the surface with protective antibodies, mostly IgA.

Other sites
- T-cells in the skin characteristically bear cutaneous lymphocyte antigen (CLA) and the chemokine receptor CCR4.

- Bone marrow is a major site of antibody production.
- The respiratory tract and the liver contain substantial numbers of lymphocytes and phagocytic cells.
- The brain, anterior chamber of the eye and testis are privileged sites in which antigens are safely sequestered.

Lymphocyte traffic into lymph nodes
- Lymphocyte recirculation between the blood and lymph nodes is guided by specialized homing receptors on the surface of the high-walled endothelium of the postcapillary venules.
- Lymphocytes are tethered and then roll along the surface of the selected endothelial cells through interactions between selectins, integrins and chemokine receptors, and their respective ligands. Arrest of the lymphocyte following LFA-1 activation results in subsequent transmigration across the endothelial cell.

The handling of antigen
- Macrophages are general antigen-presenting cells for primed lymphocytes but cannot stimulate naive T-cells.
- This is effected by dendritic cells of hematopoietic origin that process antigen, migrate to the draining lymph node and settle down as interdigitating dendritic cells. They can present antigen-derived peptides to naive T-cells, thereby powerfully initiating primary T-cell responses.
- Follicular dendritic cells in germinal centers bind immune complexes to their surface through Fc and C3b receptors. The complexes are long lived and can provide a sustained source of antigenic stimulation for B-cells.

FURTHER READING

Agace W.W. (2008) T-cell recruitment to the intestinal mucosa. *Trends in Immunology* **29**, 514–522.

Allen C.D. & Cyster J.G. (2008) Follicular dendritic cell networks of primary follicles and germinal centers: phenotype and function. *Seminars in Immunology* **20**, 14–25.

Barclay A.N. *et al.* (1997) *The Leucocyte Antigen Facts Book*, 2nd edn. Academic Press, London.

Batista F.D. & Harwood N.E. (2009) The who, how and where of antigen presentation to B cells. *Nature Reviews Immunology* **9**, 15–27.

Bajénoff M. *et al.* (2007) Highways, byways and breadcrumbs: directing lymphocyte traffic in the lymph node. *Trends in Immunology* **28**, 346–352.

Bos J.D. (ed.) (2004) *Skin Immune System (SIS): Cutaneous Immunology and Clinical Immunodermatology*, 3rd edn. Boca Raton. CRC Press.

Bromley S.K., Mempel T.R. & Luster A.D. (2008) Orchestrating the orchestrators: chemokines in control of T cell traffic. *Nature Immunology* **9**, 970–980.

Corr S.C., Gahan C.C. & Hill C. (2008) M-cells: origin, morphology and role in mucosal immunity and microbial pathogenesis. *FEMS Immunology and Medical Microbiology* **52**, 2–12.

Crispe N. (2009) The liver as a lymphoid organ. *Annual Review of Immunology* **27**, 147–163.

Gonzalez S.F., Degn S.E., Pitcher L.A., Woodruff M., Heesters B. & Carroll M.C. (2011) Trafficking of B cell antigen in lymph nodes. *Annual Review of Immunology* **29**.

Junt T., Scandella E. & Ludewig B. (2008) Form follows function: lymphoid tissue microarchitecture in antimicrobial immune defence. *Nature Reviews Immunology* **8**, 764–775.

Lefrançois L. & Puddington L. (2006) Intestinal and pulmonary mucosal T-cells: Local heroes fight to maintain the status quo. *Annual Review of Immunology* **24**, 681–704.

Ohtani O. & Ohtani Y. (2008) Structure and function of rat lymph nodes. *Archives of Histology and Cytology* **71**, 69–76.

Pillai S. & Cariappa A. (2009) The bone marrow perisinusoidal niche for recirculating B cells and the positive selection of bone marrow-derived B lymphocytes. *Immunology and Cell Biology* **87**, 16–19.

Pribila J.T., Quale A.C., Mueller K.L. & Shimizu Y. (2004) Integrins and T cell-mediated immunity. *Annual Reviews of Immunology* **22**, 157–180.

Simpson E. (2006) A historical perspective on immunological privilege. *Immunological Reviews* **213**, 12–22.

Wardlaw, A.J., Guillen C. & Morgan A. (2005) Mechanisms of T cell migration to the lung. *Clinical and Experimental Allergy* **35**, 4–7.

Wilke G., Steinhauser G., Grün J. & Berek C. (2010) *In silico* subtraction approach reveals a close lineage relationship between follicular dendritic cells and BP3(hi) stromal cells isolated from SCID mice. *European Journal of Immunology* **40**, 2165–2173.

 Now visit **www.roitt.com** to test yourself on this chapter.

CHAPTER 8
Lymphocyte activation

Key Topics

Just to Recap ...

T- and B-lymphocytes are the key effectors of adaptive immunity, using randomly generated membrane receptors to "see" antigen. In both cases, recognition of cognate antigen results in clonal expansion of the lymphocyte, which increases the numbers of cells available to mount a response and ensures that subsequent encounter with the same antigen will be met with greater force from the outset (i.e. immunological memory). While B-cell receptors (surface IgM and IgD) can directly interact with antigen, T-cells require antigen to be presented in the context of MHC molecules. Antigen presentation to naive (i.e. not previously stimulated) T-cells takes place in lymphoid tissues and is typically carried out by mature dendritic cells (DCs) that have migrated from peripheral tissues due to exposure to a maturation stimulus, such as a pathogen-derived molecular pattern (PAMP). Mature DCs present processed antigens to T-cells by displaying peptides derived from such antigens on MHC molecules. DCs also provide essential co-stimulation to T-cells in the form of B7 family ligands (CD80/CD86) and other surface molecules; the absence of co-stimulatory molecules on the DC does not productively activate the T-cell and may lead to tolerization or death of a responding T-cell. B-cell activation also occurs within lymph nodes and other

Roitt's Essential Immunology, Twelfth Edition. Peter J. Delves, Seamus J. Martin, Dennis R. Burton, Ivan M. Roitt.
© 2011 Peter J. Delves, Seamus J. Martin, Dennis R. Burton, Ivan M. Roitt. Published 2011 by Blackwell Publishing Ltd.

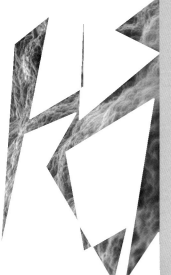

Just to Recap ... (*Continued*)

lymphoid tissues and is facilitated by specialized follicular dendritic cells that efficiently capture and concentrate antigen draining from surrounding tissues. With some exceptions, activated B-cells also require co-stimulation from T-helper cells, in the form of cytokines as well as membrane-bound CD40 ligand, to permit proliferation and differentiation. In addition to clonal expansion, activation of a B- or T-cell also results in maturation to specialized effector cells that produce antibodies (in the case of B-cells), or particular combinations of cytokines or cytotoxic molecules (in the case of T-cells).

Introduction

The adaptive immune response begins as a result of an encounter between a B- or T-lymphocyte and its specific antigen that typically results in "activation" of the lymphocyte and a radical shift in cell behavior—from a quiescent nondividing state, to a more active proliferative one. This simultaneously achieves two goals: the number of cells that are capable of responding to a particular antigen are multiplied (clonal expansion), and these new recruits are equipped with the ability to produce large quantities of cytokines or antibodies to help repel the intruder. Because of the potential dangers associated with inappropriate lymphocyte activation (to "self" or innocuous substances), signals that promote T- or B-cell activation usually require co-stimulation by other cells of the immune system. The requirement for co-stimulation raises the threshold for lymphocyte activation and provides a safeguard against autoimmunity (see Chapter 18). Failure to receive the proper co-stimulatory signals frequently results in death of the responding lymphocyte by apoptosis.

In previous chapters we learned that B- or T-cells use related, but nonetheless distinct, antigen receptors to recognize antigen. Stimulation of T- or B-cells through their respective antigen receptors initiates a cascade of signal transduction events within the responding lymphocyte that rely heavily upon **protein kinases**, proteins that can add phosphate groups to other proteins. Such phosphate groups, although puny in the overall context of the protein to which they are attached, either radically alter the activity of the target protein (in a positive or negative way), or create binding sites for other proteins to dock onto. In this way, activation of particular kinases acts as a switch to alter cell behavior. Thus, membrane receptors for antigen simply serve as the external switches for signals that permit T- and B-lymphocytes to be called into service at the appropriate time. Much of the complexity of T- and B-cell receptor signaling revolves around the issue of whether the switch should be turned on or off (i.e. when to respond or not).

While there are differences in the nature of the specific kinases that relay signals from the B- and T-cell receptors, there are also many similarities. In both cases, these signal transduction events result in the activation of many of the same transcription factors, entry into the cell division cycle, and the expression of an array of new proteins by the activated lymphocyte that equips such cells with functions characteristic of effector cells.

Clustering of membrane receptors frequently leads to their activation

All cells use plasma membrane-borne receptors to extract information from their environment. This information is propagated within the cell by signaling molecules and enables the cell to make the appropriate response; whether this is reorganization of the cell cytoskeleton (to facilitate movement), expression of new gene products, increased cellular adhesiveness, or all of the above. In many instances, occupation of the receptor with its specific ligand (whether this is a growth factor, a hormone or an antigen) results in conformational or other changes within the receptor that promotes recruitment of cytoplasmic adaptor proteins to the portion of the receptor exposed to the cytoplasm. Because many plasma membrane receptors are protein kinases, or can recruit protein kinases upon engagement with their specific ligands, stimulation of such receptors typically results in phosphorylation of regions within the receptor in contact with the cytoplasm (i.e. the cytoplasmic tail), or of associated proteins.

In the case of the B- and T-cell receptors, the receptors themselves do not have any intrinsic enzymatic activity but are associated with invariant accessory molecules (the CD3 γδε and ζ chains in the case of the T-cell receptor (TCR), and the Ig-αβ complex in the case of the B-cell receptor (BCR)) that can attract the attentions of a particular class of kinases. Central to this attraction is the presence of special motifs called **ITAMs** (*i*mmunoreceptor *t*yrosine-based *a*ctivation *m*otifs) within the cytoplasmic tails of these accessory molecules (see also p. 82, Chapter 4). Phosphorylation of ITAMs at tyrosine residues—in response to TCR or BCR stimulation—enables these motifs to interact with adaptor proteins that have an affinity for phosphorylated tyrosine motifs, thereby initiating signal transduction. We will deal, in turn, with the signaling events that take place upon encounter of a T-cell or a B-cell with antigen.

T-lymphocytes and antigen-presenting cells interact through several pairs of accessory molecules

Before we delve into the nuts and bolts of TCR-driven signaling events, it is important to recall that T-cells can only recognize antigen when presented within the peptide-binding groove of major histocompatibility complex (MHC) molecules. Furthermore, while the TCR is the primary means by which T-cells interact with the MHC–peptide complex, T-cells also express coreceptors for MHC (either CD4 or CD8) that define functional T-cell subsets. Recall that CD4 molecules act as coreceptors for MHC class II and are found on T-helper cell populations that provide "help" for activation and maturation of B-cells and cytotoxic T-cells (Figure 8.1). CD8 molecules act as coreceptors for MHC class I molecules and are a feature of cytotoxic T-cells that can kill virally infected or precancerous cells (Figure 8.1). Note, however, that the affinity of an individual TCR for its specific MHC–antigen peptide complex is relatively low (Figure 8.2). Thus, a sufficiently stable association with an antigen-presenting cell (APC) can only be achieved by the interaction of several complementary pairs of accessory molecules such as LFA-1/ICAM-1, CD2/LFA-3 and so on

(Figure 8.3). These adhesion molecules enable T-cells to associate with DCs and other APCs for the purposes of inspecting the peptides being presented within MHC molecules. However, these molecular couplings are not necessarily concerned with intercellular adhesion alone; some of these interactions also provide the necessary co-stimulation that is essential for proper lymphocyte activation.

Unstimulated lymphocytes are typically nonadherent but rapidly adhere to extracellular matrix components or other cells (such as APCs) within seconds of encountering chemokines or antigen. Integrins such as LFA-1 and VLA-4 appear to be particularly important for lymphocyte adhesion. The ease with which lymphocytes can alter their adhesiveness seems to be related to the ability of integrins to change conformation; from a closed, low-affinity state, to a more open, high-affinity, one (Figure 8.4). Thus, upon encounter of a T-cell with an APC displaying an appropriate MHC–peptide complex, signals routed through the TCR complex ensure that the affinity of LFA-1 for ICAM-1 is rapidly increased and this helps to stabilize the interaction between the T-cell and the APC. This complex has come to be known as the **immunological synapse**. Activation of the small GTPase **Rap1** by TCR stimulation appears to contribute to the rapid change in integrin adhesiveness. How Rap1 achieves this remains somewhat uncertain, but it is likely that modification of the integrin cytoplasmic tail serves to trigger a conformational change within the integrin extracellular domains; a process that has been termed "inside-out" signaling.

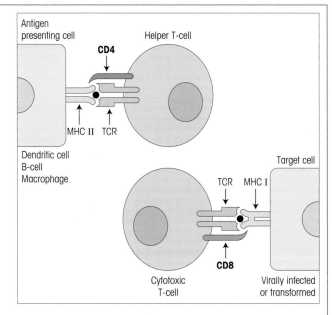

Figure 8.1. Helper and cytotoxic T-cell subsets are restricted by MHC class.

CD4 on helper T-cells acts as a coreceptor for MHC class II and helps to stabilize the interaction between the TCR and peptide–MHC complex; CD8 on cytotoxic T-cells performs a similar function by associating with MHC class I.

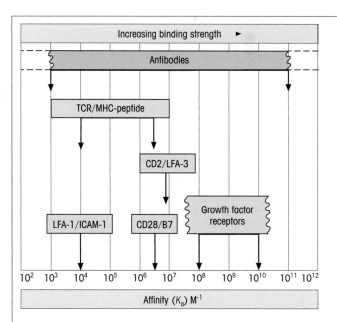

Figure 8.2. The relative affinities of molecular pairs involved in interactions between T-lymphocytes and cells presenting antigen.

The ranges of affinities for growth factors and their receptors, and of antibodies, are shown for comparison. (Based on Davies M.M. and Chien Y.-H. (1993) *Current Opinion in Immunology* **5**, 45.)

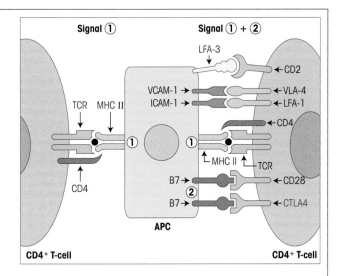

Figure 8.3. Activation of resting T-cells.

Interaction of co-stimulatory molecules leads to activation of resting T-lymphocyte by antigen-presenting cell (APC) on engagement of the T-cell receptor (TCR) with its antigen–MHC complex. Engagement of the TCR signal 1 without accompanying co-stimulatory signal 2 leads to anergy. Note, a cytotoxic rather than a helper T-cell would, of course, involve coupling of CD8 to MHC class I. Signal 2 is delivered to a resting T-cell primarily through engagement of CD28 on the T-cell by B7.1 or B7.2 on the APC. CTLA-4 competes with CD28 for B7 ligands and has a much higher affinity than CD28 for these molecules. Engagement of CTLA-4 with B7 downregulates signal 1. ICAM-1/2, *i*ntercellular *a*dhesion *m*olecule-1/2; LFA-1/2, *l*ymphocyte *f*unction-associated molecule-1/2; VCAM-1, *v*ascular *c*ell *a*dhesion *m*olecule-1; VLA-4, *v*ery *l*ate *a*ntigen-4.

The activation of T-cells requires two signals

Stimulation of the TCR by MHC–peptide (which can be mimicked by antibodies directed against the TCR or CD3 complex) is not sufficient to fully activate resting helper T-cells on their own. Upon co-stimulation via the CD28 receptor on the T-cell, however, RNA and protein synthesis is induced, the cell enlarges to a blast-like appearance, interleukin-2 (IL-2) synthesis begins and the cell moves from G0 into the G1 phase of the cell division cycle. Thus, **two signals** are required for the activation of a naive helper T-cell (Figure 8.3).

Antigen in association with MHC class II on the surface of a mature DC is clearly capable of fulfilling the requirement for both signals. Complex formation between the TCR and MHC–peptide provides signal 1, through the receptor–CD3 complex, and this is greatly enhanced by coupling of CD4 with the MHC. The T-cell is now exposed to a co-stimulatory signal (signal 2) from the mature DC. The most potent co-stimulatory molecules are the B7 family ligands (CD80/CD86) on the DC that interact with CD28 on the T-cell,

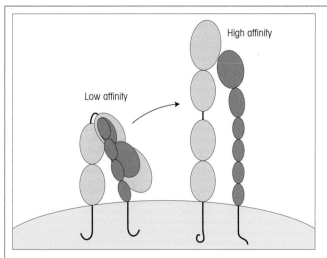

Figure 8.4. Integrin activation.

Integrins such as LFA-1 can assume different conformations that are associated with different affinities. The bent head-piece conformation has a low affinity for ligand but can be rapidly transformed into the extended high-affinity conformation by activation signals that act on the cytoplasmic tails of the integrin α and β subunits; a process known as "inside-out" signaling.

although other molecules (such as IL-1 and ligands for ICOS, CD2 and OX40) can also serve in this capacity.

Recall from Chapter 1 (p. 30) that immature DCs, that have not been exposed to PAMPs or DAMPs are incapable of productively activating T-cells. This is due to the relative absence of co-stimulatory molecules such as CD80/CD86 on the surface of immature DCs. However, a profound increase in the expression of these molecules occurs as a result of maturation of the DC subsequent to stimulation of its pattern recognition receptors with a PAMP or a DAMP. Inflammatory cytokines (such as IL-1, GM-CSF and TNFα) that are produced by macrophages and neutrophils in the initial stages of infection are also capable of converting immature, poorly co-stimulating, DCs into mature DCs capable of providing the necessary signals. Activation of resting T-cells can be blocked by anti-B7, which renders the T-cell **anergic**, i.e. unresponsive to any further stimulation by antigen. As we shall see in later chapters, the principle that two signals activate, but one may induce anergy in, an antigen-specific cell provides a potential for targeted immunosuppressive therapy. However, unlike resting T-lymphocytes, **activated T-cells proliferate in response to a *single* signal**.

Adhesion molecules such as ICAM-1, VCAM-1 and LFA-3 are not intrinsically co-stimulatory but greatly augment the effect of other signals by up to 100-fold (Figure 8.3); an important distinction. Early signaling events also involve the aggregation of **lipid rafts** composed of membrane subdomains enriched in cholesterol and glycosphingolipids. The cell membrane molecules involved in activation become concentrated within these structures.

Triggering the T-cell receptor complex

Let us now consider a situation in which a T-cell has encountered a DC displaying the correct peptide–MHC combination and has engaged with the DC such that many of the TCRs on the T-cell are engaged with a similar number of high affinity peptide–MHC molecules on the antigen-presenting cell. Such an event will greatly stabilize the interaction between the T-cell and the DC such that the duration of the encounter (the dwell time) will be sufficient to activate the T-cell. But what is the actual activating event? Put another way, how does the TCR complex register that the switch has been thrown?

Despite much investigation, we still do not have a clear answer to this question but it appears that both aggregation of the T-cell receptor complex, as well as conformational changes within the complex, play key roles in signal initiation. Recall from Chapter 4 that the T-cell receptor complex is composed of the TCR itself and the **CD3 coreceptor complex**. The CD3 coreceptor complex contains CD3γδεζ, which possess the signaling motifs (ITAMs) necessary for propagation of signals into the cell (Figure 8.5). Recent evidence suggests that in a resting T-cell the cytoplasmic tails of

the CD3ε and CD3ζ molecules are buried in the inner leaflet of the plasma membrane, which shields their ITAMs from the kinase, called Lck (which we will discuss in the next section), that is needed to get the signal transduction cascade going. Stable MHC–TCR interactions appear to be able to release the CD3ε and CD3ζ tails from the membrane, making them accessible to phosphorylation. As we shall see in the next section, the signaling cascades that result from TCR stimulation can become quite complex (Figure 8.6); but take it one step at a time and a sense of order can be extracted from the apparent chaos.

Protein tyrosine phosphorylation is an early event in T-cell signaling

Interaction between the TCR and MHC–peptide complex is greatly enhanced by recruitment of either coreceptor for MHC, CD4 or CD8, into the complex. Furthermore, because the cytoplasmic tails of CD4 and CD8 are constitutively associated with **Lck**, a protein tyrosine kinase (PTK) that can phosphorylate the three tandemly arranged ITAMs within the TCR ζ **chains**, recruitment of CD4 or CD8 to the complex results in stable association between Lck and its ζ chain substrate (Figure 8.7a).

Phosphorylation of ζ chain by Lck creates binding sites for the recruitment of another PTK, **ZAP-70 (zeta chain associated protein of 70 kDa)**, into the TCR signaling complex. Recruitment of ZAP-70 into the receptor complex results in activation of this PTK by Lck-mediated phosphorylation. ZAP-70, in turn, phosphorylates two key adaptor proteins, **LAT (linker for activation of T-cells)** and **SLP76 (SH2-domain containing leukocyte protein of 76 kDa)** that can

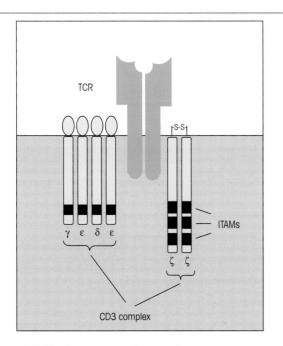

Figure 8.5. The CD3 coreceptor complex.

The TCR has no intrinsic signaling activity but signals through the associated CD3 complex. Note that the CD3 complex is thought to comprise one subunit each of CD3 γ and δ, two CD3ε subunits, and two disulfide-linked CD3ζ (zeta) subunits. As depicted in the figure, all of the CD3 coreceptor subunits contain *i*mmunoreceptor *t*yrosine-based *a*ctivation *m*otifs (ITAMs) that can become phosphorylated by kinases activated upon TCR stimulation. Phosphorylation at such motifs creates binding sites for additional signaling molecules that can propagate T-cell activation signals.

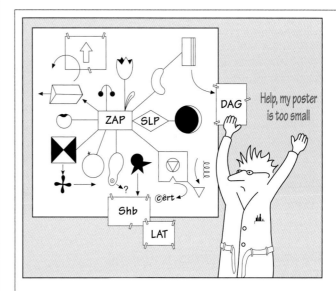

Figure 8.6. Signaling pathways can become quite complex.

(Reproduced with permission from Zolnierowicz S. & Bollen M. (2000) *EMBO Journal* **19**, 483.)

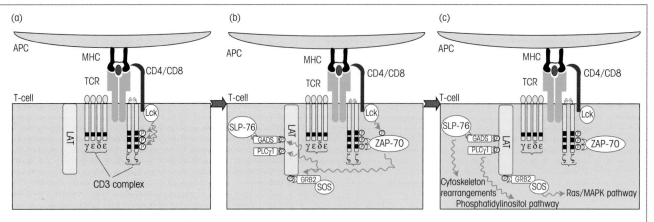

Figure 8.7. Signaling events downstream of T-cell receptor (TCR) engagement.

(a) Engagement of the TCR with the correct peptide–MHC combination leads to CD4/CD8 recruitment to the TCR complex through interactions with MHC on the antigen-presenting cell (APC) (note that, for simplicity, co-stimulation between B7 and CD28 is not depicted). Because CD4 and CD8 are constitutively associated with the Lck kinase, this brings Lck into close proximity to the ITAMs within the CD3 coreceptor complex. Lck then phosphorylates CD3ζ on multiple sites, that creates binding sites for recruitment of the ZAP-70 kinase. (b) ZAP-70 recruitment to the CD3 coreceptor complex leads to its phosphorylation and activation by Lck. Active ZAP-70 then propagates TCR signals through phosphorylation of LAT at several sites. Phosphorylated LAT serves as a platform for recruitment of multiple signaling complexes, as depicted. (c) Molecules recruited to LAT instigate three main signaling cascades, as depicted, which cooperatively achieve T-cell activation. See main text for further details.

instigate divergent signaling cascades downstream (Figure 8.7b).

LAT plays an especially significant role in subsequent events by serving as a platform for the recruitment of several additional players to the TCR complex. LAT contains many tyrosine residues that, upon phosphorylation by ZAP-70, can bind to other adaptor proteins through motifs (called SH2 domains) that bind phosphotyrosine residues. Thus, phosphorylation of LAT results in recruitment of **GADS (GRB2-related adapter protein)** that is constitutively associated with SLP76. SLP76 has been implicated in cytoskeletal rearrangements due to its ability to associate with Vav1 and NCK (Figure 8.7b). Thus, TCR stimulation induced cell shape changes are most likely due to recruitment of SLP76 into the TCR signaling complex.

Phosphorylated LAT also attracts the attentions of two additional phosphotyrosine-binding proteins; the γ1 isoform of **phospholipase C (PLCγ1)**, and the adaptor protein **GRB2 (growth factor receptor-binding protein 2)**. From this point on, at least two distinct signaling cascades can ensue; the **Ras/MAPK pathway** and the **phosphatidylinositol pathway** (Figure 8.7c).

Downstream events following TCR signaling

The Ras/MAPK pathway

Ras is a small G-protein that is constitutively associated with the plasma membrane and is frequently activated in response to diverse stimuli that promote cell division (Figure 8.8). Ras can exist in two states, GTP-bound (active) and GDP-bound (inactive). Thus, exchange of GDP for GTP stimulates Ras activation and enables this protein to recruit one of its downstream effectors, Raf. So how does TCR stimulation result in activation of Ras? One of the ways in which Ras activation can be achieved is through the activity of **GEFs (guanine-nucleotide exchange factors)** that promote exchange of GDP for GTP on Ras. One such GEF, SOS (son of sevenless), is recruited to phosphorylated LAT via the phosphotyrosine-binding protein GRB2 (Figure 8.7). Thus, phosphorylation of LAT by ZAP-70 leads directly to the recruitment of the GRB2/SOS complex to the plasma membrane where it can stimulate activation of Ras through promoting exchange of GDP for GTP.

In its GTP-bound state, Ras can recruit a kinase, **Raf (also called MAPKKK, mitogen-associated protein kinase kinase kinase!)**, to the plasma membrane that then sets in motion a series of further kinase activation events culminating in phosphorylation of the transcription factor Elk1, in addition to many other transcription factors. Elk1 phosphorylation permits translocation of this protein to the nucleus and results in the expression of Fos, yet another transcription factor. The appearance of Fos results in the formation of heterodimers with Jun to form the AP-1 complex that has binding sites on the IL-2 promoter as well as on many other genes (Figure 8.9). Deletion of AP-1 binding sites from the IL-2 promoter abrogates 90% of IL-2 enhancer activity.

The phosphatidylinositol pathway

Phosphorylation of LAT by ZAP-70 not only promotes docking of the GRB2/SOS complex on LAT, but also stimulates

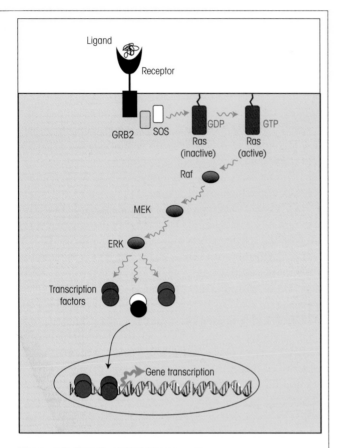

Figure 8.8. The Ras/MAP kinase pathway.

Regulation of Ras activity controls kinase amplification cascades. A number of cell surface receptors signal through Ras-regulated pathways. Ras cycles between inactive Ras–GDP and active Ras–GTP, regulated by guanine nucleotide exchange factors (GEFs) that promote the conversion of Ras–GDP to Ras–GTP, and by GTPase-activating proteins (GAPs) that increase the intrinsic GTPase activity of Ras. Upon ligand binding to receptor, receptor tyrosine kinases recruit adaptor proteins, e.g. Grb2, and GEF proteins, such as Sos ("son of sevenless"), to the plasma membrane. These events generate Ras–GTP, which can now recruit the Raf kinase (also known as *m*itogen *a*ctivated *p*rotein *k*inase, MAPK) to the plasma membrane where it becomes activated by another membrane-associated kinase. Activation of Raf then leads to a cascade of further kinase activation events downstream, culminating in the activation of a battery of transcription factors, including Elk1. The Ras/MAPK cascade is frequently invoked by growth factors and other stimuli that trigger proliferation.

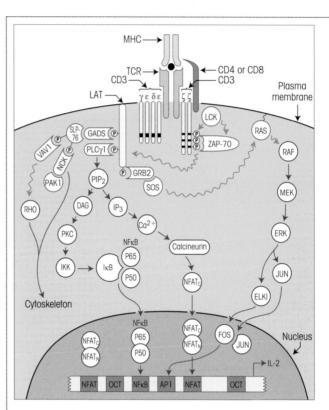

Figure 8.9. Overview of TCR-based signaling.

Signals through the MHC–antigen complex (signal 1) and B7 molecules (signal 2) initiate a cascade of protein kinase activation events and a rise in intracellular calcium, thereby activating transcription factors that control entry in the cell cycle from G0 and regulate the expression of IL-2 and many other cytokines. Stable recruitment of CD4 or CD8 to the TCR complex initiates the signal transduction cascade through phosphorylation of the tandemly arranged ITAM motifs within the CD3 ζ chains, which creates binding sites for the ZAP-70 kinase. Subsequent events are marshaled through ZAP-70-mediated phosphorylation of LAT; recruitment of several signaling complexes to LAT results in triggering of the Ras/MAPK and PLCγ1 signaling pathways. The latter pathways culminate in activation of a range of transcription factors including NFκB, NFAT and Fos/Jun heterodimers. Note that other molecules can also contribute to this pathway but have been omitted for clarity. See main body of text for further details. Abbreviations: DAG, diacylglycerol; ERK, *e*xtracellular signal *r*egulated *k*inase; IP$_3$, inositol triphosphate; LAT, *l*inker for *a*ctivated *T*-cells; NFκB, *n*uclear *f*actor κB; NFAT, *n*uclear *f*actor of *a*ctivated *T*-cells; OCT-1, octamer-binding factor; Pak1, *p*21-*a*ctivated *k*inase; PIP$_2$, phosphatidylinositol diphosphate; PKC, protein kinase C; PLC, phospholipase C; SH2, *S*rc-*h*omology domain *2;* SLAP, *SL*P-76-*a*ssociated *p*hosphoprotein; SLP-76, *S*H2-domain containing *l*eukocyte-specific 76 kDa *p*hosphoprotein; ZAP-70, ζ chain-*a*ssociated *p*rotein *k*inase. ⟶, Positive signal transduction.

recruitment of the γ1 isoform of **phospholipase C** (PLCγ1; Figure 8.7b). PLCγ1 plays a crucial role in propagating the cascade further. Phosphorylation of PLCγ1 activates this lipase that enables it to hydrolyze the membrane phospholipid, **phosphatidylinositol biphosphate (PIP$_2$)**, into diacylglycerol (DAG) and inositol triphosphate (IP$_3$) (Figure 8.9). Interaction of IP$_3$ with specific receptors in the endoplasmic reticulum triggers the release of Ca^{2+} into the cytosol that also triggers an influx of extracellular calcium. The **raised Ca^{2+}** concentration within the T-cell has at least two consequences. First, it synergizes with DAG to activate **protein kinase C** (PKC); second, it acts together with **calmodulin** to increase the activity of **calcineurin**, a protein phosphatase that can promote activation of an important transcription factor (NFAT) required for IL-2 production.

The Ca^{2+}-dependent activation of PKC by DAG is instrumental in the activation of yet another transcription factor, NFκB. NFκB is actually a family of related transcription factors that are involved in the regulation of transcription of many genes, including cytokines (such as IL-2), as well as genes that can promote cell survival by blocking signals that promote apoptosis.

Control of *IL-2* gene transcription

Transcription of IL-2 is one of the key events in preventing the signaled T-cell from lapsing into anergy and is controlled by multiple binding sites for transcriptional factors in the promoter region (Figure 8.9).

Under the influence of calcineurin, the cytoplasmic component of the *nuclear factor of activated T-cells* (**NFAT_c**) becomes dephosphorylated and this permits its translocation to the nucleus where it forms a binary complex with NFAT_n, its partner, which is constitutively expressed in the nucleus. The NFAT complex binds to two different IL-2 regulatory sites (Figure 8.9). Note here that the calcineurin effect is blocked by the anti-T-cell drugs cyclosporine and tacrolimus (see Chapter 16). PKC- and calcineurin-dependent pathways synergize in activating the multisubunit IκB kinase (IKK), which phosphorylates the inhibitor IκB thereby targeting it for ubiquitination and subsequent degradation by the proteasome. Loss of IκB from the IκB–NFκB complex exposes the nuclear localization signal on the NFκB transcription factor that then swiftly enters the nucleus. In addition, the ubiquitous transcription factor **Oct-1** interacts with specific octamer-binding sequence motifs.

We have concentrated on IL-2 transcription as an early and central consequence of T-cell activation, but more than 70 genes are newly expressed within 4 hours of T-cell activation, leading to proliferation and the synthesis of several cytokines and their receptors (see Chapter 9).

CD28 co-stimulation amplifies TCR signals and blocks apoptosis

As discussed earlier, naive T-cells typically require two signals for proper activation; one derived from TCR ligation (signal 1), and the other provided by simultaneous engagement of CD28 on the T-cell (signal 2) by CD80 (B7.1) or CD86 (B7.2) on the DC (Figure 8.3). Indeed, T-cells derived from CD28-deficient mice, or cells treated with anti-CD28 blocking antibodies, display severely reduced capacity to proliferate in response to TCR stimulation *in vitro* and *in vivo*. Moreover, CD28 deficiency also impairs T-cell differentiation and the production of cytokines required for B-cell help. Similar effects are also seen when CD80 or CD86 expression is interfered

with. So what does tickling the CD28 receptor do that is so special?

Well, the simple answer is that we do not really know what kind of signal CD28 co-stimulation produces that is radically different from the signals produced upon stimulation of the TCR complex, as several of the same signaling pathways are triggered. CD28 is expressed on the plasma membrane of naive as well as activated T-cells as a 44 kDa homo-dimer, the cytoplasmic domain of which lacks any intrinsic enzyme activity. The cytoplasmic tail of CD28 does however contain tyrosine-based motifs that, upon phosphorylation at these residues, recruit phosphatidylinositol 3-kinase (PI3K) and Grb2. Thus, upon CD28 cross-linking, signals are propagated via PI3K that can impact upon multiple signaling pathways, including cell survival, cell metabolism and protein synthesis. CD28-mediated activation of PI3K is important for the suppression of apoptosis, which appears to be achieved via the downstream target of this pathway, the PkB/Akt kinase. The latter kinase regulates transcription factors that result in increased expression of the anti-apoptotic Bcl-x_L protein. By upregulating Bcl-x_L, CD28 stimulation blocks TCR-mediated signals that would otherwise result in apoptosis (a process called **activation-induced cell death** [AICD]) (see Videoclip 2).

Grb2 docks onto the same motif within the cytoplasmic tail of CD28 as PI3K and can activate the Ras pathway via its associated guanine-nucleotide exchange factor SOS, as discussed earlier. Grb2 has also been implicated in propagating other signals during T-cell activation via recruitment of Vav, which we will discuss further below.

Recent studies also suggest that CD28 signals feed into the TCR signaling pathway at the level of the SLP-76 adaptor, delivering signals that amplify TCR signaling in a quantitative way. Although the identity of the kinase remains unknown, it has been suggested that a CD28-activated kinase phosphorylates SLP-76 during co-stimulation and this leads to enhanced recruitment and activation of Vav, a guanine nucleotide exchange factor that can promote the activation of Rac1 and c-Jun kinase (JNK) downstream. Vav activation appears to be essential for efficient proliferative responses, IL-2 production, and calcium signaling as a consequence of CD28 co-stimulation.

While early studies suggested that CD28 stimulation might result in *qualitatively* different signals to those that are generated through the TCR, many studies suggest that this might not be the case. Instead, these studies suggest that while CD28 engagement might activate pathways within the T-cell that TCR stimulation alone does not, the primary purpose of co-stimulation through CD28 may be to *quantitatively* amplify or stabilize signals through the TCR by converging on similar transcription factors such as NFκB and NFAT, which are critical for IL-2 production. In support of this view, microarray analyses of genes upregulated in response to TCR ligation alone, versus TCR ligation in the presence of CD28 co-stimulation, found, rather surprisingly, that essentially the same cohorts of genes were expressed in both cases. While signals through CD28 enhanced the expression of many of the genes switched on in response to TCR ligation, no new genes were expressed. This indicates that CD28 co-stimulation may be required in order to cross signaling thresholds that are not achievable via TCR ligation alone. One is reminded here of the choke that earlier generations of cars were supplied with to provide a slightly more fuel-rich mixture to help start a cold engine. CD28 co-stimulation of naive T-cells may serve a similar purpose, with the CD28 "choke" no longer needed when these cells have warmed up as a result of previous stimulation.

The requirement for two signals for T-cell activation is a very good way of minimizing the likelihood that T-cells will respond to self-antigens. Because T-cell receptors are generated randomly and can, in principle, recognize almost any short peptide, the immune system needs a way of letting a T-cell know that particular (i.e. nonself) peptides should be responded to while others (i.e. derived from self) should not. The fact that CD80/CD86 molecules are only upregulated on APCs that have been stimulated with a PAMP, this provides quite a clever way of ensuring that only APCs that have encountered microorganisms are able to properly present peptides to T-cells. Once again, we see the guiding hand of the innate immune system helping to qualify what represents "danger" and what does not.

Damping T-cell enthusiasm

We have frequently reiterated the premise that no self-respecting organism would permit the operation of an expanding enterprise such as a proliferating T-cell population without some sensible controlling mechanisms. There are some similarities here with regulations governing corporate takeovers in the business world, where it has been deemed prudent to ensure that no single enterprise is permitted to completely dominate the marketplace. Such monopoly practices, if allowed to occur in an unregulated way, would eventually eliminate all competition. Not a good thing for diversity or overall fitness.

In a similar vein, in order to preserve immunological diversity and the capacity to rapidly respond to new challenges of an infectious nature, it is necessary to ensure that T-cells specific for particular epitopes are not allowed to proliferate indefinitely and ultimately dominate the immune compartment. This would inevitably reduce the probability that responses to freshly encountered antigens would ever get off the ground, as naive T-cells would have to compete for access to DCs with overwhelming numbers of previously activated T-cells; with inevitable disastrous consequences for immunological fitness. For these reasons, our highly adapted immune systems have evolved ways of maintaining healthy competition between T-cells, which is achieved through downregulating immune responses upon clearance of a pathogen, along with culling of the majority of recently expanded T-cells. This is also necessary because the immune compartment is of a relatively finite size and cannot accommodate an infinite number of lymphocytes.

Damping down T-cell responses occurs via a number of mechanisms, some of which operate at the level of the activated T-cell itself, while others operate via additional T-cell subsets (**regulatory T cells**) that use a variety of strategies to rein in T-cell responses, some of which are directed at the T-cell while others are directed at DCs. Regulatory T-cells will be discussed at length in Chapter 9 (p. 242), so here we will focus primarily on molecules present on activated T-cells that serve as "off switches" for such T-cells.

Signals routed through CTLA-4 downregulate T-cell responses

Cytotoxic T-lymphocyte antigen-4 (CTLA-4) is structurally related to CD28 and also binds B7 (CD80/CD86) ligands. However, while CD28-B7 interactions are co-stimulatory, CTLA4-B7 interactions act in an opposite fashion and contribute to the termination of TCR signaling (Figure 8.10). Whereas CD28 is constitutively expressed on T-cells, CTLA-4 is not found on the resting cell but is rapidly upregulated within 3–4 hours following TCR/CD28-induced activation. CTLA-4 has a 10- to 20-fold higher affinity for both B7.1 and B7.2 and can therefore compete favorably with CD28 for binding to the latter even when present at relatively low concentrations. The mechanism by which CTLA-4 suppresses T-cell activation has been the subject of lively debate, as this receptor appears to recruit a similar repertoire of proteins (such as PI3K) to its intracellular tail as CD28 does. A number of mechanisms have been proposed to account for the inhibitory effect of CTLA-4 on T-cell activation. One mechanism is by simple competition with CD28 for binding of CD80/CD86 molecules on the DC. Another is through recruitment of SHP-1 and SHP-2 protein tyrosine phosphatases to the TCR complex that may contribute to the termination of TCR signals by dephosphorylating proteins that are required for TCR signal propagation. CTLA-4 may also antagonize the recruitment of the TCR complex to lipid rafts, which is where many of the signaling proteins that propagate TCR signals reside. Irrespective of its mechanism of action, CTLA-4 is undoubtedly critical for keeping T-cells under control and in this regard is also important for preventing responses to self-antigen. CTLA-4-deficient mice display a profound hyperproliferative disorder and die within 3 weeks of birth due to massive tissue infiltration and organ destruction by T-cells.

Cbl family ubiquitin ligases restrain TCR signals

A number of other molecules have been identified that may be involved in reigning in T-cell activation and these include the **c-Cbl family** of proteins. Members of the c-Cbl family are **protein ubiquitin ligases** that can catalyze the degradation of proteins through attaching polyubiquitin chains to such molecules, thereby targeting them for destruction via the **ubiquitin-proteasome pathway**. The ζ chain of the CD3 coreceptor complex has been identified as a target for c-Cbl-mediated ubiquitination and this can result in internalization and degradation of the TCR complex. Thus, c-Cbl proteins may raise the threshold for TCR-induced signals through destabilizing

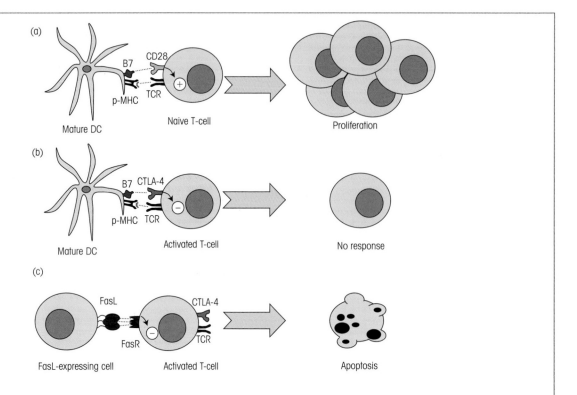

Figure 8.10. Downregulation of T-cell responses.

(a) Antigen presentation by a mature dendritic cell (DC) provides effective antigenic stimulation via peptide–MHC (signal 1) and B7 ligands (signal 2) that engage the T-cell receptor (TCR) complex and CD28 on the T-cell, respectively. (b) Antigen presentation to a previously activated T-cell that is bearing surface CTLA-4 (a CD28-related molecule that can also interact with B7 ligands) can lead to T-cell unresponsiveness due to inhibitory signals delivered through CTLA-4 co-stimulation (see main text for further details). (c) Whereas naive T-cells bearing surface Fas receptor are typically resistant to ligation of this receptor, activated T-cells acquire sensitivity to Fas receptor (FasR) engagement within a week or so of activation. Engagement of FasR on susceptible cells results in activation of the programmed cell death machinery as a result of recruitment and activation of caspase-8 within the FasR complex. Active caspase-8 the propagates a cascade of further caspase activation events to kill the cell via apoptosis.

this complex. Mice doubly deficient in c-Cbl and Cbl-b (which appear to exert somewhat redundant functions) exhibit hyper-responsiveness to TCR-induced signals, resulting in excessive proliferation and cytokine production in naive as well as differentiated effector T-cells; such mice die from autoimmune disease as a consequence. This appears to be due to a defect in downmodulation of the TCR complex in activated T-cells. Whereas, TCR complexes are normally internalized and degraded after stimulation via cognate peptide–MHC complexes (an event which contributes to the termination of TCR signals), TCR complexes fail to be internalized in Cbl/Cbl-b-deficient cells, leading to greatly extended TCR signaling and runaway T-cell expansion.

c-Cbl family proteins can also exert their influence on TCR signaling in other ways and may have an especially important role in maintaining the requirement for CD28 co-stimulation for proper T-cell activation. Surprisingly, mice deficient in Cbl-b lose the normal requirement for CD28 co-stimulation (i.e. signal 2) for T-cell proliferation; such cells make large amounts of IL-2 and proliferate vigorously in response to TCR stimulation alone. This implies that Cbl-b plays a major role

in maintaining the requirement for signal 2 for activation of naive T-cells. Although it is not yet clear exactly how this operates, activation of Vav, which occurs downstream of TCR as well as CD28 receptor stimulation, appears to be suppressed by Cbl-b in wild type cells. Thus, for effective Vav activation, signal 1 and signal 2 are normally required. However, in the absence of c-Cbl-b, a sufficient amount of Vav activation is achieved through TCR stimulation alone, bypassing the need for CD28 co-stimulation.

T-cell death occurs through stimulation of membrane Fas receptors

Another important way of standing down T-cells from active duty is to kill such cells through programmed cell death (Figure 8.10). Naive T cells, as well as recently activated T-cells express the membrane Fas (CD95) receptor but are insensitive to stimulation via this receptor as these cells contain an endogenous inhibitor (FLIP) of the proximal signaling molecule, caspase-8, that is activated as a result of stimulation through the Fas receptor. However, upon several rounds of stimulation, experienced T-cells become sensitive to stimulation via their Fas receptors, most likely due to loss of FLIP expression, and this situation results in apoptosis of these cells. Mice defective in expression of either FasR or FasL manifest a lymphoproliferative syndrome that results in autoimmune disease due to a failure to cull recently expanded lymphocytes.

Dynamic interactions at the immunological synapse

As we have described above, successful TCR triggering involves a multitude of signal transduction events that culminate in T-cell activation. But what is the probability of this occurring in an *in vivo* setting? T-cells need to be highly efficient at finding their cognate antigen and discriminating between activating and non-activating peptide–MHC complexes for several reasons.

First, the numbers of T-cells bearing the correct TCRs for productive engagement with peptide–MHC are typically small; 1 in 100 000 or fewer cells being capable of responding to a particular peptide–MHC combination is not unusual. Therefore, T-cells need to be able to efficiently recognize the correct peptide–MHC combination in a veritable sea of self-peptide–MHC and non-activating peptide–MHC molecules. Because of the need to search for the correct peptide–MHC combination, **naive T-cells are in continual motion within a lymph node**, scanning at speeds that enable them to visit up to 5000 DCs in 1 hour; quite the social networkers! Because of this ferocious rate of movement, TCR– peptide–MHC interactions are very fleeting as cells brush past each other at high speed. When an activating TCR–peptide–MHC interaction does occur, as few as 10 peptide–MHC complexes can persuade a T-cell to stop and linger, forming a more stable interaction that leads to the productive assembly of the **immunological synapse** (described below). Of course, the reader will understand that the T-cell needs to be pretty certain that this is the correct peptide–MHC complex to respond to, for if an error is made, the consequences are potentially calamitous and can result in autoimmunity.

The behavior of a T-cell within a lymph node as it searches for the correct peptide–MHC combination can be divided into several phases. Whereas T-cell movement is rapid during the seeking phase (phase I), encounter with agonistic peptide–MHC leads to stable T-cell–DC interactions lasting approximately 12 hours (phase II), during which cytokines such as IL-2 are produced. This is followed by a return to rapid movement involving further transient DC interactions (phase III), during which the T-cell divides a number of times and exits the lymph node.

A serial TCR engagement model for T-cell activation

We have already commented that the major docking forces that conjugate the APC and its T-lymphocyte counterpart must come from the complementary accessory molecules such as ICAM-1/LFA-1 and LFA-3/CD2, rather than through the relatively low affinity TCR–MHC plus peptide links (Figure 8.3). Nonetheless, cognate antigen recognition by the TCR remains a *sine qua non* for T-cell activation. Fine, but how can as few as 10 MHC–peptide complexes on a DC, through their low affinity complexing with TCRs, effect the Herculean task of sustaining a raised intracellular calcium flux for the 60 minutes required for full cell activation? Any fall in calcium flux, as may be occasioned by adding an antibody to the MHC, and NFAT$_c$ dutifully returns from the nucleus to its cytoplasmic location, so aborting the activation process.

Surprisingly, Salvatore Valitutti and Antonio Lanzavecchia have shown that as few as 100 MHC–peptide complexes on an APC can downregulate 18 000 TCRs on its cognate T-lymphocyte partner. They suggest that each MHC–peptide complex can *serially* engage up to 200 TCRs. In their model, conjugation of a MHC–peptide dimer with two TCRs activates signal transduction, phosphorylation of the CD3-associated ζ chains with subsequent downstream events, and then downregulation of those TCRs. Intermediate affinity binding favors dissociation of the MHC–peptide, freeing it to engage and trigger another TCR, so sustaining the required intracellular activation events. The model for **agonist** action would also explain why peptides giving interactions of lower or higher affinity than the optimum could behave as **antagonists** (Figure 8.11). The important phenomenon of modified peptides behaving as **partial agonists**, with differential effects on the outcome of T-cell activation, is addressed in the legend to Figure 8.11.

The immunological synapse

Experiments using peptide–MHC and ICAM-1 molecules labeled with different fluorochromes and inserted into a planar lipid bilayer on a glass support have provided evidence for the idea that T-cell activation occurs in the context of an immunological synapse. These and other imaging studies have revealed that the immunological synapse between the T-cell and the DC has a "bull's eye" pattern with a central cluster of TCR–peptide–MHC, known as the **cSMAC (central supramolecular activation complex)**, surrounded by a ring of the integrin LFA-1 interacting with its cognate ligand ICAM-1 on the DC (Figure 8.12). Initially unstable TCR–MHC interactions occur outside of integrin ring, followed by transit of the peptide–MHC molecules into the cSMAC, changing places with the adhesion molecules that now form the outer ring (Figure 8.12). It has been suggested that the generation of the immunological synapse only occurs after a certain initial threshold level of TCR triggering has been achieved, its formation being dependent upon cytoskeletal reorganization and leading to potentiation of the signal. LFA-1 engagement with ICAM-1 is essential for formation of immunological synapses for a number of reasons. In the early stages of synapse formation, these molecules serve in a predominantly adhesive capacity to tether the opposing cells to facilitate TCR and peptide–MHC

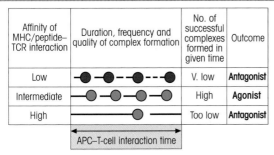

Affinity of MHC/peptide–TCR interaction	Duration, frequency and quality of complex formation	No. of successful complexes formed in given time	Outcome
Low		V. low	**Antagonist**
Intermediate		High	**Agonist**
High		Too low	**Antagonist**

APC–T-cell interaction time

Figure 8.11. Serial triggering model of T-cell receptor (TCR) activation (Valitutti S. & Lanzavecchia A. (1995) *The Immunologist* **3**, 122). Intermediate affinity complexes between MHC–peptide and TCR survive long enough for a successful activation signal to be transduced by the TCR, and the MHC–peptide dissociates and fruitfully engages another TCR. A sustained high rate of formation of successful complexes is required for full T-cell activation. Low affinity complexes have a short half-life that either has no effect on the TCR or produces inactivation, perhaps through partial phosphorylation of ζ chains (◑, successful TCR activation; ●, TCR inactivation; —, no effect: the length of the horizontal bar indicates the lifetime of that complex). Being of low affinity, they recycle rapidly and engage and inactivate a large number of TCRs. High affinity complexes have such a long lifetime before dissociation that insufficient numbers of successful triggering events occur. Thus modified peptide ligands of either low or high affinity can act as antagonists by denying the agonist access to adequate numbers of vacant TCRs. Some modified peptides act as partial agonists in that they produce differential effects on the outcomes of T-cell activation. For example, a single residue change in a hemoglobin peptide reduced IL-4 secretion 10-fold but completely knocked out T-cell proliferation. The mechanism presumably involves incomplete or inadequately transduced phosphorylation events occurring through a truncated half-life of TCR engagement, allosteric effects on the MHC–TCR partners, or orientational misalignment of the peptide within the complex. (Reproduced with permission of Hogrefe & Huber Publishers.)

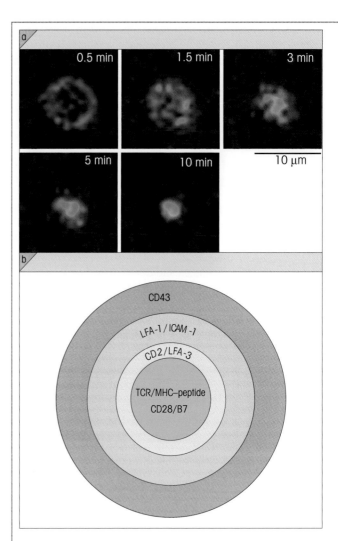

Figure 8.12. The immunological synapse.

(a) The formation of the immunological synapse. T-cells were brought into contact with planar lipid bilayers and the positions of engaged MHC–peptide (green) and engaged ICAM-1 (red) at the indicated times after initial contact are shown. (Reproduced with permission from Grakoui A., Dustin M.L. *et al.* (1999) *Science* **285**, 221. © American Association for the Advancement of Science.). (b) Diagrammatic representation of the resolved synapse in which the adhesion molecule pairs CD2/LFA-3 and LFA-1/ICAM-1, which were originally in the center, have moved to the outside and now encircle the antigen recognition and signaling interaction between T-cell receptor (TCR) and MHC–peptide and the co-stimulatory interaction between CD28 and B7. The CD43 molecule has been reported to bind to ICAM-1 and E-selectin, and upon ligation is able to induce IL-2 mRNA, CD69 and CD154 (CD40L) expression and activate the DNA-binding activity of the AP-1, NFκB and NFAT transcription factors.

interactions, thereby allowing the T-cell to scan the peptide–MHC complex on offer.

B-cells respond to three different types of antigen

B-cells typically require T-cells in order to generate high affinity antibodies and to undergo class switching. However, as we shall discuss below, certain types of antigens (called T-independent antigens) can promote B-cell activation without the help of T-cells. The antibodies thus formed are typically of low affinity and do not undergo class switching or somatic hypermutation but provide rapid protection from certain microorganisms and buy time for T-dependent B-cell responses to be made.

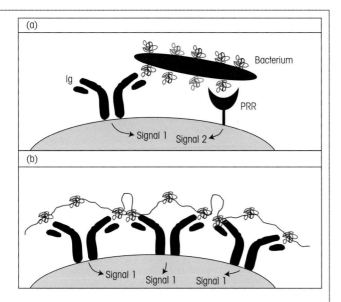

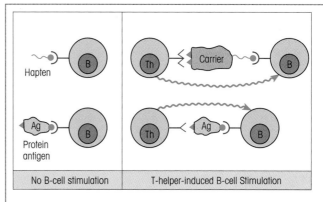

Figure 8.14. T-helper cells cooperate through protein carrier determinants to help B-cells respond to hapten or equivalent determinants on antigens (Ag) by providing accessory signals.

(For simplicity we are ignoring the MHC component and epitope processing in T-cell recognition, but we won't forget it.)

Figure 8.13. B-cell recognition of (a) type 1 and (b) type 2 thymus-independent antigens.

The complex gives a sustained signal to the B-cell because of the long half-life of this type of molecule.

1 Type 1 thymus-independent antigens

Certain antigens, such as bacterial lipopolysaccharides, when present at a sufficiently high concentration, have the ability to activate a substantial proportion of the B-cell pool polyclonally, i.e. without reference to the antigen specificity of the surface receptor hypervariable regions. They do this through binding to surface molecules, such as Toll-like receptors (TLRs) discussed in Chapter 1, which bypasses the early part of the biochemical pathway mediated by the specific antigen receptor. At concentrations that are too low to cause polyclonal activation through unaided binding to these mitogenic bypass molecules, the B-cell population with Ig receptors specific for these antigens will selectively and passively focus them on their surface, where the resulting high local concentration will suffice to drive the activation process (Figure 8.13a).

2 Type 2 thymus-independent antigens

Certain linear antigens that are not readily degraded in the body and that have an appropriately spaced, highly repeating determinant—pneumococcus polysaccharide, Ficoll, D-amino acid polymers and polyvinylpyrrolidone, for example—are also thymus-independent in their ability to stimulate B-cells directly without the need for T-cell involvement. Such antigens persist for long periods on the surface of follicular dendritic cells located at the subcapsular sinus of the lymph nodes and the splenic marginal zone, and can bind to antigen-specific B-cells with great avidity through their multivalent attachment to the complementary Ig receptors that they cross-link (Figure 8.13b).

In general, the thymus-independent antigens give rise to predominantly low affinity IgM responses, some IgG3 in the mouse, and relatively poor, if any, memory. Neonatal B-cells do not respond well to type 2 antigens and this has important consequences for the efficacy of carbohydrate vaccines in young children.

3 Thymus-dependent antigens

The need for collaboration with T-helper cells

Many antigens are thymus-dependent in that they provoke little or no antibody response in animals that have been thymectomized at birth and therefore have few T-cells (Milestone 8.1). Such antigens cannot fulfil the molecular requirements for direct stimulation; they may be univalent with respect to the specificity of each determinant; they may be readily degraded by phagocytic cells; and they may lack mitogenicity. If they bind to B-cell receptors, they will sit on the surface just like a hapten and do nothing to trigger the B-cell (Figure 8.14). Cast your mind back to the definition of a hapten—a small molecule like dinitrophenyl (DNP) that binds to preformed antibody (e.g. the surface receptor of a specific B-cell) but fails to stimulate antibody production (i.e. stimulate the B-cell). Remember also that haptens become immunogenic when coupled to an appropriate carrier protein (see p. 117). Building on the knowledge that both T- and B-cells are necessary for antibody responses to thymus-dependent antigens (Milestone 8.1), we now know that the carrier functions to stimulate T-helper cells that cooperate with B-cells to enable them to respond to the hapten by providing accessory signals (Figure 8.14). It should also be evident from Figure 8.14 that, while one determinant on a typical protein antigen is behaving as a hapten in binding to the B-cell, the other determinants subserve a carrier function in recruiting T-helper cells.

Milestone 8.1—T–B Collaboration for Antibody Production

In the 1960s, as the mysteries of the thymus were slowly unraveled, our erstwhile colleagues pushing back the frontiers of knowledge discovered that neonatal thymectomy in the mouse abrogated not only the cellular rejection of skin grafts, but also the antibody response to some but not all antigens (Figure M8.1.1). Subsequent investigations showed that both thymocytes and bone marrow cells were needed for optimal antibody responses to such **thymus-dependent antigens** (Figure M8.1.2). By carrying out these transfers with cells from animals bearing a recognizable chromosome marker (T6), it became evident that the antibody-forming cells were derived from the bone marrow inoculum, hence the nomenclature "*T*" for *T*hymus-derived lymphocytes and "*B*" for antibody-forming cell precursors originating in the *B*one marrow. This convenient nomenclature has stuck even though bone marrow contains embryonic T-cell precursors as the immunocompetent T- and B-cells differentiate in the thymus and bone marrow respectively (see Chapter 11).

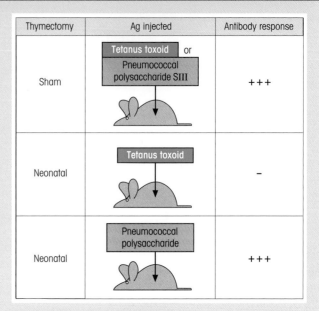

Figure M8.1.1. The antibody response to some antigens is thymus-dependent and, to others, thymus-independent.

The response to tetanus toxoid in neonatally thymectomized animals could be restored by the injection of thymocytes.

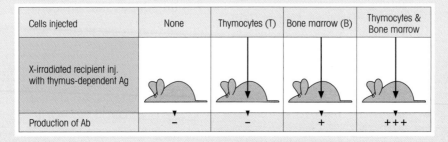

Figure M8.1.2. The antibody response to a thymus-dependent antigen requires two different T-cell populations.

Different populations of cells from a normal mouse histocompatible with the recipient (i.e. of the same H-2 haplotype) were injected into recipients who had been X-irradiated to destroy their own lymphocyte responses. They were then primed with a thymus-dependent antigen such as sheep red blood cells (i.e. an antigen that fails to give a response in neonatally thymectomized mice; Figure M8.1.1) and examined for the production of antibody after 2 weeks. The small amount of antibody (Ab) synthesized by animals receiving bone marrow alone is due to the presence of thymocyte precursors in the cell inoculum that differentiate in the intact thymus gland of the recipient.

Antigen processing by B-cells

The need for **physical linkage of hapten and carrier** strongly suggests that T-helpers must recognize the carrier determinants on the responding B-cell in order to provide the relevant accessory stimulatory signals. However, as T-cells only recognize processed membrane-bound antigen in association with MHC molecules, the T-helpers cannot recognize native antigen bound simply to the Ig receptors of the B-cell as naively depicted in Figure 8.14. All is not lost, however, as **primed B-cells can present antigen to T-helper cells**—in fact, they work at much lower antigen concentrations than conventional presenting cells because they can focus antigen through their surface receptors. Antigen bound to surface Ig is internalized in endosomes that then fuse with vesicles containing MHC class II molecules with their invariant chain. Processing of the protein antigen then occurs as described in Chapter 5 (see Figure 5.16) and the resulting antigenic peptide is recycled to

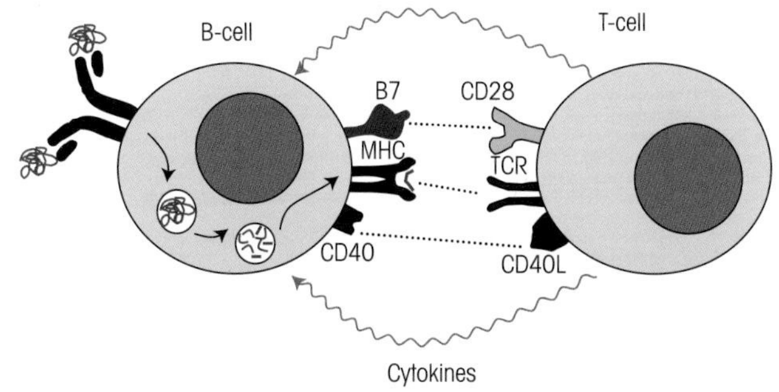

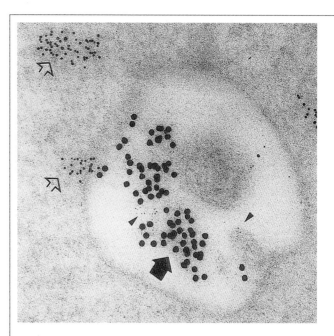

Figure 8.15. B-cell handling of a thymus-dependent antigen and presentation to an activated T-cell.

Antigen captured by the surface Ig receptor is internalized within an endosome, processed and expressed on the surface of the B-cell with MHC class II (cf. Figure 5.16). Co-stimulatory signals through the CD40–CD40L (CD154) interaction are required for the activation of the resting B-cell by the T-helper cell. In addition to CD40L-based co-stimulation, helper T-cells also provide additional stimulation to the B-cell in the form of cytokines such as IL-4.

Figure 8.16. Demonstration that endocytosed B-cell surface Ig receptors enter cytoplasmic vesicles geared for antigen processing.

Surface IgG was cross-linked with goat anti-human Ig and rabbit anti-goat Ig conjugated to 15-nm gold beads (large, dark arrow). After 2 minutes, the cell sections were prepared and stained with anti-HLA-DR invariant chain (2 nm gold; arrowheads) and an antibody to a cathepsin protease (5 nm gold; open arrows). Thus the internalized IgG is exposed to proteolysis in a vesicle containing class II molecules. The presence of invariant chain shows that the class II molecules derive from the endoplasmic reticulum and Golgi, not from the cell surface. Note the clever use of differently sized gold particles to distinguish the antibodies used for localizing the various intravesicular proteins, etc. (Photograph reproduced with permission from the authors and the publishers from Guagliardi L.E. *et al.* (1990) *Nature* **343**, 133. Copyright © 1990 Macmillan Magazines Ltd.)

the surface in association with the class II molecules where it is available for recognition by specific T-helpers (Figures 8.15 and 8.16). The need for the physical union of hapten and carrier is now revealed; the hapten leads the carrier to be processed into the cell which is programed to make anti-hapten antibody and, following stimulus by the T-helper-recognizing processed carrier, it will carry out its program and ultimately produce antibodies that react with the hapten (is there no end to the wiliness of nature?).

The nature of B-cell activation

Similar to T-cells, naive or resting B-cells are nondividing and activation through the B-cell receptor (BCR) drives these cells into the cell cycle. As is the case for the T-cell receptor, the B-cell receptor (surface Ig) does not possess any intrinsic enzymatic activity. Once again, it is the accessory molecules associated with the antigen receptor that propagate activation signals into the B-cell. It was noted in Chapter 4 that the BCR complex is composed of membrane-anchored immunoglobulin that is associated with a disulfide-linked Ig-α and Ig-β heterodimer, the cytoplasmic tails of which each contain a single ITAM motif (see Figure 4.4). As we will now discuss in more detail, antigen-driven cross-linking of the BCR results in the initiation of a PTK-driven signaling cascade, seeded by the Ig-α/β ITAMs, that awaken a panoply of transcription factors from their cellular slumber.

B-cells are stimulated by cross-linking surface Ig

B-cell activation begins with interaction between antigen and surface immunoglobulin. Recruitment of the BCR to lipid rafts is thought to play an important role in B-cell activation as surface Ig is normally excluded from lipid rafts but becomes rapidly recruited to rafts within minutes of Ig cross-linking (Figure 8.17); this event probably serves to bring the PTK **Lyn** into close proximity with the ITAMs within the cytoplasmic tails of the BCR-associated Ig-α/β heterodimer as Lyn is constitutively associated with lipid rafts. Upon recruitment, Lyn then adds phosphate groups to the tyrosine residues within the ITAMs of the cytoplasmic tails of the Ig-α/β complex. This is rapidly followed by binding of the PTK **Syk** to the ITAMs along with another kinase **Btk (Bruton's tyrosine kinase)**. Active Lyn also phosphorylates residues on CD19, a component of the B-cell coreceptor complex (discussed in detail in the next section) that reinforces signals initiated by the BCR (Figure 8.18).

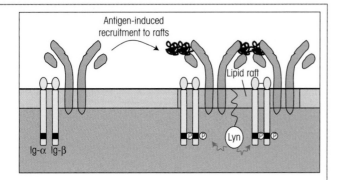

Figure 8.17. Receptor cross-linking recruits the BCR to lipid rafts.

Antigen-induced receptor cross-linking recruits the BCR, which is normally excluded from membrane cholesterol-rich lipid raft domains, to membrane lipid rafts where signaling proteins such as the protein tyrosine kinase Lyn reside. Stable recruitment of the BCR to rafts facilitates Lyn-mediated phosphorylation of ITAMs within the cytoplasmic tails of the Ig-α and Ig-β accessory molecules that initiate the BCR-driven signaling cascade.

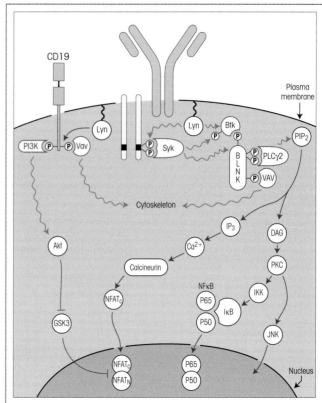

Figure 8.18. Signaling cascade downstream of antigen-driven B-cell receptor (BCR) ligation.

Upon interaction with antigen, the BCR is recruited to lipid rafts where ITAMs within the Ig-α/β heterodimer become phosphorylated by Lyn. This is followed by recruitment and activation of the Syk and Btk kinases. Phosphorylation of the B-cell adaptor protein, BLNK, creates binding sites for several other proteins, including PLCγ2 that promotes PIP_2 hydrolysis and instigates a chain of signaling events culminating in activation of the NFAT and NFκB transcription factors. The CD19 coreceptor molecule is also phosphorylated by Lyn and can suppress the inhibitory effects of GSK3 on NFAT through the PI3K/Akt pathway. BCR stimulation also results in rearrangement of the cell cytoskeleton via activation of Vav that acts as a guanine nucleotide exchange factor for small G-proteins such as Rac and Rho.

Syk fulfills a critical role within the B-cell activation process; disruption of the gene encoding Syk in the mouse has profound effects on downstream events in B-cell signaling and results in defective B-cell development. In this respect, Syk serves a similar role in B-cells to that served by ZAP-70 in T-cells. Active Syk phosphorylates and recruits **BLNK** (B-cell linker; also called SLP65, BASH and BCA) to the BCR complex. Upon phosphorylation by Syk, BLNK provides binding sites for **phospholipase Cγ2** (PLCγ2), Btk and **Vav**. Recruitment of Btk in close proximity to PLCγ2 enables Btk to phosphorylate the latter and increase its activity. Just as in the T-cell signaling pathway, activated PLCγ2 initiates a pathway that involves hydrolysis of PIP_2 to generate diacylglycerol and inositol triphosphate and results in increases in intracellular calcium and PKC activation (Figure 8.18). PKC activation, in turn, results in activation of the **NFκB** and **JNK** transcription factors and increased intracellular calcium results in **NFAT** activation, just as it does in T-cells.

The Vav family of guanine nucleotide exchange factors consists of at least three isoforms (Vav-1, -2 and -3) and is known to play a crucial role in B-cell signaling through activation of Rac1 and regulating cytoskeletal changes after BCR cross-linking; Vav-1-deficient B-cells are defective in proliferation associated with cross-linking of the BCR (Figure 8.18).

The BCR cross-linking model seems appropriate for an understanding of stimulation by type 2 thymus-independent antigens, as their repeating determinants ensure strong binding to, and cross-linking of, multiple Ig receptors on the B-cell surface to form aggregates that persist owing to the long half-life of the antigen and sustain the high intracellular calcium needed for activation. On the other hand, type 1 T-independent antigens, like the T-cell polyclonal activators, probably bypass the specific receptor and act directly on downstream molecules

such as diacylglycerol and protein kinase C as Ig-α and Ig-β are not phosphorylated.

B-cells require co-stimulation via the B-cell co-receptor complex for efficient activation

Similar to T-cells, B-cells also require **two forms of co-stimulation** to mount efficient effector responses. One form of co-stimulation takes place at the point of initial encounter of the BCR with its cognate antigen and is provided by the **B-cell coreceptor complex** that is capable of engaging with molecules such as complement that may be present in close proximity to the specific antigen recognized by the BCR. The

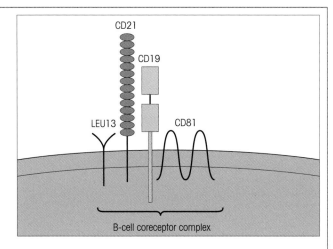

Figure 8.19. The B-cell coreceptor complex.

The B-cell coreceptor complex provides co-stimulatory signals for B-cell activation through recruitment of a number of signaling molecules, including phosphatidylinositol 3-kinase and Vav, which can amplify signals initiated through the B-cell receptor. On mature B-cells, CD19 forms a tetrameric complex with three other proteins: CD21 (complement receptor type 2), CD81 (TAPA-1) and CD225 (interferon-induced transmembrane protein 1) (LEU13). See also Figure 4.6.

other form of co-stimulation required by B-cells takes place after the initial encounter with antigen and is provided by T-cells in the form of membrane-associated **CD40 ligand that engages with CD40** on the B-cell. This form of co-stimulation requires that the B-cell has internalized antigen, followed by processing and presentation on MHC class II molecules to an appropriate T-cell. If the B-cell is displaying an MHC–peptide combination recognized by the T-cell, the latter will be stimulated to produce cytokines (such as IL-4) as well as provide co-stimulation to the B-cell in the form of CD40L. We will consider the nature of the co-stimulatory signals provided by the B-cell co-receptor complex here and deal with CD40L-based co-stimulation in a separate section below.

The mature B-cell coreceptor complex (Figure 8.19) is composed of four components: CD19, CD21 (complement receptor type 2, CR2), CD81 (TAPA-1) and CD225 (LEU13, interferon-induced transmembrane protein 1). CR2 is a receptor for the C3d breakdown product of complement and its presence within the BCR coreceptor complex enables a component of the innate immune response (complement) to synergise with the BCR to productively activate B-cells. Imagine a bacterium that has activated complement and has become coated with the products of complement activation, including C3d. If the same bacterium is subsequently captured by the BCR on a B-cell, there is now an opportunity for CR2 within the BCR coreceptor complex to bind C3d, which effectively means that the B-cell now receives two signals simultaneously. Signal one comes via the BCR and signal two via the coreceptor complex. So how does simultaneous engagement of

the coreceptor complex and the BCR lead to enhanced B-cell activation?

Well, the answer is that we don't know for sure, but it is clear that CD19 plays an especially important role in this process. **CD19** is a B-cell-specific transmembrane protein that is expressed from the pro-B-cell to the plasma-cell stage and possesses a relatively long cytoplasmic tail containing nine tyrosine residues. Upon B-cell receptor stimulation, the cytoplasmic tail of CD19 undergoes phosphorylation at several of these tyrosine residues (by kinases associated with the BCR) that creates binding sites on CD19 for several proteins, including the tyrosine kinase Lyn, Vav and phosphatidylinositol 3-kinase (PI3K). CD19 plays a role as a platform for recruitment of several proteins to the BCR complex (Figure 8.18), much in the same way that LAT functions in T-cell receptor activation.

Vav is recruited to CD19 upon phosphorylation of the latter by Lyn and, along with PI3K that is also recruited to CD19 as a result of Lyn-mediated phosphorylation (Figure 8.18), plays a role in the activation of the serine/threonine kinase **Akt**; the latter may also enhance NFAT activation through neutralizing the inhibitory effects of **GSK3 (glycogen synthase kinase 3)** on NFAT Because GSK3 can also phosphorylate and destabilize Myc and cyclin D, which are essential for cell cycle entry, Akt activation also has positive effects on proliferation of activated B-cells.

Similar to the role that CD28 plays on T-cells, the B-cell coreceptor amplifies signals transmitted through the BCR approximately 100-fold. As we have discussed above, because CD19 and CR2 (CD21) molecules enjoy mutual association, this can be brought about by bridging the Ig and CR2 receptors on the B-cell surface by antigen–C3d complexes bound to the surface of APCs. Thus, antigen-induced clustering of the B-cell coreceptor complex with the BCR lowers the threshold for B-cell activation by bringing kinases that are associated with the BCR into close proximity with the coreceptor complex. The action of these kinases on the coreceptor complex engages signaling pathways that reinforce signals originating from the BCR.

B-cells also require co-stimulation from T-helper cells

Just as T-cells require co-stimulatory signals from DCs in the form of B7 ligands for productive activation (Figure 8.3), T-dependent B-cells also require co-stimulation from T-helper cells in order to cross the threshold required for clonal expansion and differentiation to effector cells (Figure 8.15). The sequence of events goes much like this. Upon encountering cognate antigen through direct binding to a microorganism, the BCR undergoes the initial activation events described above. This culminates in the internalization of the BCR, along with captured antigen, which is then processed and presented on MHC class II molecules (Figure 8.20). To continue the process of maturation to either a plasma cell or a memory cell,

Figure 8.20. CD40–CD40L-dependent B-cell co-stimulation by a T-helper cell.

Independently activated T- and B-cells can interact if the B-cell is presenting the correct peptide–MHC complex sufficient for stimulation of the T-cell. Successful antigen presentation by a B-cell to an activated T-helper cell results in CD40L-dependent co-stimulation of the B-cell as well as the provision of cytokines, such as IL-4, by the T-cell that are essential for class switching, clonal expansion and differentiation to effector cells.

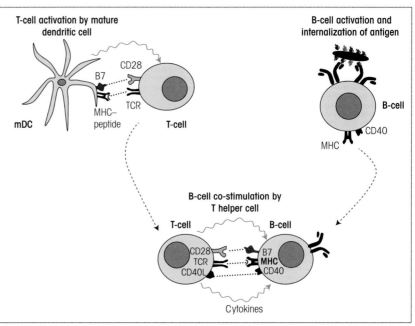

the B-cell must now encounter a T-cell capable of recognizing one of the antigenic peptides the B-cell is now presenting from the antigen it has internalized. Note that this need not be the same epitope recognized by the B-cell to undergo initial activation. Upon encountering a T-cell with the appropriate TCR, the B-cell provides stimulation to the T-cell in the form of MHC–peptide as well as co-stimulatory B7 signals (Figure 8.20). In turn, the T-cell upregulates CD40 ligand (CD40L) that can provide essential co-stimulation to the B-cell, enabling the latter to become fully activated and undergo clonal expansion and class switching. If CD40L help is not forthcoming, B-cells rapidly undergo apoptosis and are eliminated. Thus, B-cells and T-cells provide mutual co-stimulation as a means of reinforcing their initial activation signals (Figure 8.20).

In effect, the B-lymphocyte is acting as an antigen-presenting cell and, as mentioned above, it is very efficient because of its ability to concentrate the antigen by focusing onto its surface Ig. Nonetheless, although a preactivated T-helper can mutually interact with and stimulate a resting B-cell, a *resting* T-cell can only be triggered by a B-cell that has acquired the B7 co-stimulator and this is only present on activated, not resting, B-cells.

Presumably the immune complexes on follicular dendritic cells in germinal centers of secondary follicles can be taken up by the B-cells for presentation to T-helpers, but, additionally, the complexes could cross-link the sIg of the B-cell blasts and drive their proliferation in a T-independent manner. This would be enhanced by the presence of C3 in the complexes as the B-cell complement receptor (CR2) is comitogenic.

Damping down B-cell activation

We have already discussed how T-cell enthusiasm for antigen can be dissipated by engaging CTLA-4; similar mechanisms

also operate to damp down signals routed through the BCR. Several cell surface receptors, including FcγRIIB, CD22 and PIRB (paired immunoglobulin-like receptor B), have been implicated in antagonizing B-cell activation through recruitment of the protein tyrosine phosphatase SHP-1 to **ITIMs (immunoreceptor tyrosine-based *i*nhibitory *m*otifs)** in their cytoplasmic tails. SHP-1 impairs BCR signaling by antagonizing the effects of the Lyn kinase on Syk and Btk; by dephosphorylating both of these proteins SHP-1 blocks recruitment of PLCγ2 to the BCR complex. Coligation of the BCR with any of these receptors is therefore likely to block B-cell activation. CD22 appears to be constitutively associated with the BCR in resting B-cells and in this way may raise the threshold for B-cell activation. Successful formation of a B-cell receptor synapse may physically exclude CD22 from the BCR complex.

Dynamic interactions at the BCR synapse

Just as TCRs form immunological synapses during contact with specific peptide–MHC, B-cell receptors have also been found to exhibit similar behavior, particularly when antigen is presented on a membrane surface. While B-cells can be stimulated by soluble antigen, it is now widely accepted that **the primary form of antigen that triggers B-cell activation *in vivo* is localized to membrane surfaces**. The most likely culprits here are the follicular dendritic cells that are resident within lymph nodes, as well as macrophages and DCs that migrate there bearing gifts of antigen. Antigens can be immobilized on cell surfaces by complement or Fc receptors as immunocomplexes, or through direct binding to various scavenger receptors. An encounter between a B-cell and membrane-associated antigen provides the opportunity for the B-cell

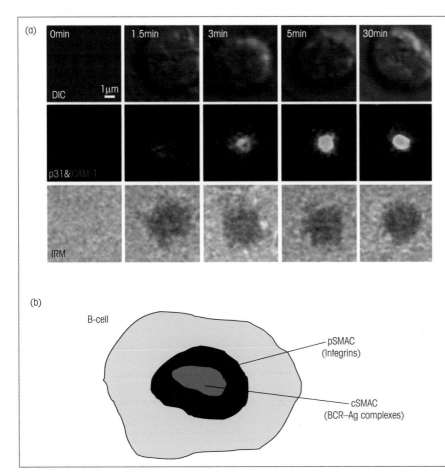

Figure 8.21. The B-cell receptor (BCR) immunological synapse.

(a) Imaging of the BCR immunological synapse. Real-time quantification of antigen and ICAM-1 recruitment to the B-cell synapse. naive B-cells were settled onto planar lipid bilayers containing glycosylphosphatidylinositol (GPI)-linked ICAM-1 (red) and p31 antigen (green). Central panels show the accumulation of the antigen p31 (green) and ICAM-1 (red) in the pattern of a mature synapse at the specified time points. Top and bottom panels show differential interference contrast and interference reflection microscopy images of the same time points. (Reproduced with permission from Carrasco Y.R., Fleire S.J., Cameron T., Dustin M.L. & Batista F.D. (2004) *Immunity* **20**, 589–599, © Elsevier). (b) Schematic representation of the BCR immunological synapse, depicting the central supramolecular activation complex (cSMAC) that is enriched in BCR–Ag microclusters, and the surrounding peripheral supramolecular activation complex (pSMAC) that is enriched in integrins such as LFA-1/ICAM-1.

membrane to spread along the opposing membrane, gathering sufficient antigen to trigger B-cell activation, as well as providing an opportunity for other contacts to be made such as those that can be provided by membrane integrins. This spreading response is driven by BCR engagement of antigen at the leading edge of the B-cell and, apart from increasing the number of BCR-antigen contacts that are then available to trigger B-cell activation, the spreading response **also increases the amount of antigen that is ultimately concentrated and internalized by the B-cell**; leading to more efficient antigen presentation to activated T-cells when the B-cell subsequently goes looking for T-cell help (Figure 8.20).

Cell spreading in response to engagement of the BCR with specific antigen is triggered in response to signals propagated via the BCR, with Lyn and Syk playing especially important roles in this process. Clearly, spreading along an antigen-bearing surface requires extensive reorganization of the cytoskeleton. Although this is not fully understood at present, activation of Vav, which as discussed earlier is involved in the regulation of the cytoskeleton via Rac and Rho, is essential here.

There is evidence that BCRs within resting B-cells are not scattered randomly within the plasma membrane but are confined to certain zones, with free diffusion restricted by contacts with the underlying actin-based cytoskeleton. In line with this,

disruption of the actin network in B-cells has been shown to lead to spontaneous BCR-dependent calcium signaling, possibly due to the spontaneous formation of **BCR microclusters**. Thus, the cytoskeleton appears to play an important role in restricting the surface distribution and behavior of BCRs in a resting B-cell. Binding of multivalent antigen to the BCR can disrupt the arrangement of BCRs in the resting B-cell resulting in the formation of BCR microclusters containing 50–500 BCRs, the formation of that also depends on an intact cytoskeleton. Indeed, the actin network within activated B-cells has been found to encircle or corral BCR microclusters within the plasma membrane.

Spreading of the B-cell across the antigen-bearing surface increases the number of BCR microclusters and eventually engages sufficient numbers of BCRs to permit crossing of the threshold for B-cell activation. Similar to T-cells, mature B-cells also express high levels of the LFA-1 and VLA-4 integrins. Interaction of these adhesion molecules with their cognate ligands, ICAM-1 and VCAM-1/fibronectin, on the cell that is displaying the immobilized antigen also promote B-cell adhesion and facilitate cell spreading along the target surface. Following spreading across an antigen-bearing surface, B-cells undergo a prolonged contraction phase that culminates in a major rearrangement of the BCR microclusters within the membrane that coalesce to form an immunological synapse, similar to that seen with T-cells (Figure 8.21). The mature BCR immunological synapse contains a central ring (cSMAC) enriched in BCR-antigen complexes, with an outer ring (pSMAC) enriched in integrins (Figure 8.21). No only do the integrin contacts promote spreading and adhesion between the interacting cell pairs, but recent evidence also suggests that such contacts lower the threshold for B-cell activation by lowering the concentration of antigen required to form a stable synapse and trigger the B-cell.

Immunocompetent T- and B-cells differ in many respects
- The antigen-specific receptors, TCR/CD3 on T-cells and surface Ig on B-cells, provide a clear distinction between these two cell types.
- T- and B-cells differ in their receptors for C3d, IgG and certain viruses.
- There are distinct polyclonal activators of T-cells (PHA, anti-CD3) and of B-cells (anti-Ig, Epstein–Barr virus).

T-lymphocytes and antigen-presenting cells interact through pairs of accessory molecules
- The docking of T-cells and APCs depends upon strong mutual interactions between complementary molecular pairs on their surfaces: MHC II–CD4, MHC I–CD8, VCAM-1–VLA-4, ICAM-1–LFA-1, LFA-3–CD2, B7–CD28 (and CTLA-4).
- B7–CTLA-4 interactions are inhibitory, whereas B7–CD28 interactions are stimulatory. CTLA-4 may antagonize the recruitment of the TCR to lipid rafts where many membrane-associated signaling proteins reside.

Activation of T-cells requires two signals
- Two signals activate T-cells, but one alone produces unresponsiveness (anergy) or death via apoptosis.
- Signal 1 is provided by the low affinity cognate TCR–MHC plus peptide interaction.
- The second co-stimulatory signal (signal 2) is mediated through ligation of CD28 by B7 (CD80/CD86) and greatly amplifies signals generated through TCR–MHC interactions.
- Previously stimulated T-cells require only one signal, through their TCRs, for efficient activation.

T-cell receptor activation
- The TCR does not possess any intrinsic enzymatic activity but is associated with accessory proteins (the CD3 coreceptor complex) that can recruit protein tyrosine kinases (PTKs).
- The TCR signal is transduced and amplified through a protein tyrosine kinase enzymic cascade.
- Recruitment of CD4 or CD8 to the TCR complex leads to phosphorylation of ITAM sequences on CD3-associated ζ chains by the CD4-associated Lck PTK. The phosphorylated ITAMs bind and then activate the ZAP-70 kinase.

Downstream events following TCR signaling
- Nonenzymic adaptor proteins form multimeric complexes with kinases and guanine nucleotide exchange factors (GEFs).
- Hydrolysis of phosphatidylinositol diphosphate by phospholipase Cγ1 or Cγ2 produces inositol triphosphate (IP$_3$) and diacylglycerol (DAG).
- IP$_3$ mobilizes intracellular calcium.
- DAG and increased calcium activate protein kinase C.
- The raised calcium together with calmodulin also stimulates calcineurin activity.
- Activation of Ras by the guanine nucleotide exchange factor Sos sets off a kinase cascade operating through Raf, the MAP kinase kinase MEK and the MAP kinase ERK. CD28 through PI3 kinase can also influence MAP kinase.
- The transcription factors Fos and Jun, NFAT and NFκB are activated by MAP kinase, calcineurin and PKC, respectively, and bind to regulatory sites in the IL-2 promoter region.
- A small number of MHC–peptide complexes can serially trigger a much larger number of TCRs thereby providing the sustained signal required for activation.
- Initial binding of integrins facilitates the formation of an immunological synapse, the core of that exchanges integrins for TCR interacting with MHC–peptide.
- Cbl family adaptor molecules are involved in negative signaling pathways.
- The phosphatase domains on CD45 are required to remove phosphates at inhibitory sites on kinases.

B-cells respond to three different types of antigen
- Type 1 thymus-independent antigens are polyclonal activators focused onto the specific B-cells by sIg receptors.
- Type 2 thymus-independent antigens are polymeric molecules that cross-link many sIg receptors and,

because of their long half-lives, provide a persistent signal to the B-cell.

■ Thymus-dependent antigens require the cooperation of helper T-cells to stimulate antibody production by B-cells.

■ Antigen captured by specific sIg receptors is taken into the B-cell, processed and expressed on the surface as a peptide in association with MHC II.

■ This complex is recognized by the T-helper cell that activates the resting B-cell.

■ The ability of protein carriers to enable the antibody response to haptens is explained by T-cell–B-cell collaboration, with T-cells recognizing the carrier and B-cells the hapten.

The nature of B-cell activation

■ Cross-linking of surface Ig receptors (e.g. by type 2 thymus-independent antigens) activates B-cells.

■ T-helper cells activate resting B-cells through TCR recognition of MHC II–carrier peptide complexes and co-stimulation through CD40L–CD40 interactions (analogous to the B7–CD28 second signal for T-cell activation).

■ B-cell co-stimulation is also provided by the B-cell coreceptor complex consisting of CD19, CD21, CD81 and LEU13.

■ B-cell receptors (BCRs) also form immunological synapses composed of numerous BCR microclusters and integrins.

FURTHER READING

Abraham R.T. & Weiss A. (2004) Jurkat T-cells and development of the T-cell receptor signaling paradigm. *Nature Reviews Immunology* **4**, 301–308.

Acuto O. & Michel F. (2003) CD28-mediated costimulation: a quantitative support for TCR signaling. *Nature Reviews Immunology* **3**, 939–951.

Batista F.D. & Harwood N.E. (2009) The who, how and where of antigen presentation to B cells. *Nature Reviews Immunology* **9**, 15–27.

Buday L. & Downward J. (2008) Many faces of Ras activation. *Biochim Biophys Acta.* **1786**, 178–187.

Bromley S.K. *et al.* (2001) The immunological synapse. *Annual Review of Immunology* **19**, 375–396.

Fooksman D.R. *et al.* (2010) Functional anatomy of T cell activation and synapse formation. *Annual Review of Immunology* **28**, 1–27.

Grakoui A. *et al.* (1999) The immunological synapse: a molecular machine controlling T-cell activation. *Science* **285**, 221–227.

Harwood N.E. & Batista F.D. (2010) Early events in B cell activation. *Annual Review of Immunology* **28**, 185–210.

Huang F. & Gu H. (2008) Negative regulation of lymphocyte development and function by the Cbl family of proteins. *Immunological Reviews* **224**, 229–238.

Jenkins M.K. *et al.* (2001) *In vivo* activation of antigen-specific CD4 T-cells. *Annual Review of Immunology* **19**, 23–45.

Kinashi T. (2005) Intracellular signaling controlling integrin activation in lymphocytes. *Nature Reviews Immunology* **5**, 546–559.

Kurosaki T. (2002) Regulation of B-cell signal transduction by adaptor proteins. *Nature Reviews Immunology* **2**, 354–363.

Mueller D.L. (2010) Mechanisms maintaining peripheral tolerance. *Nature Immunology* **11**, 21–27.

Niiro H. & Clark E.A. (2002) Regulation of B-cell fate by antigen-receptor signals. *Nature Reviews Immunology* **2**, 945–956.

Rudd C.E., Taylor A. & Schneider H. (2009) CD28 and CTLA-4 coreceptor expression and signal transduction. *Immunological Reviews* **229**, 12–26.

Smith-Garvin J.E., Koretzky G.A. & Jordan M.S. (2009) T cell activation. *Annual Review of Immunology* **27**, 591–619.

Yokosuka T. & Saito T. (2009) Dynamic regulation of T-cell costimulation through TCR–CD28 microclusters. *Immunological Reviews* **229**, 27–40.

 Now visit **www.roitt.com**
to test yourself on this chapter.

CHAPTER 9

The production of effectors

Key Topics

Just to Recap ...

The reader will be familiar with the central role of mature dendritic cells (DCs) as sources of MHC–peptide (signal 1) and co-stimulatory ligands (signal 2) for productive activation of naive T-cells; the absence of signal 2 leads to unresponsiveness or anergy. B-cells can also present antigen and co-stimulate a previously activated T-cell, for the purposes of receiving T-cell help for clonal expansion and differentiation to an effector B-cell, but DCs are typically the primary antigen-presenting cells (APCs) for activation of naive T-cells. Macrophages can also act as APCs but, due to their relatively nonmigratory behavior, have a greater role in restimulating previously activated T-cells at sites of infection rather than priming naive T-cells within secondary lymphoid tissues. The goal of antigen-driven lymphocyte activation

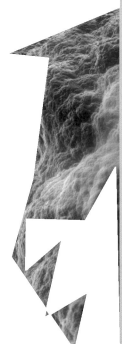

Roitt's Essential Immunology, Twelfth Edition. Peter J. Delves, Seamus J. Martin, Dennis R. Burton, Ivan M. Roitt.
© 2011 Peter J. Delves, Seamus J. Martin, Dennis R. Burton, Ivan M. Roitt. Published 2011 by Blackwell Publishing Ltd.

Just to Recap ... (*Continued*)

is to trigger clonal expansion of the correct cells so that these cells can set to work mounting an adaptive immune response. The adaptive immune response works in tandem with an ongoing innate immune response and, as we shall see, **amplifies and reinforces the innate immune response through the provision of cytokines, antibodies, and cytotoxic molecules.** Activated T-cells differentiate into **effector cells** capable of secreting diverse patterns of cytokines; similarly, activated B-cells differentiate into plasma cells capable of secreting different antibody classes. Cells of the innate immune system in general, and DCs in particular, play a key role in shaping the particular flavor of adaptive immune response that is mounted in response to antigenic stimulation. This is achieved through the secretion of different patterns of cytokines in response to the initial infection. These cytokines, in turn, influence the nature of the T- and B-cell effectors that are produced.

Introduction

Having crossed the threshold required for activation, a T-cell enters the cell division cycle and undergoes clonal proliferation and differentiation to effectors. A succession of genes is upregulated upon T-cell activation. Within the first 30 minutes, nuclear transcription factors such as Fos/Jun and NFAT, which regulate interleukin-2 (IL-2) expression and the cellular proto-oncogene c-*myc*, are expressed, but the next few hours see the synthesis of a range of cytokines and their specific receptors. Much later we see molecules like the transferrin receptor related to cell division and very late antigens such as the adhesion molecule VLA-1 that enables activated T-cells to bind to vascular endothelium at sites of infection. Collectively, these events equip activated T-cells with new functional properties, which include the ability to activate macrophages, provision of cytokine-mediated help for antibody production by B-cells, and the ability to eliminate virally infected targets by inducing apoptosis in such cells.

Activated B-cells also enter the cell cycle and undergo clonal proliferation to swell their ranks. Some of the activated B-cells eventually differentiate into plasma cells that migrate to the bone marrow where they produce and secrete large amounts of antibody for relatively long periods. Here we will consider the main issues surrounding the acquisition of effector function by T- and B-lymphocytes and the roles that effector lymphocytes play in the immune response.

Effector mechanisms

The innate immune system utilizes a number of different effector mechanisms to combat infection

In Chapter 1 we learned that **the innate immune system uses a variety of strategies** to deal with microorganisms that have successfully breached the physical barriers of the skin and mucosal surfaces. The first line of defense involves the cells and soluble factors of the innate immune system that take immediate action upon detection of nonself in the form of pathogen-associated molecular patterns (PAMPs). The steps taken by the innate immune system in dealing with a nascent infection range from direct binding of soluble pattern recognition molecules—such as complement, lysozyme and mannose-binding lectin—to orchestrate immediate destruction of a pathogen, or to enhance phagocytic uptake by macrophages and neutrophils. Macrophages and neutrophils also directly recognize and engulf pathogens via their cell associated pattern recognition receptors. Other options at the disposal of the innate immune system involve the deployment of mast cells and basophils, both of which use their granule enzymes to combat large extracellular parasites. Let us also not forget natural killer (NK) cells that are adept at killing host cells

displaying signs of viral infection or other evidence of trouble within. We also discussed the role of dendritic cells as sentinels of the innate immune system, serving to alert T-cells to an ongoing infection by presenting antigen within the context of appropriate co-stimulatory signals (i.e. ligands of the B7 family). All told, there are a number of highly effective weapons in the arsenal of the innate immune system that can be called into play for the purposes of defending the body against infection. Nonetheless, the innate immune system frequently requires assistance to deal with well adapted pathogens that deploy a range of immune evasion strategies to frustrate all of the above efforts. The cavalry comes in the form of the adaptive immune response.

Adaptive immunity also employs a range of effector mechanisms

The adaptive immune system, made up of T- and B-lymphocytes, also has a number of weapons at its disposal. In Chapter 2 we discussed the role of B-cell-derived antibodies as a means of coating microorganisms for the purposes of enhancing complement-mediated lysis via the classical pathway, or enhancing their uptake by phagocytosis via specific Fc receptors on macrophages and neutrophils, or indeed by simply aggregating infectious agents and impeding their further incursion into tissues. Antibodies can also be used to the advantage of NK cells to focus their cytotoxic actions via antibody-dependent cellular cytotoxicity (ADCC) (see p. 48). T-cells also employ a number of different strategies to defend the body from infectious agents (Figure 9.1). Recall that T-cells can be grouped into two major subdivisions: helper (Th) and cytotoxic (Tc or CTL) T-cells, that are selected to recognize antigen presented in the context of MHC class II or MHC class I molecules, respectively. Whereas T-helper cells function to help B-cells make antibodies or to activate the killing function of macrophages or NK cells, Tc cells are endowed with the ability to engage and kill virally infected cells. As we shall discuss in more detail in this chapter, **T-helper cells can be further subdivided into Th1, Th2 and Th17 cells on the basis of the cytokine profiles that these cells secrete**, as this confers different effector functions on such cells. We shall also discuss other subdivisions of T-cells (**regulatory T-cells [Tregs]**), that also differ in the cytokine profile produced, as these cells serve important regulatory functions and help to safeguard the body against inappropriate T-cell responses that are directed against self, as well as excessive or inappropriate responses directed towards nonself.

Cytokines heavily influence the generation as well as the specific function of effectors within the adaptive immune system

The production of various cytokines is central to both the maturation as well as the specific effector functions of B- and T-cells. We have already referred to the diverse roles of cytokines throughout the previous chapters and have alluded to their properties as messenger molecules that enable the disparate elements of the immune system to communicate with each other. Communication between cells of the immune system underpins the amplification of immune responses (Figure 9.1), and is also instrumental in marshalling the appropriate response (i.e. whether predominantly antibody mediated or cell mediated) depending on the nature of the infectious agent as well as its route of entry into the body. Here, we will go into more detail concerning the different categories of cytokines, how these molecules act upon their target cells, and the spectrum of responses they initiate. All of these issues are central to how the effector cells of the adaptive immune system are generated and the nature of the responses they engage in. Whereas many of the elements of the innate immune system are poised to strike with little delay upon detection of a PAMP, **the actions of T- and B-lymphocytes are heavily influenced by the cytokine environment accompanying their initial exposure to specific antigen**.

Dendritic cells and other cells of the innate immune system play a central role in the generation of effectors

As we shall discuss later in this chapter, a major influence on the type of effector cells generated in response to a pathogenic

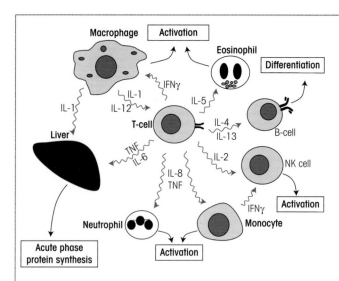

Figure 9.1. T-cells can regulate diverse elements of the immune system through the production of different cytokines.

This illustrates some, but by no means all, of the interactions that activated T-cells can have with other elements of the immune system through the directed secretion of specific cytokines. Note that not all T-cells are capable of secreting all of the cytokines indicated. Rather, specific T-cell subsets are generated that are skewed towards secretion of particular subsets of the cytokines shown.

challenge is wielded by dendritic cells that—in addition to presenting antigen (signal 1) and providing co-stimulatory signals (signal 2) to T-cells—also exert significant control over the type of T-cell response that is generated. Dendritic cells achieve this by providing additional input in the form of cytokines (signal 3) that shape the nature of the effector T-cells that are thus generated (Figure 9.2). The particular cocktail of cytokines elaborated by DCs during the initial round of T-cell stimulation in a lymph node influences whether the response will be dominated by the generation of T-cell effectors that provide help for B-cells (Th2), or alternatively, result in the generation of T-cells that activate macrophages and assist CTL function (Th1 cells). The generation of other Th subsets, characterized by particular patterns of cytokines, has also been recognized. The pattern of cytokines secreted by differentiated effector T-cells can be further influenced by local macrophages, NK cells, basophils and other cells of the innate immune system encountered by activated T-cells that migrate to sites of infection. Once again, this is through the provision of cytokines that trigger or reinforce the development of different T-cell effector subsets. This inevitably raises the question of what influences DCs to make one pattern of cytokines over another. The answer to this neatly brings us full circle, as it is the nature of the PAMPs that propel DCs into action in the first place, as well as cytokines elaborated by the other cells of the innate immune system upon encountering an infectious agent, that influence the cytokine profile adopted by an activated DC.

Before we discuss the various T- and B-lymphocyte effector cell types, let us first take a closer look at the diversity of the cytokine family and how these important cell-cell communication molecules exert their effects at a molecular level.

Cytokines act as intercellular messengers

Cytokines are structurally diverse polypeptides that function as messenger molecules that can communicate signals from one cell type to another and, amongst other things, can instruct the cell receiving the signal to proliferate, differentiate, secrete additional cytokines, migrate or die. To date, many different cytokines have been described and no doubt some remain to be discovered (Table 9.1). One of the most important cytokine groupings, to the immunologist's way of thinking, is the interleukin family as this contains cytokines that act as communicators between leukocytes. Members of the interleukin family are very diverse, belonging to different protein structural classes (Figure 9.3), because the primary qualification for membership of this family is biological (i.e. evidence of activity on leukocytes) rather than sequence or structural homology. Indeed, while additional homologs of the interleukin family are known, their status as interleukins awaits evidence that these proteins exert functional effects upon leukocytes. Approximately 34 interleukins have been described to date (IL-1 to IL-35) with the status of IL-14 as an interleukin in doubt.

Other cytokine families have been established on the basis of their ability to support proliferation of hematopoietic precursors (colony stimulating factors), or cytotoxic activity towards transformed cell types (tumor necrosis factors), or the ability to interfere with viral replication (interferons). It is

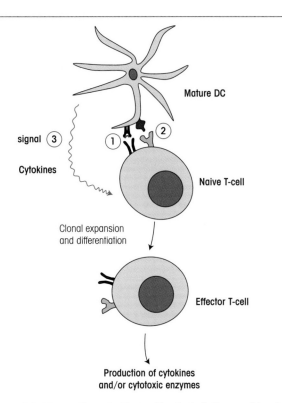

Figure 9.2. Generation of effector T-cells is influenced by the cytokine environment experienced by the T-cell at the point of initial activation.

MHC–peptide recognition by the TCR represents signal 1, co-stimulation of CD28 by B7 ligands represents signal 2, and cytokines produced by the DC represents signal 3. Note that the cytokine environment upon restimulation of a T-cell within an infected tissue will also influence the nature of the effector response made by the T-cell.

Table 9.1. Cytokines: their origin and function. APP, acute phase proteins; B, B-cell; baso, basophil; BM, bone marrow; Endo, endothelium; eosino, eosinophil; Epith, epithelium; Fibro, fibroblast; GM-CSF, granulocyte–macrophage colony-stimulating factor; IL, interleukin; LIF, leukemia inhibitory factor; Mφ, macrophage; MC, mast cell; Mono, monocyte; neutro, neutrophil; NK, natural killer; SLF, steel locus factor; T, T-cell; TGFβ, transforming growth factor-β. Note that there is not an interleukin-14. This designation was given to an activity that, upon further investigation, could not be unambiguously assigned to a single cytokine. IL-30 also awaits assignment. IL-8 is a member of the chemokine family. These cytokines are listed separately in Table 9.2.

Cytokine	Source	Effector function
Interleukins		
IL-1α, IL-1β	Mono, Mφ, DC, NK, B, Endo	Co-stimulates T activation by enhancing production of cytokines including IL-2 and its receptor; enhances B proliferation and maturation; NK cytotoxicity; induces IL-1,-6,-8, TNF, GM-CSF and PGE$_2$ by Mφ; proinflammatory by inducing chemokines and ICAM-1 and VCAM-1 on endothelium; induces fever, APP, bone resorption by osteoclasts
IL-2	Th1	Induces proliferation of activated T- and B-cells; enhances NK cytotoxicity and killing of tumor cells and bacteria by monocytes and Mφ
IL-3	T, NK, MC	Growth and differentiation of hematopoietic precursors; MC growth

Table 9.1. *Continued*

Cytokine	Source	Effector function
IL-4	Th2, Tc2, NK, NKT, γδ T, MC	Induces Th2 cells; stimulates proliferation of activated B, T, MC; upregulates MHC class II on B and Mφ, and CD23 on B; downregulates IL-12 production and thereby inhibits Th1 differentiation; increases Mφ phagocytosis; induces switch to IgG1 and IgE
IL-5	Th2, MC	Induces proliferation of eosinophils and activated B; induces switch to IgA
IL-6	Th2, Mono, Mφ, DC, BM stroma	Differentiation of myeloid stem cells and of B into plasma cells; induces APP; enhances T proliferation
IL-7	BM and thymic stroma	Induces differentiation of lymphoid stem cells into progenitor T and B; activates mature T
IL-8	Mono, Mφ, Endo	Mediates chemotaxis and activation of neutrophils
IL-9	Th	Induces proliferation of thymocytes; enhances MC growth; synergizes with IL-4 in switch to IgG1 and IgE
IL-10	Th (Th2 in mouse), Tc, B, Mono, Mφ	Inhibits IFNγ secretion by mouse, and IL-2 by human, Th1 cells; downregulates MHC class II and cytokine (including IL-12) production by mono, Mφ and DC, thereby inhibiting Th1 differentiation; inhibits T proliferation; enhances B differentiation
IL-11	BM stroma	Promotes differentiation of pro-B and megakaryocytes; induces APP
IL-12	Mono, Mφ, DC, B	Critical cytokine for Th1 differentiation; induces proliferation and IFNγ production by Th1, CD8+ and γδ T and NK; enhances NK and CD8+ T cytotoxicity
IL-13	Th2, MC	Inhibits activation and cytokine secretion by Mφ; co-activates B proliferation; upregulates MHC class II and CD23 on B and mono; induces switch to IgG1 and IgE; induces VCAM-1 on endo
IL-15	T, NK, Mono, Mφ, DC, B	Induces proliferation of T-, NK and activated B and cytokine production and cytotoxicity in NK and CD8+ T-cell; chemotactic for T-cell; stimulates growth of intestinal epithelium
IL-16	Th, Tc	Chemoattractant for CD4 T, mono and eosino; induces MHC class II
IL-17	T	Proinflammatory; stimulates production of cytokines including TNF,IL-1β,-6,-8, G-CSF
IL-17A	Th17, T-cells NK, Neutrophils	Proinflammstory, stimulates production of cytokines including TNF, IL-1β, IL-6, -8, G-CSF by epithelia, endothelia and fibroblasts.
IL-17F	Th17, T-cells NK, Neutrophils	Similar effects to IL-17A
IL-18	Mφ, DC	Induces IFNγ production by T; enhances NK cytotoxicity
IL-19	Mono	Modulation of Th1 activity
IL-20	Mono, Keratinocytes	Regulation of inflammatory responses to skin
IL-21	Th	Regulation of hematopoiesis; NK differentiation; B activation; T co-stimulation
IL-22	T	Inhibits IL-4 production by Th2
IL-23	DC	Proliferation and IFNγ production by Th1, induces expansion and survival of TH17 cells. induction of proinflammatory cytokines such as IL-1, IL-6, TNF by macrophages.
IL-24	Th2, Mono, Mφ	Induction of TNF, IL-1, IL-6, anti-tumor activity
IL-25	Th1, Mφ, Mast	Induction of IL-4, IL-5, IL-13 and Th2-associated pathologies
IL-26	T, NK	Enhanced production of IL-8 and IL-10 by epithelium

Table 9.1. *Continued*

Cytokine	Source	Effector function
IL-27	DC, Mono	Induction of TH1 responses, enhanced IFN-γ production
IL-28	Mono, DC	Type 1 IFN-like activity, inhibition of viral replication
IL-29	Mono, DC	Type 1 IFN-like activity, inhibition of viral replication
IL-30	APCs	P28 subunit of IL-27 heterodimer. Regulates 1L-12 responsiveness of naive T-cells. Synergizes with IL-12 to induce IFN-γ.
IL-31	T	Promotes inflammatory responses in skin
IL-32	NK, T	Promotes inflammation. Role in activation-induced T-cell apoptosis.
IL-33	Stroma, DC	Induction of Th2 cytokines, mediates chemotaxis of basophils and mast cells
IL-34	Stroma	Stimulates monocyte proliferation and formation of macrophage progenitors.
IL-35	Tregs	Immunosuppressive effects on Th1, Th2 and Th17 cells. Stimulates proliferation of Tregs.
Colony stimulating factors		
GM-CSF	Th, Mφ, Fibro, MC, Endo	Stimulates growth of progenitors of mono-, neutro-, eosino- and basophils; activates Mφ
G-CSF	Fibro, Endo	Stimulates growth of neutro progenitors
M-CSF	Fibro, Endo, Epith	Stimulates growth of mono progenitors
SLF	BM stroma	Stimulates stem cell division (*c-kit* ligand)
Tumor necrosis factors		
TNF (TNFα)	Th, Mono, Mφ, DC, MC, NK, B	Tumor cytotoxicity; cachexia (weight loss); induces cytokine secretion; induces E-selectin on endo; activates Mφ; antiviral
Lymphotoxin (TNFβ)	Th1, Tc	Tumor cytotoxicity; enhances phagocytosis by neutro and Mφ; involved in lymphoid organ development; antiviral
Interferons		
IFNα	Leukocytes	Inhibits viral replication; enhances MHC class II
IFNβ	Fibroblasts	Inhibits viral replication; enhances MHC class II
IFNγ	Th1, Tc1, NK	Inhibits viral replication; enhances MHC class I and II; activates Mφ; induces switch to IgG2a; antagonizes several IL-4 actions; inhibits proliferation of Th2
Others		
TGFβ	Th3, B, Mφ, MC	Proinflammatory by, e.g. chemoattraction of mono and Mφ but also anti-inflammatory by, e.g. inhibiting lymphocyte proliferation; induces switch to IgA; promotes tissue repair
LIF	Thymic epith, BM stroma	Induces APP
Eta-1	T	Stimulates IL-12 production and inhibits IL-10 production by Mφ
Oncostatin M	T, Mφ	Induces APP

important to note, however, that cytokines frequently have pleiotrophic effects, doing much more than their somewhat descriptive (and often misleading) names would suggest. Indeed, the response that many of these molecules elicit depends, to a large extent, on the context in which the cytokine signal is delivered. Thus, factors such as the differentiation stage of the cell, its position within the cell cycle (whether quiescent or proliferating) and the presence of other cytokines, can all influence the response made to a particular cytokine.

Cytokine action is transient and usually short range

Cytokines are typically low-molecular-weight (15–25 kDa) secreted proteins that mediate cell division, inflammation, cytotoxicity, differentiation, migration and repair. Because they regulate the amplitude and duration of the immune–inflammatory responses, cytokines must be produced in a transient manner tightly coupled to the presence of foreign

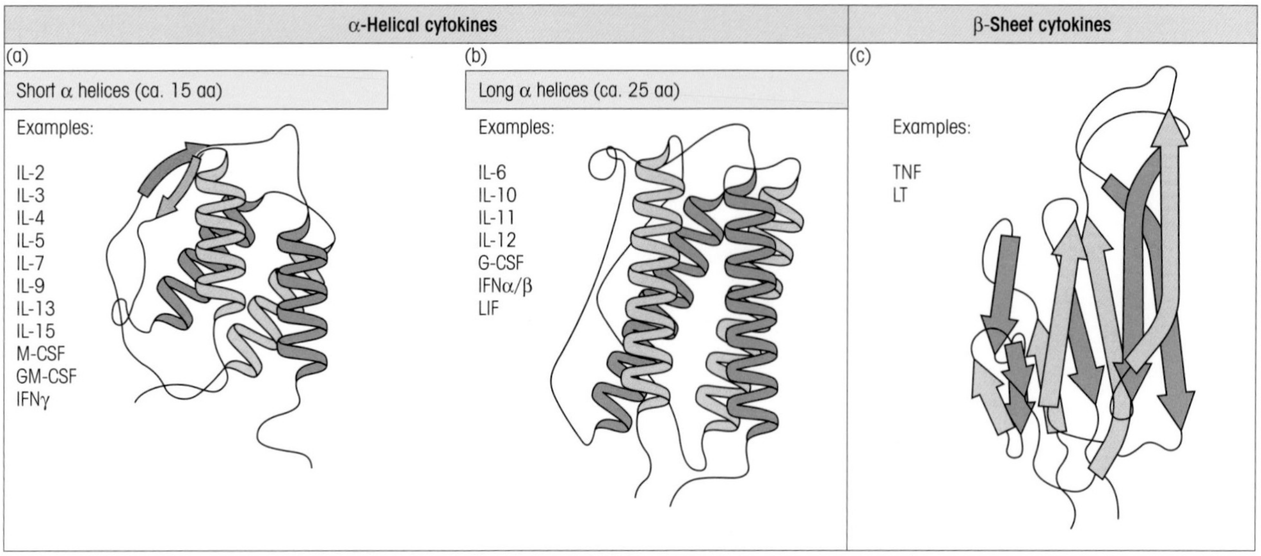

α-Helical cytokines		β-Sheet cytokines

(a)

Short α helices (ca. 15 aa)

Examples:

IL-2
IL-3
IL-4
IL-5
IL-7
IL-9
IL-13
IL-15
M-CSF
GM-CSF
IFNγ

(b)

Long α helices (ca. 25 aa)

Examples:

IL-6
IL-10
IL-11
IL-12
G-CSF
IFNα/β
LIF

(c)

Examples:

TNF
LT

Figure 9.3. Cytokine structures.

Cytokines can be divided into a number of different structural groups. Illustrated here are three of the main types of structure and some named examples of each type: (a) four short (~15 amino acids) α-helices, (b) four long (~25 amino acids) α-helices and (c) a β-sheet structure. (Reproduced with permission from Michal G. (ed.) (1999) *Biochemical Pathways: An Atlas of Biochemistry and Molecular Biology.* John Wiley & Sons, New York.)

material. Cytokine production can also occur in response to the release of endogenous "danger signals" (i.e. danger-associated molecular patterns [DAMPs]) that betray the presence of cells dying by necrosis, a mode of cell death that is typically seen in pathological situations and frequently provoked by infectious agents or tissue injury (see Chapter 1, p. 4). It is relevant that the AU-rich sequences in the 3′-untranslated regions of the mRNA of many cytokines prime these mRNAs for rapid degradation thereby ensuring that cytokine production rapidly declines in the absence of appropriate stimulation. Unlike endocrine hormones, the majority of cytokines normally act locally in a paracrine or even autocrine fashion. Thus cytokines derived from lymphocytes rarely persist in the circulation, but nonlymphoid cells such as endothelial cells and fibroblasts can be triggered by bacterial products to release cytokines that may be detected in the bloodstream, often to the detriment of the host. Septic shock, for example, is a life-threatening condition that largely results from massive overproduction of cytokines such as tumor necrosis factor (TNF) and IL-1 in response to bacterial infection and highlights the necessity to keep a tight rein on cytokine production. Certain cytokines, including IL-1 and TNF, also exist as membrane-anchored forms and can exert their stimulatory effects without becoming soluble.

Cytokines act through cell surface receptors

Cytokines are highly potent, often acting at femtomolar (10^{-15} M) concentrations, combining with small numbers of high affinity cell surface receptors to produce changes in the pattern of RNA and protein synthesis in the cells they act

upon. This is achieved through cytokine receptor-mediated activation of signal transduction cascades that culminate in the activation of transcription factors that direct the synthesis of new gene products, or increases the level of existing ones, within the cell. The end result is a **change in the behavior or functionality** of the cell as a result of these gene expression changes. Cytokine receptors typically possess specific protein–protein interaction domains or phosphorylation motifs within their cytoplasmic tails to facilitate recruitment of appropriate adaptor proteins upon receptor stimulation. A recurring theme in cytokine receptor activation pathways is the ligand-induced dimer- or trimerization of receptor subunits; this facilitates signal propagation into the cell through the interplay of the transiently associated receptor cytoplasmic tails. There are six major cytokine receptor structural families (Figure 9.4).

Hematopoietin receptors

These are the largest family, sometimes referred to simply as the cytokine receptor superfamily, and are named after the first member of this family to be defined—the hematopoietin receptor. These receptors generally consist of one or two polypeptide chains responsible for cytokine binding and an additional shared (common or "c") chain involved in signal transduction. The γc (CD132) chain is used by the IL-2 receptor (Figure 9.4a) and IL-4, IL-7, IL-9, IL-15 and IL-21 receptors, a βc (CDw131) chain by IL-3, IL-5 and granulocyte–macrophage colony-stimulating factor (GM-CSF) receptors, and gp130 (CD130) shared chain by the IL-6, IL-11, IL-12, oncostatin M, ciliary neurotrophic factor and leukemia inhibitory factor (LIF) receptors.

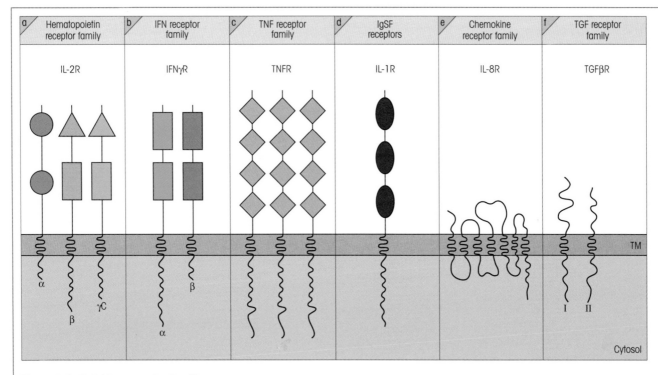

Figure 9.4. Cytokine receptor families.

One example is shown for each family. (a) The **hematopoietin receptors** operate through a common subunit (γc, βc or gp130, depending on the subfamily) that transduces the signal to the interior of the cell. In essence, binding of the cytokine to its receptor must initiate the signaling process by mediating hetero- or homodimer formation involving the common subunit. In some cases the cytokine is active when bound to the receptor either in soluble or membrane-bound form (e.g. IL-6). The IL-2 receptor is interesting with respect to its ligand binding. The α chain (CD25, reacting with the Tac monoclonal) of the receptor possesses two complement control protein structural domains and binds IL-2 with a low affinity; the β chain (CD122) has a membrane proximal fibronectin type III structural domain and a membrane distal cytokine receptor structural domain, and associates with the common γ chain (CD132) that has a similar structural organization. The β chain binds IL-2 with intermediate affinity. IL-2 binds to and dissociates from the a chain very rapidly but the same processes involving the β chain occur at two or three orders of magnitude more slowly. When the α, β and γ chains form a single receptor, the α chain binds the IL-2 rapidly and facilitates its binding to a separate site on the β chain from which it can only dissociate slowly. As the final affinity (K_d) is based on the ratio of dissociation to association rate constants, then $K_d = 10^{-4}\,\text{s}^{-1}/10^{7}\,\text{M}^{-1}\,\text{s}^{-1} = 10^{-11}\,\text{M}$, which is a very high affinity. The γ chain does not itself bind IL-2 but contributes towards signal transduction. (b) The **interferon receptor** family consists of heterodimeric molecules each of which bears two fibronectin type III domains. (c) The receptors for **TNF** and related molecules consist of a single polypeptide with four TNFR domains. The receptor trimerizes upon ligand binding and, in common with a number of other receptors, is also found in a soluble form that, when released from a cell following activation, can act as an antagonist. (d) Another group of receptors contains varying numbers of **Ig superfamily domains**, whereas (e) **chemokine receptors** are members of the G-protein-coupled receptor superfamily and have seven hydrophobic transmembrane domains. (f) The final family illustrated are the **TGF receptors** that require association between two molecules, referred to as TGFR type I and TGFR type II, for signaling to occur.

Interferon receptors

These also consist of two polypeptide chains and, in addition to the IFNα, IFNβ and IFNγ receptors (Figure 9.4b), this family includes the IL-10 receptor.

TNF receptors

Members of the TNF receptor superfamily possess cysteine-rich extracellular domains and most likely exist as preformed trimers that undergo a conformational change in their intracellular domains upon ligand binding. They include the tumor necrosis factor (TNF) receptor (Figure 9.4c) and the related Fas (CD95/APO-1) and TRAIL receptors. This family also contains the lymphotoxin (LT) and nerve growth factor (NGF) receptors, as well as the CD40 receptor, which plays an important role in co-stimulation of B-cells and dendritic cells by activated T-cells.

IgSF cytokine receptors

Immunoglobulin superfamily members are broadly utilized in many aspects of cell biology (cf. p. 309) and include the IL-1 receptor (Figure 9.4d), and the macrophage colony-stimulating factor (M-CSF) and stem cell factor (SCF/c-kit) receptors.

 ### Chemokine receptors

Chemokines (*chemo*attractant cyto*kine*) share a common functional property of promoting chemotaxis and their receptors comprise a family of approximately 20 different G-protein-coupled, seven transmembrane segment polypeptides (Figure 9.4e). Each receptor subtype is capable of binding multiple chemokines within the same family. For example, CXC receptor 2 (CXCR2) is capable of binding seven different ligands within the CXC ligand (CXCL) family.

The recruitment of T-cells, macrophages and neutrophils to an inflammatory site is greatly enhanced by the action of chemokines. These can be produced by a variety of cell types and are divided into four families based on the disposition of the first (N-terminal) two of the four canonical cysteine residues (Table 9.2). CXC chemokines have one amino acid and CX3C have three amino acids between the two cysteines. CC chemokines have adjacent cysteines at this location, whereas C chemokines lack cysteines 1 and 3 found in other chemokines. Chemokines bind to G-protein-coupled seven transmembrane receptors (Figure 9.4). Despite the fact that a single chemokine can sometimes bind to

more than one receptor, and a single receptor can bind several chemokines, many chemokines exhibit a strong tissue and receptor specificity. They play important roles in inflammation, lymphoid organ development, cell trafficking, cellular compartmentalization within lymphoid tissues, angiogenesis and wound healing.

TGF receptors

Receptors for transforming growth factors such as the TGFβ receptor (Figure 9.4f) possess cytoplasmic signaling domains with serine/threonine kinase activity.

Signal transduction through cytokine receptors

The ligand-induced homo- or heterodimerization of cytokine receptor subunits represents a common theme for signaling by cytokines. The two major routes that are utilized are the Janus kinase (JAK)–STAT and the Ras–MAP kinase pathways. We have already discussed the details of the Ras–MAP kinase pathway in Chapter 8 (see Figure 8.8) so here we will focus on the JAK–STAT pathway.

Members of the cytokine receptor superfamily (hematopoietin receptors) lack catalytic domains but are constitutively associated with one or more JAKs (Figure 9.5). There are four

Table 9.2. Chemokines and their receptors. The chemokines are grouped according to the arrangement of their cysteines (see text). The letter L designates ligand (i.e. the individual chemokine), whereas the letter R designates receptors. Names in parentheses refer to the murine homologs of the human chemokine where the names of these differ, or the murine chemokine alone if no human equivalent has been described. B, B-cell; Baso, basophil; DC, dendritic cell; Eosino, eosinophil; MEC, mucosal epithelial chemokine; Mono, monocyte; Neutro, neutrophil; NK, natural killer; T, T-cell.

Family	Chemokine	Alternative names	Chemotaxis	Receptors
CXC	CXCL1	GROα/MGSAα	Neutro	CXCR2>CXCR1
	CXCL2	GROβ/MGSAβ	Neutro	CXCR2
	CXCL3	GROγ/MGSAγ	Neutro	CXCR2
	CXCL4	PF4	Eosino,Baso, T	CXCR3-B
	CXCL5	ENA-78	Neutro	CXCR2
	CXCL6	GCP-2/(CKα-3)	Neutro	CXCR1, CXCR2
	CXCL7	NAP-2	Neutro	CXCR2
	CXCL8	IL-8	Neutro	CXCR1, CXCR2
	CXCL9	Mig	T, NK	CXCR3-A, CXCR3-B
	CXCL10	IP-10	T, NK	CXCR3-A, CXCR3-B
	CXCL11	I-TAC	T, NK	CXCR3-A, CXCR3-B
	CXCL12	SDF-1α/β	T, B, DC, Mono	CXCR4
	CXCL13	BLC/BCA-1	B	CXCR5
	CXCL14	BRAC/Bolekine	?	DC, Mono
	CXCL15	Lungkine	Neutro	?

Table 9.2. *Continued*

Family	Chemokine	Alternative names	Chemotaxis	Receptors
	CXCL16	None	T, NKT	CXCR6
C	XCL1	Lymphotactin/SCM-1α/ATAC	T	XCR1
	XCL2	SCM-1β	T	XCR1
CX3C	CX3CL1	Fractalkine/Neurotactin	T, Nk, Mono	CX3CR1
CC	CCL1	I-309/(TCA-3/P500)	Mono	CCR8
	CCL2	MCP-1/MCAF	T, NK, DC, Mono, Baso	CCR2
	CCL3	MIP-1α/LD78α	T, NK, DC, Mono, Eosino	CCR1, CCR5
	CCL4	MIP-1β	T, NK, DC, Mono	CCR5
	CCL5	RANTES	T, NK, DC, Mono, Eosino, Baso	CCR1, CCR3, CCR5
	(CCL6)	(C10/MRP-1)	Mono, Mφ, T, Eosino	CCR1
	CCL7	MCP-3	T, NK, DC, Mono, Eosino, Baso	CCR1,CCR2, CCR3
	CCL8	MCP-2	T, NK, DC, Mono, Baso	CCR3
	(CCL9/10)	(MRP-2/CCF18/MIP-1γ)	T, Mono	CCR1
	CCL11	Eotaxin-1	T, DC, Eosino, Baso	CCR3
	(CCL12)	(MCP-5)	T, NK, DC, Mono, Baso	CCR2
	CCL13	MCP-4	T, NK, DC, Mono, Eosino, Baso	CCR2, CCR3
	CCL14	HCC-1/HCC-3	T, Mono, Eosino	CCR1
	CCL15	HCC-2/Leukotactin-1/MIP-1δ	T	CCR1, CCR3
	CCL16	HCC-4/LEC/(LCC-1)	T	CCR1
	CCL17	TARC	T, DC, Mono	CCR4
	CCL18	DCCK1/PARC/AMAC-1	T, DC	?
	CCL19	MIP-3β/ELC/Exodus-3	T, B, DC	CCR7
	CCL20	MIP-3α/LARC/Exodus-1	DC	CCR6
	CCL21	6Ckine/SLC/Exodus-2/(TCA-4)	T, DC	CCR7
	CCL22	MDC/STCP-1/ABCD-1	T, DC, Mono	CCR4
	CCL23	MPIF-1	T	CCR1
	CCL24	MPIF-2/Eotaxin-2	T, DC, Eosino, Baso	CCR3
	CCL25	TECK	T, DC, Mono	CCR9
	CCL26	SCYA26/Eotaxin-3	T	CCR3
	CCL27	CTACK/ALP/ESkine	T	CCR10
	CCL28	MEC	T, B, Eosino	CCR3/CCR10

members of the mammalian JAK family: JAK1, JAK2, JAK3 and Tyk2 (tyrosine kinase 2) and all phosphorylate their downstream substrates at tyrosine residues. Genetic knockout studies have shown that the various JAKS have highly specific functions and produce lethal or severe phenotypes relating to defects in lymphoid development, failure of erythropoiesis and hypersensitivity to pathogens.

Upon cytokine-induced receptor dimerization, JAKs reciprocally phosphorylate, and thereby activate, each other. Active JAKs then phosphorylate specific tyrosine residues on the receptor cytoplasmic tails to create docking sites for members of the **STAT** (*s*ignal *t*ransducers and *a*ctivators of *t*ranscription) family of SH2 domain-containing transcription factors. STATs reside in the cytoplasm in an inactive state but, upon

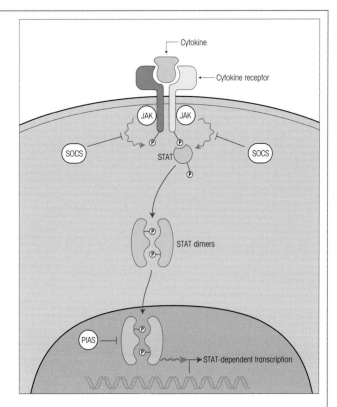

Figure 9.5. Cytokine receptor-mediated pathways for gene transcription.

Cytokine-induced receptor oligomerization activates JAK kinases that are constitutively associated with the receptor cytoplasmic tails. Upon activation, JAK kinases phosphorylate tyrosine residues within the receptor tails, thereby creating binding sites for STAT transcription factors that then become recruited to the receptor complex and are, in turn, phosphorylated by JAKs. Phosphorylation of STATs triggers their dissociation from the receptor and promotes the formation of STAT dimers that translocate to the nucleus to direct transcription of genes that have the appropriate binding motifs within their promoter regions. Members of the SOCS family of inhibitors can suppress cytokine signaling at several points, either through inhibition of JAK kinase activity directly or by promoting polyubiquitination and proteasome-mediated degradation of JAKs. The PIAS family of STAT inhibitors can form complexes with STAT proteins that either result in decreased STAT-binding to DNA or recruitment of transcriptional corepressors that can block STAT-mediated transcription. Cytokine receptors can also recruit additional adaptor proteins such as Shc, Grb2 and Sos, that can activate the MAP kinase (see Figure 8.8) and PI3 kinase signaling cascades, but these have been omitted for clarity.

recruitment to cytokine receptors (via their SH2 domains), become phosphorylated by JAKs and undergo dimerization and dissociation from the receptor. The dimerized STATs then translocate to the nucleus where they play an important role in pushing the cell through the mitotic cycle by activating transcription of various genes (Figure 9.5). Seven mammalian STATs have been described and each plays a relatively non-

redundant role in distinct cytokine signaling pathways. Individual cytokines usually employ more than one type of STAT to exert their biological effects; this is because the hematopoietin receptors are composed of two different receptor chains that are capable of recruiting distinct STAT proteins. Further complexity is achieved due to the ability of STATs to form heterodimers with each other, with the result that a single cytokine may exert its transcriptional effects via a battery of STAT combinations. JAKs may also act through src family kinases to generate other transcription factors via the Ras–MAP kinase route (see Figure 8.8). Some cytokines also activate phosphatidylinositol 3-kinase (PI3K) and phospholipase C (PLCγ).

Downregulation of JAK–STAT signaling is achieved by proteins that belong to the SOCS (*s*uppressor *o*f *c*ytokine *s*ignaling) and PIAS (*p*rotein *i*nhibitor of *a*ctivated *S*TAT) families (Figure 9.5). SOCS proteins are induced in a STAT-dependent manner and therefore represent a classical feedback inhibition mechanism where cytokine signals induce expression of proteins that dampen down their own signaling cascades. The SOCS family contains eight members (namely CIS and SOCS1–SOCS7), and these proteins utilize two distinct mechanisms to downregulate cytokine signals. On the one hand, SOCS proteins can interact with JAKs, as well as other signaling proteins such as Vav, and target these proteins for degradation by the ubiquitin-proteasome pathway (cf. p. 125). Alternatively, SOCS family proteins can interact with SH2-domain binding sites found within the activation loop of the JAK kinase domains, thereby blocking access of JAKs to their downstream substrates (Figure 9.5). Some SOCS family members, such as CIS (*c*ytokine-*i*nducible *s*rc homology domain 2 [SH2]-containing), can also directly interact with the STAT-binding SH2 domains found on cytokine receptors and by doing so can block recruitment of STAT molecules to the receptor complex. Targeted deletion of SOCS genes in the mouse has revealed the importance of these proteins for normal cytokine signaling. *SOCS-1*-deficient mice display marked growth retardation and lymphocytopenia and die from inflammation-associated multi-organ failure within 3 weeks of birth. Consistent with the role of SOCS proteins as negative regulators of cytokine signaling, lymphocytes derived from *SOCS-1*-deficient mice undergo spontaneous activation even in pathogen-free conditions. *SOCS-1*-deficient mice generated on a *RAG2*-deficient background do not display any of the phenotypes observed on a normal genetic background, confirming that SOCS-1 exerts its effects primarily within the lymphocyte compartment.

The PIAS family consists of four members (PIAS1, PIAS3, PIASX and PIASY) and can act to repress STAT-induced transcriptional activity by interacting with these proteins to either restrict their ability to interact with the DNA promoter elements they associate with, or alternatively, by recruiting transcriptional corepressor proteins such as histone deacetylase to the STAT transcriptional complexes (Figure 9.5).

JAK–STAT pathways can also be regulated by other mechanisms such as protein tyrosine phosphatase-mediated antagonism of JAK activity, for example.

Cytokines often have multiple effects

In general, cytokines are **pleiotropic**, i.e. exhibit multiple effects on a variety of cell types (Table 9.1), and there is considerable overlap and *redundancy* between them with respect to individual functions, partially accounted for by the sharing of receptor components and the utilization of common transcription factors. For example, many of the biological activities of IL-4 overlap with those of IL-13. However, it should be pointed out that virtually all cytokines have at least some unique properties.

The cytokines produced at the initial stages of T- and B-cell activation critically influence the subsequent developmental fate of the cell on the receiving end. Their roles in the generation of T- and B-cell effectors, and in the regulation of chronic inflammatory reactions (Figure 9.1), will be discussed at length later in this chapter. We should also note here the important role of cytokines in the control of hematopoiesis (Figure 9.6). The differentiation of stem cells to become the formed elements of blood within the environment of the bone marrow is carefully nurtured through the production of cytokines by the stromal cells. These include GM-CSF, G-CSF (granulocyte colony-stimulating factor), M-CSF, IL-6 and -7 and LIF (Table 9.1), and many of them are also derived from T-cells and macrophages. It is not surprising therefore that, during a period of chronic inflammation, the cytokines that are produced recruit new precursors into the hematopoietic differentiation pathway—a useful exercise in the circumstances. One of the cytokines, IL-3, should be highlighted for its exceptional ability to support the early cells in this pathway, particularly in synergy with IL-6 and G-CSF (Figure 9.6).

Network interactions

The complex and integrated relationships between the different cytokines are mediated through cellular events. The genes for IL-3, -4 and -5 and GM-CSF are all tightly linked on chromosome 5 in a region containing genes for M-CSF and its receptor and several other growth factors and receptors. Interaction may occur through a cascade in which one cytokine induces the production of another, through transmodulation of the receptor for another cytokine and through synergism or antagonism of two cytokines acting on the same cell (Figure 9.7).

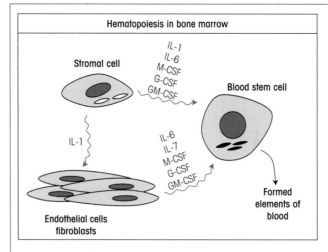

Figure 9.6. Multiple cytokines produced by effector T-cells and other cells of the immune system can influence hematopoiesis.

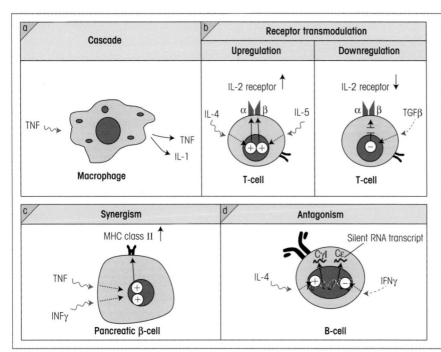

Figure 9.7. Network interactions of cytokines.

(a) Cascade: in this example TNF induces secretion of IL-1 and of itself (autocrine) in the macrophage. (Note that all diagrams in this figure are simplified in that the effects on the nucleus are due to messengers resulting from the combination of cytokine with its surface receptor.) (b) Receptor transmodulation showing upregulation of each chain forming the high affinity IL-2 receptor in an activated T-cell by individual cytokines and downregulation by TGFβ. (c) Synergy of TNF and IFNγ in upregulation of surface MHC class II molecules on cultured pancreatic insulin-secreting cells. (d) Antagonism of IL-4 and IFNγ on transcription of silent ("sterile") mRNA relating to isotype switch (cf. Figure 9.24).

Figure 9.8. Activated T-blasts expressing surface receptors for IL-2 proliferate in response to IL-2

Produced by itself or by another T-cell subset. Expansion is controlled through downregulation of the IL-2 receptor by IL-2 itself. The expanded population secretes a wide variety of biologically active cytokines of which IL-4 also enhances T-cell proliferation.

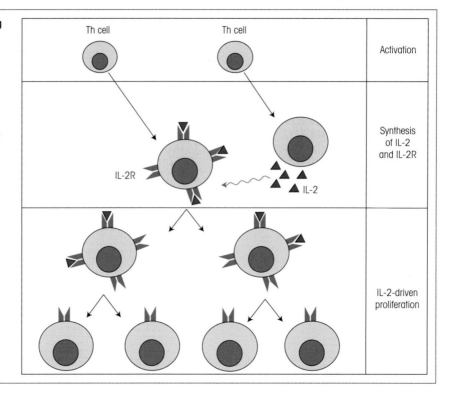

Activated T-cells proliferate in response to cytokines

In so far as T-cells are concerned, clonal proliferation following activation is critically dependent upon IL-2 (Figure 9.8). This cytokine is a single peptide of molecular weight 15.5 kDa that acts only on cells that express high affinity IL-2 receptors (Figure 9.4). These receptors are not present on resting T-cells, but are synthesized within a few hours after activation. Activated T-cells divide rapidly for 4–5 days, in an IL-2-dependent manner, and then differentiate into various effector subsets as we shall discuss below.

Separation of an activated T-cell population into those with high and low affinity IL-2 receptors showed clearly that an adequate number of high affinity receptors were mandatory for the mitogenic action of IL-2. The numbers of these receptors on the cell increase under the action of antigen and of IL-2 and, as antigen is cleared, so the receptor numbers decline and, with that, the responsiveness to IL-2. It should be appreciated that, although IL-2 is an immunologically nonspecific T-cell growth factor, it only functions appropriately in specific responses because unstimulated T-cells do not express high affinity IL-2 receptors.

As we shall see, activated T-cells also produce an impressive array of other cytokines, and the proliferative effect of IL-2 is

Because of the number of combinations that are possible and the almost yearly discovery of new cytokines, the means by which target cells integrate and interpret the complex patterns of stimuli induced by these multiple soluble factors is only slowly unfolding.

reinforced by the action of IL-4 and, to some extent, IL-6, which react with corresponding receptors on the dividing T-cells.

Different T-cell subsets can make different cytokine patterns

We have previously encountered the idea that different types of T-cells can be generated. Aside from the major subsets of CD4- and CD8-restricted T-cells, further **sub-functionalization of T-cells can be detected on the basis of the patterns of cytokines that these cells express**. As we have noted earlier, the particular pattern of cytokines secreted by an activated T-cell is influenced by the nature of the cytokines it is exposed to upon initial encounter with antigen presented by a mature DC within the secondary lymphoid organs. In a similar vein, the pattern of cytokines expressed by DCs are shaped by the nature of the pathogen-associated molecular patterns (PAMPs) that triggered maturation of the latter, as well as the prevailing cytokine environment during the initial encounter with the infectious agent. Switching our attentions back to the T-cell, **polarization** (i.e. further differentiation to a particular Th subset) of these cells can be further reinforced by cytokine signals that are encountered upon trafficking of the primed T-cell to the site of infection. In this way, T-cell responses can become tailored to the nature of the pathogen that instigated activation of the immune system in the first place. However, before we get further into the details of T-cell polarization, **we would caution the reader not to think of this process as a rigidly constraining one**, but rather as a continuum of responses that can display particularly distinct patterns at specific points within the spectrum.

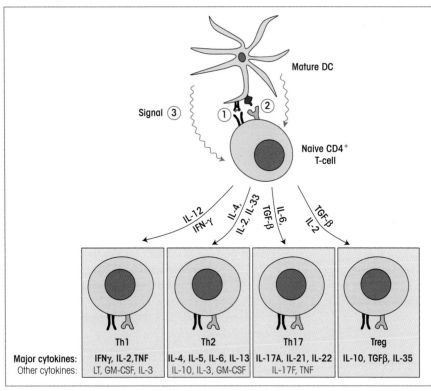

Figure 9.9. T-cells can undergo polarization to distinct subsets that secrete different cytokine combinations.

Naive T-cells can undergo activation and polarization to distinct Th subsets. Cytokines produced by dendritic cells (DCs) or other innate immune cells, representing signal 3, dictate the differentiation fate of the T-cell, as shown.

Major cytokines:	Th1	Th2	Th17	Treg
	IFNγ, IL-2, TNF	IL-4, IL-5, IL-6, IL-13	IL-17A, IL-21, IL-22	IL-10, TGFβ, IL-35
Other cytokines:	LT, GM-CSF, IL-3	IL-10, IL-3, GM-CSF	IL-17F, TNF	

Th cell polarization

Helper T-cell clones can be divided into three main subsets, Th1, Th2, and Th17, with each displaying distinct cytokine secretion profiles (Figure 9.9), which in turn, influences the range of effector functions carried out by each subset. A further subset of CD4-positive T-cells has also been identified that exerts control over the other T-cell subsets by inhibiting their effector function; such cells are called regulatory T-cells or Tregs. Let us consider some of the properties that these cytokine profiles confer on their T-cell subsets.

Th1 cells coordinate responses to intracellular pathogens

Th1 cells secrete cytokine profiles skewed towards coordinating responses to **intracellular bacterial and viral infections** (Figure 9.9). This is achieved largely through activating macrophages and assisting the expansion of cytotoxic T-lymphocytes (Tc). Because they produce high amounts of IFNγ, Th1 cells are adept at activating macrophages, which is particularly important where macrophages have become infected with intracellular bacteria that actively antagonize macrophage function. When a Th1-polarized effector cell arrives at a site of infection, it can be restimulated by local macrophages that are either infected with intracellular bacteria or that have internalized bacterial fragments. Presentation of specific antigen via MHC class II molecules on the macrophage leads to directed secretion of IFNγ by the Th1 cell to the macrophage (Figure 9.10). However, in the absence of other signals, macrophages are not very responsive to IFNγ. This problem is also solved

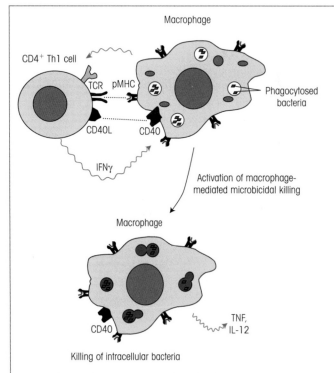

Figure 9.10. Th1 cells activate the microbicidal killing activity of macrophages.

IFNγ derived from Th1 cells is important for the activation of macrophages and can enhance the microbicidal activity of such cells to kill phagocytosed bacteria. IFNγ can also induce the secretion of IL-12 and TNF by macrophages as shown.

by the Th1 cell in the form of CD40L, which engages CD40 on the macrophage and greatly increases its sensitivity to IFNγ. Th1 cells can also enhance the microbicidal functions of the macrophage to extracellular bacteria that are engulfed via phagocytosis (Figure 9.10). Recall from Chapter 1 that macrophages greatly increase their microbicidal properties upon activation and IFNγ as well as TNFα is a very good way of achieving this. IFNγ-stimulated macrophages also produce IL-12 that leads to reinforcement of the Th1 phenotype.

Th1 cells also secrete high levels of IL-2 (Figure 9.9), which is able to support the expansion of CD8-positive cytotoxic T-cells, professional killers of virus-infected cells; we shall discuss how they kill later in this chapter. This can occur where activated T-cells have migrated to a site of infection and a Th1 cell engages an infected macrophage or DC (via MHC class II/peptide–TCR interactions) simultaneously with a CTL, which is engaged with the APC via MHC class I/peptide-TCR interactions. This creates the circumstances where a CTL can be induced to clonally expand to swell its numbers due to IL-2 produced by the Th1 cell. We will see later in this chapter that a Th1 cell can also "license" a DC for stimulation of a Tc cell after the Th1 cell has already departed.

Other cytokines secreted by Th1 cells, such as IL-3 and GM-CSF, have more distant effects on bone marrow precursors and induce the production of neutrophils and macrophages to swell the ranks of these cells, as required, during an ongoing infection.

Th2 cells coordinate responses to extracellular pathogens

Due to their ability to generate IL-4, IL-5 and IL-13 (Figure 9.9), all of which support B-cell proliferation, class switching and differentiation to effectors (Figure 9.11), Th2 cells are very good helpers for B-cells and would seem to be adapted for defense against parasites and other **extracellular pathogens** that are vulnerable to IL-4-switched IgE, IL-5-induced eosinophilia and IL-3/4-stimulated mast cell proliferation. Similar to Th1 cells, Th2 cells also produce IL-3 and GM-CSF to induce the production of neutrophils and macrophages from bone marrow precursors. IL-5 also acts at a distance and is particularly important for production of eosinophils (Figure 9.1), which, as we discussed in Chapter 1, are particularly well adapted towards combating large extracellular parasites such as parasitic worms. Due to their physical size, these infectious agents cannot be readily phagocytosed by macrophages or neutrophils. To deal with this problem, eosinophils are equipped with specialized granules containing a range of cytotoxic molecules that are released onto the surface of the parasite upon engagement of the

Figure 9.11. B-cell response to thymus-dependent (TD) antigen: clonal expansion and maturation of activated B-cells under the influence of T-cell-derived soluble factors.

Co-stimulation through the CD40L–CD40 interaction is essential for primary and secondary immune responses to TD antigens and for the formation of germinal centers and memory. c-*myc* expression, which is maximal 2 hours after antigen or anti-μ stimulation, parallels sensitivity to growth factors; transfection with c-*myc* substitutes for anti-μ.

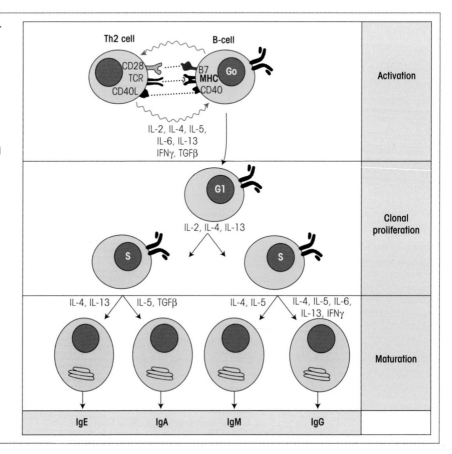

complement C3b receptors on the eosinophil with C3b-opsonized parasites.

Th17 cells promote acute inflammatory responses and recruit neutrophils

A relatively recent addition to the T-helper cell fold, Th17 cells are currently receiving considerable attention for their propensity to be involved in autoimmune reactions when the actions of these cells get out of control. Th17 cells are IL-17A-producing cells that also secrete IL-17F, IL-21 and IL-22 (Figure 9.9). These cells appear to be specialized towards mounting massive inflammatory responses towards **extracellular bacterial and fungal infections**, particularly at mucosal interfaces. This appears to be achieved through production of IL-17A, IL-17F and IL-22, which have broad effects on many nonimmune cell types, such as endothelial and epithelial cells, and elicit the production of proinflammatory cytokines and chemokines by such cells to promote neutrophil recruitment to the site of inflammation. These cytokines also induce the secretion of antimicrobial peptides, by keratinocytes for example, which strengthens their barrier function towards infection.

Cross-regulation of Th1, Th2 and Th17 subsets

Not only do the particular cytokine secreted by Th1, Th2 and Th17 cells enable them to elicit distinct biological functions, these cytokines also help to reinforce the same pattern of cytokine production, as well as inhibiting polarization to the alternative Th subset, a feature that is sometimes exploited to the benefit of certain pathogens. The ability of IFNγ, the characteristic Th1 cytokine, to inhibit the proliferation of Th2 clones, and of Th2-derived IL-4 and -10 to block both proliferation and cytokine release by Th1 cells, would seem to put the issue beyond reasonable doubt (Figure 9.12). Similarly, development of the Th1 or Th2 phenotype appears to be antagonistic to the development of Th17 cells.

Studies on the infection of mice with the pathogenic protozoan *Leishmania major* demonstrated that intravenous or intraperitoneal injection of killed promastigotes leads to protection against challenge with live parasites associated with high expression of IFNγ mRNA and low levels of IL-4 mRNA; the reciprocal finding of low IFNγ and high IL-4 expression was made after subcutaneous immunization that failed to provide protection. Furthermore, nonvaccinated mice infected with live organisms could be saved by injection of IFNγ and anti-IL-4. These results are consistent with the preferential expansion of a population of protective IFNγ-secreting Th1 cells by intraperitoneal or intravenous immunization, and of nonprotective Th2 cells producing IL-4 in the subcutaneously injected animals.

Stability versus plasticity of Th subsets

The original Mosmann–Coffman classification into Th1 and Th2 subsets was predicated on data obtained with clones that had been maintained in culture for long periods and might

have been artifacts of conditions *in vitro*. The use of cytokine-specific monoclonal antibodies for intracellular fluorescent staining, and of ELISPOT assays (cf. p. 178) for the detection of the secreted molecules, has demonstrated that the Th1 and Th2 phenotypes are also apparent in freshly sampled cells and thus also applies *in vivo*. Nonetheless, it is perhaps best not to be too rigidly constrained in one's thinking by the Th1/Th2/Th17 paradigm, but rather to look upon activated T-cells as potentially producing a whole spectrum of cytokine profiles (Th0, Figure 9.12), with possible skewing of the responses towards particular patterns depending on the nature of the antigen stimulus. Thus, other subsets may also exist, in particular the transforming growth factor-β (TGFβ) and IL-10-producing Th3/Tr1 (T-regulatory 1) cells, which are of interest because these cytokines can mediate immunosuppressive effects and may be involved in the induction of mucosally induced tolerance (cf. p. 508). Another subset that is also emerging in

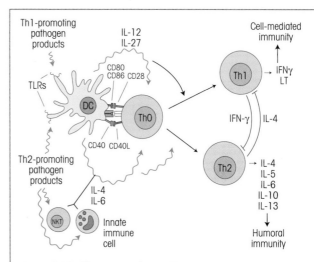

Figure 9.12. The generation of Th1 and Th2 CD4 subsets.

Following initial stimulation of T-cells, a range of cells producing a spectrum of cytokine patterns emerges. Depending on the nature of the pathogen and the response of cells of the innate immune system during the initial stages of infection, the resulting T-helper cell population can be biased towards two extremes. Th1-promoting pathogen products (such as LPS) engage Toll-like receptors (TLRs) on dendritic cells (DCs) or macrophages and induce the secretion of Th1-polarizing cytokines such as IL-12 and IL-27. The latter cytokines promote the development of Th1 cells that produce the cytokines characteristic of *cell-mediated immunity*. IL-4, possibly produced by interaction of microorganisms with the lectin-like NK1.1⁺ receptor on NKT-cells or through interaction of Th2-promoting pathogen products with TLRs on DCs, skews the development to the production of Th2 cells whose cytokines assist the progression of B-cells to antibody secretion and the provision of *humoral immunity*. Cytokines produced by polarized Th1 and Th2 subpopulations are mutually inhibitory. LT, lymphotoxin (TNFβ); Th0, early helper cell producing a spectrum of cytokines; other abbreviations as in Table 9.1.

the scientific literature is a class of Th cells that have been dubbed **follicular helper T cells (Tfh)** that appear to be important for guiding B-cell development, class switching and survival within germinal centers. Tfh cells have been found to produce high levels of IL-21 and to migrate to the follicular regions upon activation to form stable contacts with antigen-primed B cells.

It is very likely that further T-cell subsets will be identified in the coming years and current evidence suggests that rather than each subset representing highly committed and distinct T-cell "lineages," it seems that there is considerable plasticity in the spectrum of cytokines that differentiated T-cells can secrete. Furthermore, it is also apparent that **reprogramming of effector T-cells can occur**, converting differentiated T-cell subsets from one type towards another.

Cells of the innate immune system shape the Th1/Th2/Th17 response

We have already introduced the concept that the cytokine milieu that becomes established by cells of the innate immune system during the early stages of infection has a major influence on the adaptive immune response (Figures 9.2 and 9.12). In the initial stages of an infection, the innate immune responses hold the line as T-lymphocytes require priming by DCs to initiate clonal expansion and maturation to effectors. Upon migration of antigen-specific T-cells to lymph nodes where they come in contact with mature DCs fresh from their encounters with microbial pathogens, the pathogen products encountered by the DC will have polarized the latter in favor of secreting particular cytokines, as we have discussed above (Figure 9.9). Polarization of T-cells towards a Th1, Th2 or other fate is achieved via signal 3 and the nature of this signal is strongly influenced by the conditions under which the APC is primed (Figure 9.12).

Th1 polarization

IL-12 and its relatively recently discovered relatives, IL-23 and IL-27, are instrumental in polarizing towards a Th1 cell phenotype (Figure 9.12). Invasion of phagocytic cells by intracellular pathogens induces copious secretion of IL-12, which in turn stimulates IFNγ production by NK cells. Engagement of many of the known Toll-like receptors (TLRs) on DCs by microbial products (such as LPS, dsRNA and bacterial DNA) triggers DC maturation and induces IL-12 production, thereby favoring Th1 responses. Bacterial priming also induces CD40 receptor expression on DCs and induces responsiveness to CD40L, expressed by activated T-cells, for optimal IL-12 synthesis. IL-12 is also particularly effective at inducing IFNγ by activated T-cells and secretion of the latter by the T-cell further enhances IL-12 production and secretion by DCs; this acts as a classical positive feedback loop for enhancement of IL-12 production and further skews the response towards Th1.

Th2 polarization

IL-4 is pivotal for the production of a Th2 cell phenotype. While IL-12 and IFNγ promote a Th1 response, these cytokines also inhibit Th2 responses (Figure 9.12). However, IL-4 effects appear to be dominant over IL-12 and therefore the amounts of IL-4 relative to the amounts of IL-12 and IFNγ will be of paramount importance in determining the differentiation of Th0 (i.e. unpolarized) cells into Th1 or Th2. IL-4 downregulates the expression of the IL-12R β_2 subunit necessary for responsiveness to IL-12, further polarizing the Th2 dominance. It is still unclear whether signals from the innate immune system drive T-cells in the direction of a Th2 response or whether this is a default differentiation pathway for Th cells unless suppressed by Th1-polarizing signals such as IL-12 or IFNγ. A special cell population, the NKT-cells bearing the NK1.1$^+$ marker, rapidly releases an IL-4-dominated pattern of cytokines on stimulation. These cells have many unusual features. They may be CD4$^-$8$^-$ or CD4$^+$8$^-$ and express low levels of T-cell $\alpha\beta$ receptors with an invariant α chain and very restricted β, many of these receptors recognizing the nonclassical MHC-like CD1 molecule. Their morphology and granule content are intermediate between T-cells and NK cells. Although they express TCR $\alpha\beta$, there is an inclination to classify them on the fringe of the "innate" immune system with regard to their primitive characteristics and possession of the lectin-like NK1.1 receptor that may be involved in the recognition of microbial carbohydrates.

Th17 polarization

Although the precise cocktail of cytokines that triggers the production of Th17 cells is still a matter of active debate, it is clear that the pro-inflammatory cytokine IL-6 plays a particularly influential role initially. This is then reinforced by IL-23, which appears to be important for expansion and stabilization of these cells (Figure 9.9). Naive T cells do not express IL-23 receptors, but upregulate these upon productive activation, which is also enhanced by IL-6. Thus, the role of IL-23 in differentiation to Th17 cells is one of reinforcement rather than initiation. There is also evidence that TGFβ in combination with IL-6 influences the generation of Th17 cells, whereas TGFβ alone polarizes T-cells towards a Treg fate, as we shall discuss below. However, TGFβ does not appear to play an instructive role for the production of Th17 cells, rather, it appears to act by suppressing the development of either the Th1 or Th2 phenotypes, which are antagonistic to the Th17 fate.

Further thoughts on Th polarization

Whilst there is a certain amount of evidence indicating the existence of subpopulations of dendritic cells specialized for the stimulation of either Th1 or Th2 populations, it seems that DCs are relatively plastic and can adopt a Th1-, Th2- or Th17-polarizing phenotype depending on the priming signals they encounter from microbial and tissue-derived sources. However, it should be obvious from the above discussion that the cytokines produced in the immediate vicinity of the T-cell will be important.

Policing the adaptive immune system

In addition to the effector T-cell subsets that we have already discussed, there is also much evidence that T-cells can also differentiate into cells that play a **suppressive or regulatory role** in immune responses (Figure 9.9). That is to say, these cells appear to police the actions of the other classes of T-cells, stepping in to quell immune responses when this appears necessary. Such cells are called regulatory T-cells, or Tregs, and there appear to be two different categories of such cells, *natural* and *inducible* T-regs. These cells play a role in suppressing responses to self antigens, as well as inappropriate or undesirable responses to nonself antigens (such as commensal bacteria or food in the gut); indeed, it is now believed that Tregs control almost every adaptive immune response. We shall look at natural Tregs first as these appear to be the most abundant type.

Natural Tregs

Natural or thymic-derived Tregs are a population of Foxp3+CD25+CD4+ T-cells that can suppress immune responses of autoreactive T-cells by mechanisms that are still not entirely understood, but appear to involve several distinct and possibly overlapping strategies (see below). The current view is that these self-antigen-reactive T-cells develop in the thymus and are released as functionally mature cells that can act to dominantly suppress the activation of other self-reactive T-cells that escape negative selection in the thymus, possibly through competition for self-antigens presented by APCs or through CTLA4-mediated signals from the Treg to the APC.

Natural Tregs constitute 5–10% of CD4-positive T-cells and their development is critically dependent on the induction of Foxp3, a transcription factor that can repress the transcription of Th1-, Th2- and Th17-type cytokines. Loss-of-function mutations in the *FOXP3* gene result in a variety of inflammatory and autoimmune defects characterized by massive overproduction of Th1- and Th2-type cytokines, which is ultimately fatal. Tregs appear to be essential for the ongoing suppression of autoreactive T-cells, as their depletion results in the spontaneous development of autoimmune disease in otherwise normal mice. In humans, the equivalent condition resulting from mutations in the gene encoding Foxp3 is known as immune dysregulation, polyendocrinopathy, enteropathy, X-linked (IPEX). Autoimmune disease can also be provoked by adoptive transfer of Treg-depleted splenocytes from normal adult mice to syngenic recipients lacking T-cells. *In vitro* stimulation of Foxp3+Treg-depleted cells from peripheral blood of healthy individuals has revealed that T-cells reactive towards multiple self-antigens are frequently present, but proliferation of these autoreactive T-cells can be readily suppressed by adding back Tregs. Such experiments argue that self-reactive T-cells, that are not anergic, probably exist in all individuals. Thus Tregs most

likely exist to counter the actions of such cells and to prevent spontaneous autoimmunity from developing.

IL-2 is also crucial for the maintenance of natural Tregs as these T-cells are incapable of making their own IL-2, unlike activated T-cells, and rely fully on paracrine IL-2 for their survival. Consequently, the number of such cells is drastically reduced in *IL-2* and *IL-2R* knockout mice, with the result that these mice develop lymphoproliferation followed by lethal autoimmunity. The source of IL-2 for the maintenance of Tregs is unresolved but could come from autoreactive or antigen-activated T-cells that are interacting on the same DC as the Treg.

Inducible Tregs

In contrast to natural Tregs, inducible (or adaptive) Tregs (iTregs) are generated from naive T-cells in the periphery after encounter with antigen presented by DCs. These regulatory T-cells are a diverse group, although it is not yet clear whether these inducible Treg cell populations are truly distinct.

Th3 cells represent one subset of iTregs that have been found in mucosa and secrete IL-4, IL-10 and TGFβ. Such cells seem to be important for oral tolerance and Th3 cells may generally intervene to maintain tolerance towards the beneficial commensal microorganisms that populate our intestinal tract.

Tr1 cells have been described upon activation of T-cells in the presence of high concentrations of IL-10 *in vitro*. Tr1 cells secrete TGFβ and may be induced by immature DCs presenting antigen in the absence of appropriate co-stimulatory ligands.

Foxp3+-inducible Tregs have been described where TCR activation occurs in the presence of TGFβ and IL-2. Foxp3 iTreg cell differentiation also appears to be favored in particular tissue environments; gut-associated lymphoid tissues (GALT) being particularly amenable to the generation of such cells.

Tregs exert their effects through multiple mechanisms

Tregs have been reported to exert their suppressive effects via a number of different mechanisms (Figure 9.13). Some Tregs appear to stifle T-cell responses through the **production of immunosuppressive cytokines** such as IL-10, TGFβ, or IL-35. IL-10 suppresses T-cell responses by inhibiting the production of IL-2, IL-5 and TNFβ and also through inhibiting the upregulation of MHC class II as well as B7 co-stimulatory ligands on DCs and macrophages. The latter effect has the consequence of antagonizing effective antigen presentation and co-stimulation of T-cells. TGFβ also blocks cytokine production by T-cells, as well as cytoxicity and proliferation.

Treg-mediated **killing of APCs or effector T-cells** has also been reported. In this scenario, recognition of specific antigen by a Treg precipitates a cytotoxic T-cell killing reaction in which the Treg induces apoptosis in the APC presenting the Treg antigen, or in a nearby T-cell communicating with the same APC. Killing in this situation has been reported to be

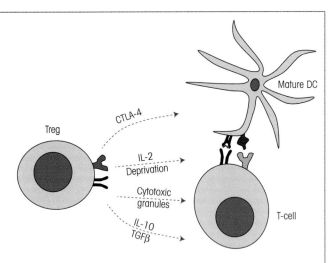

Figure 9.13. Alternative mechanisms of Treg-mediated suppression.

Regulatory T-cells (Tregs) may exert their regulatory functions on T-cells through the secretion of immunosuppressive cytokines, cytotoxic enzymes, or CTLA-4 cell-contact-dependent effects. These effects may act upon the T-cell undergoing regulation or on dendritic cells (DCs) or other antigen-presenting cells (APCs) presenting antigen to naive T-cells. See main text for further details.

dependent on granzyme B and perforin expression by the Treg. Later in this chapter we will explore the detailed mechanism of granzyme B/perforin-mediated killing (see p. 245).

Competition for IL-2 with activated T-cells has also been implicated as an effector mechanism of Tregs, as such cells can utilize but do not make their own IL-2. The strategy here appears to be that the Treg competes for IL-2 made by nearby effector cells, thereby reducing expansion of activated T-cells that are critically dependent on this cytokine for clonal proliferation (Figure 9.8).

Last, but by no means least, **CTLA-4**, the alternative receptor for B7 co-stimulatory ligands has been consistently reported to be important for Treg functions. Tregs bearing surface CTLA-4 could exert inhibitory effects on T-cell activation by a number of mechanisms. One way is through simple competition with T-cells for B7 ligands on APCs, another is by delivering negative signals to DCs via CTLA-4, which downregulates B7 ligands (i.e. CD80 and CD86) on the latter, rendering such cells incapable of productively activating naive T-cells. Indeed, Tregs have been observed to form aggregates around DCs and to suppress the upregulation of B7 ligands; such cells may also inhibit cytokine production by DCs. Importantly, Treg-specific deletion of CTLA-4 results in the spontaneous development of systemic lymphoproliferation and fatal disease in mice.

It is likely that one or more of the above mechanisms operate concurrently, depending on the context. However **a core mechanism that may be common to all Tregs appears to operate via CTLA-4**, particularly with regard to natural Tregs, as such cells express high levels of this receptor. Let us take a look at the evidence. Blockade of CTLA-4 by monoclonal antibodies provokes organ-specific autoimmune disease

and inflammatory bowel disease in otherwise healthy animals. Foxp3, along with other transcription factors, upregulates CTLA-4 via promoter-dependent effects. Mice lacking *CTLA-4*, specifically in natural Tregs succumb to a variety of autoimmune diseases in a manner similar to *FOXP3*-deficient mice.

Irrespective of the precise mechanism of action, all are agreed that Tregs are extremely important for policing the activities of potentially autoreactive T-cells, as well as for limiting excessive responses to nonself antigens. As a consequence, failure to mount effective Treg responses frequently results in autoimmune disease.

CD8$^+$ T-cell effectors in cell-mediated immunity

CD8$^+$, MHC class I-restricted, cytotoxic T-cells (Tc), also referred to as cytotoxic T-lymphocytes (CTLs), represent the other major arm of the cell-mediated immune response and are of strategic importance in the killing of virally infected cells and also contribute to the surveillance mechanisms against cancer cells (see p. 456). While some CD4$^+$ T-cells are also capable of cytotoxic killing, the majority of CTL-killing is derived from the CD8$^+$ T-cell population.

The generation of cytotoxic T-cells

CTL precursors recognize antigen on the surface of cells in association with class I major histocompatibility complex (MHC) molecules and, like B-cells, they usually require help from T-cells. The mechanism by which help is proffered may, however, be quite different to how Th2 cells stimulate B-cell proliferation and differentiation to effectors. As explained earlier (see p. 217), effective T-cell–B-cell collaboration is usually "cognate" in that the collaborating cells recognize two epitopes that are physically linked (usually on the same molecule). If we may remind the reader without causing offense, the reason for this is that the surface Ig receptors on the B-cell capture native antigen, process it internally and present it to the Th as a peptide in association with MHC class II. Although it has been shown that linked epitopes on the antigen are also necessary for cooperation between Th and the cytotoxic T-cell precursor (Tcp), the nature of T-cell recognition prevents native antigen being focused onto the Tcp by its receptor for subsequent processing, even if that cell were to express MHC II, which in its resting state it does not. It seems most likely that Th and Tcp bind to the same APC, for example a dendritic cell, which has processed viral antigen and displays processed viral peptides in association with both class II (for the Th cell) and class I (for the Tcp) on its surface; one cannot exclude the possibility that the APC could be the virally infected cell itself. Cytokines from the triggered Th will be released in close proximity to the Tcp, which is engaging the antigen–MHC signal and will be stimulated to proliferate and differentiate into a Tc under the influence of IL-2 and -6 (Figure 9.14a). However, interaction of the APC with the Th and the Tc cell can be temporally separated and, in this case, it appears that the helper T-cell "licenses" the dendritic cell for future interaction with

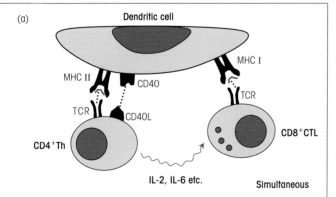

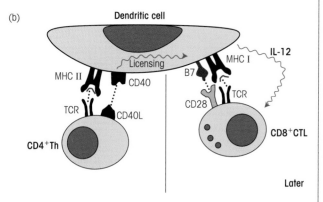

Figure 9.14. T-helper cell activation of cytotoxic T-cells.

Activation of the CD4⁺ helper T-cells (Th) by the dendritic cell involves a CD40–CD40 ligand (CD154) co-stimulatory signal and recognition of an MHC class II peptide presented by the T-cell receptor. (a) If both the Th and the cytotoxic T-lymphocyte (Tc) are present at the same time, the release of cytokines from the activated Th cells stimulates the differentiation of the CD8⁺ precursor into an activated, MHC class I-restricted Tc. However, as shown in (b), the Th and the Tc do not need to interact with the APC at the same time. In this case, the Th cell "licenses" the dendritic cell for future interaction with a Tc cell. Thus the Th cell, by engaging CD40, drives the dendritic cell from a resting state into an activated state with upregulation of co-stimulatory molecules such as B7.1 and B7.2 (CD80 and CD86, respectively) and increased cytokine production, particularly of IL-12.

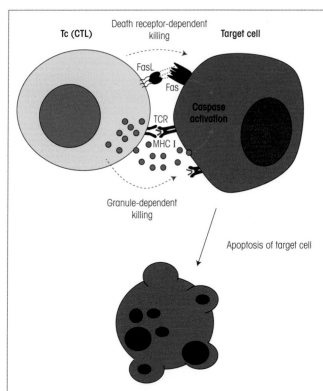

Figure 9.15. Cytotoxic T-cells (Tc, or CTL) can kill target cells via the granule-dependent or Fas ligand (FasL)-dependent, pathways to apoptosis.

Both pathways result in the activation of members of the caspase family of proteases within the target cell and these enzymes kill the target through proteolysis of hundreds of substrate proteins. See Figures 9.17 and 9.18 for further details on the mechanism of cell killing by either pathway.

the cytotoxic T-cell. It does this by activating the dendritic cell through CD40, thereby upregulating co-stimulatory molecules and cytokine production, in particular IL-12, by the dendritic cell (Figure 9.14b). An entirely Th-independent mechanism of Tc activation is also thought to occur. This has been demonstrated in, for example, the response to protein antigens given with potent adjuvants such as immunostimulatory DNA sequences (ISSs), in this case possibly involving adjuvant-induced production of proinflammatory cytokines and cell surface co-stimulatory molecules.

The lethal process

As noted above, cytotoxic T-cells are generally of the CD8 subset, and their binding to the target cell through TCR-

mediated recognition of peptide presented on class I MHC is assisted by interactions between CD8, the co-receptor for class I, and by other accessory molecules such as LFA-1 and CD2 that increase the affinity of the interaction between the CTL and the target cell (see Figure 8.3).

Upon recognition of a suitable target cell, CTLs are capable of killing via two distinct pathways; the **Fas/Fas ligand pathway** and the **perforin/granzyme pathway**, which are not mutually exclusive as both killing options may be available to an individual CTL (Figure 9.15). Both killing pathways culminate in the activation of a family of cytotoxic proteases—called caspases—within the target cell that coordinate the cell killing process from within; the only difference between the two pathways is how the caspases become activated. Comparison of T-cells lacking functional Fas ligand as well as perforin, with T cells lacking perforin alone, has demonstrated that these two pathways account for most of the killing activity of CTLs (as well as NK cells), with TNF accounting for a minor component of CTL killing. We will deal with the perforin/granzyme and Fas-dependent killing mechanisms in turn.

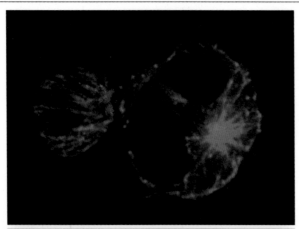

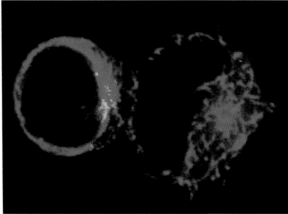

Figure 9.16. Conjugation of a cytotoxic T-cell (on left) to its target, here a mouse mastocytoma, showing polarization of the granules towards the target at the point of contact. The cytoskeletons of both cells are revealed by immunofluorescent staining with an antibody to tubulin (green) and the lytic granules with an antibody to granzyme A (red). Twenty minutes after conjugation the target cell cytoskeleton may still be intact (above), but this rapidly becomes disrupted (below). (Photographs kindly provided by Dr. Gillian Griffiths.)

Perforin/granzyme-dependent killing

CTLs contain modified lysosomes equipped with a battery of cytotoxic proteins, collectively called **cytotoxic granules**. Following activation of the CTL, the cytotoxic granules are driven at a rare old speed (up to 1.2 μm/second) along the microtubule system and delivered to the point of contact between the CTL and its target, the **immunological synapse** (Figure 9.16). Directed delivery of the cytotoxic granules towards the immunological synapse is important as this ensures the specificity of killing dictated by TCR recognition of the target and limits collateral damage to surrounding cells, as well as to the killer cell itself. As with NK cells, which have comparable granules (cf. p. 27), exocytosis of the cytotoxic granules delivers a range of cytotoxic proteins into the target cell cytosol that cooperate to promote apoptosis of the target (see Videoclip 3).

Videomicroscopy shows that CTLs are serial killers. After the "kiss of death," the T-cell can disengage and seek a further victim, there being rapid synthesis of new granules.

Cytotoxic T-cell granules contain **perforin**, a pore-forming protein similar to the C9 component of complement, and an array of cathepsin-like proteases that are collectively referred to as **granzymes**. Perforin facilitates the entry of the other granule constituents into the target cell in a manner that is still much debated. One way in which perforin may deliver granzymes into the target cell is through oligomerization into a pore on the plasma membrane of the target, thereby permitting access of the granzymes to the cytosol (Figure 9.17). Indeed, pores of up to 20 nm in diameter can be formed within lipid membranes using purified perforin. An alternative mechanism that has been proposed involves the endocytosis of the cytotoxic granules by the target cell, with perforin facilitating escape of the granzymes from the endosomes into the target cell cytosol. Irrespective of the precise way in which perforin acts, it is clear that this pore-forming protein plays an essential role in the killing process; mice deficient in perforin are severely impaired in clearing several viral pathogens. In humans, congenital perforin deficiency results in the potentially fatal immunoregulatory disorder, type 2 familial hemophagocytic lymphohistiocytosis (FHL), which is characterized by hyperactivation of T-cells and macrophages that infiltrate tissues and cause extensive damage due to overproduction of inflammatory cytokines. The latter symptoms also point towards a role for the perforin/granzyme pathway in an immunoregulatory context, such as we touched upon earlier in our discussion of the mechanism of action of Tregs (Figure 9.13).

It is not clear how all of the granzymes contribute to target cell death upon delivery into the cell cytoplasm but granzymes A and B are known to play particularly significant roles in this process. Granzyme A can promote the activation of a nuclease through proteolysis of its inhibitor and this situation results in the formation of numerous single-stranded DNA breaks within the target cell (Figure 9.17). Granzyme B can directly process and activate several members of the **caspase** family of cysteine proteases that can rapidly initiate apoptosis through restricted proteolysis of hundreds of proteins within the target cell. Granzyme B can also promote caspase activation indirectly, through activation of Bid, a protein that promotes permeabilization of mitochondria and release of mitochondrial cytochrome c into the cytosol; the latter event arms a caspase-activating complex that has been termed "the apoptosome" and this complex promotes the activation of several downstream caspases (Figure 9.17). Several additional granzymes have also been found within cytotoxic granules but their precise functional role in CTL killing remains the subject of ongoing investigation. Collectively, entry of the full spectrum of granzymes into the target cells results in very swift cell killing (within 60 minutes or so) and several parallel pathways to apoptosis are most likely engaged during this process. CTLs also express protease inhibitors, such as PI-9, that may protect them from the lethal effects of their own granule contents.

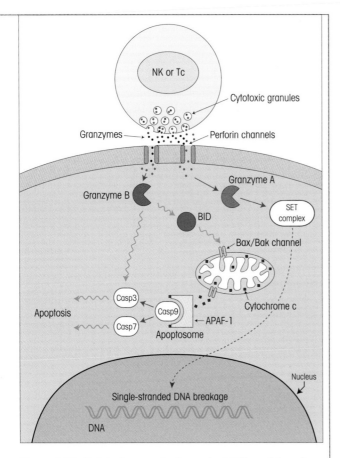

Figure 9.17. Cytotoxic granule-dependent killing of target cells by cytotoxic T-cells and NK cells.

In response to an appropriate stimulus, Tc and NK cells deliver the contents of their cytotoxic granule onto the surface of target cells. The cytotoxic granule protein perforin is thought to polymerize within the target cell membrane forming pores that permit passage of other granule constituents, which includes several serine proteases (granzymes), into the target cell. Upon entry into the target, granzyme B orchestrates apoptosis by cleaving and activating BID, which translocates to mitochondria and triggers the opening of a pore or channel within the mitochondrial outer membrane composed of Bax and/or Bak; the latter channel permits the release of cytochrome c from the mitochondrial intermembrane space into the cytoplasm where it acts as a co-factor for the assembly of a caspase-9-activating complex (the apoptosome). The apoptosome promotes activation of downstream caspases, such as caspase-3 and caspase-7, and the latter proteases coordinate apoptosis through restricted proteolysis of hundreds of substrate proteins. Granzyme B can also proteolytically process and activate caspase-3 and caspase-7 directly, providing a more direct route to caspase activation. Another granule protein, granzyme A, can cleave a protein within the SET complex (an endoplasmic reticulum-associated protein complex). This permits the translocation of a nuclease (NM23-H1) to the nuclear compartment that can catalyze single-stranded DNA breaks. Cytotoxic granules also contain other granzymes that contribute to target cell killing but substrates for these proteases have yet to be identified.

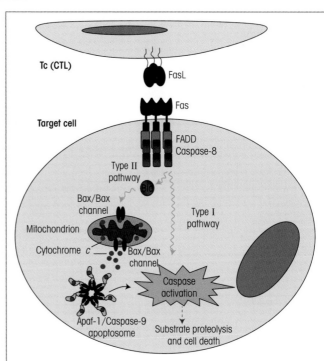

Figure 9.18. Fas–Fas ligand (FasL) route to apoptosis.

Upon encounter of a Fas ligand (FasL)-bearing cell, susceptible cells undergo apoptosis through recruitment of caspase-8 to the cytoplasmic tail of the Fas receptor, via the adaptor protein FADD. Recruitment of caspase-8 to the receptor complex results in activation of this protease, which can then amplify downstream caspase activation, either directly (type I pathway) or indirectly by cleaving Bid and provoking cytochrome c release from mitochondria (type II pathway) that activates the Apaf-1/caspase-9 "apoptosome." The apoptosome then promotes activation of downstream effector caspases that kill the cell (cf Figure 1.25).

Fas-dependent killing

CTLs are also endowed with a second killing mechanism involving Fas and its ligand (Figure 9.15). In this situation, engagement of the trimeric Fas receptor by membrane-borne Fas ligand on the CTL initiates a signaling pathway within the target cell that results in the recruitment and activation of caspase-8 at the receptor complex (Figure 9.18). Upon activation, caspase-8 can further propagate the death signal through restricted proteolysis of Bid, similar to the granzyme B pathway discussed above, or can directly process and activate downstream caspases such as caspase-3. However, the inability of perforin knockout mice to clear viruses effectively suggests that the secretory granules provide the dominant means of killing virally infected cells. One should also not lose sight of the fact that CD8 cells synthesize other cytokines, such as TNF and IFNγ, that also have potent antiviral effects.

Caspase activation coordinates target cell death from within

As we have seen, the final common pathway to cell death involves the activation of members of the caspase family of proteases within the target cell, irrespective of whether killing has been initiated via the perforin/granzyme or Fas receptor pathway. Caspases kill cells through restricted proteolysis (i.e. by cutting proteins at only one or two sites) of literally **hundreds of substrate proteins**. To date, over 600 substrates for the apoptotic caspases have been identified using global proteomic analyses. This **"death by a thousand cuts"** approach ensures that the failure to cleave a few proteins here or there is unlikely to allow a cell to escape from the clutches of these destructive enzymes once they have been set in motion. In addition to killing the target cell, caspases also trigger alterations to the plasma membrane that attract the attentions of local phagocytic cells, to promote clearance of the dying cell (Figure 9.19). Several plasma membrane alterations have been found to occur on apoptotic cells, most notably the externalization of phosphatidylserine, a phospholipid that is normally confined to the inner leaflet of the plasma membrane.

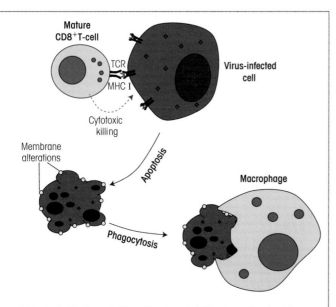

Figure 9.19. Apoptotic cells are rapidly recognized and removed by phagocytes.

Apoptotic cells acquire multiple membrane alterations (phosphatidylserine externalization on the outer leaflet of the plasma membrane being one example) that enable professional as well as nonprofessional phagocytes to recognize and engulf such cells prior to membrane rupture and release of intracellular contents. In the context of cytotoxic T-cell (Tc) killing of a virus-infected cell, this may also prevent the release of viral particles that would otherwise occur if cell death took place via necrosis (i.e. cell rupture).

Apoptotic cells are rapidly cleared through phagocytosis

The induction of apoptosis, as opposed to necrosis, by the CTL is likely to have several benefits. Apoptotic cells, by virtue of the specific alterations to their plasma membranes mentioned in the preceding section, are swiftly recognized by macrophages and other phagocytic cells and undergo phagocytosis before their intracellular contents can leak. These membrane alterations promote the selective recognition and rapid engulfment of apoptotic cells by tissue-resident macrophages, as well as nonprofessional phagocytic cells (Figure 9.19). The rapid removal of apoptotic cells from a tissue has the desirable effect of minimizing collateral damage to neighboring cells and may also prevent escape of viral particles from an infected cell. Moreover, the nucleases and caspase proteases that become activated within the target cell during apoptosis are also likely to degrade viral nucleic acids and structural proteins and may also contribute to ensuring that infectious viral particle release is kept to a minimum.

Proliferation and maturation of B-cell responses are mediated by cytokines

Upon successful activation of a T-helper cell within the T-cell areas of a lymph node, the activated T-cell then sets off, guided by chemokines, in search of a B-cell to provide help to. Within the B-cell areas of the lymph node, B-cells that have been activated through cross-linking of their surface immunoglobulin with cognate antigen presented on follicular dendritic cells require help from Th cells for full activation. To receive help, the B-cell needs to present the correct antigenic peptide to a T-cell that has already received stimulation by a DC. The activation of B-cells by Th cells, through the TCR recognition of MHC-linked antigenic peptide plus the co-stimulatory **CD40L–CD40 interaction**, leads to upregulation of the surface receptor for IL-4. Copious local release of this cytokine from the Th then drives powerful clonal proliferation and expansion of the activated B-cell population. IL-2 and IL-13 also contribute to this process (Figure 9.11).

Under the influence of IL-4 and IL-13, the expanded clones can differentiate and mature into IgE synthesizing cells. TGFβ and IL-5 encourage cells to switch their Ig class to IgA. IgM plasma cells emerge under the tutelage of IL-4 plus -5, and IgG producers result from the combined influence of IL-4, -5, -6, -13 and IFNγ (Figure 9.11).

Type 2 thymus-independent antigens can activate B-cells directly (cf. p. 217) but nonetheless still need cytokines for efficient proliferation and Ig production. These may come from accessory cells such as NK and NKT-cells that bear lectin-like receptors.

What is going on in the germinal center?

The secondary follicle with its corona or mantle of small lymphocytes surrounding the pale germinal center is a striking and unique cellular structure. First, let us recall the overall events described in Chapter 7. Secondary challenge with antigen or immune complexes induces enlargement of germinal centers, formation of new ones, appearance of memory B-cells and development of Ig-producing cells of higher affinity. B-cells entering the germinal center become **centroblasts** that divide with a very short cycle time of 6 hours, and then become nondividing **centrocytes** in the basal light zone, many of which die from apoptosis (Figure 9.20). As the surviving centrocytes mature, they differentiate either into **immunoblast plasma cell precursors**, which secrete Ig in the absence of antigen, or into **memory B-cells**.

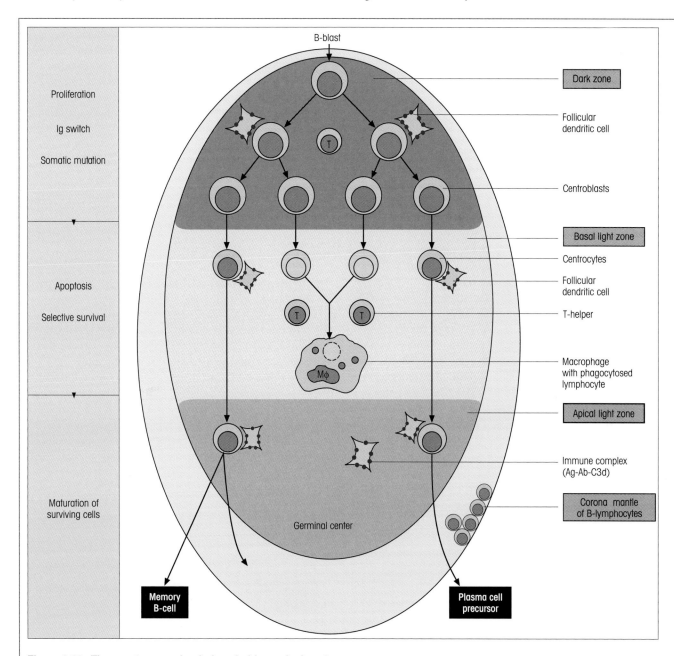

Figure 9.20. The events occurring in lymphoid germinal centers.

Germinal center B-cells can be enriched through their affinity for the peanut agglutinin lectin. They show numerous mutations in the antibody genes. Expression of LFA-1 and ICAM-1 on B-cells and follicular dendritic cells (FDCs) in the germinal center makes them "sticky." Centroblasts at the base of the follicle are strongly CD77 positive. The Th cells bear the unusual CD57 marker. The FDCs all express CD21 and CD54; those in the apical light zone are strongly CD23 positive, those in the basal light zone express little CD23. Through their surface receptors, FDCs bind immune complexes containing antigen and C3 that, in turn, are very effective B-cell stimulators as coligation of the surface receptors for antigen and C3 (CR2) lowers their threshold for activation. The co-stimulatory molecules CD40 and B7 play pivotal roles. Antibodies to CD40 prevent formation of germinal centers and anti-CD40L can disrupt established germinal centers within 12 hours. Anti-B7.2, given early in the immune response, prevents germinal center formation and, when given at the onset of hypermutation, suppresses that process.

What then is the underlying scenario? Following secondary antigen challenge, primed B-cells may be activated by para-cortical Th cells in association with interdigitating dendritic cells or macrophages, and migrate to the germinal center. There they divide in response to powerful stimuli from complexes on follicular dendritic cells (cf. p. 203) and from cytokines released by T-cells in response to antigen-presenting B-cells. During this particularly frenetic bout of cell division, **somatic hypermutation** of B-cell Ig genes occurs. The cells also undergo **Ig class switching**. Thereafter, as they transform to centrocytes, they are vulnerable and die readily, whence they are taken up as the "tingible bodies" by macrophages, unless rescued by association with antigen on a follicular dendritic cell. This could result from cross-linking of surface Ig receptors and is accompanied by expression of Bcl-x and Bcl-2 that protect against apoptosis. Interactions between BAFF (*B-cell-activating factor* of the tumor necrosis factor family; also called BLyS) on the T-helper cell and TACI (*transmembrane activator and calcium modulator and cyclophilin ligand* [CAML] *inter-actor*), its receptor on the B-cell, may also be important for the maintenance of germinal center B-cells. Signaling through CD40 and TACI, during presentation of antigen to Th cells, would also prolong the life of the centrocyte. In either case, the interactions will only occur if the mutated surface Ig receptor still binds antigen and, as the concentration of antigen gradually falls, only if the receptor is of high affinity. In other words, the system can deliver high affinity antibody by a darwinian process of high frequency mutation of the Ig genes and selection by antigen of the cells bearing the antibody that binds most strongly (Figure 9.21). This increase of affinity as the antibody level falls late in the response is of obvious benefit, as a small amount of high affinity antibody can do the job of a large amount of low affinity (as in boxing, a small "goodun" will generally be a match for a mediocre "bigun").

Further differentiation now occurs. The cells either migrate to the sites of plasma cell activity (e.g. lymph node medulla) or go to expand the memory B-cell pool depending upon the cytokine and other signals received. CD40 engagement by CD40 ligand on a T-cell guides the B-cell into the memory compartment.

The synthesis of antibody

The sequential processes by which secreted Ig arises are illustrated in Figure 9.22. In the normal antibody-forming cell there is a rapid turnover of light chains that are present in slight excess. Defective control occurs in many myeloma cells and one may see excessive production of light chains or complete suppression of heavy chain synthesis.

The variable and constant regions are spliced together in the mRNA before leaving the nucleus. Differential splicing mechanisms also provide a rational explanation for the coexpression of surface IgM and IgD with identical V regions on a single cell, and for the switch from production of membrane-bound IgM receptor to secretory IgM in the antibody-forming cell (cf. Figures 4.2 and 4.3).

Immunoglobulin class switching occurs in individual B-cells

The synthesis of antibodies belonging to the various immunoglobulin classes proceeds at different rates. Usually there is an early IgM response that tends to fall off rapidly. IgG antibody synthesis builds up to its maximum over a longer time period. On secondary challenge with antigen, the time-course of the IgM response resembles that seen in the primary. By contrast, the synthesis of IgG antibodies rapidly accelerates to a much higher titer and there is a relatively slow fall-off in serum antibody levels (Figure 9.23). The same probably holds

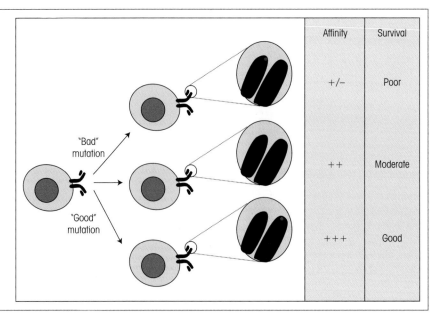

Figure 9.21. Darwinian selection by antigen of B-cells with antibody mutants of high affinity

protects against cell death in the germinal center, either through cross-linking of sIg by antigen on follicular dendritic cells, or through Th cell recognition of processed antigen and signaling through CD40. In both cases, capture of antigen, particularly as the concentration falls, will be critically affected by the affinity of the surface receptor.

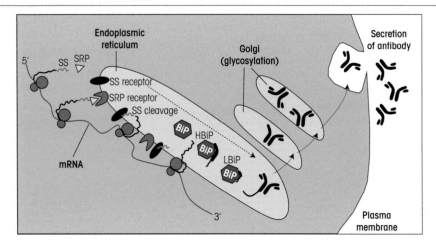

Figure 9.22. Synthesis of immunoglobulin.

As mRNA is translated on the ribosome, the N-terminal signal sequence (SS) is bound by a signal recognition particle (SRP) that docks onto a receptor on the outer membrane of the endoplasmic reticulum (ER) and facilitates entry of the nascent Ig chain into the ER lumen. The SS associates with a specific membrane receptor and is cleaved; the remainder of the chain, as it elongates, complexes with the molecular chaperone BiP (immunoglobulin-binding protein) that binds to the heavy chain C_H1 and V_L domains to control protein folding. The unassembled chains oxidize and dissociate as the full H_2L_2 Ig molecule. The assembled H_2L_2 molecules can now leave the ER for terminal glycosylation in the Golgi and final secretion. Surface receptor Ig would be inserted by its hydrophobic sequences into the membrane of the endoplasmic reticulum as it was synthesized.

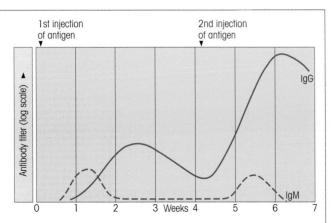

Figure 9.23. Synthesis of IgM and IgG antibody classes in the primary and secondary responses to antigen.

for IgA, and in a sense both these immunoglobulin classes provide the main immediate defense against future penetration by foreign antigens.

As we saw in chapters 3 and 4, individual B-cells can switch over from IgM to IgG production. For example, antigen challenge of irradiated recipients receiving relatively small numbers of lymphoid cells produced splenic foci of cells, each synthesizing antibodies of different heavy chain class bearing a single idiotype; the common idiotype suggests that each focus is derived from a single precursor cell whose progeny can form antibodies of different class.

Antibody synthesis in most classes shows considerable dependence upon T-cell cooperation in that the responses in T-deprived animals are strikingly deficient; such is true of mouse IgG1, IgG2a, IgA, IgE and part of the IgM antibody responses. T-independent antigens such as the polyclonal activator, lipopolysaccharide (LPS) endotoxin, induce synthesis of IgM with some IgG2b and IgG3. Immunopotentiation by complete Freund's adjuvant, a water-in-oil emulsion containing antigen in the aqueous phase and a suspension of killed tubercle bacilli in the oil phase (see p. 365), seems to occur, at least in part through the activation of Th cells that stimulate antibody production in T-dependent classes. The prediction from this, that the response to T-independent antigens (e.g. pneumococcus polysaccharide, p. 217) should not be potentiated by Freund's adjuvant, is borne out in practice; furthermore, as mentioned previously, these antigens evoke primarily IgM antibodies and poor immunological memory, as do T-dependent antigens injected into T-cell-deficient, neonatally thymectomized hosts.

Thus, in rodents at least, the switch from IgM to IgG and other classes appears to be largely under T-cell control critically mediated by CD40 and by cytokines, as we have discussed earlier in this chapter (see p. 248). Let us take another look at the stimulation of small, surface IgM-positive, B-cells by LPS. As we noted, on its own, the nonspecific mitogen evokes the synthesis of IgM, IgG3 and some IgG2b. Following addition of IL-4 to the system, there is class switching from IgM to IgE and IgG1 production, whereas IFNγ stimulates class switching from IgM to IgG2a and TGFβ induces switching from IgM to IgA or IgG2b. These cytokines induce the formation of germline sterile transcripts that start at the I (initiation) exon 5′ of the switch region for the antibody class to which

Figure 9.24. Class switching to produce antibodies of identical specificity but different immunoglobulin isotype (in this example from IgM to IgG1) is achieved by a recombination process that utilizes the specialized switch sequences (●) and leads to a loss of the intervening DNA loop (μ, δ and γ3). Each switch sequence is 1–10 kilobases in length and comprises guanosine-rich repeats of 20–100 base-pairs. Because the switch sequence associated with each C_H gene has a unique nucleotide sequence, recombination cannot occur homologously and therefore probably depends upon nonhomologous end joining. DNA repair proteins including Ku70, Ku80 and the catalytic subunit of the DNA-dependent protein kinase (DNA-PK$_{CS}$) are involved in this process.

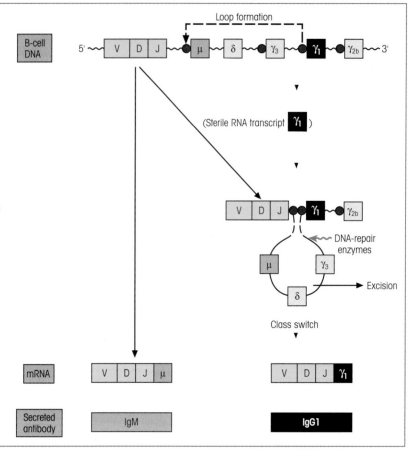

Class-switched B-cells are subject to high mutation rates after the initial response

The reader will no doubt recollect that this idea was raised in Chapters 3 and 4 when discussing the generation of diversity, and that the germinal center has been identified as the site of intense mutagenesis, which is catalyzed by activation-induced cytidine deaminase (AID). The latter removes an amino (NH$_2$) group from deoxycytidine within DNA, triggering a modified DNA-repair reaction that results in mutation of this base to any one of the four nucleotides. This reaction takes place within certain hotspots in Ig genes, guided by sequence motifs as well as chromatin modifications, such that AID-dependent mutations occur preferentially within V regions. The normal V-region mutation rate is of the order of 10^{-5}/base-pair per cell

switching will occur and terminate at the polyadenylation site 3′ of the relevant C_H gene (Figure 9.24). The transcripts are not translated but instead remain associated with the template DNA, forming RNA–DNA hybrids within the S regions of the DNA that might act as targets for enzymes involved in the recombination process. Under the influence of the recombinase, a given *VDJ* gene segment is transferred from μδ to the new constant region gene (Figure 9.24), so yielding antibodies of the same specificity but of different class.

division, but this rises to 10^{-3}/base-pair per generation in B-cells as a result of antigenic stimulation. This process is illustrated in Figure 9.25 that charts the accumulation of somatic mutations in the immunodominant V_H/V_k antibody structure during the immune response to phenyloxazolone. With time and successive boosting, the mutation rate is seen to rise dramatically and, in the context of the present discussion, it is clear that the strategically targeted hypermutations occurring within or adjacent to the complementarity determining hypervariable loops (Figure 9.26) can give rise to cells that secrete antibodies having a different combining affinity to that of the original parent cell. Randomly, some mutated daughter cells will have higher affinity for antigen, some the same or lower and others perhaps none at all (cf. Figure 9.21). Similarly, mutations in the framework regions may be "silent" or, if they disrupt the folding of the protein, give rise to non-functional molecules. Pertinently, the proportion of germinal center B-cells with "silent" mutations is high early in the immune response but falls dramatically with time, suggesting that early diversification is followed by preferential expansion of clones expressing mutations that improve their chances of reacting with and being stimulated by antigen. B-cells expressing mutated antibodies that now fail to recognize antigen undergo apoptosis, as continued antigenic stimulation via the B-cell receptor is required for B-cell survival during this phase.

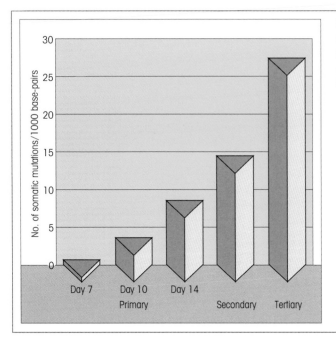

Figure 9.25. Increasing somatic mutations in the immunodominant germline antibody observed in hybridomas isolated following repeated immunization with phenyloxazolone. (Data from Berek C. & Apel M. (1989) In: Melchers F. *et al.* (eds.) *Progress in Immunology* **7**, 99, Springer-Verlag, Berlin.)

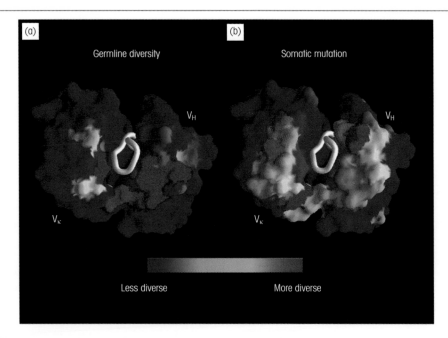

Figure 9.26. An "antigen's eye view" of sequence diversity in human antibodies.

The sequence diversity has been plotted on a scale of blue (more conserved) to red (more diverse). The V_H domain is on the right and the V_k domain on the left in both pictures. (a) Germline diversity prior to somatic hypermutation is focused at the center of the antigen-binding site. (b) Somatic hypermutation spreads diversity to regions at the periphery of the binding site that are highly conserved in the germline *V* gene repertoire. Somatic hypermutation is therefore complementary to germline diversity. The V_H CDR3, which lies at the center of the antigen-binding site, was not included in this analysis and therefore is shown in gray as a loop structure. The end of the V_k CDR3 (also excluded) lies at the center of the binding site and is not visible in this representation. (Reproduced with kind permission from Tomlinson I.M. *et al.* (1996) *Journal of Molecular Biology* **256**, 813.)

Factors affecting antibody affinity in the immune response

The effect of antigen dose

Other things being equal, the binding strength of an antigen for the surface receptor of a B-cell will be determined by the affinity constant of the reaction:

$$Ag + (surface)Ab \leftrightarrow AgAb$$

and the reactants will behave according to the laws of thermo-dynamics (cf. p. 118).

It may be supposed that, when a sufficient number of antigen molecules are bound to the receptors on the cell surface and processed for presentation to T-cells, the lymphocyte will be stimulated to develop into an antibody-producing clone. When only small amounts of antigen are present, only those lymphocytes with high affinity receptors will be able to bind sufficient antigen for stimulation to occur and their daughter cells will, of course, also produce high affinity antibody. Consideration of the antigen–antibody equilibrium equation will show that, as the concentration of antigen is increased, even antibodies with relatively low affinity will bind more antigen; therefore, at high doses of antigen, the lymphocytes with lower affinity receptors will also be stimulated and, as may be seen from Figure 9.27, these are more abundant than those with receptors of high affinity. Furthermore, there is a strong possibility that cells with the highest affinity will bind so much antigen as to become tolerized (cf. p. 304). Thus, in summary, low amounts of antigen produce high affinity antibodies, whereas high antigen concentrations give rise to an antiserum with low-to-moderate affinity.

Maturation of affinity

In addition to being brisker and fatter, secondary responses tend to be of higher affinity. There are probably two main reasons for this maturation of affinity after primary stimulation. First, once the primary response gets under way and the antigen concentration declines to low levels, only successively higher affinity cells will bind sufficient antigen to maintain proliferation. Second, at this stage the cells are mutating madly in the germinal centers, and any mutants with an adventitiously higher affinity will bind well to antigen on follicular dendritic cells and be positively selected for by its persistent clonal expansion. Modification of antibody specificity by somatic point mutations allows gradual diversification on which positive selection for affinity can act during clonal expansion.

It is worth noting that responses to thymus-independent antigens, which have poorly developed memory with very rare mutations, do not show this phenomenon of affinity maturation. Overall, the ability of Th to facilitate responses to nonpolymeric, nonpolyclonally activating antigens, to induce expansive clonal proliferation, to effect class switching

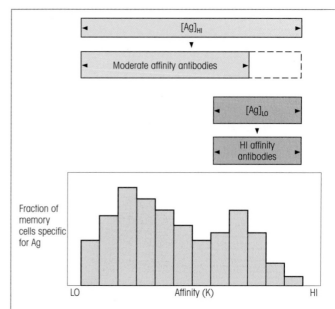

Figure 9.27. Relationship of antigen concentration to affinity of antibodies produced.

Low concentrations of antigen ([Ag]$_{LO}$) bind to and permit stimulation of a range of high affinity memory cells and the resulting antibodies are of high affinity. High doses of antigen ([Ag]$_{HI}$) are able to bind sufficiently to the low affinity cells and thereby allow their stimulation, whilst the highest affinity cells may bind an excess of antigen and be tolerized (dashed line); the resulting antiserum will have a population of low-to-moderate affinity antibodies.

and, lastly, to fine-tune responses to higher affinity has provided us with bigger, better and more flexible immune responses.

Memory cells

As the immune response subsides, the majority of recently expanded effector cells are culled by large-scale induction of apoptosis in this population. In chapter 8, we discussed the important role of Fas–Fas ligand interactions in this process and how activated effector T-cells become susceptible to Fas ligand-bearing cells as they age. The source of Fas ligand that is responsible for eliminating recently expanded T-cells can be the T-cell itself, thus activated T-cells can kill themselves in an autocrine (i.e. suicidal) manner, or can be killed by neighboring T-cells bearing Fas ligand in a paracrine (i.e. fratricidal) manner. Whereas both naive as well as activated T-cells express the Fas receptor, the former are protected from the cell-killing effects of Fas ligand due to the expression of a molecule (FLIP) that disrupts the signaling cascade downstream of receptor stimulation that would otherwise activate the cell-killing properties of this cascade. B-cells are also susceptible to Fas ligand-dependent killing, particularly if they fail to receive CD40L-dependent stimulation from a cognate Th2 cell.

However, a subpopulation of cells escape the culling process and these form the **memory compartment** that live to mount a more rapid and efficient secondary immune response upon re-exposure to the same antigen. It is possible that the memory cell population represents a subpopulation of cells that bypass the effector cell stage entirely, but this concept remains controversial. The process of memory cell generation is central to the concept of vaccination and memory cells have been the subjects of much investigation as a consequence.

The generation of memory

It is not clear whether memory cells and effector cells are derived from the same cell compartment or represent distinct differentiation trajectories of activated lymphocytes. It has been suggested that memory and effector cells may be demarcated through **asymmetric division** of T-cells upon productive stimulation with antigen (Figure 9.28). In this model, the cell pole nearest to the immunological synapse (i.e. the point at which the T-cell and DC or target cell make productive TCR–peptide/MHC interactions) may have a distribution of **cell fate determinants** (i.e. transcription factors) different to the opposite cell pole. The distribution of cell fate determinants within a cell can be regulated by polarity complex proteins. Subsequent division of the activated T-cell may distribute such cell fate determinants asymmetrically between daughter cells, and this could set up the subsequent effector versus memory cell differentiation trajectories (Figure 9.28). There is some evidence to support such a model, with the polarity complex protein Scribble, associating with the immunological synapse, whereas another polarity complex protein, PKCζ, has been found to associate with the opposite cell pole. Furthermore, some studies have reported that the daughter cell inheriting the immunological synapse had greater expression levels of LFA-1 and became effector cells, with the other cell pole becoming memory cells (Figure 9.28). However, there is also evidence that effector cells can become memory cells, so the issue is not clear-cut.

Is antigen persistence required for the maintenance of memory?

Antibodies encoded by unmutated germline genes represent a form of evolutionary memory, in the sense that they tend to include specificities for commonly encountered pathogens and are found in the so-called "natural antibody" fraction of serum. Memory acquired during the adaptive immune response requires contact with antigen and expansion of antigen-specific memory cells, as seen for example in the 20-fold increase in cytotoxic T-cell precursors after immunization of females with the male H-Y antigen.

Memory of early infections such as measles is long-lived and **the question arises as to whether the memory cells are long-lived or are subject to repeated antigen stimulation from persisting antigen or subclinical reinfection.** Peter Panum in 1847 described a measles epidemic on the Faroe

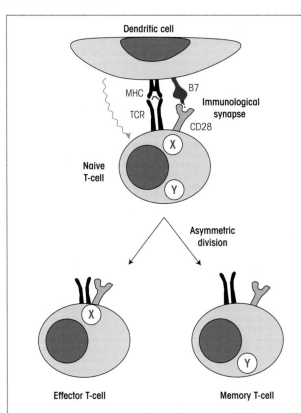

Figure 9.28. Asymmetric cell divsion may contribute to the generation of effector versus memory cells.

A possible mechanism for the generation of effector versus long-lived memory T-cells is through asymmetric division of activated naive T-cells due to unequal distribution of cell fate determinants, designated "X" and "Y" here for illustrative purposes, that can influence cell fate commitment. Cell fate determinants could be transcription factors that can commit cells to distinct differentiation pathways and may be unequally segregated within cells as a result of tethering to different polarity complex proteins that restrict their free diffusion. In the diagram above, cell fate determinant "X" is tethered close to the immunological synapse and specifies an effector cell fate upon subsequent cell division. In contrast, cell fate determinant "Y" is tethered at the opposite pole and commits the cell to a memory fate upon subsequent division.

Islands in the previous year in which almost the entire population suffered from infection except for a few old people who had been infected 65 years earlier. While this evidence favors the long half-life hypothesis, memory function of B-cells transferred to an irradiated syngeneic recipient is lost within a month unless antigen is given or the donor is transgenic for the *bcl-2* gene (remember that signals in the germinal center that prevent apoptosis of centrocytic B-cells also upregulate *bcl-2* expression). It is envisaged that B-cell memory is a dynamic state in which survival of the memory cells is maintained by recurrent signals from follicular dendritic cells in the germinal centers, the only long-term repository of antigen.

Evidence from mouse models strongly suggests that **memory T-cells can, at least in principle, persist in the absence of antigen**. T-cells isolated from mice several months after they were immunized with lymphocytic choriomeningitis virus (LCMV) were transferred into two groups of genetically modified mice that lacked endogenous T-cells, one of the groups additionally lacking MHC class I expression. T-cells were parked in these mice for 10 months and then analysed *in vitro*. Functional virus-specific CD8+ CTLs were still present in both groups of mice, and in similar numbers, even though those from the class I⁻ mice could not have had antigen presented to their TCR. Indeed, these memory T-cells undergo antigen- and MHC-independent proliferation *in vivo*, their numbers controlled, at least in part, by a balance between proliferation-inducing signals from IL-15 and cell death-inducing signals from IL-2 released in the local environment, both cytokines binding to the IL-2R β chain (cf. Figure 9.4). Other recent findings indicate that helper T-cell memory also does not require the continued presence of antigen or MHC and, at least in some cases, Th memory is maintained in the absence of cell division.

However, we should not lose sight of the fact that, while these experiments in transgenic and knockout animals clearly demonstrate that immunological memory *can* be maintained in the absence of antigen, usually antigen persists as complexes on follicular dendritic cells. Therefore, there is the potential for antigen-presenting cells within the germinal center to capture and process this complexed antigen and then present it to memory T-cells. Some evidence, again recent, suggests that it is a type of dendritic cell, and not the germinal center B-cells, that may subserve this function. To add complexity, there is also accumulating evidence that the mechanisms used to maintain memory T-cells in the mouse, a relatively short-lived animal, may differ significantly from those employed by the human immune system. **Specific antigen may play a much more important role in maintaining T-lymphocyte memory in man, not least because ongoing entry of new memory cells specific for diverse antigens to the memory compartment will generate competition between memory cells.** Because the naive and memory cell pools are maintained at a relatively constant size, it is likely that memory cells that receive periodic re-stimulation with antigen are likely to persist for longer than those that fail to re-encounter antigen. Competition may be absent or diminished in mouse models where animals are typically maintained in artificially clean environments; such cosseting is likely to reduce the rate of entry of new T-cell specificities to the memory compartment and therefore reduce competition between memory cell populations. In support of this view, while there is evidence that T-cell memory in humans can persist for decades after exposure to particular antigens, immunity does indeed decline over time and estimates of the half-life of T-cell responses have put this between 8 and 15 years. In addition, because the lifespan of the laboratory mouse is far shorter than the average human, the problems associated with retention of memory cells in the

human are likely to be greater than those faced by laboratory mice. Ongoing attrition of memory T-cells, in the absence of antigenic re-stimulation, may contribute to the increased rate and severity of infectious diseases in the elderly and may also explain why latent viruses, such as varicella zoster (human herpesvirus 3), may reactivate many years after initial infection.

The memory population is not simply an expansion of corresponding naive cells

In general, memory cells are more readily stimulated by a given dose of antigen because they have a higher affinity. In the case of B-cells, we are satisfied by the evidence that links mutation and antigen-driven selection, occurring within the germinal centers of secondary lymph node follicles, to the creation of high affinity memory cells. The receptors for antigen on memory T-cells also have higher affinity but, as they do not undergo significant somatic mutation during the priming response, it would seem that cells with **pre-existing receptors of relatively higher affinity in the population of naive cells proliferate selectively through preferential binding to the antigen**.

Intuitively one would not expect to improve on affinity to the same extent that somatic hypermutation can achieve for the B-cells, but nonetheless memory T-cells augment their binding avidity for the antigen-presenting cell through increased expression of accessory adhesion molecules, CD2, LFA-1, LFA-3 and ICAM-1. As several of these molecules also function to enhance signal transduction, the memory T-cell is more readily triggered than its naive counterpart. Indeed, memory cells enter cell division and secrete cytokines more rapidly than naive cells, and there is some evidence that they may secrete a broader range of cytokines than do naive cells.

A phenotypic change in the isoform of the leukocyte common antigen CD45R, derived by differential splicing, allows some distinction to be made between naive and memory cells. Expression of CD45RA has been used as a marker of naive T-cells and of CD45RO as a marker of memory cells capable of responding to recall antigens. However, most of the features associated with the CD45RO subset are in fact manifestations of **activated cells** and CD45RO cells can revert to the CD45RA phenotype. Memory cells, perhaps in the absence of antigenic stimulation, may therefore lose their activated status and join a resting pool. Another marker used for differentiating naive from memory cells takes one step back on the CD ladder and utilizes differences in the relative expression of the adhesion molecule CD44; naive T-cells seem to express low levels of CD44 whilst memory T-cells express high levels.

A role for CD44 in antagonizing Fas-dependent signals for apoptosis

Recent evidence suggests that CD44 may be important for entry into the memory cell compartment through the

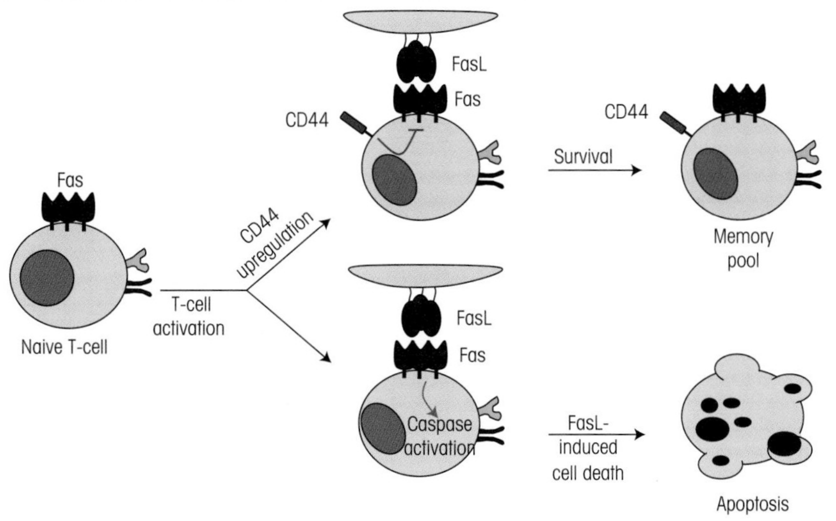

Figure 9.29. CD44 can antagonize Fas–Fas ligand-dependent apoptosis of expanded T-cells.

T-cells become susceptible to apoptosis-triggering signals routed through surface Fas receptors within a few days after activation. The source of Fas ligand (FasL) can be from the activated T-cell itself (autocrine), a neighboring activated T-cell (paracrine), a cytotoxic T-cell, or a dendritic cell. Upregulation of surface CD44 appears to be able to interfere with Fas-dependent signals for apoptosis, via a mechanism that remains to be defined, and this may protect activated T-cells from deletion and permit entry into the memory compartment. Note that this mechanism may only apply to Th1 cells.

inhibition of Fas-dependent signals for apoptosis (Figure 9.29). As we discussed above, Fas–FasL interactions play an important role in the elimination of a sizable proportion of recently activated lymphocytes. In addition to becoming susceptible to FasL-driven apoptosis, activated T-cells upregulate surface expression of CD44 and maintain high expression thereafter but the role of CD44 in T-cell function was somewhat unclear; however, recent observations implicate CD44 as having a role in dictating entry into the memory compartment. Influenza-specific CD44-deficient versus wild type Th1 cells were adoptively transferred into wild type mice and subsequent antigenic challenge found that whereas robust antigen recall responses could be found in the CD44-positive cells, CD44-deficient cells failed to respond to antigen. CD44 deficiency did not appear to impact on either T-cell activation, expansion in response to antigen, or acquisition of effector function. However, such cells were susceptible to Fas-dependent apoptosis during the later stages of expansion unlike their CD44-expressing counterparts, although the mechanisms for this effect remain unclear. A caveat is that CD44-mediated protection appears to apply only to Th1 cells and thus different mechanisms may operate in different T-cell subsets.

Lanzavecchia and colleagues have proposed that the CCR7 chemokine receptor allows a distinction to be made between CCR7+ "central memory" T-cells, which differentiate from naive T-cells, and CCR7− "effector memory" T-cells, which subsequently arise from the central memory T-cells (Figure 9.30). Both populations are long-lived. The central memory cells provide a clonally expanded pool of antigen-primed cells that can travel to secondary lymphoid organs under the influence of the CCL21 (SLC) chemokine (cf. Table 9.2) and, following re-encounter with antigen, can stimulate dendritic cells, help B-cells and generate effector cells. In contrast, effector memory T-cells possess CCR1, CCR3 and CCR5 receptors

for proinflammatory chemokines and constitute tissue-homing cells that mediate inflammatory reactions or cytotoxicity.

Maintenance of memory cells

Recently, IL-7 has emerged as a key regulator of peripheral T-cell survival and homeostatic turnover. Unlike most other cytokines that use receptors containing the common γ-chain (CD132), IL-7 is produced constitutively at low levels, is detectable in human serum, and may contribute to the antigen-independent maintenance of CD4 and CD8 memory T-cells by stimulating homeostatic division of these cells. Whereas studies using MHC-deficient mice have shown that peptide–MHC interactions are not essential for the persistence of memory T-cells, CD4 T-cells decline rapidly in the absence of IL-7. The expression of IL-7R is highest on resting cells, ensuring that these cells compete more effectively for available IL-7 than activated effector T-cells. Indeed, stimulation via the TCR induces downregulation of the receptor for IL-7 as effector T-cells come under the influence of cytokines produced during immune responses (such as IL-2, IL-4, IL-7, IL-15 and IL-21). As the response subsides, T-cells become dependent on IL-7 for their continued survival once more. Thus, the current view is that IL-7 contributes to the antigen-independent maintenance of T-cells by permitting homeostatic division of these cells in the absence of antigenic stimulation (Figure 9.31). IL-15 also appears to be more important for the maintenance of CD8 memory T-cells as mice deficient in either IL-15 or IL-15Rα chain display reduced CD8 T-cell memory that can be rescued by transfer of these cells to normal mice. Thus, IL-7 and IL-15 appear to act in concert to maintain the memory T-cell pool, the latter being particularly important for the maintenance of CD8 memory T-cells (Figure 9.31).

The persistence of memory cells may also be influenced by physical factors, such as the length of **chromosomal**

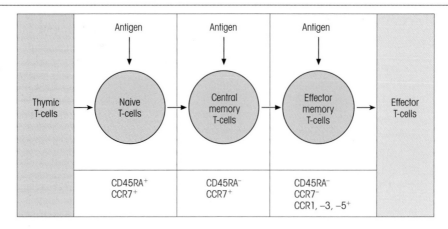

Figure 9.30. Central and effector memory T-cells.

Naive T-cells bear the CD45RA splice variant of the CD45 molecule and are attracted from the thymus into secondary lymphoid tissue under the influence of CCR7-binding chemokines such as CCL19 (MIP-3β) and CCL21 (6Ckine/SLC). Upon encounter with antigen, some of these cells become effectors of the primary immune response, whilst others differentiate into central memory T-cells that retain the CCR7 chemokine receptor but lose expression of CD45RA. Subsequent re-encounter with antigen will push these cells into the effector memory compartment with replacement of CCR7 by other chemokine receptors such as CCR1, CCR3 and CCR5. This changes the homing characteristics of these cells that can now relocate as cytokine-secreting or cytotoxic T-cells to inflammatory sites under the influence of a number of chemokines including CCL3 (MIP-1α), CCL4 (MIP-1β) and CCL5 (RANTES) (see Table 9.2). Note that whilst the activation and subsequent differentiation of these cells is dependent on antigen, both central memory and effector memory T-cells are thought to be long-lived in the absence of antigen.

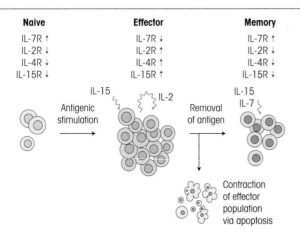

Figure 9.31. Cytokine receptor expression and cytokine availability control T-cell proliferation and survival.

Naive CD4 and CD8 T-cells express high levels of IL-7R and low levels of receptors for other cytokines, such as IL-2, IL-4 and IL-15, which can influence T-cell proliferation and survival. Antigenic stimulation induces downregulation of IL-7R and upregulation of receptors for IL-2, IL-4 and IL-15 as these cytokines sustain T-cell clonal expansion and survival during the effector phase of the immune response. During resolution of the immune response, massive apoptosis occurs within the effector cell compartment leaving only the "fittest" cells to become memory cells. The memory cell compartment appears to rely upon IL-7 for long-term survival with IL-15 also thought to be required, particularly for the maintenance of memory CD8 T-cells.

telomeres, that impose limits on the number of divisions that most mammalian cells can undergo; the so-called **Hayflick limit**. The progressive erosion of chromosomal telomeres during each cell division can result in cells entering a state of senescence from which they cannot exit. In this situation, cells are unable to divide further and are likely to be functionally compromised and therefore of little further use to the immune system. For many cell types, the Hayflick limit is typically reached within 40–50 cell divisions, but lymphocytes may be permitted somewhat more cell divisions than this due to the upregulation of the telomere-lengthening enzyme, **telomerase**, within activated lymphocytes. It has been reported that CD8 T-cells fail to upregulate telomerase after four restimulations with antigen while CD4 T-cells may retain this ability for longer.

Virgin B-cells lose their surface IgM and IgD and switch receptor isotype on becoming memory cells, and the differential expression of these surface markers has greatly facilitated the separation of B- and T-cells into naive and memory populations for further study. The co-stimulatory molecules B7.1 (CD80) and B7.2 (CD86) are rapidly upregulated on memory B-cells, and the potent ability of these cells to present antigen to T-cells could well account for the brisk and robust nature of secondary responses. A scheme similar to that outlined in Figure 9.30 for T-cells may also exist for the B-lymphocyte compartment, with an initial population of memory cells possessing the B220 marker developing into B220⁻ memory B-cells that then go on to generate antibody-secreting effector cells.

A succession of genes is upregulated by T-cell activation

- Within 15–30 minutes, genes for transcription factors concerned in the progression G0 to G1 and in the control of IL-2 are expressed.
- Up to 14 hours, cytokines and their receptors are expressed.
- Later, a variety of genes related to cell division and adhesion are upregulated.
- Activated T-cells differentiate to effector cells after 4–5 days of clonal expansion.

Effector mechanisms

- The innate immune system utilizes a number of different effector mechanisms (such as phagocytosis, complement activation and deployment of cells containing cytotoxic granules, such as NK cells and eosinophils) to combat infection
- Similarly, adaptive immunity also employs a range of effector mechanisms, including the deployment of cytotoxic T-cells (Tc or CTL), T helper cells (Th) and antibody-secreting B-cells. Th cells can be further subdivided into Th1, Th2 and Th17 cells on the basis of the cytokine profiles that these cells produce and this confers different effector functions on such cells.
- Cytokines heavily influence the generation as well as the specific function of effectors within the adaptive immune system.
- Dendritic cells, with contributions from other cells of the innate immune, system play a central role in the generation of effectors through the provision of signal 3, which represents distinct patterns of cytokines that have polarizing influences on the effector cells subsequently generated.

Cytokines act as intercellular messengers

- Cytokines act transiently and usually at short range, although circulating IL-1 and IL-6 can mediate release of acute phase proteins from the liver.
- Cytokines are mostly small proteins that act through surface receptors belonging to six structural families.
- Cytokine-induced dimerization of individual subunits of the main (hematopoietin) receptor family activates protein tyrosine kinases, including JAKs, and leads to phosphorylation and activation of STAT transcription factors.
- Cytokine signaling can be downregulated by members of the SOCS and PIAS family of inhibitors that act to suppress JAK activity or STAT-dependent transcription, respectively.
- Cytokines are pleiotropic, i.e. have multiple effects in the general areas of: (i) control of lymphocyte growth, (ii) activation of innate immune mechanisms

(including inflammation), and (iii) control of bone marrow hematopoiesis (cf. Figure 9.4).
- Cytokines may act sequentially, through one cytokine inducing production of another or by transmodulation of the receptor for another cytokine; they can also act synergistically or antagonistically.
- The roles of cytokines *in vivo* can be assessed by gene "knockout," transfection or inhibition by specific antibodies.

Activated T-cells proliferate in response to cytokines

- IL-2 acts as an autocrine growth factor for Th1 and paracrine for Th2 cells that have upregulated their IL-2 receptors.
- Cytokines act on cells that express the appropriate cytokine receptor.

Different T-cell subsets can make different cytokines

- The cytokine milieu that is established within the initial stages of infection has a significant influence on the pattern of cytokines secreted by Th cell populations.
- As immunization proceeds, Th tend to develop into three subsets: Th1 cells concerned in inflammatory processes, macrophage activation and delayed sensitivity make IL-2 and -3, IFNγ, TNF, lymphotoxin and GM-CSF; Th2 cells help B-cells to synthesize antibody and secrete IL-3, -4, -5, -6 and -13, TNF and GM-CSF; Th17 cells mount massive inflammatory responses to fungi and extracellular bacteria, especially at mucosal surfaces. Th17 cells make IL-17A, IL-21, IL-22 and IL-17F and elicit the production of pro-inflammatory cytokines and chemokines by nonimmune cells, such as endothelial cells and fibroblasts, to promote neutrophil recruitment to the site of inflammation.
- Interaction of antigen with macrophages or dendritic cells, via their Toll-like receptors (TLRs) and other pattern recognition receptors, leads to production of IL-12 and IL-27 that skews T-cell responses to the Th1 type, or IL-4 that will skew the responses to the Th2 pole. IL-6 in combination with TGFβ initially, followed by IL-23 later, is important for the production of Th17 cells.
- Other subsets may exist, including natural Foxp3+ inducibleTregs and inducible Foxp3+ Tregs or TGFβ-secreting Th3 (Tr1) regulatory cells.

CD4-positive T-cell effectors in cell-mediated immunity

- Cytokines mediate chronic inflammatory responses and induce the expression of MHC class II on endothelial cells, a variety of epithelial cells and many tumor cell lines, so facilitating interactions between T-cells and nonlymphoid cells.

■ Differential expression of chemokine receptors permits selective recruitment of neutrophils, macrophages, dendritic cells and T- and B-cells.

■ TNF synergizes with IFNγ in killing cells.

■ T-cell-mediated inflammation is strongly downregulated by IL-4 and IL-10.

Regulatory T cells (Tregs) police the actions of T helper cells

■ Different classes of Tregs exist. Natural Tregs are thymus-generated Foxp3+ T-cells that can dominantly antagonize the actions of self-reactive T-cells.

■ Inducible T-regs can be produced through suboptimal TCR-mediated stimulation especially in the presence of IL-10 or TGFβ.

■ Tregs exert their effects through multiple mechanisms, including the secretion of immunosuppressive cytokines IL-10, TGFβ and IL-35, the killing of autoreactive T-cells through granzyme B/perforin, competition for IL-2, or CTLA-4-mediated effects.

■ CTLA-4-mediated antagonism of efficient antigen presentation and co-stimulation of DCs by Tregs may be a core mechanism of action.

CD8+ T-cell effectors in cell-mediated immunity

■ Cytotoxic T-cells are generated against cells (e.g. virally infected) that have intracellularly derived peptide associated with surface MHC class I. They kill using lytic granules containing perforin and granzymes or via the Fas–Fas ligand pathway.

■ CTLs contain modified lysosomes equipped with a battery of cytotoxic proteins, collectively called cytotoxic granules. The cytotoxic granule-dependent pathway to apoptosis is orchestrated by granzyme B, a serine protease that can process and activate the mitochondrial-permeabilizing protein, Bid, as well as members of the caspase family of cell death proteases. Granzyme A also plays an important role in granule-dependent killing.

■ Fas-dependent killing is routed through caspase-8, which kills in a manner very similar to granzyme B by activating downstream caspases that then coordinate death of the cell in the manner of apoptosis.

■ Caspase activation coordinates target cell death from within. Upon activation, caspases cleave literally hundreds of cellular proteins to coordinate apoptosis.

■ Apoptotic cells are rapidly cleared through phagocytosis as a result of the appearance of membrane changes that enable phagocytes to selectively recognize and remove these cells.

Proliferation of B-cell responses is mediated by cytokines

■ Early proliferation is mediated by IL-4 that also aids IgE synthesis.

■ IgA producers are driven by TGFβ and IL-5.

■ IL-4 plus IL-5 promote IgM and IL-4, -5, -6 and -13 plus IFNγ stimulate IgG synthesis.

Events in the germinal center

■ There is clonal expansion, isotype switch and mutation in the dark zone centroblasts.

■ The B-cell centroblasts die through apoptosis unless rescued by certain signals that upregulate *bcl-2*. These include cross-linking of surface Ig by complexes on follicular dendritic cells and engagement of the CD40 receptor that drives the cell to the memory compartment.

■ The selection of mutants by antigen guides the development of high affinity B-cells.

The synthesis of antibody

■ RNA for variable and constant regions is spliced together before leaving the nucleus.

■ Differential splicing allows coexpression of IgM and IgD with identical V regions on a single cell and the switch from membrane-bound to secreted IgM.

Ig class switching occurs in individual B-cells

■ IgM produced early in the response switches to IgG, particularly with thymus-dependent antigens. The switch is largely under T-cell control.

■ IgG, but not IgM, responses improve on secondary challenge.

Antibody affinity during the immune response

■ Low doses of antigen tend to select high affinity B-cells and hence antibodies as only these can be rescued in the germinal center.

■ For the same reasons, affinity matures as antigen concentration falls during an immune response.

Memory cells

■ Upon disappearance of the source of antigen that initiated their production, the vast majority of effector lymphocytes are eliminated via apoptosis. A fraction of antigen-responsive cells are retained, possibly those with the highest affinity for antigen, and these form the memory compartment.

■ Apoptosis of activated effector lymphocytes occurs in large measure via the Fas–Fas ligand-dependent pathway. FasL may be supplied in an autocrine or paracrine manner.

■ Asymmetric division of activated lymphocytes may contribute to the generation of memory versus effector cells through the unequal distribution of cell fate determinants that influence their subsequent differentiation.

■ Murine memory T-cells can be maintained in the absence of antigen but human T-cell memory may require periodic restimulation with antigen.

■ Immune complexes on the surface of follicular dendritic cells in the germinal centers provide a long-term source of antigen.

■ Memory cells have higher affinity than naive cells, in the case of B-cells through somatic mutation, and in the case of T-cells through selective proliferation of cells with higher affinity receptors and through upregulated expression of associated molecules such as CD2 and LFA-1, that increase the avidity (functional affinity) for the antigen-presenting cell.

■ Activated memory and naive T-cells are distinguished by the expression of CD45 isoforms, the former having the CD45RO phenotype, the latter CD45RA. It seems likely that a proportion of the CD45RO population reverts to a CD45RA pool of resting memory cells. CD45RA⁻ memory cells can be divided into CCR7⁺ central memory and CCR7⁻ effector memory cells.

■ High levels of CD44 expression are also characteristic of memory T-cells, low level expression being associated with naive T-cells.

■ CD44 may participate in the generation of memory through antagonizing Fas-dependent signals for apoptosis.

■ IL-7 appears to be critical for the long-term survival of CD4 T-cell populations and is preferentially bound by resting T-cells. Memory CD8 T-cells require IL-15 for their long-term survival.

FURTHER READING

Barnes M.J. & Powrie F. (2009) Regulatory T cells reinforce intestinal homeostasis. *Immunity* **31**, 401–411.

Batista F.D. & Harwood N.E. (2009) The who, how and where of antigen presentation to B cells. *Nature Reviews Immunology* **9**, 15–27.

Beverly P.C.L. (2004) Kinetics and clonality of immunological memory in humans. *Seminars in Immunology* **16**, 315–321.

Bradley L.M., Haynes L. & Swain S.L. (2005) IL-7: maintaining T-cell memory and achieving homeostasis. *Trends in Immunology* **26**, 172–176.

Camacho S.A., Kosco-Vilbois M.H. & Berek C. (1998) The dynamic structure of the germinal center. *Immunology Today* **19**, 511–514.

Cullen S.P. & Martin S.J. (2008) Mechanisms of granule-dependent killing. *Cell Death and Differentiation* **15**, 251–62.

Fazilleau N. *et al.* (2009) Follicular helper T cells: lineage and location. *Immunity* **30**, 324–335.

Fujimoto M. & Naka T. (2003) Regulation of cytokine signaling by SOCS family molecules. *Trends in Immunology* **24**, 659–666.

Kapsenberg M.L. (2003) Dendritic cell control of pathogen-driven T-cell polarization. *Nature Reviews Immunology* **3**, 984–993.

Kinoshita K. & Honjo T. (2000) Unique and unprecedented recombination mechanisms in class switching. *Current Opinion in Immunology* **12**, 195–198.

Korn T., Bettelli E., Oukka M. & Kuchroo V.K. (2009) IL-17 and Th17 Cells. *Annual Review of Immunology* **27**, 485–517.

Lanzavecchia A. & Sallusto F. (2002) Progressive differentiation and selection of the fittest in the immune response. *Nature Reviews Immunology* **2**, 982–987.

Littman D.R. & Rudensky A.Y. (2010) Th17 and regulatory T cells in mediating and restraining inflammation. *Cell* **140**, 845–58.

Mills K.H.G. (2004) Regulatory T-cells: friend or foe in immunity to infection? *Nature Reviews Immunology* **4**, 841–855.

Mitchell D.M. & Williams M.A. (2010) An activation marker finds a function. *Immunity* **32**, 9–12.

Moser B. & Loetscher P. (2001) Lymphocyte traffic control by chemokines. *Nature Immunology* **2**, 123–128.

O'Garra A. & Murphy K.M. (2009) From IL-10 to IL-12: how pathogens and their products stimulate APCs to induce T_H1 development. *Nature Immunology* **10**, 929–932.

O'Shea J.J. & Paul W.E. (2010) Mechanisms underlying lineage commitment and plasticity of helper CD4+ T cells. *Science* **327**, 1098–1102.

Sallusto F., Mackay C.R. & Lanzavecchia A. (2000) The role of chemokine receptors in primary, effector, and memory immune responses. *Annual Review of Immunology* **18**, 593–620.

Schluns K.S. & Lefrançois L. (2003) Cytokine control of memory T-cell development and survival. *Nature Reviews Immunology* **3**, 269–279.

Shuai K. & Liu B. (2003) Regulation of JAK–STAT signalling in the immune system. *Nature Reviews Immunology* **3**, 900–911.

Sprent J. & Surh C.D. (2001) Generation and maintenance of memory T-cells. *Current Opinion in Immunology* **13**, 248–254.

Strasser A., Jost, P.J. & Nagata S. (2009) The many roles of FAS receptor signaling in the immune system. *Immunity* **30**, 180–92.

Taylor R.C., Cullen S.P. & Martin S.J. (2008) Apoptosis: controlled demolition at the cellular level. *Nature Reviews Molecular Cell Biol.* **9**, 231–241

Trinchieri G. (2003) Interleukin-12 and the regulation of innate resistance and adaptive immunity. *Nature Reviews Immunology* **3**, 133–146.

Wing K. & Sakaguchi S. (2010) Regulatory T cells exert checks and balances on self tolerance and autoimmunity. *Nat Immunol.* **11**, 7–13.

Zlotnik A. & Yoshie O. (2000) Chemokines: a new classification system and their role in immunity. *Immunity* **12**, 121–127.

Now visit **www.roitt.com**
to test yourself on this chapter.

CHAPTER 10
Control mechanisms

Key Topics

Just to Recap ...

The broadly specific phagocytic and inflammatory cells of the innate response need to migrate to the site of the infection. The lymphocytes of the adaptive response have to proliferate in organized secondary lymphoid tissues (the lymph nodes, spleen and mucosa-associated lymphoid tissues) in order to generate sufficient numbers of antigen-specific cells. T-cells must be activated by professional antigen-presenting cells, with most B-cell responses requiring help from T-cells that have specificity for the same antigen. Multiple levels of control exist to ensure that these responses are both quantitatively and qualitatively appropriate.

Introduction

Upon contact with an infectious agent the appropriate antigen-specific cells of the acquired immune response proliferate, often to form a sizable proportion of the lymphocytes in the local lymphoid tissues. However, it is crucial that this process does not become excessive as this could lead to the immune response itself causing substantial damage to our own tissues. Furthermore, it is important that responses only occur as a reaction to foreign pathogens and that once the pathogen has been eliminated the immune system returns to its resting state. It makes sense for **antigen** to be a major regulatory factor and for lymphocyte responses to be driven by the presence of an infection, falling off in intensity as the pathogen is eliminated (Figure 10.1).

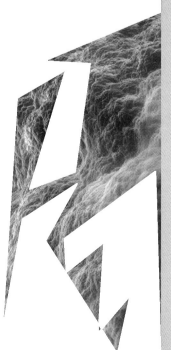

Roitt's Essential Immunology, Twelfth Edition. Peter J. Delves, Seamus J. Martin, Dennis R. Burton, Ivan M. Roitt.
© 2011 Peter J. Delves, Seamus J. Martin, Dennis R. Burton, Ivan M. Roitt. Published 2011 by Blackwell Publishing Ltd.

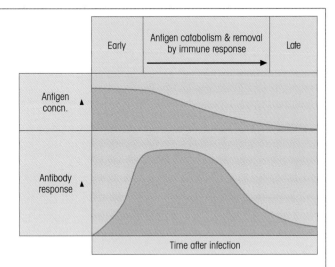

Figure 10.1. Antigen drives the immune response.

As antigen concentration falls due to catabolism and elimination by antibody, the intensity of the immune response declines, but is maintained for some time at a lower level by antigen trapped on germinal center follicular dendritic cells.

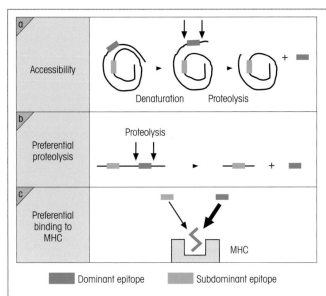

Dominant epitope   Subdominant epitope

Figure 10.2. Mechanisms of epitope dominance at the MHC level.

There is a clear hierarchy of epitopes with respect to competitive binding based on: (a) differential accessibility to proteases as the molecule unfolds; (b) the presence or absence of particular amino acid sequences that constitute protease sensitive sites; and (c) the relative affinity of the generated peptides for the MHC. Thus, dominant epitopes bag the lion's share of the available MHC grooves, subdominant epitopes are less successful, and cryptic epitopes generate miserably low concentrations of peptide–MHC that are ignored by potentially reactive naive T-cells. The other factor that can influence dominance is the availability of reactive T-cells; if these have been eliminated, e.g. through tolerization by cross-reacting self-antigens, even a peptide that dominates the MHC groove would be unable to provoke an immune response.

Antigens can interfere with each other

The presence of one antigen in a mixture of antigens can drastically diminish the immune response to the others. This is true even for epitopes within a given molecule; for example certain epitopes within the pre-S2 region of the hepatitis B surface antigen are highly immunogenic whereas others only induce relatively weak immune responses. Clearly, the possibility that certain antigens in a mixture, or particular epitopes in a given antigen, may compromise a desired protective immune response has implications for vaccine design. Factors that determine immunodominance include the precursor frequency of the T- and B-cells bearing antigen receptors for different epitopes on the antigen, the relative affinity of the B-cell receptors for their respective epitopes, the degree to which the surface membrane antibody protects the epitope from proteolysis following endocytosis of the antibody–antigen complex by the B-cell, and the ability to generate processed antigenic peptides that have a strong affinity for the *m*ajor *h*istocompatibility *c*omplex (MHC) groove (Figure 10.2).

Complement and antibody help regulate immune responses

Innate immune mechanisms are usually first on the scene and activation of the alternative pathway of complement will lead to C3b and C3d deposition on the microbe. When C3d-coated antigens are recognized by the B-cell, cross-linking of the B-cell receptor (BCR) and the CD21 complement receptor, with its associated signal-transducing molecule CD19, enhances B-cell activation (Figure 10.3a). IgM and IgG3

(which is produced relatively early following class switching in many immune responses) can also enhance the antibody response in a complement-dependent manner, and therefore presumably by the same mechanism but involving the classical pathway of complement activation. The other IgG subclasses can enhance not only antibody production but also CD4[+] T-cell responses via binding of immune complexes to activating FcγR such as FcγRI, FcγRIIA and FcγRIII and the resulting increased antigen uptake and presentation by dendritic cells. IgE antibodies can also enhance production of all antibody isotypes and promote CD4[+] T-cell responses. Here the mechanism involves FcεRII (CD23), the low affinity receptor for IgE, and probably depends on the enhancement of antigen presentation by B-cells.

Paradoxically, IgG antibodies of all subclasses can not only stimulate but also inhibit the antibody response. One mechanism by which this is known to occur for most IgG subclasses is by cross-linking of the BCR with FcγRIIb (cf. p. 64), which then delivers a negative signal by suppressing tyrosine

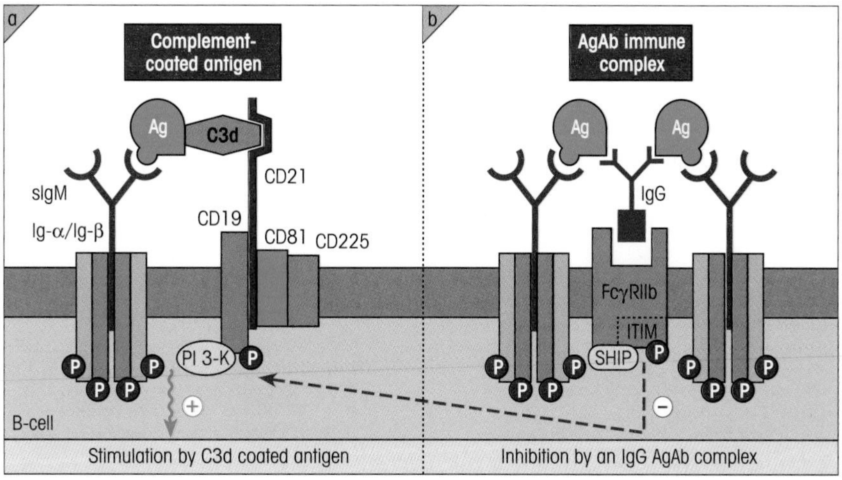

Figure 10.3. Cross-linking of surface IgM antigen receptor to the CD21 complement receptor stimulates, and to the Fcγ receptor FcγRIIb inhibits, B-cells.

(a) Following activation of complement, C3d becomes covalently bound to the microbial surface. The CD21 complement receptor, which together with its associated CD19–CD81–CD225 (Leu13) signaling complex forms the B-cell coreceptor (cf. p. 221), binds C3d. The complement-coated antigen cross-links this complex to the surface IgM (sIgM) of the BCR, leading to tyrosine phosphorylation of CD19 and subsequent binding of phosphatidylinositol 3-kinase (PI 3-K), which results in activation of the B-cell. (b) The FcγRIIb molecule possesses a cytoplasmic immunoreceptor tyrosine-based inhibitory motif (ITIM) and, upon cross-linking to membrane Ig, becomes phosphorylated and binds the inositol polyphosphate 5′-phosphatase SHIP. This suppresses phosphorylation of CD19 and thus inhibits B-cell activation.

phosphorylation of CD19 (Figure 10.3b). However, murine IgG3, which is not recognized by FcγRIIb, can also inhibit antibody production. Furthermore, inhibition can be obtained using F(ab')$_2$ fragments of polyclonal IgG and is seen in knock-out mice lacking FcγRIIb. Thus it seems that epitope masking by antibody can also inhibit antibody responses by preventing the B-cell from seeing the relevant epitopes on the antigen. Indeed it would be logical if early on when the concentration and affinity of specific antibody is low there is stimulation of the response, but later when there is an excess of antibody the combination of epitope masking and negative feedback together with antigen elimination by phagocytosis and digestion downregulates the response. Multiple considerations, including antigen concentration, antibody affinity, epitope specificity, subclass distribution, and expression levels of the relevant FcγR, probably determine whether IgG plays a stimulatory or inhibitory role during the course of an immune response.

Activation-induced cell death

Clearly the removal of antigen from the body by the immune system will lead to a downregulation of lymphocyte proliferation due to the absence of signals through the antigen receptor. However, even in the presence of antigen the potential for excessive proliferation is limited by a process referred to as *activation-induced cell death* (AICD). Subsequent to their activation, T-cells upregulate death receptors and their ligands (Figure 10.4a). The death receptors are members of the tumor necrosis factor receptor (TNF-R) family and include TNFRI, Fas (CD95), *TNF-related apoptosis-inducing ligand receptor 1* (TRAIL-R1, *death receptor* DR4) and TRAIL-R2 (DR5). If the ligands are present on cell surfaces they can activate apoptosis in adjacent cells. However, they are often released from the cell surface by proteases, producing soluble forms that in some cases retain activity; for example the soluble version of TRAIL retains the ability to signal through TRAIL-R1. Such soluble ligands can potentially mediate either paracrine or autocrine cell death *in vivo,* and show promise as tumor therapeutics. Apoptosis induction through death receptors initially involves cleavage of the inactive cysteine protease procaspase-8 to yield active caspase-8 (Figure 10.4a). Ultimately, this activation pathway converges with the mitochondrial apoptosis pathway induced by cellular stress (Figure 10.4b), both leading to the activation of downstream effector caspases.

Although the death receptor and mitochondrial pathways are activated by different stimuli they are interconnected in that caspase-8 can cleave the Bcl-2 family member Bid to produce a truncated form (tBid), which then activates Bax leading to mitochondrial outer membrane permeabilization. This allows pro-apoptotic molecules such as cytochrome *c* to be released from the space between the outer and inner

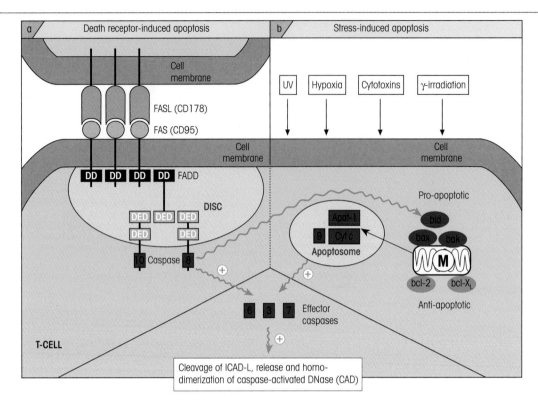

Figure 10.4. Activation-induced cell death involving death receptors and their ligands.

(a) Receptor-based induction of apoptosis involves the trimerization of TNF-R family members (e.g. Fas) by trimerized ligands (e.g. Fas-ligand). This brings together cytoplasmic death domains (DD) that can recruit a number of death effector domain (DED)-containing adaptor molecules to form the death-inducing signaling complex (DISC). The different receptors use different combinations of DED-containing adaptors; Fas uses FADD (*Fas*-associated protein with *death domain*). The DISC, which also includes caspase-10, induces the cleavage of inactive procaspase-8 into active caspase-8 with subsequent activation of downstream effector caspases. This process eventually leads to the caspase-3 mediated cleavage of the long version of the inhibitor of caspase-activated DNase (ICAD-L). Cleavage of ICAD-L results in the release of CAD, which then homodimerizes to form the active endonuclease that cleaves internucleosomal DNA. (b) A second pathway of apoptosis induction, often triggered by cellular stress, involves a number of mitochondrion (M)-associated proteins including cytochrome *c* and pro-apoptotic (Bax, Bak, Bid) and anti-apoptotic (Bcl-2, Bcl-X_L) members of the Bcl-2 family. Caspase-9 activation is the key event in this pathway and requires the formation of the "apoptosome" complex formed when cytochrome *c* is released upon Bax- and Bak-mediated permeabilization of the mitochondrial outer membrane in response to pro-apoptotic signals. Following its association with cytochrome *c* and the cofactor Apaf-1, the procaspase-9 is activated and cleaves procaspase-3. M, mitochondrion (cf. Figures 9.18 and 9.19).

mitochondrial membranes. Other members of the Bcl-2 family, such as Bcl-2 itself and Bcl-x_L, act as watchdogs to inhibit unwanted apoptosis by preventing the stimulation of outer membrane permeabilization.

Of particular relevance to death receptor-mediated AICD is the molecule FLIP, which exists in various forms. The long form of FLIP (FLIP$_L$) bears structural similarity to caspase-8, and therefore when expressed at high levels competitively inhibits recruitment of caspase-8 into the *death-inducing signaling complex* (DISC). Thus, FLIP levels can determine the fate of the cell when the death receptor is engaged by its ligand but does not affect apoptosis induced by the stress-activated mitochondrial pathway (Figure 10.5).

Immunoregulation by T-cells

Helper T-cell specialization

There is abundant evidence to suggest that helper T-cells (Th) can be divided into different subsets, with different functional activities, based upon the cytokines they produce. The three major subpopulations that have so far been defined are IFNγ-secreting Th1 cells, IL-4-secreting Th2 cells and IL-17-secreting Th17 cells. Don't worry that you have missed something because, although there are also cells referred to as Th3 cells (see below) as well as IL-9 producing Th9 cells, there aren't (as yet!) any Th cells with other numbers until you get to Th17.

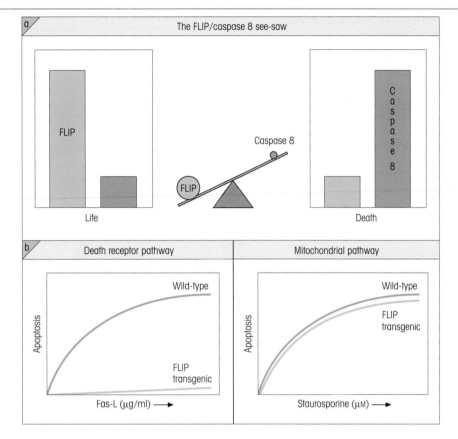

Figure 10.5. Life and death decisions.

(a) The relative amounts of anti-apoptotic FLIP and pro-apoptotic caspase-8 can determine the fate of the cell. (b) Experiments involving overexpression of FLIP in transgenic mice indicate that this protein protects T-cells from activation-induced cell death (AICD) stimulated through the death receptor pathway by Fas-ligand, but not from cell death triggered via the mitochondrial pathway using the drug staurosporine. (Based on data obtained by J. Tschopp and colleagues.)

Note, however, that although Th1 and Th2 cells are "helper" cells they can also be viewed as "suppressor" cells with respect to the fact that they mutually antagonize each other's activity (Figure 10.6a). Indeed, it is a recurrent theme in immunology that individual cells and molecules can enhance some responses whilst inhibiting others in order to maintain immune homeostasis.

The Th17 subset share with the Foxp3⁺ regulatory T-cells (Tregs, shortly to be discussed) the fact that they are induced by the cytokine TGFβ. However, Th17 cells are only induced when certain other cytokines are present (in the human IL-1β and/or IL-23, in the mouse IL-6 and/or IL-21) and therefore precursor T-cells will differentiate into **either** Tregs (in the presence of TGFβ but absence of these particular cytokines) **or** Th17 cells, leading at least in part to a reciprocal relationship between these two populations (Figure 10.6b). This situation is reinforced by the ability of the transcription factor Foxp3 in Tregs to bind to, and thereby inhibit, the RORγt transcription factor required for Th17 cell activity. Unlike the suppressive Treg cells, Th17 cells are mostly concerned with promoting tissue inflammation.

T-cell-mediated suppression

It is perhaps inevitable that nature, having evolved a functional set of T-cells that promote immune responses, should also develop a regulatory set whose job would be to modulate the helpers. T-cell mediated suppression was first brought to the serious attention of the immunological fraternity by a phenomenon colorfully named by its discoverer, Dick Gershon, as "infectious tolerance." Quite surprisingly it was shown that, if mice were made unresponsive by injection of a high dose of sheep red blood cells (SRBC), their T-cells would suppress specific antibody formation in normal recipients to which they had been transferred (Figure 10.7). It may not be apparent to the reader why this result was at all surprising, but at that time antigen-induced tolerance was regarded essentially as a negative phenomenon involving the depletion or silencing of clones

Figure 10.6. Antagonism between T-cell subpopulations.

(a) Th1 cells are generated under the direction of IL-12 production by dendritic cells. Once they are generated they can suppress the generation of Th2 cells by secreting the cytokine IFNγ, which prevents the expression of the GATA3 and STAT6 transcription factors required for the Th2 phenotype, whereas the production of IL-4 and IL-13 by Th2 cells limits the expression of the T-bet and STAT4 transcription factors associated with Th1 activity. (b) The Foxp3 transcription factor acts antagonistically against the RORγT transcription factor required for Th17 activity. Thus either Foxp3⁺ regulatory T cells (Treg) or RORγt⁺ Th17 cells will tend to dominate depending on which of these two transcription factors becomes most strongly expressed. This is at least to some extent controlled by the local cytokine environment.

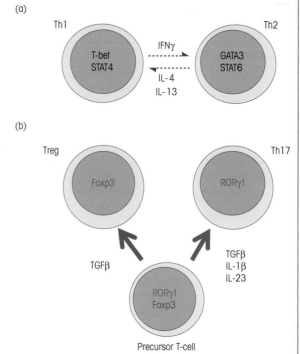

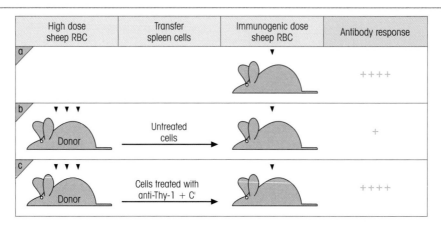

Figure 10.7. Demonstration of T-suppressor cells.

(a) A mouse of an appropriate strain immunized with an immunogenic dose of sheep erythrocytes makes a strong antibody response. However, if spleen cells from a donor of the same strain previously injected with a high dose of antigen (b) are first transferred to the syngeneic animal, they depress the antibody response to a normally immunogenic dose of the antigen. The effect is lost if the spleen cells are first treated with a T-cell-specific antiserum (anti-Thy-1) plus complement (c), showing that the suppressors are T-cells. (After Gershon R.K. & Kondo K. (1971) *Immunology* **21**, 903–914.)

rather than a state of active suppression. Over the years, T-cell-mediated suppression has been shown to modulate a variety of humoral and cellular responses, the latter including delayed-type hypersensitivity, cytotoxic T-cells and antigen-specific T-cell proliferation. However, the existence of dedicated professional T-suppressor cells was a question that generated a great deal of heat.

Suppressor and helper epitopes can be discrete

Detailed analysis of murine responses to antigens such as hen egg-white lysozyme tells us that certain determinants can evoke very strong suppression rather than help depending on the mouse strain, and also that T-cell-mediated suppression directed to one determinant can switch off helper and antibody

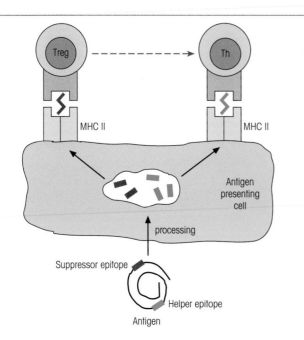

Figure 10.8. Possible mechanism to explain the need for a physical linkage between suppressor and helper epitopes.

The helper (Th) and regulatory/suppressor (Treg) cells can interact by binding close together on the surface of an antigen-presenting cell, which processes the antigen and displays the different epitopes on separate MHC class II molecules on its surface.

responses to other determinants on the same molecule. Thus mice of *H-2^b* haplotype respond poorly to lysozyme because they develop dominant suppression; however, if the three N-terminal amino acids are removed from the antigen, these mice now make a splendid response, showing that the T-regulation directed against the determinant associated with the N-terminal region has switched off the response to the remaining determinants on the antigen. Similar results have been obtained in several other systems. This situation must imply that the antigen itself acts as a form of bridge to allow communication between regulatory/suppressor T-cells and cells reacting to the other determinants, as might occur through these cells binding to an antigen-presenting cell expressing several different processed determinants of the same antigen on its surface (Figure 10.8).

Characteristics of suppression

Originally, suppressor T-cells in mice were found to possess Ly2 (now called CD8a) and Ly3 (CD8b) on their surface. As researchers began to characterize these CD8⁺ T-suppressor cells they were described as expressing a molecule called I-J encoded within the MHC region and were able to produce soluble suppressor factors that were frequently antigen-specific. These suppressor factors proved impossible to define biochemically, and when the entire murine MHC was cloned it was found

that I-J didn't exist! There then, perhaps not unsurprisingly under the circumstances, followed a period of extreme skepticism regarding the very existence of suppressor T-cells. However, during the last decade or so they have made a dramatic comeback, although it is now appreciated that the majority of these cells belong to the CD4 rather than the CD8 T-cell lineage, and the current vogue is to refer to them as **regulatory T-cells**. The characterization of these cells has itself, however, not been without its problems and there seem to be several different types of Tregs. Whilst some require cell–cell contact in order to suppress, others depend upon soluble cytokines to mediate their effect.

Both CD4⁺ and CD8⁺ T-cells can suppress immune responses

Let us first look at CD8⁺ T suppressors. One experimental example relates to the B10.A (2R) mouse strain, which has a low immune response to lactate dehydrogenase β (LDHβ) associated with the possession of the H-2Eβ gene of the k rather than b haplotype. Lymphoid cells taken from these animals after immunization with LDHβ proliferate poorly *in vitro* in the presence of antigen, but if CD8⁺ cells are depleted, the remaining CD4⁺ cells give a much higher response. Adding back the CD8⁺ cells reimposes the active suppression. Human suppressor T-cells can also belong to the CD8 subset. Thus, for example, CD8⁺CD28⁻ suppressor cells can prevent antigen-presenting B-cells from upregulating co-stimulatory B7 molecules thereby leading to an inability of these B-cells to elicit T-cell help for antibody production.

Although it is clear from such experiments that CD8⁺ T-cells can mediate suppression, the current view is that CD4⁺CD25⁺Foxp3⁺ Treg cells are the major effectors of suppression and are able to suppress the activity of CD4⁺ T-cells, CD8⁺ T-cells, dendritic cells and B-cells. If anti-CD25 and complement are used to deplete CD25⁺ cells from the lymph nodes or spleen of BALB/c mice and then the remaining CD25⁻ cells transferred into athymic (nude) BALB/c mice, the recipients develop multiple autoimmune diseases. However, if CD4⁺CD25⁺ cells are subsequently given shortly after the CD25⁻ cells the mice do not develop autoimmune disease, suggesting that the CD4⁺CD25⁺ population contains Tregs that quash autoreactive T-cells. Many similar experiments have established that CD4⁺CD25⁺ T-cells do indeed include Tregs able to mediate suppression of autoimmunity, allograft rejection and allergic responses. Because CD25 (the α chain of the IL-2 receptor) is a general marker of cell activation, it is not possible to use this as a defining characteristic of regulatory T-cells. Rather it is their expression of Foxp3 that most closely defines them as regulatory T-cells. Foxp3 is a forkhead transcription factor that controls the expression of a number of genes involved in determining the suppressive phenotype (Figure 10.9). Indeed, if the *Foxp3* gene is introduced into naive CD4⁺CD25⁻ T-cells they are converted into cells capable of suppressing T-cell proliferation (Figure 10.10). Such trans-

Figure 10.9. Role of the Foxp3 transcription factor in mediating suppression.

Foxp3 binds to the promotor regions of the *CD25*, *CTLA4* and *GITR* genes and recruits histone acetyltransferase enzymes thereby causing acetylation of histones in that area of the DNA and thus facilitating activation of gene transcription. However, when Foxp3 binds to promotors associated with the IL-2 and IFNγ genes it recruits histone deacetylase enzymes with resulting repression of gene transcription.

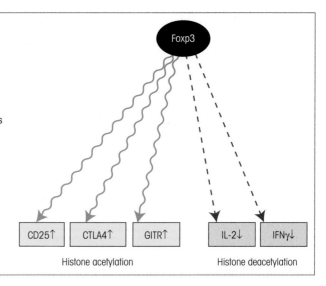

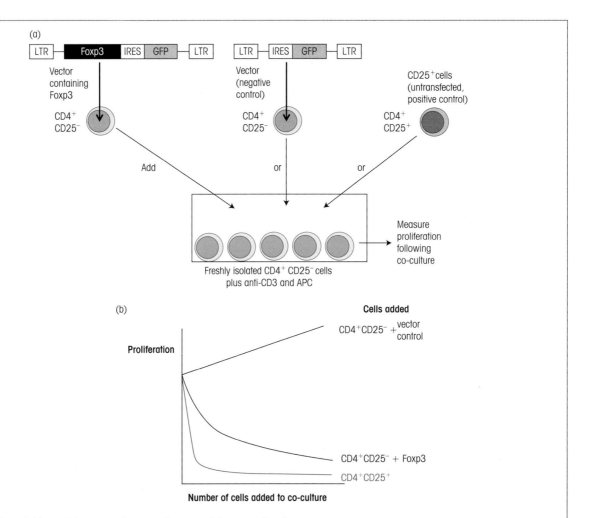

Figure 10.10 Acquisition of Foxp3 confers regulatory activity upon T-cells.

(a) The *Foxp3* gene was introduced into a retroviral vector composed of 5′ and 3′ long terminal repeats (LTR), an internal ribosome entry site (IRES) and green fluorescent protein (GFP). This construct, or the vector without Foxp3, was then transfected into CD4⁺CD25⁻ cells (which are known to lack regulatory T-cell activity). Varying numbers (up to 2.5×10^4) of the transfected T-cells, or of nontransfected freshly isolated CD4⁺CD25⁺ Treg cells (as a positive control, red), were added to a culture of 2.5×10^4 freshly isolated CD4⁺CD25⁻ cells stimulated with an anti-CD3 mAb in the presence of antigen-presenting cells. (b) Proliferation (as measured by ³H-labeled TdR incorporation) was inhibited by Foxp3-transfected CD25⁻ T-cells to an extent comparable with that observed with the freshly isolated CD4⁺CD25⁺ Treg cells, indicating that Foxp3 confers suppressive activity on T-cells. (Based on Hori S., Nomura T. & Sakaguchi S. (2003) *Science* **299**, 1057–1061.)

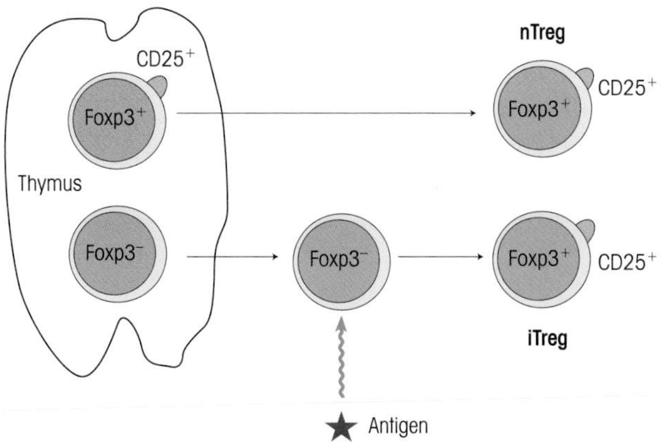

Figure 10.11. **Naturally occuring and inducible regulatory T-cells.**

Naturally occurring regulatory T-cells (nTregs) already express Foxp3 and CD25 upon becoming mature in the thymus and can immediately act to suppress immune responses upon their entry into the periphery. In contrast, the inducible regulatory T-cells (iTregs) initially lack expression of Foxp3 and CD25, and the ability to suppress immune responses. However, they can convert into functional Foxp3⁺CD25⁺ Tregs following stimulation by antigen in the secondary lymphoid tissues.

fected cells with newly acquired Foxp3 are, just like freshly isolated Tregs, able to protect mice against the development of autoimmune disease in various animal models.

Tregs can occur naturally or be induced by antigen

CD4⁺CD25⁺ Tregs comprise two major populations, **naturally occurring Tregs** (nTregs), which express Foxp3 from the time they are produced in the thymus, and **inducible Tregs** (iTregs), which arise in the periphery from CD4⁺CD25⁻ precursors and express Foxp3 and CD25 upon activation (Figure 10.11). The naturally occurring Tregs also express CTLA-4, OX40, GITR (*g*lucocorticoid-*i*nduced *T*NF receptor family *r*elated molecule), L-selectin and cell surface TGFβ. The activation of these cells is usually antigen specific, but they can subsequently suppress the responses to other antigens, a situation referred to as linked suppression. The precise mechanism they use to suppress immune responses to either the initiating antigen or to other antigens is still being established, but usually requires cell–cell contact between the regulator and the regulated. Proposed mechanisms include perforin/granzyme-mediated apoptosis of the regulated T-cell, interaction of galactin-1 on the surface of the Treg with its receptor on the regulated T-cell leading to cell cycle arrest, or interference with the activation of dendritic cells. Some induced Tregs have a very similar phenotype and are also thought to suppress via cell contact-dependent mechanisms.

Other types of suppressor/regulatory cells also exist

Regulatory T-cells that do not require cell–cell contact have also been described. Thus, human CD4 cells stimulated with antigen in the presence of IL-10 can develop into CD25⁺ CTLA-4⁺GITR⁺Foxp3⁺Tr1 cells that themselves secrete IL-10, a cytokine that can mediate immunosuppressive functions (Figure 10.12). A further population of iTregs with a similar phenotype to Tr1 cells are the Th3 cells, which are defined by the fact that they secrete TGFβ, another cytokine with the capacity to be immunosuppressive. It should be noted that the various different subsets of CD4⁺ T-cells (Tregs, Th1, Th2, Th17, etc.) may not be locked into remaining as that cell type for their entire life, and that therefore a cell belonging to one subset may be able to convert into a different subset under certain microenvironmental conditions.

Various types of immunoregulatory γδ T-cells have also been described but they remain relatively poorly characterized. However, the ability of these cells to produce IL-10 and TGFβ certainly suggests that they have the potential to inhibit immune responses. Some γδ T-cells are Foxp3⁺ and, despite secreting substantial amounts of TGFβ they suppress T-cell proliferation by a cell contact-dependent mechanism. Another type of potentially regulatory cell is the NKT cell that bears an invariant TCR, responds to the synthetic glycolipid α-galactosylceramide presented by CD1d (cf. p. 133), and is able to produce both the Th1 cytokine interferon-γ (IFNγ) and the Th2 cytokine IL-4.

Several studies have recently shown that populations of granulocytic and monocytic cells that are able to inhibit T-cell activation are present in pathological situations including cancer, chronic infection, inflammation, trauma, sepsis and transplantation. These **myeloid-derived suppressor cells** (MDSC) can directly affecting signaling through the T-cell receptor and may also be capable of inducing Foxp3⁺ Tregs. Their role, if any, in the normal physiological regulation of immune responses is somewhat unclear at present. However, it is possible that following infection these suppressor cells transiently appear as part of the normal differentiation into mature (nonsuppressive) myeloid cells. The cells with transient MDSC activity may serve to limit T-cell-mediated immuno-pathology that might otherwise cause excessive damage to the host.

Ongoing research will hopefully help clarify the roles of the various types of suppressor/regulatory cells.

Some of the main factors controlling the immune response that have been discussed so far are summarized in Figure 10.13.

Idiotype networks

Jerne's network hypothesis

In 1974 the Nobel laureate Neils Jerne published a paper entitled "Towards a network theory of the immune system" in which he proposed that structures formed by the variable

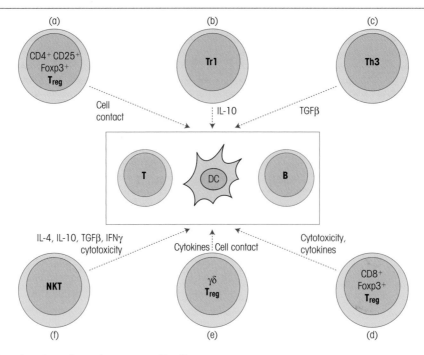

Figure 10.12. The diversity of regulatory/suppressor T-cells.

A number of different types of regulatory/suppressor T-cells have been described that can act, to varying extents, to inhibit effector T-cells, B-cells and dendritic cells. These include: (a) the naturally occurring and induced Tregs already discussed that generally suppress using mechanisms that require cell–cell contact;

(b) IL-10-secreting Tr1 cells; (c) TGFβ-secreting Th3 cells; (d) CD8 cells that may suppress using cytotoxicity or cytokines; (e) immunosuppressive T-cells bearing a γδ TCR; and (f) NKT cells for which cytokine- and cytotoxicity-mediated modes of operation have been proposed.

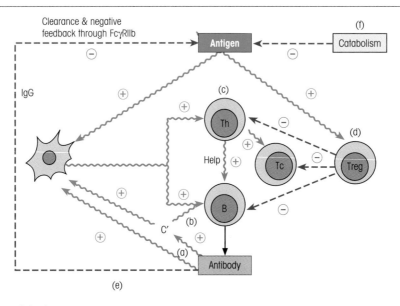

Figure 10.13. Regulation of the immune response.

(a) Antibodies are able to stimulate immune responses by coating antigen for enhanced uptake by MHC class II⁺ professional antigen-presenting cells and subsequent processing and presentation to helper T-cells, by forming Ab–Ag complexes that bind to Fc receptors on follicular dendritic cells for presentation of intact antigen to B-cells, and by activating complement via the classical pathway and thereby generating both C3b, which acts as an opsonin, and C3d (b), which is involved in B-cell co-stimulation. Helper T-cells (c) will provide assistance for the activation of B-cells and cytotoxic T-cells. Under some

circumstances antigen will preferentially stimulate regulatory/suppressor T-cells (d), which will downregulate T- and B-cell responses. In addition to activating the response, antibodies are also able to downregulate immune responses (e) by facilitating the clearance of antigen from the body, by epitope masking, and, for IgG antibodies, by negative feedback through the FcγRIIb on B-cells. The catabolism (f) of the antigen by both the successful immune response and by the normal degradative processes of the body will clearly also lead to a loss of stimulation of the immune system.

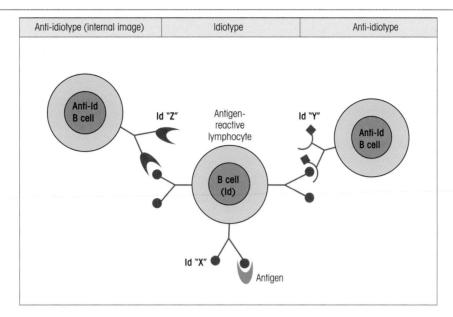

Figure 10.14. Antigen receptor variable regions connect lymphocytes via idiotypic interactions.

Idiotypes (Id) are essentially "shapes" generated by the folding of amino acid sequences in the variable region of the antigen receptor. The receptors on one lymphocyte have the potential to reciprocally recognize an idiotype on the receptors of another lymphocyte if the two shapes "fit," just like conventional antibody–antigen binding. Although these are mutual interactions between two different idiotypes, one of these idiotypes will usually be referred to as the anti-idiotype and the other as the idiotype. In practice they are both idiotypes and simultaneously both anti-idiotypes, an excellent example of the chicken and egg conundrum! Interaction through idiotype–idiotype recognition can potentially lead to stimulation or suppression of lymphocyte activity. B-cell–B-cell, B-cell–T-cell and T-cell–T-cell interactions are all possible. For example, T-cell–T-cell interactions can occur through direct recognition of one T-cell receptor (TCR) by the other, or more usually by recognition of a processed TCR peptide associated with MHC. Out of the many different possible "anti-idiotype" structures some may by chance bear an idiotype of similar shape to the antigen (i.e. provide an **internal image**, represented by one of our own molecules, of a structure found in the external world—for example an antigen on a pathogen). This situation is illustrated by idiotype "Z" on the left of the figure that not only recognizes the antigen-specific idiotype "X" but also bears a structure similar to that of the antigen that is recognized by Id "X." Idiotype "Y" on the right of the figure also recognizes idiotype "X" but does not bear any resemblance to the antigen. Note that receptors of different antigen specificity can sometimes bear the same idiotype (these are referred to as cross-reactive idiotypes) and that the network can be much more extensive than illustrated in the figure with anti-anti-Id, anti-anti-anti-Id and so on.

regions of antibodies (i.e. the antibody idiotype, p. 68) could recognize other antibody variable regions in such a way that they would form a network based upon mutual idiotype-anti-idiotype interactions. Because B-cells use the antibody molecule as their antigen receptor this would provide a connectivity between different clones of B-cells, and therefore the potential for regulation of the individual clones that are members of the network (Figure 10.14). This concept was later extended to include the idiotypes present on the T-cell receptors of both CD4[+] and CD8[+] T-cells. There is no doubt that the elements that can form an idiotypic network are present in the body, and autoanti-idiotypes occur during the course of antigen-induced responses. For example, certain strains of mice injected with pneumococcal vaccines make an antibody response to the phosphorylcholine groups in which the germ-line-encoded idiotype T15 dominates. Waves of T15[+] and of anti-T15 (i.e. autoanti-idiotype) cells are demonstrable. Anti-idiotypic reac-tivity has also been demonstrated in T-cell populations using various experimental systems. The extent to which idiotypic interactions contribute to the regulation of immune responses is still debated among immunologists, but clearly there is the potential for such interactions to both stimulate and inhibit the lymphocytes that contribute to the network.

Internal image anti-idiotypes

Given the almost infinite amino acid sequences, and therefore structures, that can be generated within antibody variable regions, it is not too surprising that occasionally an anti-idiotype will have a similar shape to an antigen. These antibodies can therefore sometimes provide an "**internal image**" of an external antigen in that a component of our own body (the anti-idiotype) resembles a structure on a foreign antigen (Figure 10.14). As we know that under suitable conditions anti-Id can be used as "antigen" to stimulate antibody production, it might be possible to use internal image monoclonal anti-Ids as "surrogate" antigens for immunization in cases where the antigen is difficult to obtain in bulk—for example, antigens from parasites such as filaria or the weak embryonic antigens associated with some cancers. Another example is where protein antigens obtained by chemical synthesis or gene cloning fail to fold into the configuration of the native molecule; this is not a problem with the anti-Id, which by definition has been selected to have the shape of the antigenic epitope.

The influence of genetic factors

Some genes affect general responsiveness

Biozzi and colleagues showed that mice can be selectively bred for high or low antibody responses through several generations to yield two lines, one of which consistently produces high-titer antibodies to a variety of antigens, and the other, antibodies of relatively low titer (Figure 10.15). Out of the ten or so different genetic loci involved, some influence T-cell and B-cell proliferation and differentiation, whilst others affect dendritic cell and macrophage behavior.

Antigen receptor genes are linked to the immune response

Clearly, the Ig and TCR V, D and J genes encoding the specific recognition sites of the lymphocyte antigen receptors are of fundamental importance to the acquired immune response. However, as the mechanisms for generating receptor diversity from the available genes are so powerful (cf. p. 90), immunodeficiency is unlikely to occur as a consequence of a poor Ig or TCR variable region gene repertoire. Nevertheless, just occasionally, we see holes in the repertoire due to the absence of a gene; failure to respond to the sugar polymer $\alpha1$–6 dextran is a feature of animals without a particular immunoglobulin V gene, and mice lacking the $V\alpha_2$ TCR gene cannot mount a cytotoxic T-cell response to the male H-Y antigen.

Immune responses are influenced by the MHC

There was much excitement when it was first discovered that the antibody responses to a number of thymus-dependent antigenically simple substances are determined by genes mapping to the MHC. For example, mice of the H-2^b haplotype respond well to the synthetic branched

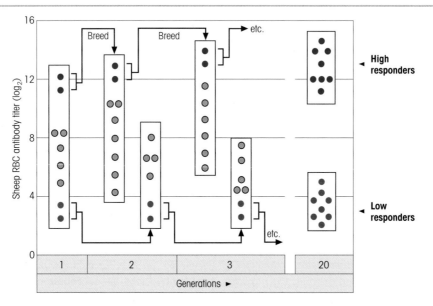

Figure 10.15. Selective breeding of high and low antibody responders

A foundation population of wild mice (with diverse genetic makeup and great variability in antibody response) is immunized with sheep red blood cells (SRBC), a multideterminant antigen. The antibody titer of each individual mouse is shown by a circle. The male and female giving the highest titer antibodies (●) were bred and their litter challenged with antigen. Again, the best responders were bred together and so on for 20 generations when all mice were high responders to SRBC and a variety of other antigens. The same was done for the poorest responders (●), yielding a strain of low responder animals. The two lines are comparable in their ability to clear carbon particles or sheep erythrocytes from the blood by phagocytosis, but macrophages from the high responders present antigen more efficiently (cf. p. 200). On the other hand, the low responders survive infection by *Salmonella typhimurium* better and their macrophages support much slower replication of *Listeria* (cf. p. 325), indicative of an inherently more aggressive macrophage microbicidal ability.

Table 10.1. H-2 haplotype linked to high, low and intermediate immune responses to synthetic peptides. (T,G)-A–L, polylysine with polyalanine side-chains randomly tipped with tyrosine and glutamine; (H,G)-A–L, the same with histidine in place of tyrosine.

ANTIGEN	H-2 HAPLOTYPE				
	b	k	d	a	s
(T,G)-A–L	Hi	Lo	Int	Lo	Lo
(H,G)-A–L	Lo	Hi	Int	Hi	Lo

Table 10.2. Mapping of the Ir gene for (H,G)-A–L responses by analysis of different recombinant strains.

Strain	H-2 region				(H,G)-A–L Response
	K	A	E	D	
A	k	k	k	b	Hi
A.TL	s	k	k	b	Hi
B.IO.A (4R)	k	k	b	b	Hi
B.IO	b	b	b	b	Lo
A.SW	s	s	s	s	Lo

polypeptide (T,G)-A–L, whereas $H\text{-}2^k$ mice respond poorly (Table 10.1). It was said that mice of the H-2^b haplotype (i.e. a particular set of H-2 genes) are **high responders** to (T,G)-A–L because they possess the appropriate immune response (Ir) gene. With another synthetic antigen, (H,G)-A–L, having histidine in place of tyrosine, the position is reversed, the "poor (T,G)-A–L responders" now giving a good antibody response and the "good (T,G)-A–L responders" a weak one, showing that the capacity of a particular strain to give a high or low response varies with the individual antigen (Table 10.1). These relationships are only apparent when antigens of highly restricted structure are studied because the response to each single determinant is controlled by an Ir gene and it is less likely that the different determinants on a complex antigen will all be associated with consistently high or consistently low responder Ir genes; however, although one would expect an average of randomly high and low responder genes, as the various determinants on most thymus-dependent complex antigens are structurally unrelated, the outcome will be biased by the dominance of one or more epitopes (cf. p. 264).

With complex antigens, in most but not all cases, H-2 linkage is usually only seen when the dose administered is so low that just one immunodominant determinant is recognized by the immune system. In this way, reactions controlled by MHC genes are distinct from the overall responsiveness to a variety of complex antigens that is a feature of the Biozzi mice (above).

The Ir genes map to the mouse H-2I region and control antigen presentation to αβ T-cells

Table 10.2 gives some idea of the type of analysis used to map the *Ir* genes. The three high responder strains have individual *H-2* genes derived from prototypic pure strains (B.10 and A. SW) that have been interbred to produce recombinations within the H-2 region. The only genes the high responders have in common are A^k and D^b; as the B.10 strain bearing the D^b gene is a low responder, high response must be linked in this case to possession of A^k. The I region (I-A and I-E) molecules are the murine class II MHC molecules, and polymor-

phisms within these genes affect the peptide-binding groove and therefore their ability to present antigen to CD4$^+$ helper T-cells. They thus directly influence the responsiveness of the mice with respect to their thymus-dependent antibody response to antigen *in vivo*. Indeed, there is a good correlation between antigen-specific T-cell proliferation and the antibody responder status of the animal. This also explains why these *H-2* gene effects are seen with thymus-dependent but not T-independent B-cell antigens.

Three mechanisms can account for class II-linked high and low responsiveness:

1 *Defective presentation.* In a high responder, processing of antigen and its recognition by a corresponding T-cell lead to lymphocyte triggering and clonal expansion (Figure 10.16a). Although there is (and has to be) considerable degeneracy in the specificity of the class II groove for peptide binding, as alluded to above the variation in certain key residues can alter the strength of binding to a particular peptide (cf. p. 129) and convert a high to a low responder because the MHC fails to present antigen to the reactive T-cell (Figure 10.16b). Sometimes the natural processing of an antigen in a given individual does not produce a peptide that fits well into their MHC molecules. One study showed that a cytotoxic T-cell clone restricted to HLA-A2, which recognized residues 58–68 of influenza A virus matrix protein, could cross-react with cells from an HLA-A69 subject pulsed with the same peptide; nonetheless, the clone failed to recognize HLA-A69 cells *infected* with influenza A virus. Interestingly, individuals with the HLA-A69 class I MHC develop immunity to a different epitope on the same protein.

2 *Defective T-cell repertoire.* T-cells with moderate to high affinity for self-MHC molecules and their complexes with processed self-antigens are tolerized (cf. p. 293), so creating a "hole" in the T-cell repertoire. If there is a cross-reaction, i.e. similarity in shape at the T-cell recognition level between a foreign antigen and a self-molecule that has already

Figure 10.16. Different mechanisms can account for low T-cell response to antigen in association with MHC class II.

(a) For the activation of CD4⁺ T-cells it is necessary for peptide to bind with a high affinity to the binding groove formed from the α_1 and β_1 domains of an MHC class II molecule and then for the TCR to bind to the peptide–MHC complex. (b) If the peptide is unable to bind to the MHC groove then clearly there is no possibility of a T-cell response. (c) During negative selection in the thymus T-cells will become tolerized to peptides derived from self antigens and this tolerance will extend to any similar (cross-reactive) peptides derived from foreign antigens. (d) Even if the peptide binds the MHC and the T-cell bears an appropriate TCR, under some circumstances responsiveness may be blocked by the presence of Tregs.

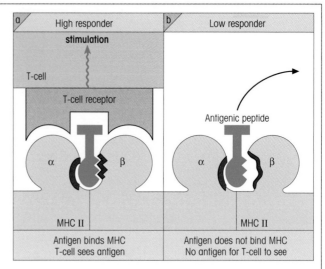

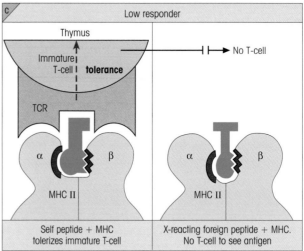

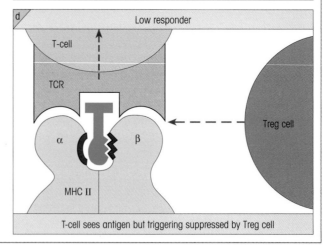

induced unresponsiveness, the host will lack T-cells specific for the foreign antigen and therefore be a low responder (Figure 10.16c). To take a concrete example, mice of DBA/2 strain respond well to the synthetic peptide polyglutamyl, polytyrosine (GT), whereas BALB/c mice do not, although both have identical class II genes. BALB/c B-cell blasts express a structure that mimics GT and the presumption would be that self-tolerance makes these mice unresponsive to GT. This was confirmed by showing that DBA/2 mice made tolerant by a small number of BALB/c hematopoietic cells were changed from high to low responder status. To round off the story in a very satisfying way, DBA/2 mice injected with BALB/c B-blasts, induced by the polyclonal activator lipopolysaccharide, were found to be primed for GT.

3 *T-cell-mediated suppression.* We would like to refer again to the transferable suppression that can occur to relatively complex antigens (see p. 268), as it illustrates the notion that low responder status can arise as a result of regulatory cell activity (Figure 10.16d). Low response can be dominant in class II heterozygotes, indicating that suppression can act against Th restricted to any other class II molecule. In this it differs from models 1 and 2 above where high response is dominant in a heterozygote because the factors associated with the low responder gene (defective presentation or defective T-cell repertoire) cannot influence the activity of a high responder gene if also present.

The genetic contributions to the immune response are summarized in Figure 10.17.

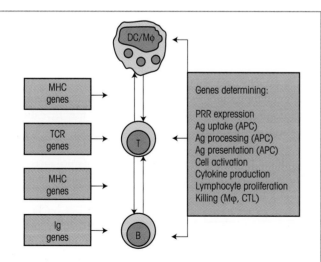

Figure 10.17. Genetic control of the immune response.

Multiple genes determine immune responsiveness, including those that recombine to generate the antigen-specific receptors of lymphocytes, the highly polymorphic MHC genes, and genes determining a variety of activities of immune system cells. APC, professional antigen-presenting cells (dendritic cells [DC], macrophages [Mφ], B-cells); PRR, pattern recognition receptors.

Regulatory immunoneuroendocrine networks

There is a danger, as one focuses more and more on the antics of the immune system, of looking at the body as a collection of myeloid and lymphoid cells roaming around in a big sack and of having no regard to the integrated physiology of the organism. Within the wider physiological context, attention has been drawn increasingly to interactions between immunological and neuroendocrine systems.

Immunological cells have the receptors that enable them to receive signals from a whole range of hormones: corticosteroids, insulin, growth hormone, estradiol, testosterone, prolactin, β-adrenergic agents, acetylcholine, endorphins and enkephalins. By and large, glucocorticoids and androgens depress immune responses, whereas estrogens, growth hormone, thyroxine and insulin do the opposite.

A neuroendocrine feedback loop affecting immune responses

The secretion of **glucocorticoids** is a major response to stresses induced by a wide range of stimuli, such as extreme changes of temperature, fear, hunger and physical injury. They are also released as a consequence of immune responses and limit those responses in a neuroendocrine feedback loop. Thus, IL-1 (Figure 10.18), IL-6 and TNF are capable of stimulating

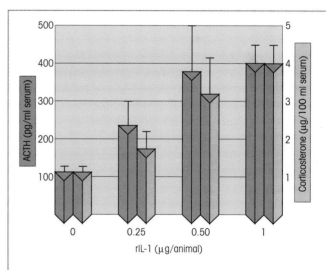

Figure 10.18. Enhancement of ACTH and corticosterone blood levels in C3H/HeJ mice 2 hours after injection of recombinant IL-1.

Values are means ± standard error of the mean (SEM) for groups of seven or eight mice. The significance of the mouse strain used is that it lacks receptors for bacterial lipopolysaccharide (LPS), and so the effects cannot be attributed to LPS contamination of the IL-1 preparation. (Reprinted from Besedovsky H., del Rey A., Sorkin E. & Dinarello C.A. (1986) *Science* **233**, 652–654, with permission. Copyright © 1986 by the AAAS.)

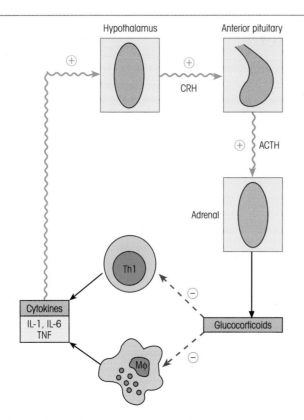

Figure 10.19. Glucocorticoid negative feedback on cytokine production.

Additional regulatory circuits based on neuroendocrine interactions with the immune system are almost certain to exist given that lymphoid and myeloid cells in both primary and secondary lymphoid organs can produce hormones and neuropeptides, and classical endocrine glands as well as neurons and glial cells can synthesize cytokines and appropriate receptors. Production of prolactin and its receptors by peripheral lymphoid cells and thymocytes is worthy of attention. Lymphocyte expression of the prolactin receptor is upregulated following activation and, in autoimmune disease, witness the beneficial effects of bromocriptine, an inhibitor of prolactin synthesis, in the NZB × NZW model of murine systemic lupus erythematosus (cf. p. 480). ACTH, adrenocorticotropic hormone; CRH, corticotropin-releasing hormone.

glucocorticoid synthesis and do so through the hypothalamic–pituitary–adrenal axis. This, in turn, leads to the downregulation of Th1 and macrophage activity, so completing the negative feedback circuit (Figure 10.19). Although glucocorticoids also inhibit Th2 cells, the mechanisms by which they inhibit Th1 and Th2 cells are different, and their inhibition of Th1 cells is much more potent. They strongly repress the T-bet transcription factor that is necessary for differentiation into the Th1 phenotype, but less vehemently inhibit the GATA3 transcription factor required for differentiation into Th2 cells. The immunosuppressive effects of glucocorticoids are reinforced by the induction of regulatory T-cells. Thus, incubating dendritic cells with the glucocorticoid dexamethasone results in expression of GILZ (glucocorticoid-induced leucine zipper), which causes the DCs to promote expression of Foxp3 in inducible Tregs.

It has been shown that adrenalectomy prevents spontaneous recovery from *e*xperimental *a*llergic *e*ncephalomyelitis (EAE). This demyelinating disease is associated with progressive paralysis and is produced by immunization with myelin basic protein in complete Freund's adjuvant. Induction of the disease can be blocked by implants of corticosterone. Spontaneous recovery from EAE in intact animals is associated with a dominance of Th2 autoantigen-specific clones, supporting the view that glucocorticoids more powerfully suppress Th1 responses. Individuals with a genetic predisposition to high levels of stress-induced glucocorticoids might therefore be expected to have increased susceptibility to infections with intracellular pathogens such as *Mycobacterium leprae* that require effective Th1 cell-mediated immunity for their eradication.

Neonatal exposure to bacterial endotoxin (LPS) not only exerts a long-term influence on endocrine and central nervous system development, but substantially affects predisposition to inflammatory disease and therefore appears to program or "reset" the functional development of both the endocrine and immune systems. Thus, in adult life, rats that had been exposed to endotoxin during the first week of life had higher basal levels of corticosterone compared with control animals, and showed a greater increase in corticosterone levels in response to noise stress and a more rapid rise in corticosterone levels following challenge with LPS.

The effect of gender

Females often mount stronger immune responses than males and are far more susceptible to autoimmune disease, an issue that will be discussed in greater depth in Chapter 18. It is noteworthy that both estrogen receptors and androgen receptors are present on various cell types in the immune system, including lymphocytes and macrophages. Although investigations into the role of estrogen in immune responses have often led to apparently contradictory data, it has often been found to enhance lymphocyte responses. Likewise, androgen deprivation induced by castration of postpubertal male mice increases the levels of T-cells in secondary lymphoid tissues and enhances T-cell proliferation.

Although estrogen can have a beneficial effect on helper T-cell, B-cell and NKT cell responses (Figure 10.20) it should be noted that it can also cause expansion of clones of CD4⁺CD25⁺ T-cells and that it upregulates both Foxp3 and IL-10 expression in these suppressor cells. With respect to NKT cells, substantially enhanced levels of IFNγ are produced by these cells when they are stimulated with antigen in the presence of physiological concentrations of estrogen, providing a possible explanation for the observation that female mice produce higher levels of this cytokine in response to antigen challenge.

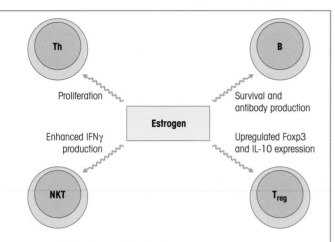

Figure 10.20. Some effects of estrogen on lymphocyte function.

The pituitary hormone prolactin also has immunostimulatory activity for a variety of cells of the immune system including T-cells, B-cells, NK cells, macrophages and dendritic cells. It has been shown to enhance antibody responses by both decreasing B-cell clonal deletion and by lowering the threshold for breaking anergy in B-cells, and increased levels of this hormone have been described in a number of systemic autoimmune diseases.

"Psychoimmunology"

Both primary and secondary lymphoid tissues are richly innervated by the sympathetic nervous system. The enzyme dopamine β-hydroxylase catalyses the conversion of dopamine to the catecholamine neurotransmitter norepinephrine, which is released from sympathetic neurons in these tissues. Mice in which the gene for this enzyme has been deleted by homologous recombination exhibited enhanced susceptibility to infection with *Mycobacterium tuberculosis* and impaired production of the Th1 cytokines IFNγ and TNF in response to this intracellular pathogen. Although these animals showed no obvious developmental defects in their immune system, impaired Th1 responses were also found following immunization of these mice with the hapten TNP coupled to KLH. These observations suggest that norepinephrine can play a role in determining the potency of the immune response.

Denervated skin shows greatly reduced leukocyte infiltration in response to local damage, implicating cutaneous neurons in the recruitment of leukocytes. Sympathetic nerves that innervate lymphatic vessels and lymph nodes are involved in regulating the flow of lymph and may participate in controlling the migration of β-adrenergic receptor-bearing dendritic cells from inflammatory sites to the local lymph nodes. Mast cells and nerves often have an intimate anatomical relationship and nerve growth factor causes mast cell degranulation. The gastrointestinal tract also has extensive innervation and a high

number of immune effector cells. In this context, the ability of substance P to stimulate, and of somatostatin to inhibit, proliferation of Peyer's patch lymphocytes may prove to have more than a trivial significance.

There seems to be an interaction between inflammation and nerve growth in regions of wound healing and repair. Mast cells are often abundant, IL-6 induces neurite growth and IL-1 enhances production of nerve growth factor in sciatic nerve explants. IL-1 also increases slow-wave sleep when introduced into the lateral ventricle of the brain, and both IL-1 and interferon produce pyrogenic effects through their action on the temperature-controlling center.

Although it is not clear just how these diverse neuroendocrine effects fit into the regulation of immune responses, at a more physiological level, stress and circadian rhythms modify the functioning of the immune system. Factors such as restraint, noise and exam anxiety have been observed to influence a number of immune functions including phagocytosis, lymphocyte proliferation, NK activity and IgA secretion. Amazingly, it has been reported that the delayed-type hypersensitivity Mantoux reaction in the skin can be modified by hypnosis. An elegant demonstration of nervous system control is provided by studies showing suppression of immune responses by Pavlovian conditioning. In the classic Pavlovian paradigm, a stimulus such as food that unconditionally elicits a particular response, in this case salivation, is repeatedly paired with a neutral stimulus that does not elicit the same response. Eventually, the neutral stimulus becomes a conditional stimulus and will elicit salivation in the absence of food. Rats were given cyclophosphamide (an immunosuppressive drug) as an unconditional and saccharin as a conditional stimulus repeatedly; subsequently, there was a depressed antibody response when the animals were challenged with antigen together with just the conditional stimulus, saccharin. As more and more data accumulate, it is becoming clearer how immunoneuroendocrine networks could play a role in allergy and in autoimmune diseases such as rheumatoid arthritis, type 1 diabetes and multiple sclerosis.

Effects of diet, pollutants and trauma on immunity

Malnutrition diminishes the effectiveness of the immune response

The greatly increased susceptibility of undernourished individuals to infection can be attributed to many other factors: poor sanitation and personal hygiene, overcrowding and inadequate health education. But, in addition, there are gross effects of **protein–calorie malnutrition** on immunocompetence. The widespread atrophy of lymphoid tissues and a substantial reduction in circulating CD4 T-cells underlie serious impairment of cell-mediated immunity. Antibody responses may be intact but they are of lower affinity; phagocytosis of bacteria is relatively normal but the subsequent intracellular destruction is compromised. Deficiencies in pyridoxine, folic acid and vitamins C and E result in generally impaired immune responses.

Zinc deficiency is rather interesting, reducing the activity of the thymus and thymic hormones, shifting the Th1/Th2 balance towards Th2-dominated responses, decreasing the effectiveness of vaccination and leading to a decline in the activity of phagocytic cells and NK cells. Meanwhile, iron deficiency impairs the oxidative burst in neutrophils as the flavocytochrome NADP oxidase is an iron-containing enzyme.

Of course there is another side to all this in that moderate restriction of total calorie intake and/or marked reduction in fat intake ameliorates autoimmune disease, at least in animal models. Omega-3 polyunsaturated fatty acids (PUFAs), as found in fish oils, have been shown to be protective in some but not all clinical trials involving patients with rheumatoid arthritis. This fact is perhaps not too surprising given the now well established observation that PUFAs are able to downregulate the production of a number of proinflammatory cytokines, including TNF.

Vitamins A and D exhibit immunomodulatory effects

Retinoic acid, a **vitamin A** metabolite, stimulates the development of regulatory T-cells and Th2 cells, but inhibits the production of Th17 cells. Among the cells that produce retinoic acid are dendritic cells in the gut, leading to imprinting of T-cells with the CCR9 chemokine receptor and the $\alpha_4\beta_7$ integrin, the ligand for the mucosal addressin MadCAM-1. This situation ensures that the appropriate lymphocytes home to the gut-associated lymphoid tissues. **Vitamin D** is also an important regulator. It is produced not only by the UV-irradiated dermis, but also by activated macrophages, the hypercalcemia associated with sarcoidosis being attributable to production of the vitamin by macrophages in the active granulomas. The vitamin is a potent inhibitor of T-cell proliferation and of Th1 cytokine production. This generates a neat feedback loop at sites of inflammation where macrophages activated by IFNγ produce vitamin D, which suppresses the T-cells making the interferon. It also downregulates antigen presentation by macrophages and promotes multinucleated giant cell formation in chronic granulomatous lesions. Just like vitamin A, it promotes Th2 activity, especially at mucosal surfaces, stimulates Treg activity and downregulates differentiation of Th17 cells: quite a busy little vitamin.

Other factors

Given the overdue sensitivity to the importance of environmental contamination, it is important to monitor the nature and levels of **pollution** that may influence immunity. Here is just one example: polyhalogenated organic compounds (such as polychlorinated biphenyls) steadily pervade the environ-

ment and, being stable and lipophilic, accumulate readily in the aquatic food chain where they largely resist metabolic breakdown. It was shown that Baltic herrings with relatively high levels of these pollutants, as compared with uncontaminated Atlantic herrings, were immunotoxic when fed to captive harbor seals, suggesting one reason why seals along the coasts of northwestern Europe succumbed so alarmingly to infection with the otherwise nonvirulent phocine distemper virus in 1988.

Multiple traumatic injury, surgery and major burns are also immunosuppressive and so contribute to the increased risk of sepsis. Corticosteroids produced by stressful conditions, the immunosuppressive prostaglandin E_2 released from damaged tissues and bacterial endotoxin derived from the disturbance of gut flora are all factors that influence the outcome after trauma.

Effects of aging

The elderly are more susceptible to infection and have decreased responses to vaccines compared with younger folk. Spurred by improved longevity, attention is increasingly focused on understanding how our immune system wears out with age. There is now clear evidence that both the adaptive and innate arms of the immune response decline (Figure 10.21).

The thymic involution that occurs at puberty leads to a decreased output of T-cells and a reduction in thymic hormone production. As aging progresses there is a decline in the absolute numbers of both T-cells and B-cells but an increase in the absolute number of NK cells. Although both CD4+ and CD8+ T-cell populations decline, perhaps the most profound changes occur in the CD8 compartment. After repeated division CD8+

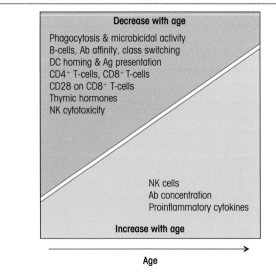

Figure 10.21. Age trends in some immunological parameters.

cells lose expression of the CD28 molecule required for co-stimulation. A lifetime of making immune responses, coupled with the aforementioned reduced thymic output, lead eventually to T-cell clonal exhaustion. This exhaustion is a consequence of the fact that lymphocyte responses rely upon clonal proliferation. There is a finite number of times a cell can divide, the Hayflick limit, and this is associated with a shortening of the length of the telomeres at the ends of the chromosomes. Once this limit is reached the cells reach senescence and can no longer divide. Senescent lymphocytes, which are known to possess a memory phenotype, may take up niches that could otherwise be occupied by T-cells proliferating in response to infection.

With regard to B-cells, there is a decline in cell number and a decrease in the ability of both peripheral blood and splenic B-cells to class switch. There are reduced levels of the enzyme activation-induced cytidine deaminase in B-lymphocytes isolated from the elderly; this enzyme is required for both class switching and affinity maturation. Rather paradoxically, not only IgM levels but also IgG and IgA antibody levels are increased in the aged. However, at least some of these antibodies are of relatively low affinity. The increase in total IgG and IgA antibody levels may reflect secretion by bone marrow plasmablasts of antibodies with limited somatic hypermutation.

Regarding innate responses, the phagocytic activity of both neutrophils and macrophages decreases, as does their microbicidal activity. Dendritic cells appear to have both a reduced ability to home to lymph nodes and ability to stimulate T-cells. Not everything declines with age. Proinflammatory cytokines, including IL-1, IL-6 and TNF, are increased, and as already mentioned so are NK cell numbers. However, the proliferative response of these NK cells to IL-2 and their killing ability are impaired.

Control by antigen
- Immune responses are largely antigen driven. As the level of antigen falls due to an effective immune response, so does the intensity of the response.
- Antigens can compete with each other: particularly as a result of competition between processed peptides for the available MHC grooves.

Feedback control by complement and antibody
- Antigens coated with C3d can boost antibody responses by cross-linking the CD21 complement receptor with the BCR.
- IgM, IgG and IgE antibodies are able to boost antibody responses, either by activating complement via the classical pathway (IgM, IgG) or by facilitating FcR-mediated uptake of antigen by APCs.
- IgG is also able to limit antibody responses via a negative feedback mechanism through the inhibitory FcγRIIb on B-cells and also by Fc-independent effects that probably involve epitope masking so that the antigen is no longer able to be seen by the BCR on the B-cell.

T-cell regulation
- Activated T-cells express members of the TNF receptor family, including Fas, which act as death receptors and restrain unlimited clonal expansion by promoting activation-induced cell death (AICD).
- Regulatory T-cells (Tregs) can suppress the activity of both helper **and cytotoxic** T-cells as well as dendritic cell and B-cell activity.
- Suppressor and helper epitopes can exist on the same molecule.
- Effectors of suppression include naturally occurring CD4⁺CD25⁺Foxp3⁺ Treg, which arise directly in the thymus, and inducible Tregs, which express Foxp3 only after their activation in the periphery. These both seem to act via cell-contact dependent mechanisms.
- Other types of regulatory T-cells act by secreting immunosuppressive cytokines, with Tr1 cells producing IL-10 and Th3 cells that release TGFβ. Immunoregulatory γδ T-cells, CD8⁺ T-suppressor cells, and myeloid-derived suppressor cells can also contribute to the inhibition of immune responses.
- Th1 and Th2 cells mutually inhibit each other through production of their respective cytokines IFNγ and IL-4/-10.
- Tregs and Th17 cells also exhibit a reciprocal relationship. The Foxp3 transcription factor associated with regulatory T-cell activity blocks the RORγt transcription factor required for Th17 cell activity.

Idiotype networks
- Antigen-specific receptors on lymphocytes can interact with the idiotypes on the receptors of other lymphocytes to form a network (Jerne) that may naturally regulate immune responses.
- T-cell idiotypic interactions can also be demonstrated.
- The network offers the potential for therapeutic intervention to manipulate immunity.
- "Internal image" anti-idiotypes can be used to mimic antigens.

Genetic factors influence the immune response
- Multiple genes control the overall antibody response to complex antigens: some affect macrophage antigen processing and microbicidal activity and

some the rate of proliferation of differentiating B-cells.

■ Immunoglobulin and TCR genes are very adaptable because they rearrange to create the antigen receptors, but "holes" in the repertoire can occur.

■ Immune response genes are located in the MHC class II locus and control the interactions between professional antigen-presenting cells and T-cells.

■ Class II-linked high and low responsiveness may be due to defective presentation by MHC, a defective T-cell repertoire caused by tolerance to MHC + self-peptides, and T-suppression.

Immunoneuroendocrine networks

■ Immunological, neurological and endocrinological systems interact, forming regulatory circuits.

■ Feedback by cytokines augments the production of corticosteroids and is important because this shuts down Th1 and macrophage activity.

■ Estrogens can enhance both T- and B-cell responses, but can also promote the activity of regulatory cells.

Effects of diet and other factors on immunity

■ Protein-calorie malnutrition grossly impairs cell-mediated immunity and phagocyte microbicidal potency.

■ Trauma and environmental pollution can both act to impair immune mechanisms.

■ Polyunsaturated fatty acids downregulate the production of pro-inflammatory cytokines. Both vitamin A and vitamin D stimulate Th2 and Treg cells and thereby also inhibit Th1 and Th17 cells, respectively.

Aging and the immune response

■ The elderly are more prone to infection and respond less effectively to vaccines.

■ The ability of phagocytic cells to both engulf and kill microorganisms decreases with age, as does the efficiency of dendritic cell homing to lymph nodes and their activation of T-cells.

■ Involution of the thymus at puberty results in a reduced output of T-cells.

■ CD4$^+$ T-cell, CD8$^+$ T-cell and B-cell numbers all decline with age, although NK cell numbers increase.

■ The concentration of circulating antibody is often elevated in later life, but these antibodies tend to be of rather low affinity.

■ Levels of the proinflammatory cytokines TNF, IL-1 and IL-6 also increase with age.

FURTHER READING

Behn U. (2007) Idiotypic networks: toward a renaissance? *Immunological Reviews* **216**, 142–152.

Cohen I.R. (2000) *Tending Adam's Garden*. Academic Press, London.

Feuerer M. *et al.* (2009) Foxp3$^+$ regulatory T cells: differentiation, specification, subphenotypes. *Nature Immunology* **10**, 689–695.

Gabrilovich D.I. & Nagaraj S. (2009) Myeloid-derived suppressor cells as regulators of the immune system. *Nature Reviews Immunology* **9**, 162–174.

Hjelm F. *et al.* (2006) Antibody-mediated regulation of the immune response. *Scandinavian Journal of Immunology* **64**, 177–184.

Korn T. *et al.* (2009) IL-17 and Th17 cells. *Annual Review of Immunology* **27**, 485–517.

Nikolich-Zugich J. & Rudd B.D. (2010) Immune memory and aging: an infinite or finite resource? *Current Opinion in Immunology* **22**, 535–540.

Shevach E.M. (2009) Mechanisms of Foxp3$^+$ T regulatory cell-mediated suppression. *Immunity* **30**, 636–645.

Taub D.D. (2008) Neuroendocrine interactions in the immune system. *Cellular Immunology* **252**, 1–6.

Now visit **www.roitt.com** to test yourself on this chapter.

CHAPTER 11
Ontogeny and phylogeny

Key Topics

Just to Recap ...

The immune system relies upon the cells of the innate and adaptive responses. Innate responses, which are not antigen specific and lack immunological memory, involve neutrophils, eosinophils, mast cells, basophils, monocytes, macrophages, NK cells and various types of interdigitating dendritic cell. In contrast the highly antigen-specific adaptive response, which characteristically develops immunological memory, is based upon lymphocytes. These lymphocytes, which recombine antigen-receptor genes in order to generate a quite incredible diversity of antigen recognition, comprise the helper, regulatory and cytotoxic T-cells and the antibody-producing B-cells.

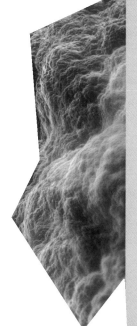

Roitt's Essential Immunology, Twelfth Edition. Peter J. Delves, Seamus J. Martin, Dennis R. Burton, Ivan M. Roitt.
© 2011 Peter J. Delves, Seamus J. Martin, Dennis R. Burton, Ivan M. Roitt. Published 2011 by Blackwell Publishing Ltd.

Introduction

In this chapter we will look at the development (ontogeny) of the cells of the immune system in the individual, and the evolution (phylogeny) of the immune response from primitive species through to mammals.

Virtually all cells of the immune response, with the exception of the follicular dendritic cell, are derived from pluripotent hematopoietic stem cells. These stem cells differentiate down various developmental pathways, with those that are destined to become T-lymphocytes having first to migrate to the thymus.

CD antigens

Analysis of the cells of the immune system often involves detection of cell surface molecules that allow scientists to differentiate one cell type from another. Indeed the expression of such molecules is very often association with the differentiation of individual cells along developmental pathways. The detection of these so-called "cell surface markers" usually relies on using antibodies as probes for their expression. Immunologists from the far corners of the world who have produced monoclonal antibodies directed to surface molecules on B- and T-cells, macrophages, neutrophils, natural killer (NK) cells, and so on, get together every so often to compare the specificities of their reagents in international workshops whose spirit of cooperation should be a lesson to most politicians. When a cluster of monoclonal antibodies are found to react with the same polypeptide, they clearly represent a series of reagents defining a given marker and are assigned a CD (**cluster of differentiation**) number that defines the particular cell surface antigen recognized by these antibodies. By 2011 there were 363 designated CD antigens assigned, with some of them subdivided into different variants. Those listed in Table 11.1 are most relevant to our discussions. It is important to appreciate that the expression level of cell surface molecules often changes as cells differentiate or become activated and that "subpopulations" of cells exist that differentially express particular molecules. When expressed at a low level the "presence" or "absence" of a given CD antigen may be rather subjective, but be aware that low level expression does not necessarily imply biological irrelevance.

Hematopoietic stem cells

Hematopoiesis originates in the early yolk sac but, as embryogenesis proceeds, this function is taken over by the fetal liver and finally by the bone marrow where it continues throughout life. The pluripotent **hematopoietic stem cell** (**HSC**) gives rise to the erythrocytes (red blood cells), the leukocytes (white blood cells) and the megakaryocytes, which generate platelets. These various cell types are often collectively referred to as the "formed elements of the blood" (Figure 11.1). The HSCs have a relatively unlimited capacity to renew themselves through the creation of further stem cells. Thus an animal can be completely protected against the lethal effects of high doses of irradiation by injection of bone

marrow cells that will repopulate its lymphoid and myeloid systems. The capacity for self-renewal is not absolute and declines with age in parallel with a shortening of the telomeres (p. 449).

The bone marrow contains at least two types of stem cell, the HSC mentioned above and a minority population of bone marrow stromal stem cells (also called the bone marrow mesenchymal stem cell), which give rise to the bone marrow stroma and under appropriate signals can differentiate into adipocytes (fat cells), osteocytes (bone cells), chondrocytes (cartilage cells) and, possibly, myocytes (muscle cells) and hepatocytes (liver cells). The HSC in the mouse is $CD34^{low/-}$, $Sca\text{-}1^+$, $Thy\text{-}1^{+/low}$, $CD38^+$, c-kit $(CD117)^+$ and lin^-, whereas the surface phenotype of the equivalent cell in human is $CD34^{+,}$ $CD59^+$, $Thy\text{-}1^+$, $CD133^+$, $CD38^{low/-}$, $c\text{-kit}^{-/low}$ and lin^-. Impressively, as few as 10 HSCs can prevent death in lethally irradiated SCID mice.

The HSCs differentiate within the microenvironment of the stromal cells, which produce various growth factors including IL-2, -3, -4, -5, -6, -7, -11 and -15, G-CSF, granulocyte macrophage colony-stimulating factor (GM-CSF), stem cell factor (SCF), flt3 ligand, erythropoietin (EPO), thrombopoietin (TPO) and so on. SCF remains associated with the extracellular matrix and acts on primitive stem cells through its receptor, the tyrosine kinase membrane receptor c-kit, to promote survival of HSCs by preventing their apoptosis. Hematopoiesis needs to be kept under tight control, for example by transforming growth factor β (TGFβ), which exerts a cytostatic effect on HSCs.

Mice with *s*evere *c*ombined *i*mmuno*d*eficiency (SCID) provide a happy environment for fragments of human fetal liver and thymus that, if implanted contiguously, will produce formed elements of the blood for 6–12 months.

The thymus provides the environment for T-cell differentiation

The thymus is organized into a series of lobules based upon meshworks of epithelial cells derived embryologically from an outpushing of the gut endoderm of the third pharyngeal pouch and that form well-defined cortical and medullary zones (Figure 11.2). This framework of epithelial cells provides the microenvironment for T-cell differentiation. In both neonatal and adult mice $c\text{-kit}^+$ $CD44^+$ T-cell progenitors arrive from the bone marrow in waves of immigration that appear to be regu-

Table 11.1. Some of the major clusters of differentiation (CD) markers on human cells. A complete list can be found on the Browse section of the Human Cell Differentiation Molecules database: http://www.hcdm.org/ MoleculeInformation/tabid/54/Default.aspx. *, activated; B, B-lymphocytes; FDC, follicular dendritic cells; G, granulocytes; IDC, interdigitating dendritic cells; LBP, LPS-binding protein; LPS, lipopolysaccharide; Mast, mast cells; Mφ, macrophages; Mo, monocytes; NK, natural killer cells; T, T-lymphocytes.

CD	Expression	Functions
CD1	IDC, B subset	Presents glycolipid and other nonpeptide antigens to T-cells
CD2	T, NK	Receptor for CD58 (LFA-3) co-stimulator
CD3	T	Transducing elements of T-cell receptor
CD4	MHC class II restricted T, IDC, Mo, Mφ	Receptor for MHC class II
CD5	T, B subset	Involved in antigen receptor signaling
CD8	MHC class I restricted T	Receptor for MHC class I
CD14	G, Mo, Mφ	Receptor for LPS/LBP complex
CD16	G, NK, B, Mφ, IDC	FcγRIII (medium-affinity IgG receptor)
CD19	B, FDC	Part of B-cell antigen receptor complex
CD20	B	Provides signals for B cell activation and proliferation
CD21	B, FDC	CR2. Receptor for C3d and Epstein–Barr virus. Part of B-cell antigen receptor complex
CD23	B, Mo, FDC	FcεRII (low affinity IgE receptor)
CD25	*T, *B, *Mo, *Mφ	IL-2 receptor α chain
CD28	T, *B	Receptor for CD80/CD86 (B7.1 and B7.2) co-stimulators
CD32	Mo, Mφ, IDC, FDC, G, NK, B	FcγRII (low-affinity IgG receptor)
CD34	Progenitors	Adhesion molecule. Stem cell marker
CD40	B, Mφ, IDC, FDC	Receptor for CD154 (CD40L) co-stimulator
CD45RA	Resting/Naive T-cells, B, G, Mo, NK	Phosphatase, cell activation
CD45RO	Effector T-cell, Mo, Mφ, IDC	Phosphatase, cell activation
CD64	Mo, Mφ, IDC	FcγRI (high-affinity IgG receptor)
CD79a/CD79b	B	Igα/Igβ-transducing elements of B-cell receptor
CD80	*B, *T, Mφ, IDC	B7.1 receptor for CD28 co-stimulator and for CTLA4 inhibitory signal
CD86	B, IDC, Mo	B7.2 receptor for CD28 co-stimulator and for CTLA4 inhibitory signal
CD95	Widespread	Fas receptor for FasL (CD178). Transmits apoptotic signals

lated by the accessibility of developmental niches in the thymus. There are subtle interactions between the extracellular matrix proteins and a variety of adhesion/homing molecules that, in addition to CD44, include the laminin-specific α_6 integrin. Several chemokines also play an essential role, with CXCL12 (stromal cell-derived factor-1, SDF-1) being a particularly potent chemoattractant for the CXCR4$^+$ progenitor cells in man.

Thymic hormones

The thymic epithelial cells produce a series of peptide hormones that are capable of promoting the appearance of T-cell differen-

tiation markers and a variety of T-cell functions on culture with bone marrow cells *in vitro*. The circulating levels of these hormones *in vivo* begin to decline from puberty onwards, reaching vanishingly small amounts by the age of 60 years. Several have been well characterized and sequenced, including thymulin, thymosin α_1, *t*hymic *h*umoral *f*actor (THF) and thymopoietin (and its active pentapeptide thymopontin, TP-5). Of these, only thymulin is of exclusively thymic origin. This zinc-dependent nonapeptide tends to normalize the balance of immune responses: it restores antibody avidity and antibody production in aged mice and yet stimulates suppressor activity in animals with autoimmune hemolytic anemia induced by

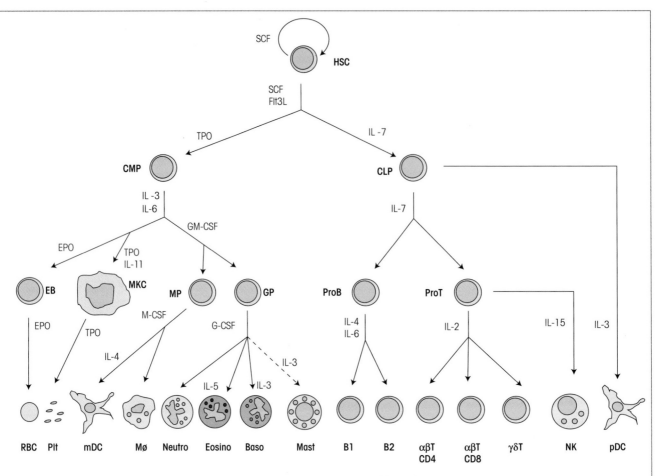

Figure 11.1. The multipotential hematopoietic stem cell and its progeny which differentiate under the influence of a series of soluble cytokines and growth factors within the microenvironment of the bone marrow.

The expression of various nuclear transcription factors (not shown) directs the differentiation process. For example, the *Ikaros* gene encodes a zinc-fingered transcription factor critical for driving the development of a common myeloid/lymphoid precursor into a lymphoid-restricted progenitor giving rise to T-, B- and NK cells. Growth factors/cytokines: EPO, erythropoietin; Flt3L, FMS-like tyrosine kinase-3 ligand; G-CSF, granulocyte colony-stimulating factor; GM-CSF, granulocyte–macrophage colony-stimulating factor (so-called because it promotes the formation of mixed colonies of these two cell types from bone marrow progenitors either in tissue culture or on transfer to an irradiated recipient where they appear in the spleen); IL-3, interleukin-3 (often termed the multi-CSF because it stimulates progenitors of platelets, erythrocytes, all the types of myeloid cells, and also plasmacytoid dendritic cells); M-CSF, monocyte colony-stimulating factor; SCF, stem cell factor; TPO, thrombopoietin; Cells: B1 and B2, B-cell subpopulations; Baso, basophil; EB, erythroblast, CLP, common lymphoid progenitor; CMP, common myeloid progenitor; Eosino, eosinophil; GP, granulocyte progenitor; HSC, hematopoietic stem cell, Mφ, macrophage; Mast, mast cell; mDC, myeloid dendritic cell; MKC, megakaryocyte; MP, monocyte/macrophage/DC progenitor; Neutro, neutrophil; NK, natural killer; Plt, platelets; pDC, plasmacytoid dendritic cell; RBC, red blood cell.

cross-reactive rat red cells (cf. p. 489). Thymulin may be looked upon as a true hormone, secreted by the thymus in a regulated fashion and acting at a distance from the thymus as a fine physiological immunoregulator contributing to the maintenance of T-cell subset homeostasis.

Cellular interactions in the thymus

Specialized large epithelial cells in the outer cortex, known as "nurse" cells (Figure 11.2b), are associated with large numbers of lymphocytes that lie within pockets produced by the long membrane extensions of these cells. The epithelial cells of the deep cortex have branched processes, rich in class II MHC, and connect through specialized cell junctions called desmosomes to form a network through which cortical lymphocytes must pass on their way to the medulla. The cortical lymphocytes are densely packed compared with those in the medulla (Figure 11.2a), many are in division and large numbers of them are undergoing apoptosis. On their way to the medulla, the lymphocytes pass a cordon of "sentinel" macrophages at

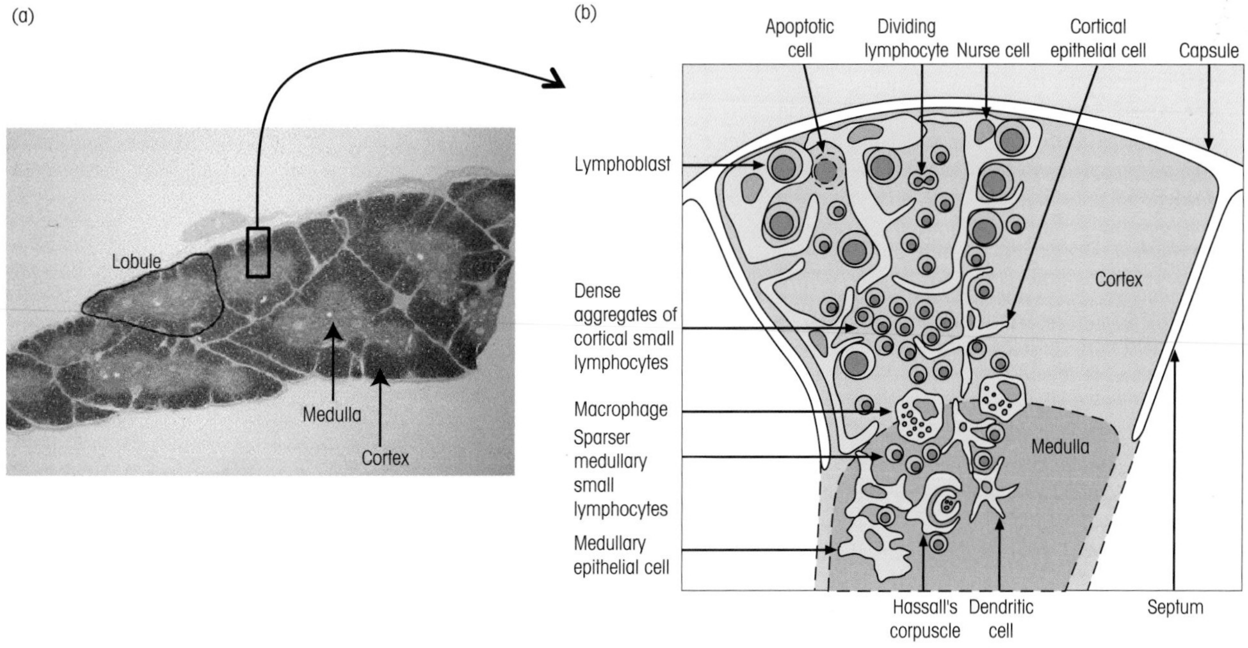

Figure 11.2. The thymus.

(a) The thymus is partially divided into lobules by connective tissue septa. Note the discrete outer cortex and inner medulla apparent within each lobule. (Kindly provided by Rand S. Swenson, Dartmouth Medical School, http://www.dartmouth.edu/~anatomy/Histo) (b) Cellular features of a thymus lobule. See text for description. (Adapted from Hood L.E., Weissman I.L., Wood W.B. & Wilson J.H. (1984) *Immunology*, 2nd edn, p. 261. Benjamin Cummings, California.)

the corticomedullary junction. Bone marrow-derived dendritic cells are present in the medulla and the epithelial cells have broader processes than their cortical counterparts and express high levels of both class I and class II MHC. Whorled keratinized epithelial cells in the medulla form the highly characteristic Hassall's corpuscles (Figure 11.2b) beloved of histopathology examiners. These structures serve as a disposal system for dying thymocytes, perhaps following their phagocytosis by dendritic cells, and are the only location where apoptotic cells are found in the medulla.

A fairly complex relationship with the nervous and endocrine systems exists; the thymus is richly innervated with both adrenergic and cholinergic fibers. Both thymocytes and thymic stromal cells express receptors for a number of neurotransmitters and neuropeptides. Somatostatin is expressed by both cortical and medullary thymic epithelial cells and is able to induce the migration of thymocytes that express the receptor for this neuropeptide. Glucocorticoid hormones, such as hydrocortisone (cortisol) and cortisone, are classically associated with the adrenal gland but are also produced by thymic epithelial cells. During stress the output of these hormones increases and directly provokes thymic involution and apoptosis of thymocytes. The sex hormones testosterone, estrogen and progesterone can also promote thymic involution.

In the human thymic involution commences naturally within the first 12 months of life, the thymic epithelial space, where T-cells are generated, reducing. This decline continues throughout life, with an estimated reduction of around 3% a year through middle age (35–45 years) and by 1% thereafter. Indeed the first 12 months of life is when T-cell production is at its most vigorous. The size of the organ gives no clue to these changes because there is replacement by connective and adipose tissue. In a sense, the thymus is progressively disposable because, as we shall see, it establishes a long-lasting peripheral T-cell pool that enables the host to withstand its loss without catastrophic failure of immunological function— witness the minimal effects of thymectomy in the adult compared with the **dramatic influence in the neonate** (Milestone 11.1). Nevertheless, the adult thymus retains a residue of corticomedullary tissue containing a normal range of thymocyte subsets with a broad spectrum of TCR gene rearrangements. Adult patients receiving either T-cell-depleted bone marrow or peripheral blood hematopoietic stem cells following ablative therapy are able to generate new naive T-cells at a rate that is inversely related to the age of the individual. These observations establish that new T-cells are generated in adult life, albeit at a lower rate than during the first few years of life.

Bone marrow stem cells become immunocompetent T-cells in the thymus

The evidence for this comes from experiments on the reconstitution of irradiated hosts. An irradiated animal is restored

⦿ Milestone 11.1—The Immunological Function of the Thymus

Ludwig Gross had found that a form of mouse leukemia could be induced in low-leukemia strains by inoculating filtered leukemic tissue from high-leukemia strains provided that this was done in the immediate neonatal period. As the thymus was known to be involved in the leukemic process, Jacques Miller decided to test the hypothesis that the Gross virus could only multiply in the neonatal thymus by infecting neonatally thymectomized mice of low-leukemia strains. The results were consistent with this hypothesis but, strangely, animals of one strain died of a wasting disease that Miller deduced could have been due to susceptibility to infection, as fewer mice died when they were moved from the converted horse stables, which served as an animal house to "cleaner" quarters.

Autopsy showed the animals to have atrophied lymphoid tissue and low blood lymphocyte levels, and Miller therefore decided to test their immunocompetence before the onset of wasting disease. To his astonishment, skin grafts, even from rats (Figure M11.1.1) as well as from other mouse strains, were fully accepted. These phenomena were not induced by thymectomy later in life and, in writing up his preliminary results in 1961 (Miller J.F.A.P., *Lancet* **ii**, 748–749), Miller suggested that "during embryogenesis the thymus would produce the originators of immunologically competent cells, many of which would have migrated to other sites at about the time of birth." All in all a superb example of the scientific method and its application by a top-flight scientist.

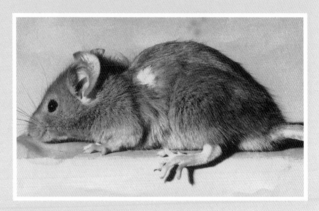

Figure M11.1.1. Acceptance of a rat skin graft by a mouse that had been neonatally thymectomized.

by bone marrow grafts through the immediate restitution of granulocyte precursors; in the longer term, also through reconstitution of the T- and B-cells destroyed by irradiation. However, if the animal is thymectomized before irradiation, bone marrow cells will not reconstitute the T-lymphocyte population (cf. Figure 6.42).

By days 11–12 in the mouse embryo, lymphoblastoid stem cells from the bone marrow begin to colonize the periphery of the epithelial thymus rudiment. If the thymus is removed at this stage and incubated in organ culture, a whole variety of mature T-lymphocytes will be generated. This generation is not seen if 10-day thymuses are cultured, and shows that the lymphoblastoid colonizers give rise to the immunocompetent small lymphocyte progeny.

T-cell ontogeny

Differentiation is accompanied by changes in surface markers

T-cell progenitors arriving from the bone marrow enter the thymus through venules at the corticomedullary junction. The developing T-cells in the thymus are referred to as thymocytes. The newly arrived early thymocytes lack both the CD4 and CD8 coreceptors and are therefore referred to as **double-negative** (DN) cells (Figure 11.3). They do, however, express the chemokine receptor CCR7 and, under the influence of chemokines such as CCL19 and CCL21, they migrate through the thymic cortex towards the outer subcapsular zone before they express a randomly generated TCR and also switch on expression of both CD4 and CD8 to become **double-positive** (DP) cells. They then undergo a process referred to as thymic

education, which comprises two steps—positive selection and negative selection (Figure 11.3)—to ensure that the **single-positive** (SP) CD4 or CD8 cells that exit the thymus bear a TCR that can recognize peptides derived from foreign antigens presented by that individual's own MHC variants.

The earliest of these progenitors, the DN1 cells (Figure 11.4), retain pluripotentiality, still express the stem cell marker CD34, and also express high levels of the adhesion molecule CD44 and the stem cell factor (SCF) receptor (c-kit, CD117) (p. 284). As they mature into DN2 cells they lose CD34 expression and begin to express the IL-2 receptor α chain (CD25). These cells are restricted to producing T-cells and lymphoid dendritic cells. T-cell development is severely impaired in *Notch-1*$^{-/-}$ knockout mice, Notch-1 signaling being necessary for T-cell lineage commitment of the DN1 and DN2 cells. Indeed, the Notch-1 ligands with the rather exotic names of Jagged-1, Jagged-2, δ-like-1 and δ-like-4 are expressed on thymic epithelial cells in a highly regulated way. Further differentiation into DN3 cells and a downregulation of CCR7 expression accompanies their arrival in the subcapsular zone. Transient expression of the recombinase-activating genes *RAG-1* and *RAG-2*, together with an increase in chromatin accessibility, permits recombination of TCR γ-chain and δ-chain or of the TCR β-chain genes during the DN2 and DN3 stages, resulting in commitment to the T-cell lineage. Expression of CD3, the invariant signal transducing complex of the TCR, occurs at this stage, whilst CD44 and c-kit molecules are lost. The γδ T-cells branch off at this point. The loss of CD25 signifies passage of αβ T-cell precursors into the DN4 population, which subsequently differentiate into the CD4$^+$ (the marker for MHC class II recognition) **and** CD8$^+$ (class I recognition)

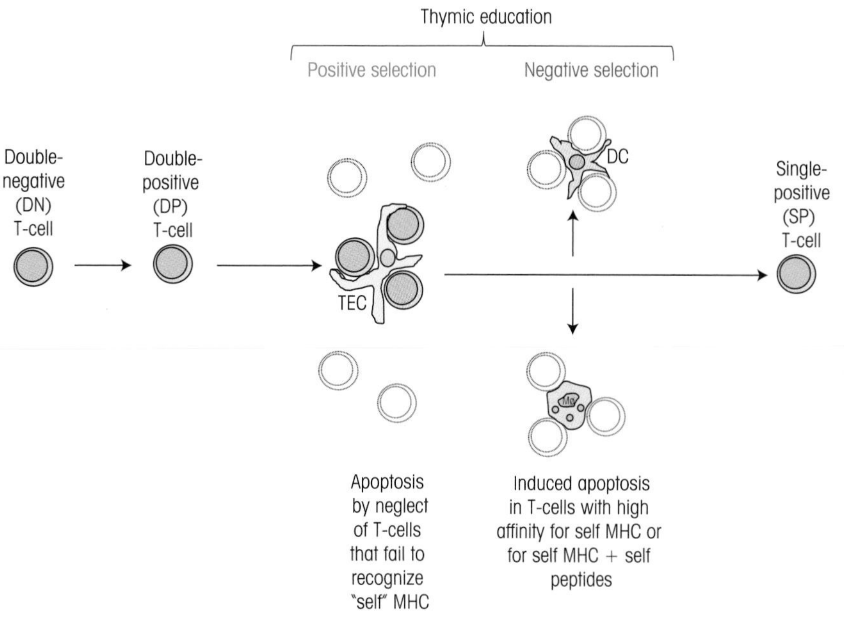

Figure 11.3. Thymic education.

Following a productive recombination of their T-cell receptor (TCR) α-chain and TCR β-chain genes they express a cell surface TCR together with both CD4 and CD8 to become double-positive (DP) cells. Positive selection on thymic epithelial cells (TEC) that express both MHC class I and MHC class II, rescues cells from a "default" pathway of apoptosis, which would occur due to neglect of these cells. As long as they have generated a TCR able to recognize "self" MHC with a low or intermediate affinity they are saved from neglect and these rescued cells are then protected from apoptosis unless they undergo negative selection due to high affinity interaction of their TCR with self MHC or self MHC + self peptides present on dendritic cells (DC) and macrophages (Mφ). The CD4$^+$CD8$^-$ and CD4$^-$CD8$^+$ single-positive (SP) T-cells that exit the thymus therefore possess a TCR with the potential to detect foreign peptides presented by "self" MHC.

double-positive (DP) thymocytes. TCR α-chain gene rearrangement occurs when RAG-1 and RAG-2 are again transiently expressed immediately following expression of CD4 and CD8. The DP thymocytes then begin to re-express high amounts of CCR7 causing them to migrate back through the cortex, eventually crossing the corticomedullary junction into the medulla. The CD4 and CD8 markers segregate in parallel with differentiation into separate immunocompetent populations of **single-positive (SP) CD4$^+$** (mostly **T-helpers**) and **CD8$^+$** (mostly **cytotoxic**) **T-cell precursors**.

In addition to the factors mentioned above, thymocyte development is critically dependent on IL-7, which is produced locally by the thymic epithelial cells and is necessary for the transition to the DN3 stage. Signaling through the IL-7 receptor and c-kit also help drive the early extensive proliferation that occurs in thymocytes prior to the rearrangement of the TCR genes, with thymic stromal lymphopoietin (TSLP) acting as an additional ligand for the IL-7 receptor α-chain. SCF, IL-7 and TSLP are aided and abetted in this task by Wnt family soluble molecules produced by the thymic epithelium that are recognized by receptor complexes on the thymocytes consisting of Frizzled family receptors together with low-density lipoprotein receptor-related proteins LRP5 or LRP6. This stimulation also aids thymocyte differentiation and causes the upregulation of adhesion molecules required for the ordered migration of the chemokine-responsive thymocytes through the thymus. The γδ cells remain double negative, i.e. CD4$^-$8$^-$, except for a small subset that express CD8.

The factors that determine whether the double-positive cells become single-positive CD4$^+$ class II-restricted cells or CD8$^+$ class I-restricted cells in the thymus are still not fully established. Two major scenarios have been put forward. The **stochastic/selection** hypothesis suggests that expression of either the CD4 or CD8 coreceptor is randomly switched off and then cells that have a TCR–coreceptor combination capable of recognizing an appropriate peptide–MHC are selected for survival. By contrast, the **instructive** hypothesis declares that interaction of the TCR with MHC–peptide results in signals that instruct the T-cells to switch off expression of the "useless" coreceptor incapable of recognizing that particular class of MHC. In order to reconcile the fact that there is supporting data for both hypotheses, various other models have been put forward including proposals that stronger **signal strength** or longer **signal duration** favors CD4 cell development. These various models are still the subject of debate amongst the immunological community. What is fairly clear, however, is that expression of the transcription factors Th-POK, TOX and GATA-3 are important for CD4$^+$ T-cell development whereas production of the transcription factor RUNX3 favors CD8$^+$ T-cell development.

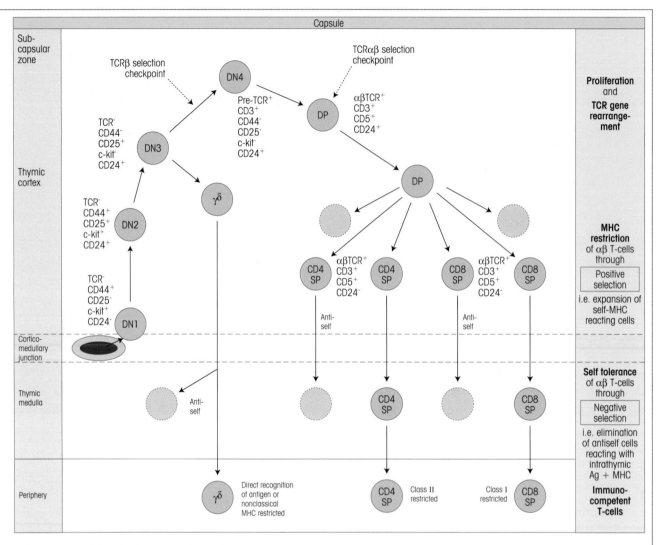

Figure 11.4. Differentiation of T-cells within the thymus.

T-cell precursors arriving from the bone marrow enter the thymus via blood vessels at the cortico-medullary junction. The transition between the different populations of CD4⁻CD8⁻ (double-negative, DN) T-cell precursors in the thymus is marked by the differential expression of CD44, CD25, c-kit and CD24. DN3 cells are unable to progress to the DN4 stage unless they successfully rearrange one of their two T-cell receptor (TCR) β-chain gene loci. Successful rearrangement of the TCR α-chain to form the mature receptor is obligatory for differentiation beyond the early CD4⁺CD8⁺ (double-positive, DP) stage. The double-positive T-cells that bear an αβ TCR are subjected to positive and negative selection events, the "useless" T-cells (i.e. those unable to recognize self MHC) that die by neglect during positive selection and the self-reactive negatively selected cells

are indicated in gray. Autoreactive cells with specificity for self-antigens not expressed in the thymus may be tolerized by extrathymic peripheral contact with antigen. γδ T-cells, which develop from the DN3 T-cell precursors, mainly appear to recognize antigen directly, in a manner analogous to the antibody molecule on B-cells, although some may be restricted by nonclassical MHC-like molecules. Details and location of positive and negative selection events for γδ T-cells are not well characterized. NKT cells, which are not shown in the diagram for the sake of clarity, arise from the double-positive T-cells to become CD4⁺CD8⁻, CD4⁻CD8⁺ or CD4⁻CD8⁻cells bearing an invariant αβ TCR and the NK1.1 marker (cf. p. 135). They usually recognize antigens presented by CD1d.

NKT cells constitute a distinct subset of αβ T-cells

These cells, which branch from conventional T-cells at the double-positive stage of thymocyte development, express markers associated with both T-cells and NK cells, such as a

TCR and the C-lectin-type receptor NK1.1, respectively. The TCR of NKT cells is mostly composed of an invariant TCR α chain (Vα14Jα18 in mice, Vα24J18 in human) together with a Vβ8 (mouse) or Vβ11 (human) β chain. They recognize glycolipids such as the endogenous lysosomal isoglobotrihexosylceramide (iGb3) and the microbial antigen phosphatidyli-nositol mannoside from mycobacteria. These antigens are presented to the invariant TCR by the nonpolymorphic MHC class I-like CD1d molecule, and when activated the NKT cells secrete large amounts of cytokines including IFNγ and IL-4, i.e. both Th1 and Th2-type cytokines. It has been proposed that NKT cells may function primarily as regulatory cells.

Receptor rearrangement

Rearrangement of *V*-, *D*- and *J*-region genes are required to generate the TCR (see p. 87). By day 15 of fetal development cells with the γδ TCR can be detected in the mouse thymus followed soon by the appearance of a "**pre-TCR**" version of the αβ TCR. Notch-1 signals (again!) appear to play a role in αβ versus γδ lineage commitment, although the details are still being worked out.

The development of αβ receptors

The TCR β-chain gene is usually rearranged at the DN3 stage and associates with an invariant pre-α chain, pTα, to form a "pre-TCR," functional rearrangement of the β-chain being required for transition to the DN4 stage (Figure 11.4). Signaling through the pre-TCR occurs in a ligand-independent manner whereby the pre-TCR molecules constitutively target to lipid rafts. Activation of signaling cascades involving Ras/MAPK and phospholipase Cγ1 pathways recruit Ets-1 and other transcription factors, stimulating the proliferation and differentiation of DN3 cells into DN4 and subsequently into DP cells, as well as mediating feedback inhibition on further TCR Vβ gene rearrangement. Subsequent development of pre-T-cells requires rearrangement of the **Vα** gene segments so allowing formation of the mature αβ TCR.

Rearrangement of the Vβ genes on the sister chromatid is suppressed following the expression of the pre-TCR (remember each cell contains two chromosomes for each α and β cluster). Thus each cell only expresses a single TCR β chain and the process by which the homologous genes on the sister chromatid are suppressed is called **allelic exclusion**. This exclusion is at least partially due to the methylation of histones maintaining a closed chromatin structure that prevents access of the recombinases to the TCR gene segments on the excluded allele.

The α chains are not always allelically excluded, so that many immature T-cells in the thymus have two antigen-specific receptors, each with their own α chain but sharing a common β chain. However, expression of one of the α chains is usually lost during T-cell maturation, leaving the cell with a single specificity αβ TCR. Nonetheless, around 1–8% of peripheral T-cells in both mice and humans have cell surface TCRs that all have the same β chain but can employ one of two different α chains. These dual specificity T-cells may extend the TCR repertoire to include recognition of foreign antigen peptides that would not otherwise be selected in the thymus.

The development of γδ receptors

Unlike the αβ TCR, the γδ TCR in many cases seems to be able to bind directly to antigen without the necessity for antigen presentation by MHC or MHC-like molecules, i.e. it recognizes antigen directly in a manner similar to antibody. The γδ lineage does not produce a "pre-receptor" and mice expressing rearranged γ and δ transgenes do not rearrange any further γ or δ gene segments, indicating allelic exclusion of sister chromatid genes.

γδ T-cells in the mouse, unlike the human, predominate in association with epithelial cells. A curious feature of the cells leaving the fetal thymus is the restriction in V gene utilization. Virtually all of the first wave of fetal γδ cells express Vγ5 and colonize the skin; the second wave predominantly utilizes Vγ6 and seed the uterus in the female. In adult life, there is far more receptor diversity due to a high degree of junctional variation (cf. p. 91), although the intraepithelial cells in the intestine preferentially use Vγ4 and those in encapsulated lymphoid tissue tend to express Vγ4, Vγ1.1 and Vγ2. It should be noted that, just to confuse everyone, other nomenclatures are also currently in circulation regarding the numbering of the individual murine Vγ genes. The Vγ set in the skin readily proliferates and secretes IL-2 on exposure to heat-shocked keratinocytes, implying a role in the surveillance of trauma signals. The γδ T-cells in peripheral lymphoid tissue respond well to the tuberculosis antigen PPD ("purified protein derivative") and to conserved epitopes from mycobacterial and self-heat-shock protein hsp65. However, evidence from γδ TCR knockout mice suggests that overall, in the adult, γδ T-cells may make a minor contribution to pathogen-specific protection. It has therefore been proposed that their primary role may be in the regulation of αβ T-cells, with most γδ T-cells biased towards a Th1 cytokine secretion pattern.

Two major γδ subsets predominate in the human, Vγ9,Vδ2 and Vγ1,Vδ2. The Vγ9 set rises from 25% of the total γδ cells in cord blood to around 70% in adult blood; at the same time, the proportion of Vγ1 falls from 50% to less than 30%. The majority of the Vγ9 set have the activated memory phenotype CD45RO, probably as a result of stimulation by common ligands for the Vγ9,Vδ2 TCR, such as nonproteinaceous phosphate-bearing antigenic components of mycobacteria, *Plasmodium falciparum* and the superantigen staphylococcal enterotoxin A.

Cells are positively selected for self-MHC restriction in the thymus

The ability of T-cells to recognize antigenic peptides in association with self-MHC is developed in the thymus. If an (H-2^k × H-2^b) F1 animal is sensitized to an antigen, the primed T-cells can recognize that antigen on presenting cells of either *H-2^k* or *H-2^b* haplotype, i.e. they can use either parental haplotype as a recognition restriction element. However, if bone marrow cells from the (H-2^k × H-2^b) F1 are used to reconstitute an irradiated F1 that had earlier been thymectomized and

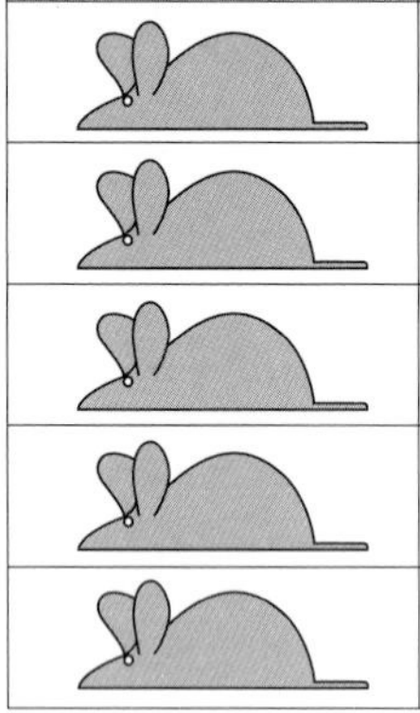

Thymectomize *b* x *k* mice	Graft with thymus of haplotype	Irradiate and reconstitute with *b* x *k* bone marrow	Prime with KLH	Proliferative response of primed T-cells to KLH on antigen-presenting cells of haplotype	
				*H-2^b^*	*H-2^k^*
	b x *k*	→		++	++
	b	→		++	-
	dGuo-treated *b*	→		++	-
	k	→		-	++
	dGuo-treated *k*	→		-	++

Figure 11.5. Imprinting of H-2 T-helper restriction by the haplotype of the thymus.

Host mice were F1 crosses between strains of haplotype *H-2^b^* and *H-2^k^*. They were thymectomized and grafted with 14-day fetal thymuses, irradiated and reconstituted with F1 bone marrow. After priming with the antigen keyhole limpet hemocyanin (KLH), the proliferative response of lymph node T-cells to KLH on antigen-presenting cells of each parental haplotype was assessed. In some experiments, the thymus lobes were cultured in deoxyguanosine (dGuo), which destroys intrathymic cells of macrophage/dendritic cell lineage, but this had no effect on positive selection. (From Lo D. & Sprent J. (1986) *Nature* **319**, 672–675.)

given an H-2^k thymus, the subsequently primed T-cells can only recognize antigens in the context of H-2^k, not of H-2^b (Figure 11.5). Thus it is **the phenotype of the thymus that imprints H-2 restriction** on the differentiating T-cells.

It will also be seen in Figure 11.5 that incubation of the thymus graft with deoxyguanosine, which destroys the cells of macrophage and dendritic cell lineage, has no effect on imprinting, suggesting that this function is carried out by epithelial cells. Confirmation of this comes from a study showing that lethally irradiated H-2^k mice, reconstituted with (b × k) F1 bone marrow and then injected intrathymically with an H-2^b thymic epithelial cell line, developed T-cells restricted by the *b* haplotype. The epithelial cells are rich in both MHC class I and class II cell surface molecules and the current view is that double-positive (CD4$^+$8$^+$) T-cells bearing receptors that recognize self-MHC on the epithelial cells are positively selected for differentiation to CD4$^+$8$^-$ or CD4$^-$8$^+$ single-positive cells. The evidence for this comes largely from studies in transgenic mice. As this is a very active area, we would like to cite some experimental examples; nonprofessionals may need to hang on to their haplotypes, put on their ice-packs and concentrate.

One highly sophisticated study starts with a cytotoxic T-cell clone raised in H-2^b females against male cells of the same strain. The clone recognizes the male antigen, H-Y, and this is seen in association with the H-2D^b self-MHC molecules, i.e. it reacts with the H-2^b/Y complex. The α and β chains for the T-cell receptor of this clone are now introduced as transgenes into SCID mice, which lack the ability to rearrange their own germline variable region receptor genes; thus the only TCR that could possibly be expressed is that encoded by the transgenes, provided of course that we are looking at females rather than males, in whom the clone would be eliminated by self-reactivity. If the transgenic SCID females bear the original *H-2^b^* haplotype (e.g. F1 hybrids between *b* × *d* haplotypes), then the anti-H-2^b/Y receptor is amply expressed on CD8$^+$ cytotoxic precursor cells (Table 11.2a), whereas H-2^d transgenics lacking H-2^b produce only double-positive CD4$^+$8$^+$ thymocytes with no single-positive CD4$^+$8$^-$ or CD4$^-$8$^+$ cells. Thus, as CD4$^+$8$^+$ cells express their TCR transgene, they only differentiate into CD8$^+$ immunocompetent cells if they come into contact with thymic epithelial cells of the MHC haplotype recognized by their receptor. We say that such self-recognizing thymocytes are being **positively selected**. Positive intracellular events accompany the positive selection process as the protein tyrosine kinases fyn and lck are activated in double-positive CD4$^+$8$^+$ thymocytes maturing to single-positive CD8$^+$ cells in the *b* haplotype background, but are low in cells that fail to differentiate into mature cells in the nonselective *d* haplotype.

In another example, genes encoding an αβ receptor from a T-helper clone (2B4), which responds to moth cytochrome *c* in association with the class II molecule H-2Eα^k,β^b (remember H-2E has an α and β chain), are transfected into H-2^k and H-2^b mice. For irrelevant reasons, H-2^k mice express the H-2E molecule on the surface of their antigen-presenting cells, but

Table 11.2. Positive and negative selection in SCID transgenic mice bearing the αβ receptors of an H-2D^b T-cell clone cytotoxic for the male antigen H-Y, i.e. the clone is of _H-2^b_ haplotype and is female anti-male. (a) The only T-cells are those bearing the already rearranged transgenic TCR, as SCID mice cannot rearrange their own _V_ genes. The clones are only expanded beyond the CD4$^+$8$^+$ stage when positively selected by contact with the MHC haplotype (_H-2^b_) recognized by the original clone from which the transgene was derived. Also, as the TCR recognized class I, only CD8$^+$ cells were selected. (b) When the anti-male transgenic clone is expressed on intrathymic T-cells in a male environment, the strong engagement of the TCR with male antigen-bearing cells eliminates them. (Based on data from von Boehmer H. _et al._ (1989) In: Melchers F. _et al._ (eds.) _Progress in Immunology 7_, p. 297. Springer-Verlag, Berlin.) +, crude measure of the relative numbers of T-cells in the thymus having the phenotype indicated.

Phenotype of thymocytes	(a) Positive selection		(b) Negative selection	
	Haplotype of transgenic females		Transgenic H-2^b mice	
	_H-2$^{b/d}$_	_H-2$^{d/d}$_	Males	Females
CD4$^-$8$^-$ TCR$^-$	+	++	+++	+
CD4$^+$8$^+$ TCR$^\pm$	++	+	−	+++
CD4$^-$8$^+$ TCR^{++}	+	−	−	+
CD4$^-$8$^-$ TCR^{++}	−	−	−	−

Table 11.3. Induction of tolerance in bone marrow stem cells by incubation with deoxyguanosine (dGuo)-sensitive macrophages or dendritic cells in the thymus. Clearly, the bone marrow cells induce tolerance to their own haplotype. Thus the thymic tolerance-inducing cells can be replaced by progenitors in the bone marrow inoculum (Jenkinson E.J., Jhittay P., Kingston R. & Owen J.J. (1985) _Transplantation_ 39, 331) or by adult dendritic cells from spleen, showing that it is the stage of differentiation of the immature T-cell rather than any special nature of the thymic antigen-presenting cell which leads to tolerance (Matzinger P. & Guerder S. (1989) _Nature_ 338, 74).

Bone marrow cells	Incubate with H-2^d thymus	Tolerance induction to _H-2_ haplotype		
		_k_	_d_	_b_
k	Untreated	+	+	−
k	dGuo-treated	+	−	−
k + d	dGuo-treated	+	+	−

H-2^b do not. In the event, the frequency of circulating CD4$^+$ T-cells bearing the 2B4 receptor was 10 times greater in the H-2^k relative to H-2^b strains, again speaking for positive selection of double-positive thymocytes that recognize their own thymic MHC. In a further twist to the story, positive selection only occurred in mice manipulated to express H-2E on their cortical rather than their medullary epithelial cells, showing that this differentiation step is effected before the developing thymocytes reach the medulla. ("Read it again Sam" as Humphrey Bogart might have said!)

T-cell tolerance

The induction of immunological tolerance is necessary to avoid self-reactivity

In essence, lymphocytes use receptors that recognize foreign antigens through complementarity of shape (see p. 114). To a large extent the building blocks used to form microbial and host molecules are the same, and so it is the assembled shapes of _self_ and _nonself_ molecules that must be discriminated by the immune system if potentially disastrous autoreactivity is to be avoided. The restriction of each lymphocyte to a single specificity makes the job of establishing self-tolerance that much easier, simply because it just requires a mechanism that functionally deletes self-reacting cells and leaves the remainder of the repertoire unscathed. The most radical difference between self and nonself molecules lies in the fact that, in early life, the developing lymphocytes are surrounded by self and normally only meet nonself antigens at a later stage and then within the context of the adjuvanticity and cytokine release usually associated with infection. Evolution has exploited these differences to establish the mechanisms of **immunological tolerance to host constituents** (Milestone 11.2).

Self-tolerance can be induced in the thymus

As developing T-cells are to be found in the thymus, one might expect this to be the milieu in which exposure to self-antigens on the surrounding cells would induce tolerance. The expectation is reasonable. If stem cells in bone marrow of _H-2^k_ haplotype are cultured with fetal thymus of H-2^d origin, the maturing cells become tolerant to H-2^d, as shown by their inability to give a mixed lymphocyte proliferative response when cultured with stimulators of H-2^d phenotype; third-party responsiveness is not affected. Further experiments with deoxyguanosine-treated thymuses showed that the cells responsible for tolerance induction were deoxyguanosine-sensitive, bone marrow-derived macrophages or dendritic cells that are abundant at the corticomedullary junction (Table 11.3).

Intrathymic clonal deletion leads to self-tolerance

There seems little doubt that strongly self-reactive T-cells can be physically deleted within the thymus. If we look at the

Milestone 11.2—The Discovery of Immunological Tolerance

Over 60 years ago, Owen made the intriguing observation that nonidentical (dizygotic) twin cattle, which shared the same placental circulation and whose circulations were thereby linked, grew up with appreciable numbers of red cells from the other twin in their blood; if they had not shared the same circulation at birth, red cells from the twin injected in adult life would have been rapidly eliminated by an immunological response. From this finding, Burnet and Fenner conceived the notion that potential antigens that reach the lymphoid cells during their developing immunologically immature phase can in some way specifically suppress any future response to that antigen when the animal reaches immunological maturity. This, they considered, would provide a means whereby unresponsiveness to the body's own constituents could be established and thereby enable the lymphoid cells to make the important distinction between "self" and "nonself." On this basis, any foreign cells introduced into the body during immunological development should trick the animal into treating them as "self"-components in later life, and the studies of Medawar and his colleagues have shown that **immunological tolerance**, or unresponsiveness, can be artificially induced in this way. Thus neonatal injection of CBA mouse cells into newborn A strain animals suppresses their ability to reject a CBA graft immunologically in adult life (Figure M11.2.1). Tolerance can also be induced with soluble antigens; for example, rabbits injected with bovine serum albumin without adjuvant at birth fail to make antibodies on later challenge with this protein.

Persistence of antigen is required to maintain tolerance. In Medawar's experiments, the tolerant state was long lived because the injected CBA cells survived and the animals continued to be chimeric (i.e. they possessed both A and CBA cells). With nonliving antigens, such as soluble bovine serum albumin, tolerance is gradually lost because in the absence of antigen, newly recruited immunocompetent cells that are being generated throughout life are not being rendered tolerant. As recruitment of newly competent T-lymphocytes is drastically curtailed by removal of the thymus, it is of interest to note that the tolerant state persists for much longer in thymectomized animals.

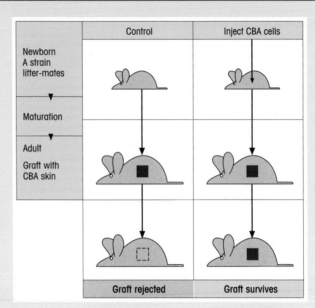

Figure M11.2.1. Induction of tolerance to foreign CBA skin graft in A strain mice by neonatal injection of antigen.

The effect is antigen specific as the tolerant mice can reject third-party grafts normally. (After Billingham R., Brent L. & Medawar P.B. (1953) *Nature* **172**, 603–606.)

The vital importance of the experiments by Medawar and his team was their demonstration that a state of immunological tolerance can result from exposure to an antigen. As will be discussed in the text, there is a window of susceptibility to clonal deletion of self-reacting T-lymphocytes at an immature phase in their ontogenic development within the thymus (and in the case of B-cells within the bone marrow). Although in animal models it is often easier to impose tolerance during the neonatal period when there is extensive production of naive lymphocytes, tolerance can be induced throughout life. Note that resting T-cells are generally more readily tolerizable than memory cells.

experiment in Table 11.2b, we can see that SCID males bearing the rearranged transgenes coding for the αβ receptor reacting with the male H-Y antigen do not possess any immunocompetent thymic cells expressing this receptor, whereas the females that lack H-Y do. Thus, when the developing T-cells react with self-antigen in the thymus, they are deleted. In other words, self-reactive cells undergo a **negative selection** process in the thymus, a process that constitutes **central tolerance** of the T-cells. Expression of the *AIRE* (*au*toimmune *re*gulator) gene in medullary thymic epithelial cells acts as a master switch directing the transcriptional activation of the genes for a number of organ-specific self antigens. The ectopic expression of these antigens provokes the elimination of the correspond-

ing self-reactive thymocytes. Confirmation of the importance of AIRE expression for such clonal deletion has come from experiments using a double transgenic model developed by Goodnow and colleagues. In these mice a membrane-bound version of hen egg lysozyme (HEL) is transgenically expressed as a "neo-self" antigen (because it is always present it becomes essentially a self antigen), and high numbers of thymocytes specific for this antigen are also generated by introduction of the relevant TCR as the other transgene. When the HEL transgene is linked to the tissue-specific *rat insulin promoter* (RIP), expression of the "self" antigen occurs in both the β-cells in the islets of Langerhans of the pancreas *and* in the thymus. In the absence of AIRE the RIP-driven expression of

HEL fails to occur in thymic epithelium, but still occurs in the pancreatic islets. The developing transgenic T-cells that are normally deleted in the thymus escape deletion in the AIRE deficient mice and kill the β-cells in the pancreas (Figure 11.6).

Deletion of thymocytes also occurs when thymic cells bear certain self-components that act as superantigens (cf. p. 136), in this case because the antigen reacts with a whole family of Vβ receptors through recognition of nonvariable structures on a Vβ segment. For example, mice of the *Mls^a* genotype delete Vβ6-bearing cells, the *Mls* being a locus encoding a B-cell superantigen that induces strong proliferation in Vβ6 T-cells from a strain bearing a different *Mls* allele (cf. p. 136). Even exogenous superantigens, such as staphylococcal enterotoxin B that activates the Vβ3 and Vβ8 T-cell families in the adult, can induce apoptosis in early immature thymocytes utilizing these receptor families.

Factors affecting positive or negative selection in the thymus

T-cells that either fail to express a TCR at all, or which express a TCR of very low affinity, do not receive survival signals and die from neglect. For the remaining cells the engagement of the TCR by MHC–peptide underlies both positive and negative selection. But how can the same MHC–peptide signal have two totally different outcomes? Well, positive and negative selection may occur at low and high degrees of TCR ligation, respectively. For example, high concentrations of antibody to the TCR-associated CD3 induce apoptosis in thymocytes (Figure 11.7), whereas low concentrations do not. Furthermore, many examples have been published showing that the same peptide will induce positive selection at low concentration and negative selection at high concentration. This has led to the avidity model, which postulates that no interaction or a very low avidity interaction between T-cell and peptide–MHC will lead to death by neglect, a low/intermediate avidity interaction will positively select double-positive CD4+8+ thymocytes, while a high avidity interaction will lead to clonal deletion. Thus, engagement of the TCR with self-MHC on cortical epithelial cells leads to expansion and positive selection for clones that recognize self-MHC, perhaps with a whole range of affinities, but that engagement of the TCR with high affinity for self-MHC (+ self-peptide) on medullary epithelial cells and dendritic cells will lead to elimination and hence negative

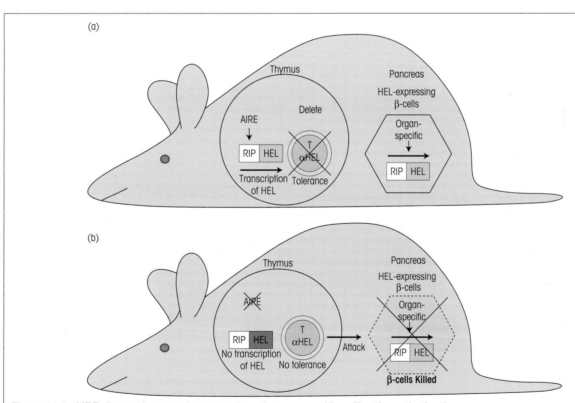

Figure 11.6. AIRE directs the ectopic expression of organ-specific self antigens in the thymus.

Double transgenic mice were generated by crossing transgenic mice expressing a membrane-bound form of hen egg lysozyme (HEL) under the control of the rat insulin promoter (RIP) with mice expressing the transgenic 3A9 αβ TCR specific for the amino acid 46–61 peptide from HEL presented by the I-A^k MHC class II molecule. These mice normally tolerize the transgenic T-cells in the thymus (a), but this did not occur if the mice were backcrossed to mice in which the AIRE gene had been knocked out (b). The incidence of type 1 diabetes was dramatically increased in the absence of AIRE expression. (Based on data from Liston A. *et al.* (2004) *Journal of Experimental Medicine* **200**, 1015–1026.)

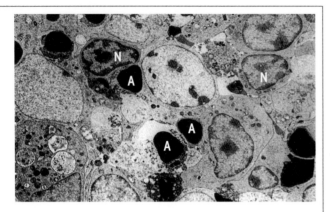

Figure 11.7. Electron micrograph of cells induced to undergo apoptosis in intact fetal thymus lobes after short-term exposure to anti-CD3.

A and N indicate representative apoptotic and normal lymphocytes, respectively. Note the highly condensed state of the nuclei of the apoptotic lymphocytes. (Photograph kindly donated by Professor J.J.T. Owen, from Smith *et al.* (1989) *Nature* **337**, 181–184. Reproduced by permission from Macmillan Journals Ltd, London.)

selection. Although still not fully worked out, there are also obvious differences in the biochemical pathways used for positive and negative signaling. Positive selection is cyclosporine sensitive and dependent on the Ras–MEK–ERK pathway (cf. p. 211), whereas negative selection is cyclosporine resistant and independent of this pathway. Different intensities of signaling from the TCR, Notch and other receptors may influence which pathway is utilized. The Ikaros transcription factor seems to be important in regulating signaling thresholds during selection events in the thymus, and also appears to help determine whether DP thymocytes become CD4 or CD8 SP cells during positive selection. Thus, thymocytes in Ikaros knockout mice preferentially develop into CD4 SP cells compared with thymocytes in wild-type mice. Let us finish on a cautionary note: the avidity model may be substantially correct but it could be an oversimplification. For instance, certain superantigens, which can cause clonal deletion of certain Vβ families, fail to expand them even at very low concentrations when the model would have indicated positive selection. This finding has spawned other models involving conformational changes at the TCR–peptide–MHC binding interface. Given the complex interactions of peptides behaving as agonists, partial agonists and antagonists it is likely that the last word has not yet been spoken (not that it ever is in science!).

T-cell tolerance can also be due to clonal anergy

We have already entertained the idea that engagement of the TCR plus a co-stimulatory signal from an antigen-presenting cell are both required for T-cell stimulation, but, when the co-stimulatory signal is lacking, the T-cell becomes tolerized or anergic, or, if you prefer, paralyzed. T-cell tolerance occurring

outside the thymus is referred to as **peripheral tolerance**. Thus, anergy can be induced in T-cells by peripheral antigens *in vivo* when presented by cells lacking co-stimulatory molecules. The anergic T-cells are unable to produce IL-2, even if subsequently given signals through their TCR with concomitant co-stimulation by cross-linking CD28 on their cell surface. In some experimental models, anergy can be broken by providing high levels of exogenous IL-2, i.e. anergy is a potentially reversible tolerance whereas clonal deletion by apoptosis clearly is not, as the deleted cells no longer exist.

The anergic state can even be passed on to surrounding cells, a process referred to as **infectious anergy**. If a clone of T-helpers is subject to a limiting dilution experiment (p. 175), the minimal unit of proliferation in response to peptide on an APC is usually several cells not just one. This implies that triggering only occurs in small groups or clusters of cells and suggests that paracrine or multicellular interactions between potential responders bound to a single APC are needed to drive the cells into division (Figure 11.8a). It will be appreciated that, if a naive T-cell binds to its antigen, even on a professional APC in secondary lymphoid tissues, it will not be stimulated if its neighbors in the cluster have already been made anergic. Indeed, instead of being triggered, it will itself become anergic, so perpetuating the infectious anergic process (Figure 11.8b). CD4⁺CD25⁺Foxp3⁺ Treg cells, which often naturally exhibit a state of profound anergy, may be the critical cell here. It is thought that such cells can downregulate MHC class II and the co-stimulatory CD80 (B7.1) and CD86 (B7.2) molecules on the APC, generating an infectious anergy that does not require the simultaneous presence of the Tregs and the cells that will themselves be made anergic (Figure 11.8c). Anergic regulatory T-cells might also be capable of inducing apoptosis in dendritic cells via CD95–CD95L interactions, or cause the dendritic cells to induce apoptosis in responder T-cells, again by the CD95 pathway. We shall see later in Chapter 16 that the induction of transplantation immunosuppression with a nondepleting anti-CD4 can be long-lasting because the production of anergic regulatory T-cells prevents the priming of newly immunocompetent T-lymphocytes by the transplantation antigen(s).

Lack of communication can cause unresponsiveness

It takes two to tango: if the self-molecule cannot engage the TCR, there can be no response. The anatomical isolation of molecules, like the lens protein of the eye and myelin basic protein in the brain, virtually precludes them from contact with lymphocytes, except perhaps for minute amounts of breakdown metabolic products that leak out and may be taken up by antigen-presenting cells, but at concentrations way below that required to trigger the corresponding naive T-cell.

Even when a tissue is exposed to circulating lymphocytes, the concentration of processed peptide on the cell surface may be insufficient to attract attention from a potentially auto-

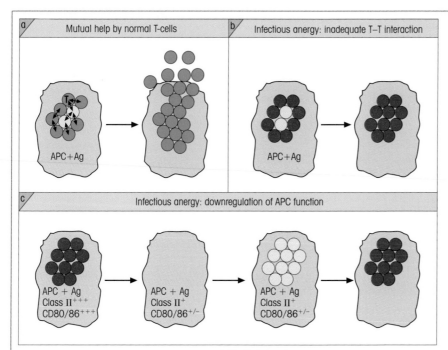

Figure 11.8. Infectious anergy.

(a) Clusters of normal T-cells (green) around newly immunocompetent cells (gray) reacting with the same APC mutually support activation and proliferation. (b) Newly immunocompetent cells surrounded by anergic T-cells (red) receive no stimulatory signals from their neighbors and are themselves rendered anergic. (c) The anergic T-cells can act as regulatory T-cells whereby they downregulate expression of MHC class II, CD80 (B7.1) and CD86 (B7.2) molecules on the APC. This effect requires cell–cell contact between the anergic T-cells and the APC. Subsequent encounter of newly immunocompetent cells with this APC will lead to anergy.

reactive cell in the absence of co-stimulatory B7. This situation was demonstrated rather elegantly in animals bearing two transgenes: one for the TCR of a CD8 cytotoxic T-cell specific for lymphocytic choriomeningitis (LCM) virus glycoprotein, and the other for the glycoprotein itself expressed on pancreatic β-cells through the insulin promoter. The result? A deafening silence: the T-cells were not deleted or tolerized, nor were the β-cells attacked. If these mice were then infected with LCM virus, the naive transgenic T-cells were presented with adequate concentrations of the processed glycoprotein within the adjuvant context of a true infection and were now stimulated. Their *primed* progeny, having an increased avidity (cf. p. 486) and thereby being able to recognize the low concentrations of processed glycoprotein on the β-cells, attacked their targets even in the absence of B7 and caused diabetes (Figure 11.9). This may sound a trifle tortuous, but the principle could have important implications for the induction of autoimmunity by cross-reacting T-cell epitopes.

Molecules that are specifically restricted to particular organs that do not normally express MHC class II represent another special case, as they would not have the opportunity to interact with organ-specific CD4 T-helper cells.

Immunological silence would also result if an individual has no genes coding for lymphocyte receptors directed against particular self-determinants; analysis of the experimentally induced autoantibody response to cytochrome c suggests that only those parts of the molecule that show species variation are autoantigenic, whereas the highly conserved regions where the genes have not altered for a much longer time appear to be silent, supposedly because the autoreactive specificities have had time to disappear during evolution.

B-cells differentiate in the fetal liver and then in bone marrow

A series of differentiation markers are associated with B-cell maturation (Figure 11.10). The B-lymphocyte precursors, pro-B-cells, are present among the islands of hematopoietic cells in fetal liver by 8–9 weeks of gestation in humans and 14 days in the mouse. Production of B-cells wanes in newborn and neonatal liver and is mostly taken over by the bone marrow for the remainder of life. Stromal reticular cells, which express adhesion molecules and secrete IL-7, extend long dendritic processes making intimate contact with IL-7 receptor-positive B-cell progenitors.

Pax5 is a major determining factor in B-cell differentiation

Development of hematopoietic cells along the B-cell lineage requires expression of E2A and of early B-cell factor (EBF); the absence of either of these prevents pro-B-cells progressing to the pre-B-cell stage (Figure 11.11). Also required is expression of the *Pax5* gene that encodes the BSAP (*B*-cell-*s*pecific *a*ctivator *p*rotein) transcription factor. Thus, in *Pax5*$^{-/-}$ knockout mice, early pre-B-cells (containing partially rearranged immunoglobulin heavy chain genes) fail to differentiate into mature, surface Ig⁺, B-cells (Figure 11.11). However, if the pre-B-cells from *Pax5*$^{-/-}$ knockout mice are provided with the appropriate cytokines *in vitro,* they can be driven to produce T-cells, NK cells, macrophages, dendritic cells, granulocytes and even osteoclasts! These unexpected findings clearly demonstrated that the early pre-B-cell has the potential to be diverted from its

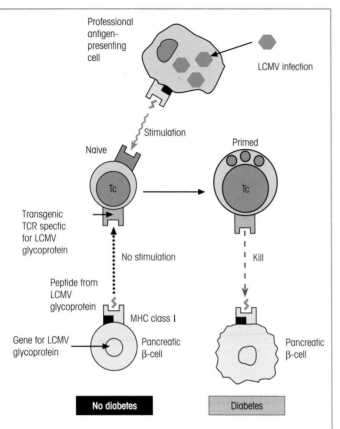

Figure 11.9. Mutual unawareness of a naive cytotoxic precursor T-cell and its B7-negative cellular target bearing epitopes present at low concentrations.

Priming of the naive cell by a natural infection and subsequent attack by the higher avidity primed cells on the target tissue. LCMV, lymphocytic choriomeningitis virus. (From Ohashi P.S. *et al.* (1991) *Cell* **65**, 305–317.)

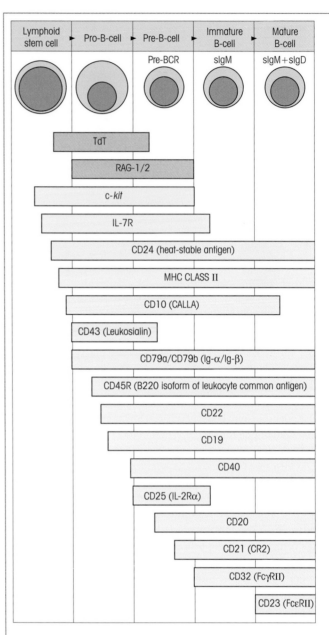

Figure 11.10. Some of the differentiation markers of developing B-cells.

The time of appearance of enzymes involved in Ig gene rearrangement and diversification (blue boxes) and of surface markers defined by monoclonal antibodies (orange boxes, see Table 11.1 for list of CD members) is shown.

chosen path and instead provide a source of cells for many other hematopoietic lineages. However, these pre-B-cells are not pluripotent as, unlike bone marrow hematopoietic stem cells, they are unable to rescue lethally irradiated mice. It is clear that *Pax5* acts as a critical master gene by directing B-cell development along the correct pathway, and does this by repressing expression of genes, such as those encoding Notch-1, myeloperoxidase and monocyte/macrophage colony-stimulating factor receptor, that are associated with other lineages, whilst activating B-cell-specific genes including Ig-α, CD19 and the adaptor protein BLNK.

B-1 and B-2 cells represent two distinct populations

There exists a subpopulation of B-cells (referred to as **B-1 cells**) that, in addition to surface IgM, express CD5. The progenitors of this subset move from the fetal liver to the peritoneal cavity fairly early in life, at which stage they are the most abundant B-cell type and predominate in their contribution to the idi-

otype network and to the production of low affinity, multispecific IgM autoantibodies and the so-called "natural" antibodies to bacterial carbohydrates, which seemingly arise slightly later in the neonatal period without obvious exposure to conventional antigens.

The **B-1 phenotype, high surface IgM, low surface IgD, CD43⁺ and CD23⁻**, is shared by a minority subpopulation

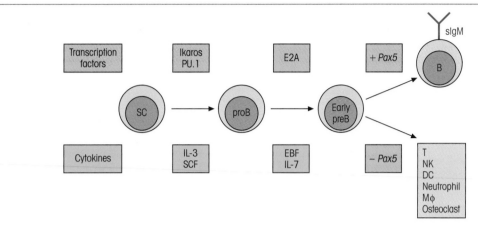

Figure 11.11. *Pax5* is required for B-cell differentiation.

Hematopoietic stem cells (SC) under the influence of stem cell factor (SCF), IL-3 and the Ikaros and PU.1 transcription factors can differentiate into pro-B-cells. Further differentiation into pre-B-cells requires the E2A transcription factor together with early B-cell factor (EBF) and IL-7. Homozygous E2A mutant mice lack pre-B-cells, there being a block to $D_H J_H$ rearrangement in the Ig heavy chain locus plus severe reduction in RAG-1, Ig-α, CD19 and λ_5 transcripts. If at the early pre-B stage *Pax5* is not expressed, then differentiation along the B-cell lineage pathway comes to an abrupt halt. These early pre-B-cells have rearranged Ig D_H to J_H indicating their intention to become B-cells. However, even at this late stage, they can make other lineage choices as evidenced by the fact that, in the absence of *Pax5* expression, they can give rise to a number of other cell types if they are provided with appropriate cytokines. Indeed, *Pax5*$^{-/-}$ clones are able to develop into T-cells if transferred to immunodeficient mice, in which case they express rearranged TCR genes in addition to their initial Ig heavy chain gene rearrangement.

that is, however, CD5$^-$; these two populations are referred to as B-1a and B-1b respectively (Figure 11.12). Conventional B-cells (**B-2 cells**), have the **phenotype low surface IgM, high surface IgD, CD5$^-$, CD43$^-$ and CD23$^+$**, reflecting the fact that they represent a separate developmental lineage. Some general comments may be in order. At least in mice, B-1a, B1-b and B-2 cells are each derived from distinct progenitors. Although B-1 cells can shift to a B-2 phenotype, and possibly vice versa, there is minimal conversion between the two lineages under normal circumstances. B-1 cells are particularly prevalent in the peritoneal and pleural cavities, maintain their numbers by self-replenishment and limit their *de novo* production from progenitors by feedback regulation. B-1a cells can express both CD5 and its ligand CD72 on their surface, which should encourage mutual interaction, but a major factor influencing self-renewal could be the constitutive production of IL-10, as treatment of mice with anti-IL-10 from birth virtually wipes out the B-1 subset. The predisposition for self-renewal may underlie their undue susceptibility to become leukemic, with the malignant cells in chronic lymphocytic leukemia being almost invariably CD5$^+$.

B-1 cells tend to use particular germline *V* genes and respond to type 2 thymus-independent antigens (cf. p. 217). Furthermore, they may be involved in the generation of an idiotype network concerned in self-tolerance, the response to conserved microbial antigens, and possibly the idiotypic

regulation of B-2 responses. They are certainly the source of "natural antibodies" that provide a pre-existing first line of IgM defense against common microbes.

Development of B-cell specificity

The sequence of immunoglobulin gene rearrangements

There is an orderly sequence of Ig gene rearrangements during early B-cell differentiation (Figure 11.13):

■ **Stage 1.** Initially, the *D–J* segments on both alleles of the Ig heavy chain gene loci (one from each parent) rearrange so that one *D* segment is placed next to one *J* segment. The random nature of this rearrangement process will usually result in the *DJ* combination on one allele being different to that on the other allele.

■ **Stage 2.** A *V–DJ* recombinational event now occurs on just one of the two heavy chain alleles, whereby a randomly picked *V* segment is placed next to the already recombined *DJ* segment. If this proves to be a *nonproductive* rearrangement (i.e. adjacent segments are joined in an incorrect reading frame or in such a way as to generate a termination codon downstream from the splice point), then a second *V–DJ* rearrangement will occur on the sister heavy chain

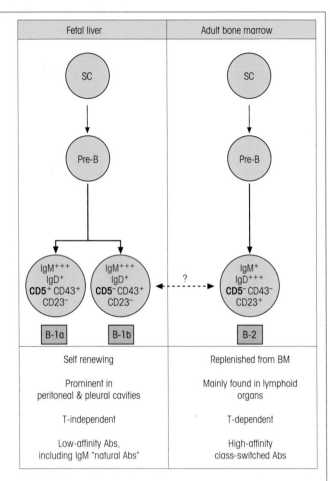

Fetal liver		Adult bone marrow
SC		SC
Pre-B		Pre-B
IgM+++ IgD+ **CD5+** CD43+ CD23−	IgM+++ IgD+ **CD5−** CD43+ CD23−	IgM+ IgD+++ **CD5−** CD43− CD23+
B-1a	B-1b	B-2
Self renewing		Replenished from BM
Prominent in peritoneal & pleural cavities		Mainly found in lymphoid organs
T-independent		T-dependent
Low-affinity Abs, including IgM "natural Abs"		High-affinity class-switched Abs

Figure 11.12. The development of separate B-cell subpopulations.

B-1 cells particularly produce IgM lower affinity "natural antibody." By contrast, B-2 cells give rise to the higher affinity IgG antibody produced by helper T-cell-dependent class-switched B-cells. It is thought that, although these subsets might be able to give rise to each other under some circumstances, generally they are maintained as separate lineages.

locus. If a productive rearrangement is not achieved, we can wave the pre-B-cell a fond farewell.

- **Stage 3.** If a productive rearrangement is made, the *VDJ* segment in the pre-B-cell utilizes the heavy chain constant (C_H) region $C\mu$ gene to synthesize μ heavy chains. At around the same time, two genes, V_{preB} (*CD179a*) and λ_5 (*CD179b*), with homology for the V_L and C_L segments of λ light chains respectively, are temporarily transcribed to form a "pseudo-light chain" that associates with the conventional μ heavy chains to generate a surface surrogate "IgM" receptor, together with the Ig-α (CD79a) and Ig-β (CD79b) chains conventionally required to form a functional B-cell

receptor. This surrogate receptor closely parallels the pre-$T\alpha/\beta$ receptor on pre-T-cell precursors of $\alpha\beta$ TCR-bearing cells.

- **Stage 4.** The surface receptor is signaled upon cross-linking possibly involving the positive charges on an arginine rich segment of λ_5 interacting with negatively charged regions of undefined ligands on stromal cells. Signaling by the pre B-cell receptor through Igα/β causes **allelic exclusion** whereby there is suppression of any further rearrangement of heavy chain genes on a sister chromatid.

- **Stage 5.** Expression of the *i*nterferon *r*egulatory *f*actors IRF-4 and IRF-8 downregulates the production of V_{pre-B} and λ_5 and induces rearrangement of the conventional light-chain genes. This involves *V–J* recombinations on first one and then the other κ allele until a productive $V\kappa$–J rearrangement is accomplished. If this fails, an attempt is made to achieve productive rearrangement of the λ alleles. Subsequent expression of a productively rearranged light chain is thought to involve binding of IRF-4, IRF-8 andE2A transcription factors to the κ or λ enhancers. Synthesis of conventional surface IgM now proceeds.

- **Stage 6.** The surface IgM molecule prohibits any further gene shuffling by allelic exclusion of any nonrearranged light chain genes. Surface IgD bearing an identical VDJ sequence to the IgM heavy chain is produced by alternative splicing of the heavy chain RNA transcript and the naive IgM⁺IgD⁺ B-cell is now ready for its encounter with antigen.

Upon antigenic stimulation IgD is lost and, in the presence of appropriate T-cell help, class switching from IgM to IgG, IgA or IgE antibody production can occur. At the terminal stages in the life of a fully mature plasma cell, virtually all surface Ig is shed.

The importance of allelic exclusion

As each cell has chromosomes derived from each parent, the differentiating B-cell has four light (two kappa, two lambda) and two heavy chain gene clusters to choose from. We have described how, once the *VDJ* DNA rearrangement has occurred within one heavy and *VJ* rearrangement in one light chain cluster, the *V* genes on the other four chromosomes are held in the germline (i.e. inherited) state by an allelic exclusion mechanism so that the cell is able to express only one heavy and one light chain. This is essential for clonal selection to work as the cell is then only programed to make the one antibody it uses as its cell surface receptor for antigen. Furthermore, this gene exclusion mechanism prevents the formation of molecules containing two different light or two different heavy chains that would have nonidentical combining sites and therefore be functionally monovalent with respect to the majority of antigens; such antibodies would be nonagglutinating and would tend to have low avidity as the bonus effect of multivalency could not operate.

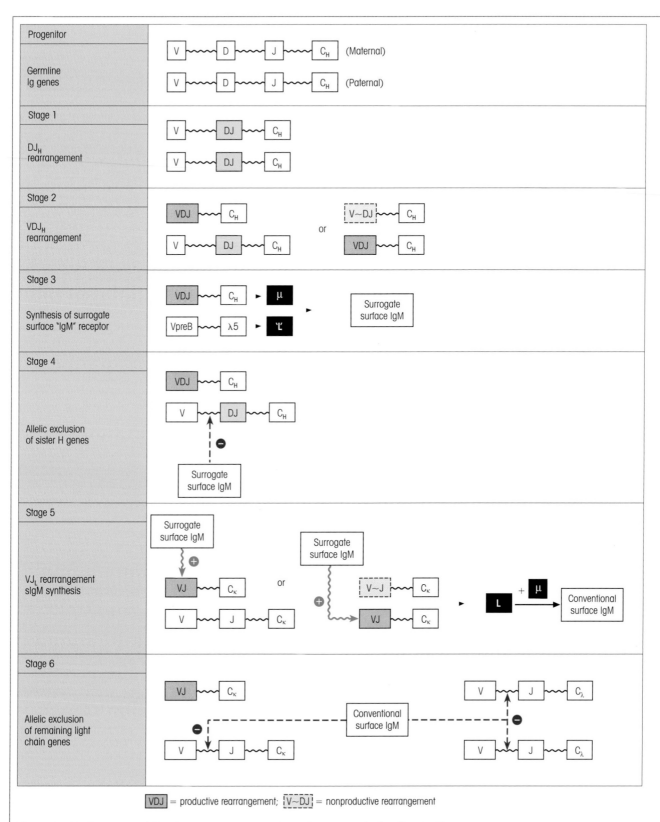

VDJ = productive rearrangement; V~DJ = nonproductive rearrangement

Figure 11.13. Sequence of B-cell gene rearrangements and allelic exclusion (See text.)

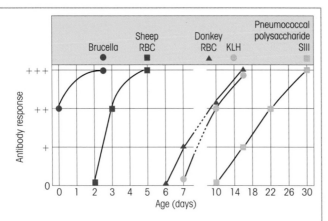

Figure 11.14. Sequential appearance of responsiveness to different antigens in the neonatal rat.

RBC, red blood cell; KLH, keyhole limpet hemocyanin.

Different specific responses can appear sequentially

The responses to given antigens in the neonatal period appear sequentially, suggesting a programed rearrangement of V genes in a definite order (Figure 11.14). Early in ontogeny there is a bias favoring the rearrangement of the V_H genes most proximal to the *DJ* segment.

The induction of tolerance in B-lymphocytes

Tolerance can be caused by clonal deletion and clonal anergy

Just as for T-cells, so both deletion and anergy can operate on B-cells to prevent the reaction to self. Excellent evidence for deletion comes from mice bearing transgenes coding for IgM, which binds to H-2K molecules of all *H-2* haplotypes except *d* and *f*. Mice of *H-2ᵈ* haplotype express the transgenic IgM abundantly in the serum, while 25–50% of total B-cells bear the transgenic antibody. (*d* × *k*) F1 crosses completely failed to express the transgene, i.e. B-cells programed for anti-H-2Kᵏ were expressed in *H-2ᵈ* mice but deleted in mice positive for H-2Kᵏ that in these circumstances acts as an autoantigen.

Tolerance through B-cell anergy was clearly demonstrated in another study in which double transgenic mice were made to express both soluble lysozyme and a high affinity antibody to lysozyme. The animals were completely tolerant and could not be immunized to make anti-lysozyme; nor did the transgenic antibody appear in the serum although it was abundantly present on the surface of B-cells. These anergic cells could bind antigen to their surface receptors but could not be activated. Like the aged *roué*, wistfully drinking in the visual attractions of some young belle, these tolerized lymphocytes can "see" the antigen but lack the ability to do anything about it.

Whether deletion or anergy is the outcome of the encounter with self probably depends upon the concentration and ability to cross-link Ig receptors. In the first of the two B-cell tolerance models above, the H-2Kᵏ autoantigen would be richly expressed on cells in contact with the developing B-lymphocytes and could effectively cause cross-linking. In the second case, the lysozyme, masquerading as a "self"-molecule, is essentially univalent with respect to the receptors on an anti-lysozyme B-cell and would not readily bring about cross-linking. The hypothesis was tested by stitching a transmembrane hydrophobic segment onto the lysozyme transgene so that the antigen would be multiply inserted into the cell membrane. Result? B-cells expressing the high affinity anti-lysozyme transgene were eliminated.

Another self-censoring mechanism, receptor editing, can come into play. We have already discussed one type of receptor editing (cf. p. 92) in which secondary rearrangements substitute another *V* gene onto an already rearranged *V(D)J* segment. However, receptor editing can also occur by wholesale replacement of an entire light chain. This can best be explained by an example. If the heavy and light chain Ig genes encoding a high affinity anti-DNA autoantibody are introduced as transgenes into a mouse, a variety of light chains are produced by genetic reshuffling until a combination with the heavy chain is achieved that no longer has anti-DNA activity, i.e. the autoreactivity is edited out. This will often involve replacement of a κ light chain with a new rearrangement made on the λ light chain locus and is associated with re-expression of the *RAG-1/2* genes.

Once peripheralized, the bulk of the B-cell pool is stable; lymph node B- (and T-) cells from unprimed mice survived comfortably for at least 20 months on transfer to H-2 identical SCID animals.

Tolerance may result from helpless B-cells

With soluble proteins at least, T-cells are more readily tolerized than B-cells (Figure 11.15) and, depending upon the circulating protein concentration, a number of self-reacting B-cells may be present in the body that cannot be triggered by T-dependent self-components as the T-cells required to provide the necessary T–B help are already tolerant—you might describe the B-cells as helpless. If we think of the determinant on a self-component that combines with the receptors on a self-reacting B-cell as a hapten and another determinant that has to be recognized by a T-cell as a carrier (cf. Figure 8.14), then tolerance in the T-cell to the carrier will prevent the provision of T-cell help and the B-cell will be unresponsive. Take C5 as an example; this is normally circulating at concentrations that tolerize T- but not B-cells. Some strains of mice are congenitally deficient in C5 and their T-cells can help C5-positive strains to make antibodies to C5, i.e. the C5-positive strains still have inducible B-cells but they are helpless and need non-tolerized T-cells from the C5-negative strain (Figure 11.16).

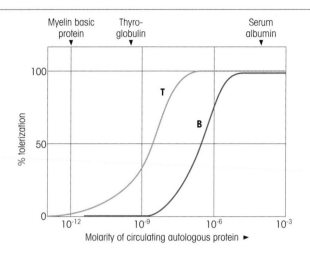

Figure 11.15. Relative susceptibility of T- and B-cells to tolerance by circulating self-antigens.

Those circulating at low concentration induce no tolerance; at intermediate concentration, e.g. thyroglobulin, T-cells are moderately tolerized; molecules such as albumin which circulate at high concentrations tolerize both B- and T-cells.

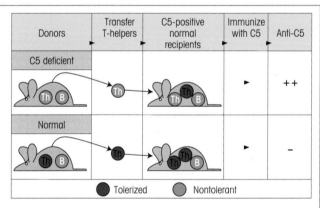

Figure 11.16. Circulating C5 tolerizes T- but not B-cells leaving them helpless.

Animals with congenital C5 deficiency do not tolerize their T-helpers and can be used to break tolerance in normal mice.

It is worth noting the observation that injection of high doses of a soluble antigen without adjuvant, even when given several days after primary immunization with that antigen, prevented the emergence of high-affinity mutated antibodies. Transfer experiments showed the T-cells to be tolerant. This tells us that, even when an immune response is well underway, T-helpers in the germinal center are needed to permit the mutations that lead to affinity maturation of antibody and, as a further corollary, that soluble self-antigens in the extracellular fluids can act to switch off autoreactive B-cells arising in the germinal centers by hypermutation.

Presumably, self-tolerance in both B- and T-cells involves all the mechanisms we have discussed to varying degrees and these are summarized in Figure 11.17. Remember that, throughout the life of an animal, new stem cells are continually differentiating into immunocompetent lymphocytes and what is early in ontogeny for them can be late for the host; this means that self-tolerance mechanisms are still acting on early lymphocytes even in the adult, although it is always comforting to note that the threshold concentration for tolerance induction is very much lower for pre-B-cells relative to mature B-cells.

Natural killer (NK) cell ontogeny

Natural killer cells mainly differentiate in the bone marrow from hematopoietic stem cells (HSC), although some NK cells also may arise in the thymus from early lymphoid precursors (ELP). These HSC and ELP give rise to NK precursors that can either remain in the primary lymphoid organs or seed to lymph nodes, spleen and liver. The precursors are stimulated to proliferate and differentiate by IL-2 and IL-15. At this stage they lack many of the markers of mature NK cells such as CD16 (FcγRIII) and the NK inhibitory and stimulatory receptors. Upon expression of the inhibitory receptors and their subsequent engagement by self MHC molecules, a process referred to as "education" or "licensing" of NK cells occurs that is critical for their development into mature fully functional NK cells. The mature NK cells can then relocate to other locations in the body including mucosal tissues such as the respiratory tract, GI tract and uterus.

The overall response in the neonate

Lymph node and spleen remain relatively underdeveloped in the human at the time of birth, except where there has been intrauterine exposure to antigens as in congenital infections with rubella or other organisms. Although the ability to reject grafts and to mount an antibody response is reasonably well developed by birth the immune system is still relatively immature and therefore not fully immunocompetent. Overall, there is a skewing towards Th2 responses in the newborn. Nonetheless, the immunoglobulin levels, with one exception, are low, particularly in the absence of intrauterine infection. The exception is the IgG acquired by placental transfer from the mother using the neonatal Fc-receptor, FcRn (cf. Figure 3.17a). The combination of immune immaturity and the presence of potentially "blocking" maternal antibodies that might limit access of antigen to the B-cell receptors could compromise the generation of immunological memory to natural infections and to vaccines in the newborn. However, the maternal IgG is catabolized with a half-life of approximately 3–4 weeks and there is therefore a fall in IgG concentration over the first 3 months accentuated by the increase in blood volume of the growing infant. Thereafter, the rate of IgG synthesis by the newborn's own B-cells overtakes the rate of breakdown of maternal IgG

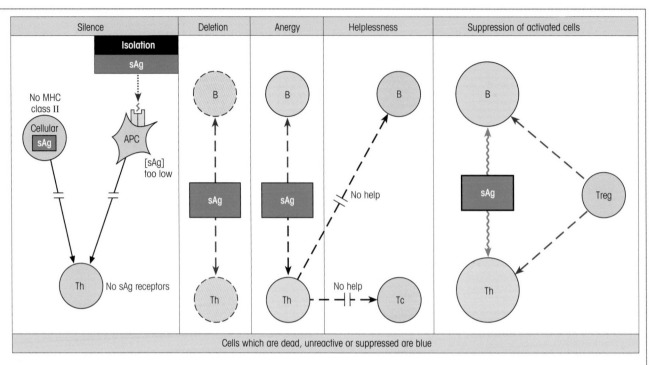

Figure 11.17. Mechanisms of self-tolerance

(See text.) sAg, self-antigen; APC, antigen-presenting cell; Th, T-helper; Treg, regulatory T-cell; Tc, cytotoxic T-cell precursor.

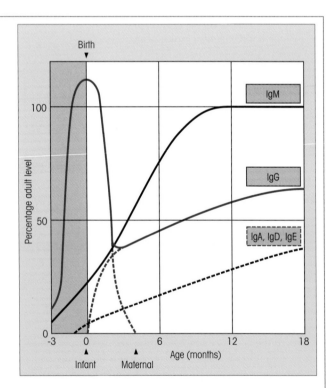

Figure 11.18. Development of serum immunoglobulin levels in the human.

(After Hobbs J.R. (1969) In Adinolfi M. (ed.) *Immunology and Development*, p. 118. Heinemann, London.)

and the overall concentration increases steadily. The other immunoglobulins do not cross the placenta and the low but significant levels of IgM in cord blood are synthesized by the baby (Figure 11.18). IgM reaches adult levels by 9 months of age. Only trace levels of IgA, IgD and IgE are present in the circulation of the newborn.

The evolution of the immune response

Earliest defences

Virtually all living organisms have mechanisms that have evolved to protect them against infection. Restriction endonucleases did not arise to make the life of the molecular geneticist easier, they provide protection to the prokaryotes (bacteria and archaea) against infection with bacteriophage viruses by chopping up foreign DNA. Amoeba are single celled eukaryotes that are able to engulf and subsequently break down particulate matter by phagocytosis, a process that evolved into a defence strategy of importance throughout the animal kingdom (cf. Milestone 1.1). Mechanisms for the recognition and subsequent **rejection of nonself** can be identified in invertebrates as far down the evolutionary scale as marine sponges (Figure 11.19).

Plant defenses against infection

Immune responses in plants have so far only been investigated in a relatively small number of species, and much of the

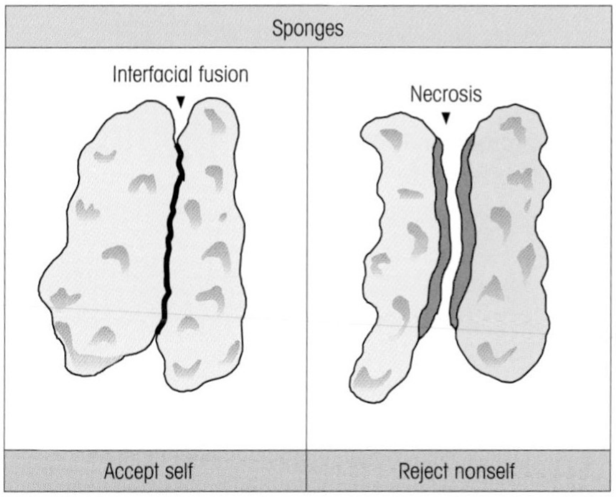

Figure 11.19. Recognition and rejection of nonself.

Parabiosed fingers of a marine sponge from the same colony are permanently united but members of different colonies reject each other by 7–9 days.

research has focused on the model higher plant *Arabidopsis,* a member of the mustard family, and its response to infection with the bacterium *Pseudomonas syringae.* Nonetheless, it is clear that plants can detect pathogen-associated molecular patterns (PAMPs; cf. p. 4) using pattern recognition receptors (PRRs) that initiate a MAP kinase signaling cascade that switches on a respiratory burst to generate reactive oxygen species. Furthermore, activation of a number of immunity genes results in the production of molecules such as defensins with potent antimicrobial activity. One such PRR is FLS2 (flagellin sensitive 2), which is present in the plasma membrane and detects bacterial flagellin. Because plants lack a mobile defence system, this **PAMP-triggered immunity (PTI)** is a feature of each individual plant cell. If pathogens manage to evade PTI responses then a second type of defence system, the faster and stronger **effector-triggered immunity (ETI)**, is deployed. These ETI responses depend upon direct or indirect recognition of pathogen effector proteins in the plant cell by cytoplasmic NB-LRR (nucleotide binding—leucine rich repeat) proteins encoded by *R* (resistance) genes. ETI results in the generation of some of the same antimicrobial compounds that are produced during PTI but also initiates an immediate hypersensitive response (HR) leading to localized apoptosis thereby rapidly curtailing the growth of the infectious agent. The HR also induces an "immune state" of **systemic acquired resistance** (SAR) that persists for several weeks and extends to a broad range of bacterial, viral and fungal pathogens beyond the initiating infective agent. A series of SAR genes encode a wide variety of microbicidal proteins that can be induced through endogenous chemical mediators such as salicylic acid, jasmonic acid and azelaic acid. Jasmonic acid also contributes to resistance against herbivorous insects.

Invertebrate microbial defense mechanisms

In many phyla, phagocytosis is augmented by coating with agglutinins and bactericidins capable of binding to PAMPs on the microbial surface so providing the basis for the recognition of "nonself." It is notable that infection very rapidly induces the synthesis of an impressive battery of antimicrobial peptides in higher insects following activation of transcription factors that bind to promoter sequence motifs homologous to regulatory elements involved in the mammalian acute phase response. Thus, the toll molecule in drosophila is a receptor for PAMPs that activate NFκB in these flies. *Drosophila* with a loss-of-function mutation in *toll* is susceptible to fungal infections. Antimicrobial peptides produced by insects include disulfide-bridged cyclic peptides such as the anti-Gram-positive defensins and the antifungal peptide, drosomycin. Linear peptides inducible by infection include the cecropins and a series of anti-Gram-negative glycine- or proline-rich polypeptides. Cecropins, which have also been identified in mammals, are strongly cationic peptides with amphipathic α-helices causing lethal disintegration of bacterial membranes by creating ion channels.

Elements of a primordial complement system also exist among the lower orders. A protease inhibitor, a β_2-macroglobulin structurally homologous to C3 with internal thiolester, is present in the horseshoe crab. Conceivably this might represent an ancestral version of C3 that is activated by proteases released at a site of infection, deposited onto the microbe and recognized there as a ligand for the phagocytic cells. The complement receptor CR3 is an integrin, and related integrins in insects may harbor common ancestors. Mention of the horseshoe crab may have stirred a neuronal network in readers with good memories, to recall its synthesis of limulin (cf. p. 24), which is homologous with the mammalian acute phase C-reactive protein (CRP); presumably, it acts as a lectin to opsonize bacteria and is likely to be a product of the evolutionary line leading ultimately to C1q, mannose-binding lectin and lung surfactant protein.

The other major strategy effectively deployed by invertebrates is to wall off an invading microorganism. This is achieved, for example, through proteolytic cascades which produce a coagulum of "gelled" hemolymph around the offender.

Adaptive immune responses appear with the vertebrates

Lower vertebrates

The jawless vertebrates, today comprising only the lamprey and hagfish, possess lymphocyte-like cells that express a transmembrane-only variable lymphocyte receptor A (VLRA) on cells that may mediate cellular responses and a VLRB on cells that mediate humoral responses that is also produced as a secreted molecule. These VLRs are not members of the immunoglobulin superfamily but contain variable and constant regions and use a gene conversion-like mechanism to generate diversity. Lymphocytes and genuine adaptive T- and B-responses do not emerge in the phylogenetic tree until we reach the jawed vertebrates.

T-cells appear

Cartilaginous fishes have well defined T- and B-cells together with 18S and 7S immunoglobulins with heavy and light chains, but the responses are *T-independent*. The toad, *Xenopus*, is a pliable, if unlovely, species for study as it is possible to make transgenics and cloned tadpoles fairly readily, and it has a less complex lymphoid system than mammals, characterized by a small number of lymphocytes and a restricted antibody repertoire not subject to somatic mutation. Furthermore, positive and negative thymic selection have been demonstrated in frogs.

The emergence of a thymus in the teleosts (bony fishes), amphibians, reptiles, birds and mammals was of course associated with MHC molecules, cell-mediated immunity, cytotoxic T-cells and allograft rejection. It could be argued that we also see phylogenetically more ancient, T-independent B-1 (CD5-positive) cells joined by a new T-dependent B-2 population. However, T-dependent, high affinity, heterogeneous, rapid secondary antibody responses are only seen with warm-blooded vertebrates such as birds and mammals, and these correlate directly with the evolution of germinal centers.

Generation of antibody diversity

Mechanisms for the generation of antibody diversity receive quite different emphasis as one goes from one species to another. We are already familiar with the mammalian system where recombinational events involve multiple *V, D* and *J* gene segments. The horned shark also has many *V* genes, but the opportunities for combinatorial joining are tightly constrained by close linkage between individual *V, D, J* and *C* segments and this may be a factor in the restricted antibody response of this species. In sharp contrast, there is only one operational *V* gene at the light chain locus in the chicken, but this undergoes extensive somatic diversification utilizing nonfunctional adjoining *V* pseudogenes in a gene conversion-like process. Camel lovers should note that not only do they get by on little water but, like the llamas, a proportion of their functional antibodies lack light chains. The especially long CDR3 loop in the heavy chain variable region compensates for the lack of a light chain in these antibodies.

The evolution of distinct B- and T-cell lineages was accompanied by the development of separate sites for differentiation

The differential effects of neonatal bursectomy and thymectomy in the chicken on subsequent humoral and cellular responses paved the way for our eventual recognition of the separate lymphocyte lineages that subserve these functions (Figure 11.20). Like the thymus, the bursa of Fabricius develops as an embryonic outpushing of the gut endoderm, this time from hindgut as distinct from foregut, and provides the microenvironment to cradle incoming stem cells and direct their differentiation to immunocompetent B-lymphocytes. Neonatal bursectomy had a profound effect on overall immunoglobulin levels and on specific antibody production following immunization, but did not unduly influence the cell-mediated delayed-type hypersensitivity (DTH) response to tuberculin or affect graft rejection or graft-versus-host

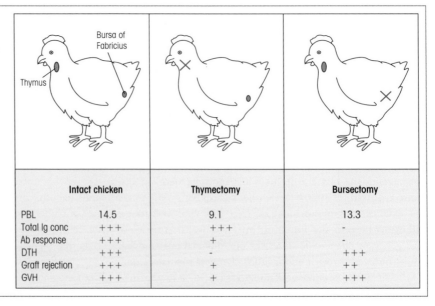

Figure 11.20. Effect of neonatal bursectomy and thymectomy on the development of immunologic competence in the chicken.

PBL, Peripheral blood lymphocyte count ×10⁻³; Total Ig conc, concentration of circulating immunoglobulins; Ab response, antibody response to immunization with specific antigen; DTH, delayed-type hypersensitivity; GVH, graft-versus-host reaction. (From Cooper M.D., Peterson R.D.A., South M.A. & Good R.A. (1966) *Journal of Experimental Medicine* **123**, 75, with permission of the editors.)

	Intact chicken	Thymectomy	Bursectomy
PBL	14.5	9.1	13.3
Total Ig conc	+++	+++	-
Ab response	+++	+	-
DTH	+++	-	+++
Graft rejection	+++	+	++
GVH	+++	+	+++

responses. On the other hand, thymectomy grossly impaired cell-mediated reactions and inhibited antibody production to most protein antigens.

The distinctive anatomical location of the B-cell differentiation site in a separate lymphoid organ in the chicken was immensely valuable to progress in this field because it allowed the above types of experiments to be carried out. However, many years went by in a fruitless search for an equivalent bursa in mammals before it was realized that the primary site for B-cell generation was in fact the bone marrow itself.

Cellular recognition molecules exploit the immunoglobulin gene superfamily

When nature fortuitously chances upon a protein structure ("motif" is the buzz word) that successfully mediates some useful function, the selective forces of evolution make sure that it is widely exploited. Thus, the molecules involved in antigen recognition that we have described in Chapters 3 and 4 are members of a gene superfamily related by sequence and presumably a common ancestry. All polypeptide members of this family, which includes heavy and light Ig chains, T-cell receptor chains, MHC molecules and β_2-microglobulin, are composed of one or more immunoglobulin homology units. Each Ig-type domain is roughly 110 amino acids in length and is characterized by certain conserved residues around the two cysteines found in each domain and the alternating hydrophobic and hydrophilic amino acids that give rise to the familiar antiparallel β-pleated strands with interspersed short variable lengths having a marked propensity to form reversed turns—the "**immunoglobulin fold**" (cf. p. 58).

A very important feature of the Ig domain structure is mutual complementarity, which allows strong interdomain noncovalent interactions, such as those between V_H and V_L and the two C_H3 regions. Gene duplication and diversification can create mutual families of interacting molecules, such as CD4 with MHC class II, CD8 with MHC class I and IgA with the poly-Ig receptor (Figure 11.21). Likewise, the intercellular adhesion molecules ICAM-1 and N-CAM (Figure 11.21) are richly endowed with these domains, and the long evolutionary history of N-CAM strongly suggests that these structures made an early appearance in phylogeny as mediators of intercellular recognition. In marine sponges, Ig superfamily structures are found both on the extracellular portion of the receptor tyrosine kinases (RTKs) and in the cell recognition molecules (CRMs), both thought to be involved in allograft rejection. A recent trawl of the protein sequence database revealed hundreds of known members of the Ig superfamily. Some family!

The **integrins**, whose members include the leukocyte function-associated antigen-1 (LFA-1) and the very late antigens (VLAs), form another structural superfamily that contains a number of hematopoietic cell surface molecules concerned with adhesion to extracellular matrix proteins and to cell surface ligands; their function is to direct leukocytes to particular tissue sites (see discussion on p. 190).

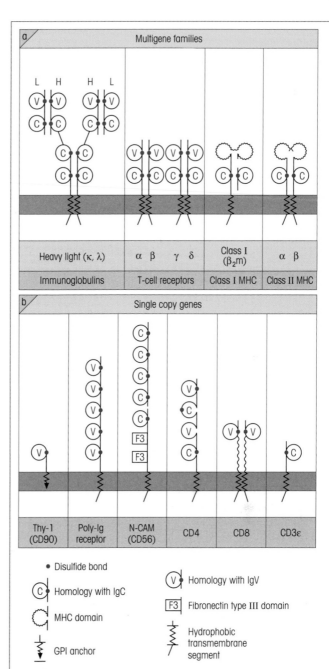

Figure 11.21. The immunoglobulin superfamily

This superfamily comprises a large number of surface molecules that all share a common structure, the immunoglobulin-type domain, suggesting evolution from a single primordial ancestral gene. Just a few examples are shown. (a) Multigene families involved in antigen recognition (the single copy β_2-microglobulin [β_2m] is included because of its association with class I). (b) Single copy genes. Thy-1 is present on T-cells and neurons. The poly-Ig receptor transports secretory IgA across mucosal membranes. N-CAM is an adhesion molecule on neuronal cells, NK cells and a subpopulation of T-cells. (Reprinted by permission from *Nature* **323**, 15. Copyright © 1986, Macmillan Magazines Ltd with some updating.)

CD antigens help distinguish different populations of leukocytes

- Cell surface molecules defined by monoclonal antibodies are assigned CD numbers that can act as "markers" of cell differentiation.

Multipotential hematopoietic stem cells from the bone marrow give rise to all the formed elements of the blood

- Expansion and differentiation are driven by soluble growth (colony-stimulating) factors and contact with reticular stromal cells.

The differentiation of T-cells occurs within the microenvironment of the thymus

- Precursor T-cells arising from stem cells in the bone marrow travel to the thymus under the influence of chemokines in order to become immunocompetent T-cells.

T-cell ontogeny

- Differentiation to immunocompetent T-cell subsets is accompanied by changes in the surface phenotype that can be recognized with monoclonal antibodies.
- TCR genes rearrange in the thymus cortex, producing a $\gamma\delta$ TCR or a pre-$\alpha\beta$ TCR, consisting of an invariant pre-Tα associated with a conventional Vβ, before final rearrangement of the Vα to generate the mature $\alpha\beta$ TCR.
- Double-negative CD4$^-$8$^-$ pre-T-cells are driven and expanded by Notch-mediated and other signals to become double-positive CD4$^+$8$^+$.
- The thymus epithelial cells **positively select** CD4$^+$8$^+$ T-cells with avidity for their MHC haplotype so that single-positive CD4$^+$ or CD8$^+$ T-cells develop that are restricted to the recognition of antigen in the context of the epithelial cell haplotype.
- NKT cells, which express both a TCR and NK cell markers such as NK1.1, have highly restricted TCR variable regions and recognize glycolipid antigens presented by the MHC-like molecule CD1d. They secrete IL-4 and IFNγ and may function as regulatory cells.

T-cell tolerance

- The induction of immunological tolerance is necessary to avoid self-reactivity.
- High avidity T-cells that react with self-antigens presented by medullary dendritic cells and macrophages are eliminated by **negative selection**. The paradigm that low avidity binding to MHC–peptide produces positive selection and high avidity

negative, is probably broadly true but may need some amendment.
- The autoimmune regulator (AIRE) directs the ectopic expression of several organ-specific self antigens in the thymic medullary epithelial cells leading to deletion of the relevant T-cells.
- Self-tolerance can also be achieved by anergy.
- Anergic cells attached to a dendritic cell can downregulate the antigen-presenting ability of that cell, resulting in infectious anergy.
- Regulatory T-cells normally suppress the activities of self-reactive T-cells that escape the deletional or anergy processes.
- A state of what is effectively self-tolerance also arises when there is a failure to adequately present a self-antigen to lymphocytes, either because of sequestration, lack of class II on the antigen-presenting cell or low concentration of peptide–MHC (cryptic self).

B-cells differentiate in the fetal liver and then in the bone marrow

- They become immunocompetent B-cells after passing through pro-B-, pre-B- and immature B-cell stages.
- *Pax5* expression is essential for progression from the pre-B- to immature B-cell stage.

B-1 and B-2 represent two distinct subpopulations of B-cells

- B-1 cells represent a minor population expressing high sIgM and low sIgD. B-1a cells are CD5$^+$, B-1b are CD5$^-$. The majority of conventional B-cells, the B-2 population, are sIgM^{lo}, sIgD^{hi}, CD5$^-$. The B-1 population predominates in early life, shows a high level of idiotype–anti-idiotype connectivity, and produces low affinity IgM polyreactive antibodies, many of them autoantibodies, and T-independent "natural" IgM antibacterial antibodies that appear spontaneously.

Development of B-cell specificity

- The sequence of Ig variable gene rearrangements is *DJ* and then *VDJ*.
- *VDJ* transcription produces μ chains that associate with $V_{preB}.\lambda_5$ chains to form a surrogate surface IgM-like receptor.
- This receptor signals allelic exclusion of nonrearranged heavy chains and initiates rearrangement of $V–J_\kappa$ and, if unproductive, $V–J_\lambda$
- If the rearrangement at any stage is unproductive, i.e. does not lead to an acceptable gene reading frame, the allele on the sister chromosome is rearranged.

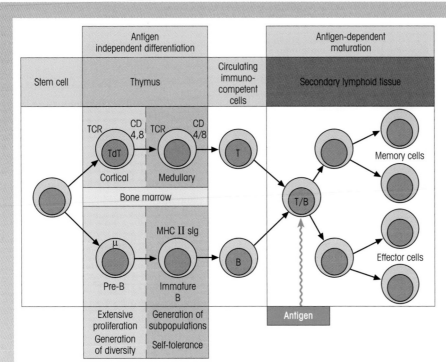

Figure 11.22. Antigen-independent differentiation and antigen-dependent maturation of T- and B-cells.

Cortical thymocytes are positively selected to recognize self-MHC haplotype. TdT, terminal deoxynucleotidyl transferase.

- The mechanisms of allelic exclusion ensure that each lymphocyte is programed for only one antibody.
- Responses to different antigens appear sequentially with age.

The induction of tolerance in B-lymphocytes

- B-cell tolerance is induced by clonal deletion, clonal anergy, receptor editing and "helplessness" due to preferential tolerization of T-cells needed to cooperate in B-cell stimulation.

Natural killer (NK) cell ontogeny

- NK cells develop in the bone marrow and express inhibitory receptors for MHC class I and stimulating receptors recognizing a variety of cell surface ligands.

The overall response in the neonate

- Maternal IgG crosses the placenta and provides a high level of passive immunity at birth.
- The antigen-independent differentiation within primary lymphoid organs and antigen-driven maturation in secondary lymphoid organs are summarized in Figure 11.22.

The evolution of the immune response

- Even prokaryotic organisms need to defend themselves from infection, for example by using restriction endonucleases to destroy foreign DNA.
- Plants utilize PAMP-triggered immunity (PTI) backed up by effector-triggered immunity (ETI), which can lead to systemic acquired resistance (SAR) to infection which shows broad specificity and lasts for several weeks.
- Recognition of self is of fundamental importance for multicellular organisms, even lowly forms like marine sponges.
- Invertebrates have defense mechanisms based on phagocytosis, killing by a multiplicity of microbicidal peptides, and imprisonment of the invader by coagulation of the hemolymph.
- B- and T-cell responses are well defined in the vertebrates and the evolution of these distinct lineages was accompanied by the development of separate sites for differentiation.
- The success of the immunoglobulin domain structure, possibly through its ability to give noncovalent mutual binding, has been exploited by evolution to produce the very large Ig superfamily of recognition molecules, including Ig, TCRs, MHC class I and II, β_2-microglobulin, CD4, CD8, the poly-Ig receptor and Thy-1. Another superfamily, the integrins, which includes LFA-1 and the VLA molecules, is concerned with leukocyte binding to endothelial cells and extracellular matrix proteins.

FURTHER READING

Bains I. *et al.* (2009) Quantifying thymic export: combining models of naive T cell proliferation and TCR excision circle dynamics gives an explicit measure of thymic output. *Journal of Immunology* **183**, 4329–4336.

Blom B. & Spits H. (2006) Development of human lymphoid cells. *Annual Review of Immunology* **24**, 287–320.

Boehm T. & Bleul C.C. (2007) The evolutionary history of lymphoid organs. *Nature Immunology* **8**, 131–135.

Cumano A. & Godin I. (2007) Ontogeny of the hematopoietic system. *Annual Review of Immunology* **25**, 745–785.

He X., Park K. & Kappes D.J. (2010) The role of ThPOK in control of CD4/CD8 lineage commitment. *Annual Review of Immunology* **28**, 295–320.

Huntington N.D., Vosshenrich C.A.J. & Di Santo J.P. (2007) Developmental pathways that generate natural-killer-cell diversity in mice and humans. *Nature Reviews Immunology* **7**, 703–714.

Jones J.D.G. & Dangl J.L. (2006) The plant immune system. *Nature* **444**, 323–329.

Kaushansky K. (2006) Lineage-specific hematopoietic growth factors. *The New England Journal of Medicine* **354**, 2034–2045.

Majeti R., Park C.Y. & Weissman I.L. (2007) Identification of a hierarchy of multipotent hematopoietic progenitors in human cord blood. *Cell Stem Cell* **1**, 635–645.

Pancer Z. & Cooper M.D. (2006) The evolution of adaptive immunity. *Annual Review of Immunology* **24**, 497–518.

Roozendaal R. & Mebius R.E. (2011) Stromal cell–immune cell interactions. *Annual Review of Immunology* **29**.

Ruddle N.H. & Akirav E.M. (2009) Secondary lymphoid organs: responding to genetic and environmental cues in ontogeny and the immune response. *Journal of Immunology* **183**, 2205–2212.

Singer A., Adoro S. & Park J.H. (2008) Lineage fate and intense debate: myths, models and mechanisms of CD4- versus CD8-lineage choice. *Nature Reviews Immunology* **8**, 788–801.

Vera Göhre V. & Robatzek S. (2008) Breaking the barriers: microbial effector molecules subvert plant immunity. *Annual Review of Phytopathology* **46**, 189–215.

Zhang C.C. & Lodish H.F. (2008) Cytokines regulating hematopoietic stem cell function. *Current Opinion in Hematology* **15**, 307–311.

Now visit **www.roitt.com**
to test yourself on this chapter.

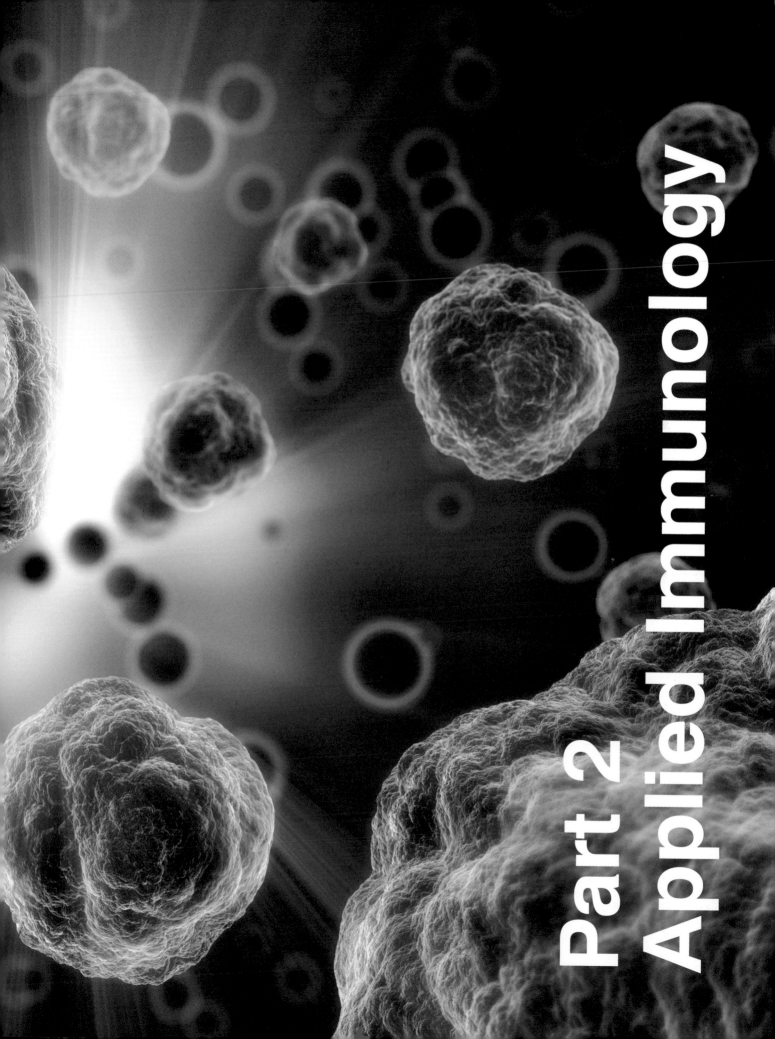

Part 2
Applied Immunology

CHAPTER 12
Adversarial strategies during infection

Key Topics

Just to Recap ...

The immune system has a wide range of cells and molecules at its disposal to fight infection. Phagocytes engulf small pathogens such as bacteria, viruses and fungi and then use a broad range of microbicidal components to destroy the trapped organism. Pathogens that are too large to be engulfed, for example parasitic worms, can be destroyed by the release of toxic substances from cells such as eosinophils. Antibody is also effective against extracellular pathogens and acts predominantly through its effects as an opsonin for phagocytosis and by initiating the classical pathway of complement activation. Complement can also be directly activated by extracellular pathogens, either via the alternative or lectin pathways. The immune system must employ different strategies for intracellular pathogens as these are not generally susceptible to phagocytic cells or humoral immunity. Cytotoxic T-lymphocytes and NK cells will kill virus-infected host cells thereby depriving the pathogen of the ability to replicate. In the case of intracellular bacteria such as *Mycobacterium tuberculosis* residing in macrophages, the macrophage-activating properties of IFNγ is of value.

Introduction

We are engaged in constant warfare with the microbes that surround us and the processes of mutation and evolution have tended to select microorganisms that have evolved means of evading our defense mechanisms. Pathogens

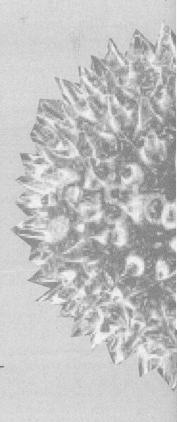
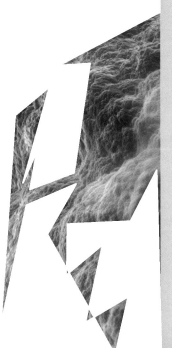

Roitt's Essential Immunology, Twelfth Edition. Peter J. Delves, Seamus J. Martin, Dennis R. Burton, Ivan M. Roitt.
© 2011 Peter J. Delves, Seamus J. Martin, Dennis R. Burton, Ivan M. Roitt. Published 2011 by Blackwell Publishing Ltd.

Introduction (*Continued*)

continue to take a terrifying toll (Figure 12.1), particularly in the developing world. Newly emerged infections including H1NI and H5NI influenza A variants, *E. coli* O157:H7, *Clostridium difficile*, prions, *Legionella pneumophila*, *Chlamydia trachomatis*, HIV and Ebola virus are stretching healthcare resources. Furthermore, old adversaries have re-emerged, such as dengue, West Nile virus, cholera, plague, Rift Valley fever and Lyme disease. Over half of all human pathogens are zoonoses, infections that are present in species other than man but that can be transmitted from animals to humans. Climate changes that are currently occurring due to global warming may lead to an increase in vector-borne infectious diseases such as malaria in many areas of the world including the USA and Europe. In this chapter, we look at the varied, often ingenious, adversarial strategies that we and our enemies have developed.

Infection remains a major healthcare problem

During the middle of the last century it had seemed that the introduction of antibiotics had finally beaten infectious disease, but now multidrug resistance has become an extremely worrying development, as seen with tuberculosis, malaria, *Streptococcus pneumoniae*, *Enterococcus faecalis*, *Pseudomonas aeruginosa* and methicillin-resistant *Staphylococcus aureus* (MRSA). Resistance to sulfa drugs occurred in *S. aureus* in the 1940s, to penicillin in the 1950s, to methicillin in the 1980s and to vancomycin in 2002.

Infections arising after 48 hours of hospital admission may well have been acquired in the hospital and are then referred to as "nosocomial" infections; MRSA and other multidrug-resistant organisms often lurk in such institutions, as does *Clostridium difficile* type 027, which carries a mutation resulting in high levels of toxin production. It is also becoming increasingly appreciated that infectious agents are related to many "noninfectious" diseases, such as the association of *Helicobacter pylori* with gastric ulcers and gastric cancer, and of various viruses with other cancers.

Inflammation revisited

The initial reaction to pathogens that breach the external protective barriers (p. 6) is usually an acute inflammatory response involving an influx of leukocytes, complement, antibody and other plasma proteins into a site of infection or injury. This was discussed in the introductory chapters but let's now re-examine the mechanisms of inflammation in greater depth. The reader may find it helpful to have another look at the relevant sections in Chapters 1 and 2, particularly those relating to Figures 1.21 and 1.22.

Mediators of inflammation

A complex variety of mediators are involved in acute inflammatory responses (Figure 12.2). Some act directly on the smooth muscle wall surrounding the arterioles to alter blood flow. Others act on the venules to cause contraction of the endothelial cells with transient opening of the interendothelial junctions and consequent transudation of plasma. The migration of leukocytes from the bloodstream is facilitated by mediators that upregulate the expression of adherence molecules on both endothelial and white cells and others that lead the leukocytes to the inflamed site through chemotaxis.

Leukocytes bind to endothelial cells through paired adhesion molecules

Redirecting the leukocytes charging along the blood into the site of inflammation is somewhat like having to encourage bulls stampeding down the Pamplona main street to move quietly into the side roads. The adherence of leukocytes to the endothelial vessel wall through the interaction of complementary binding of cell surface molecules is an absolutely crucial step. Several classes of molecule subserve this function, some acting as lectins to bind a carbohydrate ligand on the complementary partner.

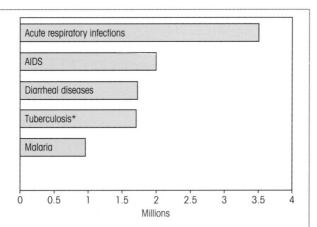

Figure 12.1. Estimated annual deaths from infectious disease.

These five diseases cause almost 90% of the deaths from infectious disease worldwide. Data are based on estimates for the year 2008. *Excludes deaths from tuberculosis in patients infected with HIV. For more information, see http://www.who.int/topics/infectious_diseases/en

Mediator action					
	Dilatation	Increase permeability	Upregulate adhesion mol.		Neutrophil chemotaxis
			Endothelium	Neutrophil	
Histamine	+	+	+ +		
Bradykinin	+	+ +			
PGE$_2$	+ + +	Potentiates other mediators			
C5a		+ +	+	+ +	+ + +
Leukotriene-B$_4$		+ +		+ +	+ + +
f.Met.Leu.Phe		+ +		+	+
Platelet-activating factor	+	+ +		+ +	
IL-8 (CXCL8)				+ + +	+ + +
NAP-2 (CXCL7)				+ +	+ +
IL-1β			+ +	+ +	
TNF			+ +	+ +	

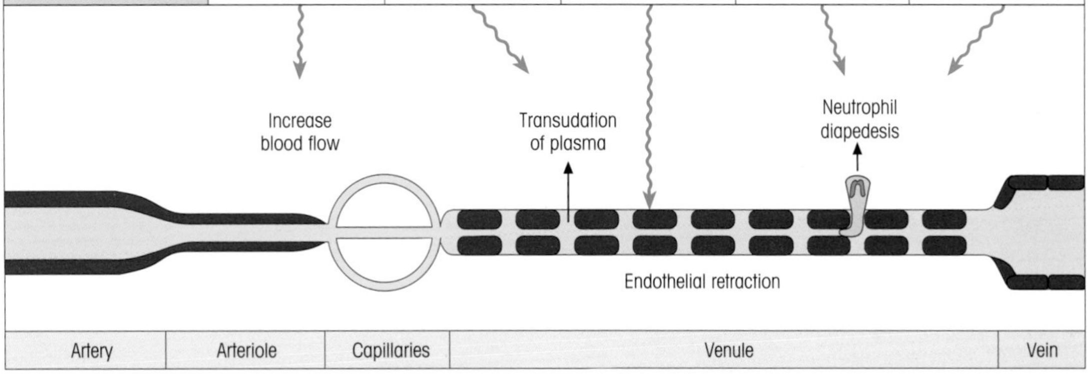

Increase blood flow

Transudation of plasma

Neutrophil diapedesis

Endothelial retraction

Artery	Arteriole	Capillaries	Venule	Vein

Figure 12.2. The principal mediators of acute inflammation.

The reader should refer back to Figure 1.21 to recall the range of products generated by the mast cell. The later acting cytokines such as the interleukin IL-1β are largely macrophage-derived and these cells also secrete prostaglandin E$_2$ (PGE$_2$), leukotriene B$_4$ and the neutrophil-activating chemokine NAP-2 (CXCL7).

Initiation of the acute inflammatory response

A very early event is the upregulation of P-selectin and platelet-activating factor (PAF) on the endothelial cells lining the venules by histamine or thrombin released by the original inflammatory stimulus. Recruitment of these molecules from intracellular storage vesicles ensures that they appear within minutes on the cell surface. Engagement of the lectin-like domain at the tip of the P-selectin molecule with sialyl Lewis^x carbohydrate determinants borne by the P-selectin glycoprotein ligand-1 (PSGL-1) on the neutrophil surface causes the cell to slow and then **roll** along the endothelial wall and helps PAF to dock onto its corresponding receptor. This, in turn, increases surface expression of the integrins leukocyte function-associated molecule-1 (LFA-1) and Mac-1, which bind the neutrophil very firmly to the endothelial surface (Figure 12.3).

Activation of the neutrophils also increases their responsiveness to chemotactic agents and, under the influence of C5a and leukotriene B$_4$, they exit from the circulation by moving purposefully through the gap between endothelial cells, across the basement membrane (**diapedesis**) and up the chemotactic gradient to the inflammation site. Here they phagocytose the microorganisms and use their various killing mechanisms to destroy the pathogen (cf. p. 13). Additionally, they release *n*eutrophil *e*xtracellular *t*raps (NETs), which act like a spider's web to ensnare the prey and thereby prevent them from spreading (Figure 12.4). The NETs contain a number of antimicrobial agents including elastase, proteinase 3, gelatinase, tryptase, bactericidal permeability-increasing protein (BPI), cathepsin G, myeloperoxidase, lactoferrin, and the cathelicidin LL-37, thereby also contributing directly to destruction of the microorganisms.

Damage to vascular endothelium, which exposes the basement membrane, and bacterial toxins such as lipopolysaccharide (LPS), trigger the blood coagulation and fibrinolysis pathways. Activation of platelets, for example by contact with basement membrane collagen or induced endothelial PAF, leads to the release of many inflammatory mediators including

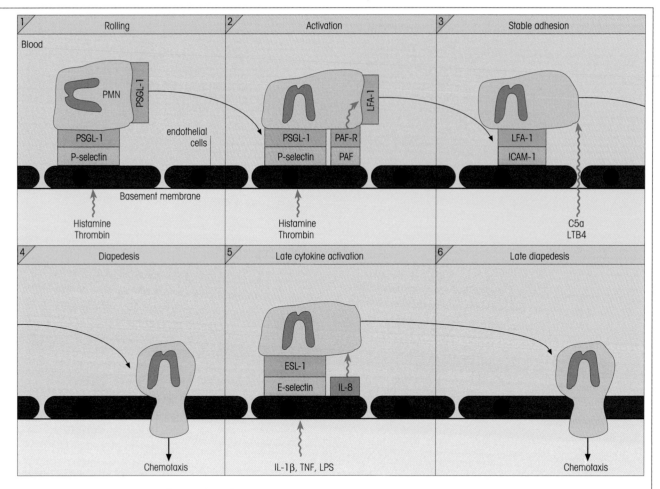

Figure 12.3. Early events in inflammation affecting neutrophil margination and diapedesis.

(1) Mediators such as histamine and thrombin induce the upregulation of P-selectin on the vessel wall. Leukocyte–endothelial interaction (rolling) occurs following binding to ligands on the polymorphonuclear neutrophil (PMN) such as P-selectin glycoprotein ligand-1 (PSGL-1, CD162). (2) Subsequent induction of platelet-activating factor (PAF) and its engagement with the PAF receptor on the neutrophil activates the leukocyte, resulting in expression of integrins such as leukocyte functional antigen-1 (LFA-1). (3) Intercellular adhesion molecule-1 (ICAM-1) also becomes expressed on the endothelium, permitting stable adhesion via interaction with the LFA-1. A chemotactic gradient is provided by C5a and leukotriene B$_4$ (LTB$_4$), leading to (4) diapedesis of the activated neutrophils. (5) Subsequent expression of endothelial E-selectin (promoted by IL-1β, TNF and LPS) and of IL-8 induce binding and activation of more neutrophils and (6) their diapedesis into the tissues. (Compare events involved in homing and transmigration of lymphocytes, Figure 7.6.)

histamine and a number of chemokines that are stored in granules. Some newly synthesized mediators such as IL-1β are translated from mRNA in the anucleate platelets. Aggregation of the activated platelets occurs and **thrombus** formation is initiated by adherence through platelet glycoprotein Ib to von Willebrand factor on the vascular surface. Such platelet plugs are adept at stemming the loss of blood from a damaged artery, but in the venous system the damaged site is sealed by a **fibrin clot** resulting from activation of the intrinsic clotting system via contact of Hageman factor (factor XII) with the exposed surface of the basement membrane. Activated Hageman factor also triggers the kinin and plasmin systems and several of the resulting products influence the inflammatory process, including bradykinin and fibrinopeptides that, together with comple-

ment components C3a and C5a, increase vascular permeability and thrombin, which contributes towards activation of endothelium.

The ongoing inflammatory process

One must not ignore the role of the tissue macrophage that, under the stimulus of local infection or injury, secretes an imposing array of mediators. In particular, the cytokines IL-1β and TNF act at a later time than histamine or thrombin to stimulate the endothelial cells and maintain the inflammatory process by upregulating E-selectin and sustaining P-selectin expression. Thus, expression of E-selectin occurs 2–4 hours after the initiation of acute inflammation, being dependent

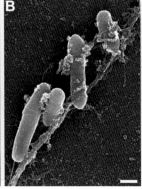
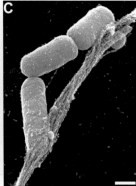

Figure 12.4. Neutrophil extracellular traps.

Release of granule proteins and chromatin from neutrophils leads to the formation of neutrophil extracellular traps (NETs), which prevent bacterial spreading and ensure that microbicidal substances released from the neutrophils are kept in the immediate vicinity of the bacteria for optimal killing of the microbe and minimal collateral damage to host tissues.

Scanning electron micrograph of NETs from IL-8 activated neutrophils trapping: (A) *Staphylococcus aureus;* (B) *Salmonella typhimurium;* (C) *Shigella flexneri.* The bar indicates 500 nm. (Reproduced from Brinkman V. *et al.* (2004) *Science* **303**, 1532, with permission from the publishers.)

upon activation of gene transcription. The E-selectin engages the glycoprotein E-selectin ligand-1 (ESL-1) on the neutrophil. Other later acting components are the **chemokines** (chemotactic cytokines) IL-8 (CXCL8) and neutrophil-activating peptide-2 (NAP-2, CXCL7) that are highly effective neutrophil chemoattractants. IL-1β and TNF also act on endothelial cells, fibroblasts and epithelial cells to stimulate secretion of another chemokine, MCP-1 (CCL2), which attracts mononuclear phagocytes to the inflammatory site to strengthen and maintain the defensive reaction to infection.

Perhaps this is a good time to remind ourselves of the important role of chemokines (Table 9.2) in selectively attracting multiple types of leukocytes to inflammatory foci. Inflammatory chemokines are typically induced by microbial products such as lipopolysaccharide (LPS) and by proinflammatory cytokines including IL-1β, TNF and IFNγ. As a very broad generalization, chemokines of the CXC subfamily, such as IL-8, are specific for neutrophils and, to varying extents, lymphocytes, whereas chemokines with the CC motif are chemotactic for T-cells, monocytes, dendritic cells, and variably for natural killer (NK) cells, basophils and eosinophils. Eotaxin (CCL11) is chemotactic for eosinophils, and the presence of significant concentrations of this mediator together with RANTES (*r*egulated upon *a*ctivation *n*ormal *T*-cell *e*xpressed and *s*ecreted, CCL5) in mucosal surfaces contribute towards the enhanced population of eosinophils in those tissues. The different chemokines bind to particular heparin and heparan sulfate glycosaminoglycans so that, after secretion, the chemotactic gradient can be maintained by attachment to the extracellular matrix as a form of scaffolding.

Clearly, this whole operation serves to focus the immune defenses around the invading microorganisms. These become coated with antibody, C3b and certain acute phase proteins and are ripe for phagocytosis by the neutrophils and macro-

phages; under the influence of the inflammatory mediators these have upregulated complement and Fc receptors, enhanced phagocytic responses and hyped-up killing powers, all adding up to bad news for the microbe.

Of course it is beneficial to recruit lymphocytes to sites of infection and we should remember that endothelial cells in these areas express VCAM-1 (cf. p. 193), which acts as a homing receptor for VLA-4-positive activated memory T-cells, while many chemokines (cf. Table 9.2) are chemotactic for lymphocytes.

Regulation and resolution of inflammation

With its customary prudence, evolution has established regulatory mechanisms to prevent inflammation from getting out of hand. At the humoral level we have a series of complement regulatory proteins: C1 inhibitor, C4b-binding protein, the C3 control proteins factors H and I, complement receptor CR1 (CD35), *d*ecay *a*ccelerating *f*actor (DAF, CD55), *m*embrane *c*ofactor *p*rotein (MCP, CD46), immunoconglutinin and homologous restriction factor 20 (HRF20, CD59) (cf. p. 373). Some of the acute phase proteins derived from the plasma transudate, including α-1 antichymotrypsinogen, α-1 antitrypsin, heparin cofactor-2 and plasminogen-activator inhibitor-1, are protease inhibitors.

At the cellular level, PGE$_2$, transforming growth factor-β (TGFβ) and glucocorticoids are powerful regulators. PGE$_2$ is a potent inhibitor of lymphocyte proliferation and cytokine production by T-cells and macrophages. TGFβ deactivates macrophages by inhibiting the production of reactive oxygen intermediates, inhibiting the class II MHC transactivator (CIITA) and thus downregulating class II expression, and quelling the cytotoxic enthusiasm of both macrophages and NK cells. Endogenous glucocorticoids produced via the hypothalamic–pituitary–adrenal axis exert their anti-inflammatory effects both through the repression of a number of genes for proinflammatory cytokines and adhesion molecules, and the induction of the inflammation inhibitors lipocortin-1, secretory leukocyte proteinase inhibitor (SLPI, an inhibitor of neutrophil elastase) and IL-1 receptor antagonist. IL-10 inhibits antigen presentation, cytokine production and nitric oxide (NO) killing by macrophages, the latter inhibition being greatly enhanced by synergistic action with IL-4 and TGFβ.

Once the agent that has provoked the inflammatory reaction has been cleared, these regulatory processes will normalize the site. When the inflammation traumatizes tissues through its intensity and extent, TGFβ plays a major role in the subsequent wound healing by stimulating fibroblast division and the laying down of new extracellular matrix elements.

Chronic inflammation

If an inflammatory agent persists, either because of its resistance to metabolic breakdown or through the inability of a deficient immune system to clear an infectious microbe, the character of the cellular response changes. The site becomes dominated by macrophages with varying morphology: many have an activated appearance, some form what are termed "epithelioid" cells and others fuse to form giant cells. Lymphocytes in various guises are also often present. This characteristic **granuloma** walls off the persisting agent from the remainder of the body (see type IV hypersensitivity in Chapter 15, p. 414).

Protective responses against bacteria

Most bacteria have an extracellular existence making them susceptible to phagocytic cells and complement. Neutrophils and macrophages can employ their pattern recognition receptors to directly recognize pathogen-associated molecular patterns on the microbe. Complement can be activated by the alternative or lectin pathways. However, things get positively uncomfortable for the microorganisms when antibody arrives on the scene, as then complement can also be activated via the classical pathway not to mention the fact that the bacteria will become very effectively opsonized for enhanced phagocytosis. However, the organisms don't take all this lying down and there are a vast array of strategies that they have developed in order to avoid being destroyed.

Bacterial survival strategies

As with virtually all infectious agents, if you can think of a possible avoidance strategy, some microbe will already have used it (Table 12.1).

Evading phagocytosis

The cell walls of bacteria are not all the same (Figure 12.5) and in some cases are inherently resistant to microbicidal agents; but many other strategies are used to evade either phagocytic (Figure 12.6) or complement-mediated (Figure 12.7) defences. A common mechanism by which virulent forms escape phagocytosis is by synthesis of an outer **capsule**, which does not

Table 12.1. Examples of mechanisms used by bacteria to avoid the host immune response. (Partly based on Merrell D.S. and Falkow S. (2004) *Nature* **430**, 250.)

Immune process	Example	Mechanism
Phagocytosis	*Yersinia*	Inhibition of actin skeleton in phagocytes by YopT cleavage of RhoA (see Figure 12.8)
	Legionella	Dot/icm intracellular multiplication genes inhibit phagolysosome fusion
Complement	*Streptococcus pyogenes*	M protein binding of C4b-binding protein reduces C3 convertase activity
Apoptosis	*Shigella flexneri*	IpaB-mediated activation of Caspase-1 induces apoptosis (see Figure 12.8)
	Mycobacterium tuberculosis	Increased expression of *bcl2* and Rb inhibits apoptosis
Cytokine production	*Vibrio cholerae*	Cholera toxin inhibition of IL-12 secretion
	Bordetella pertussis	Pertussis toxin induction of IL-1 and IL-4
Antibody	*Staphylococcus aureus*	IgG opsonization for phagocytosis blocked by protein A binding the antibody the 'wrong way' round
	Neisseria gonorrhoeae	Antigenic variation by recombination within *pilE* gene
T-cell activation	*Helicobacter pylori*	VacA vacuolating cytotoxin inhibits calcineurin signaling pathways

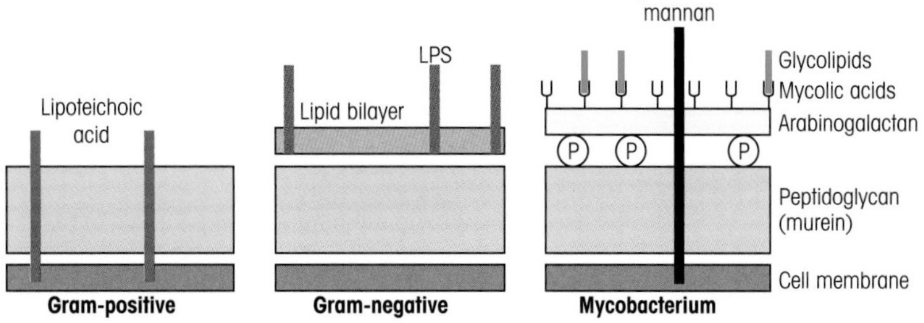

Lipoarabino-
mannan

LPS

Lipoteichoic
acid

Lipid bilayer

Glycolipids
Mycolic acids
Arabinogalactan

Peptidoglycan
(murein)

Cell membrane

Gram-positive   **Gram-negative**   **Mycobacterium**

Figure 12.5. The structure of bacterial cell walls.

All types have an inner cell membrane and a peptidoglycan wall that can be cleaved by lysozyme. The outer lipid bilayer of Gram-negative bacteria, which is susceptible to the action of complement or cationic proteins, sometimes contains lipopolysaccharide (LPS; also known as endotoxin; composed of a membrane-distal hydrophilic polysaccharide [which forms the highly polymorphic O-specific antigens] attached to a basal core polysaccharide, itself linked to the hydrophobic membrane-anchoring lipid A). One hundred and seventy-nine O antigen variants of *Escherichia coli* are known. The mycobacterial cell wall is highly resistant to breakdown. Gram-positive and Gram-negative bacteria sometimes also possess fimbriae or flagellae. All three types of bacterial cell wall may or may not be covered by an outer capsule. When present, outer capsules often protect the bacteria from phagocytosis.

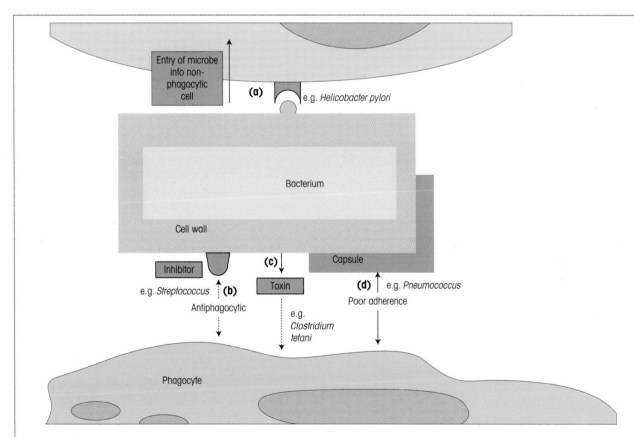

Figure 12.6. Phagocytosis avoidance strategies by extracellular bacteria.

(a) Microbe attaches to surface component to enter nonphagocytic cell; (b) surface inhibitor of phagocytosis; (c) exotoxin poisons phagocyte; (d) capsule gives poor phagocyte adherence.

Figure 12.7. Complement avoidance strategies by extracellular bacteria.

(a) Accelerated breakdown of complement by action of microbial products;
(b) complement effectors are deviated from the microbial cell wall; (c) capsule provides nonstabilizing surface for alternative pathway convertase; (d) capsule impervious to complement membrane attack complex (MAC).

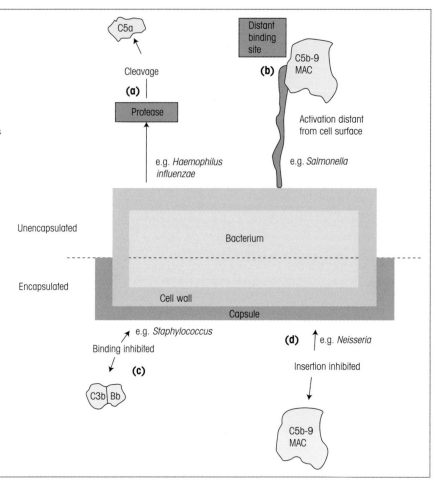

adhere readily to phagocytic cells and covers carbohydrate molecules on the bacterial surface that could otherwise be recognized by phagocyte receptors. For example, as few as 10 encapsulated pneumococci can kill a mouse but, if the capsule is removed by treatment with hyaluronidase, 10 000 bacteria are required for the job. Many pathogens evolve capsules that physically prevent access of phagocytes to C3b deposited on the bacterial cell wall.

Other organisms have actively **antiphagocytic** cell surface molecules and some go so far as to secrete **exotoxins**, which actually poison the leukocytes. Yet another ruse is to gain entry into a nonphagocytic cell and thereby hide from the professional phagocyte. Presumably, some organisms try to avoid undue provocation of phagocytic cells by adhering to and *colonizing the external mucosal surfaces* of the intestine.

Challenging the complement system

Poor activation of complement. Normal mammalian cells are protected from complement destruction by regulatory proteins such as MCP and DAF, which cause C3 convertase breakdown (see p. 373 for further discussion). Microorganisms lack these regulatory proteins so that, even in the absence of antibody, most of them would activate the alternative complement pathway by stabilization of the $\overline{C3bBb}$ convertase on their

surfaces and/or triggering the lectin pathway following interaction with microbial sugars. However, bacterial capsules in general tend to be poor activators of complement and selective pressures have favored the synthesis of capsules whose surface components do not permit stable binding of the convertase.

Acceleration of complement breakdown. Members of the regulators of complement activation (RCA) family that diminish C3 convertase activity include C4b-binding protein (C4BP), factor H and factor H-like protein 1 (FHL-1). Certain bacterial surface molecules, notably those rich in sialic acid, bind factor H, which then acts as a focus for the degradation of C3b by the serine protease factor I (cf. p. 19). This is seen, for example, with *Neisseria gonorrhoeae*. Similarly, the hypervariable regions of the M-proteins of certain *Streptococcus pyogenes* (group A streptococcus) strains are able to bind FHL-1, whereas other strains downregulate complement activation by interacting with C4BP, this time acting as a cofactor for factor I-mediated degradation of the C4b component of the classical pathway C3 convertase $\overline{C4b2a}$. *Haemophilus influenzae*, all group A streptococci, and group B, C and G streptococci of human origin, produce a C5a peptidase that acts as a virulence factor by proteolytically cleaving and thereby inactivating C5a.

Complement deviation. Some species manage to avoid lysis by deviating the complement activation site either to a secreted decoy protein or to a position on the bacterial surface distant from the cell membrane.

Resistance to insertion of terminal complement components. Gram-positive organisms (cf. Figure 12.5) have evolved thick peptidoglycan layers that prevent the insertion of the lytic C5b–9 membrane attack complex into the bacterial cell membrane. Many capsules do the same (Figure 12.7).

Interfering with internal events in the macrophage

Enteric Gram-negative bacteria in the gut have developed a number of ways of influencing macrophage activity, including inducing apoptosis, preventing phagosome–lysosome fusion and affecting the actin cytoskeleton (Figure 12.8).

Antigenic variation

Individual antigens can be altered in the face of a determined host antibody response. Examples include variation of surface lipoproteins in the Lyme disease spirochete *Borrelia burgdorferi*, of enzymes involved in synthesizing surface structures in *Campylobacter jejuni*, and of the pili in *Neisseria meningitidis*. In addition, new strains can arise, as has occurred with the life-threatening *E. coli* O157:H7 that can cause hemolytic uremic syndrome and appears to have emerged about 50 years ago by incorporation of shigella toxin genes into the *E. coli* O55 genome.

The host counter-attack

Antibodies can defeat these devious attempts to avoid engulfment by neutralizing the antiphagocytic molecules and by binding to the surface of the organisms to focus the site for fixation of complement, so "opsonizing" them for ingestion by neutrophils and macrophages or preparing them for the terminal membrane attack complex (Milestone 12.1). However, antibody production by B-cells usually requires T-cell help, and the T-cells need to be activated by antigen-presenting cells.

As already discussed in Chapter 1, but so important that it is worth repeating, pathogen-associated molecular patterns (PAMPs), such as the all-important lipopolysaccharide (LPS) endotoxin of Gram-negative bacteria, peptidoglycan, lipoteichoic acids, mannans, bacterial DNA, double-stranded RNA and glucans, are molecules that are broadly expressed by microbial pathogens but not present on host tissues. Thus these molecules serve as an alerting service for the immune system, which detects their presence using pattern recognition receptors (PRRs) expressed on the surface of antigen-presenting cells. It will be recalled that such receptors include the mannose receptor (CD206), which facilitates phagocytosis of microorganisms by macrophages, and the scavenger receptor (CD204) which mediates clearance of bacteria from the circulation. LPS-binding protein (LBP) transfers LPS to the CD14 PRR on monocytes, macrophages, dendritic cells and B-cells. This leads to the recruitment of the Toll-like receptor 4 (TLR4) molecule, which triggers expression of proinflammatory genes, including those for IL-1, IL-6, IL-12 and TNF, and the upregulation of

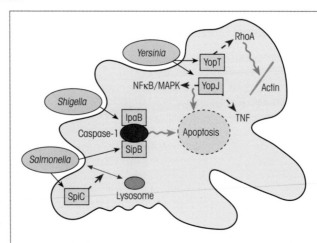

Figure 12.8. Evasion of macrophage defenses by enteric bacteria.

The IpaB (*invasion plasmid antigen B*) and SipB (*Salmonella invasion protein B*) molecules secreted by *Shigella* and *Salmonella*, respectively, can activate caspase 1 and thereby set off a train of events that will lead to the death of the macrophage by apoptosis. The SpiC (*salmonella pathogenicity island C*) protein from *Salmonella* inhibits the trafficking of cellular vesicles, and therefore is able to prevent lysosomes fusing with phagocytic vesicles. *Yersinia* produces a number of Yop molecules (*yersinia outer proteins*) able to interfere with the normal functioning of the phagocyte. For example, YopJ inhibits tumor necrosis factor (TNF) production and downregulates nuclear factor κB (NFκB) and MAP kinases, thereby facilitating apoptosis by inhibiting anti-apoptotic pathways. YopT prevents phagocytosis by modifying the GTPase RhoA involved in regulating the actin cytoskeleton. (Based on Donnenberg M.S. (2000) *Nature* **406**, 768.)

the CD80 (B7.1) and CD86 (B7.2) co-stimulatory molecules. Although each of the 13 or so Toll-like receptors so far characterized recognize broadly expressed microbial structures, it has been suggested that collectively they are able to some extent to discriminate between different pathogens by detection of particular combinations of PAMPS in a "bar-code"-type approach.

Toxin neutralization

Circulating antibodies can neutralize the soluble antiphagocytic molecules and other exotoxins (e.g. phospholipase C of *Clostridium perfringens*) released by bacteria. Combination near the biologically active site of the toxin would stereochemically block reaction with the substrate, whereas combination distant from the active site may also cause inhibition through allosteric conformational changes. In its complex with antibody, the toxin may be unable to diffuse away rapidly and will be susceptible to phagocytosis.

Opsonization of bacteria

Independently of antibody. Differences between the carbohydrate structures on bacteria and self are exploited by the

⊙ Milestone 12.1—The Protective Effects of Antibody

The pioneering research that led to the recognition of the antibacterial protection afforded by antibody clustered in the last years of the 19th century. A good place to start the story is the discovery by Roux and Yersin in 1888, at the Pasteur Institute in Paris, that the exotoxin of diphtheria bacillus could be isolated from a bacteria-free filtrate of the medium used to culture the organism. Von Behring (Figure M12.1.1) and Kitasato at Koch's Institute in Berlin in 1890 then went on to show that animals could develop an immunity to such toxins that was due to the development of specific neutralizing substances referred to generally as **antibodies** (anti-foreign bodies) (Figure M12.1.2). They further succeeded in passively transferring immunity to another animal with serum containing the antitoxin. The dawning of an era of serotherapy came in 1894 with Roux's successful treatment of patients with diphtheria by injection of immune horse serum.

Sir Almroth Wright (Figure M12.1.3) in London in 1903 proposed that the main action of the increased antibody produced after infection was to reinforce killing by the phagocytes. He called the antibodies **opsonins** (Gk. *opson*, a dressing or relish), because they prepared the bacteria as food for the phagocytic cells, and amply verified his predictions by showing that antibodies dramatically increased the phagocytosis of bacteria *in vitro*, thereby cleverly linking *innate* to *adaptive* immunity.

George Bernard Shaw even referred to Almroth Wright's proposal in his play *The Doctor's Dilemma*. In the preface he gave an evocative description of the function of opsonins: "the

white corpuscles or phagocytes that attack and devour disease germs for us do their work only when we butter the disease germs appetizingly for them with a natural sauce that Sir Almroth named opsonins ..." (A more extended account of immunology at the turn of the 19th century may be found in Silverstein A.M. (2009) *A History of Immunology*. 2nd edn. Elsevier.)

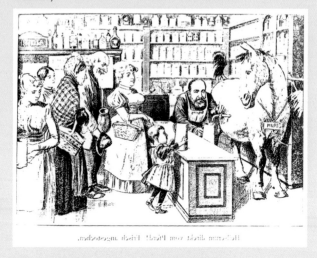

Figure M12.1.2. Von Behring extracting serum using a tap.

Caricature by Lustigen Blättern, 1894. (Legend: "Serum direct from the horse! Freshly drawn.")

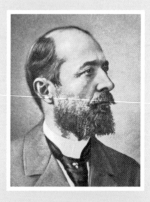

Figure M12.1.1. Emil von Behring (1854–1917).

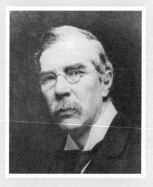

Figure M12.1.3. Sir Almroth Wright (1861–1947).

(Images kindly supplied by The Wellcome Collection, London.)

collectins (cf. p. 25), a series of molecules with similar ultrastructure to C1q and that bear C-terminal lectin domains. These include mannose-binding lectin (MBL) that, on binding to terminal mannose on the bacterial surface, initiates antibody-independent complement activation (cf. p. 25). Other collectins, lung surfactant proteins SP-A and SP-D and, in cattle, conglutinin, also recognize carbohydrate ligands and can all act as opsonins (see Milestone 12.1) mediating phagocytosis by virtue of their binding to the C1q receptor.

Augmented by antibody. Encapsulated bacteria that resist phagocytosis become extremely attractive to neutrophils and macrophages when coated with antibody and their rate of clearance from the bloodstream is strikingly enhanced (Figure 12.9). The less effective removal of coated bacteria in complement-deficient animals emphasizes the synergism between antibody and complement for opsonization, which is mediated through specific receptors for immunoglobulin Fc and complement on the phagocyte surface (Figure 12.10). It is clearly advantageous that the IgG subclasses that bind strongly to the IgG Fc receptors (e.g. IgG1 and IgG3 in the human) also fix complement well, it being appreciated that C3b bound to IgG is a very efficient opsonin because it engages two receptors simultaneously. Complexes containing C3b and C4b may show immune adherence to the CR1 complement receptors on erythrocytes to provide aggregates that are extremely rapidly transported to the liver and spleen for phagocytosis.

Some elaboration on **complement receptors** may be pertinent at this stage. The CR1 receptor (CD35) for C3b is also present on neutrophils, eosinophils, monocytes, B-cells and lymph node follicular dendritic cells (FDC). Together with the CR3 receptor (CD11b/CD18), it has the main responsibility for clearance of complexes containing C3. The *CR1* gene is linked in a cluster with C4b-binding protein and factor H, all of which subserve a regulatory function by binding to C3b or C4b to disassemble the C3/C5 convertases, and act as cofactors for the proteolytic inactivation of C3b and C4b by factor I.

CR2 receptors (CD21) for iC3b, C3dg and C3d are present on B-cells and FDC, and transduce accessory signals for B-cell activation especially in the germinal centers (cf. p. 248). They act as the receptor for Epstein–Barr virus (EBV), binding to the gp350 major viral envelope glycoprotein and thereby facilitate entry of the virus into B-cells, with MHC class II molecules acting as a coreceptor binding to viral gp42.

CR3 receptors (CD11b/CD18 on neutrophils, eosinophils, monocytes and NK cells) bind iC3b, C3dg and C3d. They are related to LFA-1 and CR4 (CD11c/CD18, binds iC3b and C3dg) in being members of the β_2 integrin subfamily (cf. Table

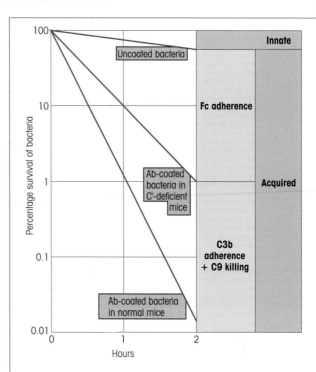

Figure 12.9. Effect of opsonizing antibody and complement on rate of clearance of virulent bacteria from the blood.

The uncoated bacteria are phagocytosed rather slowly (*innate immunity*) but, on coating with antibody (Ab) (*acquired immunity*), adherence to phagocytes is increased many-fold. The adherence is less effective in complement-deficient animals. This situation is hypothetical but realistic; the natural proliferation of the bacteria has been ignored.

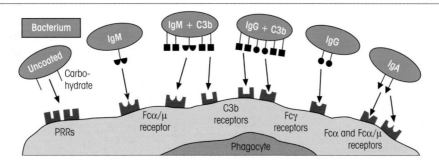

Figure 12.10. Immunoglobulin and complement greatly increase the adherence of bacteria (and other antigens) to macrophages and neutrophils.

Uncoated bacteria adhere to pattern recognition receptors (PRRs) such as various Toll-like receptors (TLR) and the mannose-binding receptor. The Fcα/μR on macrophages binds to IgM (⌣)-coated bacteria. High affinity receptors for IgG Fc (●) and for C3b (CR1) and iC3b (CR3) (■) on the macrophage and neutrophil surface considerably enhance the strength of binding. The augmenting effect of complement is due to the fact that two adjacent IgG molecules can fix many C3b molecules, thereby increasing the number of links to the macrophage (cf. "bonus effect of multivalency"; p. 121). Bacteria opsonized with IgA (▼) can adhere to the phagocyte via the Fcα/μR already mentioned, or via FcαRI (CD89), which is present on the surface of both macrophages and neutrophils.

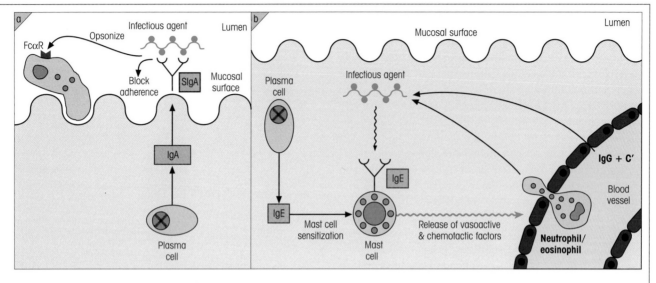

Figure 12.11. Defense of the mucosal surfaces.

(a) IgA opsonizes organisms and prevents adherence to the mucosa. (b) IgE recruits agents of the immune response by firing the release of mediators from mast cells.

7.1). CR5 is found on neutrophils and platelets and binds C3d and C3dg. A number of other complement receptors have been described including some with specificity for C1q, for C3a and C4a, and the CD88 molecule with specificity for C5a.

Some further effects of complement

Some strains of Gram-negative bacteria that have a lipoprotein outer wall resembling mammalian surface membranes in structure are susceptible to the bactericidal action of fresh serum containing antibody. The antibody initiates the development of a complement-mediated lesion that is said to allow access of serum lysozyme to the inner peptidoglycan wall of the bacterium to cause eventual cell death. Activation of complement through union of antibody and bacterium will also generate the C3a and C5a anaphylatoxins leading to extensive transudation of serum components, including more antibody, and to the chemotactic attraction of neutrophils to aid in phagocytosis, as described earlier under the acute inflammation umbrella (cf. Figures 2.18 and 12.3).

The secretory immune system protects the external mucosal surfaces

We have earlier emphasized the critical nature of the mucosal barriers where there is a potentially hostile interface with the microbial hordes. With an area of around $400\,m^2$, give or take a tennis court or two, the epithelium of the adult mucosae represents the most frequent portal of entry for common infectious agents and allergens. The need for well marshaled, highly effective mucosal immunity is glaringly obvious.

The gut mucosal surfaces are defended by both antigen-specific and nonantigen-specific mechanisms. Among the non-specific mechanisms, antimicrobial peptides are produced not only by neutrophils and macrophages but also by mucosal epithelium. As described in Chapter 1, the group of antimicrobial peptides called defensins lyse bacteria via disruption of their surface membranes. Specific immunity is provided by secretory IgA and IgM, with IgA1 predominating in the upper areas and IgA2 in the large bowel. Most other mucosal surfaces are also protected predominantly by IgA with the exception of the reproductive tract tissues of both male and female, where the dominant antibody isotype is IgG. The size of the task is highlighted by the fact that 80% of the Ig-producing B-cells in the body are present in the secretory mucosae and exocrine glands. IgA antibodies afford protection in the external body fluids, tears, saliva, nasal secretions and those bathing the surfaces of the intestine and lung by coating bacteria and viruses and preventing their adherence to the epithelial cells of the mucous membranes, which is essential for viral infection and bacterial colonization. Secretory IgA molecules themselves have very little innate adhesiveness for epithelial cells, but high affinity Fc receptors for this Ig class are present on macrophages and neutrophils and can mediate phagocytosis (Figure 12.11a).

If an infectious agent succeeds in penetrating the IgA barrier, it comes up against the next line of defense of the secretory system (see p. 196), which is manned by IgE. Indeed, most serum IgE arises from plasma cells in mucosal tissues and their local draining lymph nodes. Although present in low concentration, IgE is firmly bound to the Fc receptors of the mast cell (see p. 395) and contact with antigen leads to the release of mediators that effectively recruit agents of the immune response and generate a local acute inflammatory reaction. Thus histamine, by increasing vascular permeability, causes the transudation of IgG and complement into the area, while chemotactic factors for neutrophils and eosinophils attract the effector cells needed to dispose of the infectious organism coated with specific IgG and C3b (Figure 12.11b). Engagement of the Fcγ and C3b receptors on local macrophages by such complexes will lead to secretion of factors that further reinforce these vascular permeability and chemotactic events. Broadly, one would say that immune exclusion in the gut is noninflammatory, but immune elimination of organisms that penetrate the mucosa is proinflammatory.

Where the opsonized organism is too large to be engulfed, phagocytes can employ antibody-dependent cellular cytotoxicity (ADCC, p. 48) and there is evidence for its involvement in parasitic infections (see p. 17).

The mucosal tissues contain various T-cell populations, but their role and that of the mucosal epithelial cells, other than in a helper function for local antibody production, is of less relevance for the defense against extracellular bacteria.

Some specific bacterial infections

First let us see how these considerations apply to defense against infection by common organisms such as streptococci and staphylococci. The β-hemolytic **streptococci** were classified by Lancefield according to their carbohydrate antigen, the most important for human disease belonging to group A. *Streptococcus pyogenes* most commonly causes acute pharyngitis (strep sore throat) and the skin condition impetigo, but is also responsible for scarlet fever and has emerged as a cause of the much rarer but often fatal toxic shock syndrome and of the always alarming necrotizing fasciitis (flesh-eating disease). Rheumatic fever and glomerular nephritis sometimes occur as serious postinfection sequelae.

The most important virulence factor is the surface M-protein (variants of which form the basis of the Griffith typing). This protein is an acceptor for factor H that facilitates C3b breakdown, and binds fibrinogen and its fragments that cover sites that could act as complement activators. It thereby inhibits opsonization and the protection afforded by antibodies to the M-component is attributable to the striking increase in phagocytosis, which they induce. The ability of group A streptococci to elicit cross-reactive autoantibodies that bind to cardiac myosin results in poststreptococcal autoimmune disease. High titer antibodies to the streptolysin O exotoxin (ASO), which damages membranes, indicate recent streptococcal infection. The streptococcal pyrogenic exotoxins SPE-A, -C and -H, and the streptococcal mitogenic exotoxin SMEZ-2, are superantigens associated with scarlet fever and toxic shock syndrome. The toxins are neutralized by antibody and the erythematous intradermal reaction to injected toxin (the Dick reaction) is only seen in individuals lacking antibody. Antibody can also neutralize bacterial enzymes like hyaluronidase that act to spread the infection.

The mutans streptococci (*Streptococcus mutans* and *S. sobrinus*) are an important cause of dental caries. The organisms possess a glucosyltransferase enzyme that converts sucrose to glucose polymers (glucans) that aid adhesion to the tooth surface. Small-scale clinical trials with vaccines based upon the glucosyltransferase, usually together with components of the surface antigen I/II fibrillar adhesins, have shown that salivary IgA against mutans streptococci can be increased and, in some cases, interfere with colonization.

Virulent forms of **staphylococci**, of which *Staphylococcus aureus* is perhaps the most common, resist phagocytosis. Both staphylococci and streptococci express surface proteins that bind to the Fc region of the IgG heavy chain (protein A and protein G, respectively) and serve to limit antibody-mediated effector functions by binding the antibodies the "wrong way" round. Virulence factors encoded by *S. aureus* genes also include adhesins and cell wall teichoic acid on the surface of the bacterium, toxic shock syndrome toxin-1, enterotoxins and enzymes. The penicillin-binding protein 2a is able to synthesize peptidoglycan even in the presence of β-lactam antibiotics. Other virulence factors are acquired from lysogenic bacteriophages, including Panton-Valentine leucocidin and chemotaxis inhibitory protein (CHIP). Although *S. aureus* is readily phagocytosed in the presence of *adequate* amounts of antibody, a small proportion of the ingested bacteria survives and they are difficult organisms to eliminate completely. Where the infection is inadequately controlled, severe lesions may occur in the immunized host as a consequence of type IV delayed hypersensitivity reactions. Thus, staphylococci were found to be avirulent when injected into mice passively immunized with antibody, but caused extensive tissue damage in animals previously given sensitized T-cells. The methicillin-resistant *S. aureus* (MRSA) "superbug," which was already also resistant to all the β-lactam antibiotics, has now become vancomycin resistant following transfer of drug resistance from *Enterococcus*. New drugs such as linezolid and daptomycin can be used to treat MRSA infections but there are rare instances of resistance developing to these antibiotics as well—pretty scary stuff.

Other examples where antibodies are required to overcome the inherently antiphagocytic properties of **bacterial capsules** are seen in immunity to pneumococci, meningococci and *Haemophilus influenzae*. *Bacillus anthracis* possesses an antiphagocytic capsule composed of a γ-polypeptide of D-glutamic acid but, although anticapsular antibodies effectively promote uptake by neutrophils, the exotoxin is so potent that vaccines are inadequate unless they also stimulate antitoxin immunity. In addition to releasing such lethal exotoxins, *Pseudomonas aeruginosa* also produces an elastase that inactivates C3a and C5a; as a result, only minimal inflammatory responses are made in the absence of neutralizing antibodies.

The ploy of **diverting complement activation** to insensitive sites is seen rather well with different strains of Gram-negative salmonella and *E. coli* organisms that vary in the number of O-specific oligosaccharide side-chains attached to the lipid-A-linked core polysaccharide of the endotoxin (cf. Figure 12.5). Variants with long side-chains are relatively insensitive to killing by serum through the alternative complement pathway (see p. 19); as the side-chains become shorter and shorter, the serum sensitivity increases. Although all variants activate the alternative pathway, only those with short or no side-chains allow the cytotoxic membrane attack complex to be inserted near to the outer lipid bilayer. On the other hand, antibodies focus the complex to a more vulnerable site.

The destruction of gonococci by serum containing antibody is dependent upon the formation of the membrane attack complex, and rare individuals lacking C8 or C9 are susceptible to neisseria infection. *N. gonorrhoeae* (gonococci) specifically binds complement proteins and prevents their insertion in the outer membranes, but antibody, like a ubiquitous "Mr Fixit," corrects this situation, at least so far as the host is concerned. With respect to the infective process itself, IgA and IgG produced in the genital tract in response to these organisms inhibits the attachment of the bacteria, through their pili, to mucosal cells, but seems unable to afford adequate protection against reinfection. This seems to be due to a very effective antigenic shift mechanism that alters the sequence of the expressed pilin by gene conversion. Gonococcal colony *op*acity-*a*ssociated (Opa) proteins bind to the *i*mmunoreceptor *t*yrosine-based *i*nhibitory *m*otif (ITIM)-containing long tail isoform of CD66a on CD4+ T-cells and thereby inhibit their activation and proliferation. Failure to achieve good protection might also be a reflection of the ability of the gonococci to produce a protease that cleaves a proline-rich sequence present in the hinge region of IgA1 (but not of IgA2), although the presence in most individuals of neutralizing antibodies against this protease may interfere with its proteolytic activity. Meningococci, which frequently infect the nasopharynx, *H. influenzae* and *Streptococcus pneumoniae* have similar IgA1 proteases.

Cholera is caused by the colonization of the small intestine by *Vibrio cholerae* and the subsequent action of its enterotoxin. The B subunits of the toxin bind to GM1 monosialoganglioside receptors and translocate the A subunit across the membrane where it activates adenyl cyclase. The increased cAMP then causes fluid loss by inhibiting uptake of sodium chloride and stimulating active Cl⁻ secretion by intestinal epithelial cells. Locally synthesized IgA antibodies against *V. cholerae* lipopolysaccharide and the toxin provide independent protection against cholera, the first by inhibiting bacterial adherence to the intestinal wall, the second by blocking attachment of the toxin to its receptor. In accord with this analysis are the epidemiological data showing that children who drink milk with high titers of IgA antibodies specific for either of these antigens are less likely to develop clinical cholera.

The ways in which antibody can help overcome the different facets of bacterial invasion are summarized in Figure 12.12.

The habitat of intracellular bacteria allows avoidance of many of the host defenses

A number of different bacterial species have evolved to reside inside the host's cells. Here they are hidden from many of the

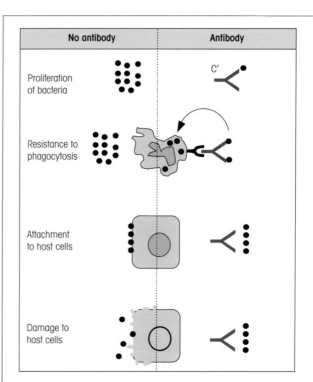

Figure 12.12. Antibody defenses against bacterial invasion.

Antibodies are able to prevent the proliferation of bacteria by, e.g. blocking metabolic transport mechanisms such as receptors for iron-chelating compounds and by activating complement. Resistance to phagocytosis can be overcome by opsonizing the bacteria for subsequent recognition by Fc receptors on neutrophils and macrophages. The production of antibodies against fimbriae, lipoteichoic acid and capsules can prevent attachment of bacteria to host cells. Neutralizing antibodies to bacterial toxins can prevent damage to host cells.

defences, such as antibodies, that the immune system regularly employs against pathogens. However, all is not lost because the host has a number of strategies that it can use to deal with such bacteria including various cell-mediated responses.

Bacterial survival strategies

Yersinia and *Salmonella* are among the select number of bacterial pathogens that have evolved special mechanisms to enter, survive and replicate within normally **nonphagocytic host cells**. The former gains entry through binding of its outer membrane protein, invasin, to multiple β₁-integrin receptors on the host cell. For *Salmonella* a number of bacterial proteins including *s*almonella *i*nvasion *p*rotein A (SipA) and the *s*almonella *o*uter *p*roteins SopA, SopB, SopD and SopE₂ stimulate events such as cytoskeletal rearrangements and membrane ruffling to facilitate entry into host cells.

Some strains of bacteria, such as the tubercle and leprosy bacilli and listeria and brucella organisms, escape the wrath of

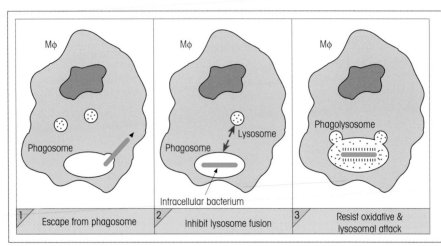

Figure 12.13. Evasion of phagocytic death by intracellular bacteria residing in macrophages (Mϕ).

the immune system by cheekily fashioning an intracellular life within one of its strongholds, the macrophage no less. Mononuclear phagocytes are a good target for such organisms in the sense that they are very mobile and allow wide dissemination throughout the body. Entry of bacteria is facilitated by phagocytic uptake after attachment to pattern recognition receptors and, following opsonization, to Fcγ and C3b receptors. Once inside, many of them defy the mighty macrophage by subverting their killing mechanisms in a variety of ways. Organisms such as *Mycobacterium tuberculosis* neutralize the pH in the phagosome and inhibit subsequent fusion with the lysosomes (Figure 12.13). Mycobacterial cell wall peptidoglycan and glycolipids, such as lipoarabinomannan, inhibit macrophage activation. *Listeria monocytogenes* uses a lysin, listeriolysin O, to escape from its phagosomal prison to lie happily free within the cytoplasm; some rickettsiae and the protozoan *Trypanosoma cruzi* can do the same using other lysins. Certain bacteria, although primarily extracellular in habit, can invade nonphagocytic cells. An example is *Helicobacter pylori*, which is able to reside in epithelial cells that then serve as a reservoir for re-infection.

Defense against intracellular bacteria needs to recruit T-cell-mediated immunity (CMI)

In an elegant series of experiments, Mackaness demonstrated the importance of CMI reactions for the killing of intracellular parasites and the establishment of an immune state. Animals infected with moderate doses of *M. tuberculosis* overcome the infection and are immune to subsequent challenge with the bacillus. The immunity can be transferred to a normal recipient with T-lymphocytes but not macrophages or serum from an immune animal. Supporting this view, that specific immunity is mediated by T-cells, is the greater susceptibility to infection with tubercle and leprosy bacilli of mice in which the T-lymphocytes have been depressed by thymectomy plus anti-T-cell monoclonals, or in which the TCR genes have been disrupted by homologous gene recombination (knockout mice).

Activated macrophages kill intracellular parasites

When monocytes first settle down in the tissue to become "resident" macrophages they are essentially in a resting state with minimal microbicidal capability. However, the development of an inflammatory environment will partially activate them and the subsequent recruitment of pathogen-specific Th1 cells will lead to full activation. The production of macrophage activating factors such as IFNγ, TNF and lymphotoxin by these Th1 cells results in the macrophages now being able to kill obligate intracellular microbes (Figure 12.14). Foremost among the killing mechanisms that are upregulated are those mediated by reactive oxygen intermediates and NO· radicals. The activated macrophage is undeniably a formidable cell, capable of secreting the 60 or so substances that are concerned in chronic inflammatory reactions (Figure 12.15)—not the sort to meet in an alley on a dark night!

The mechanism of T-cell-mediated immunity in the Mackaness experiments now becomes clear. Specifically primed T-cells react with processed antigen derived from the intracellular bacteria present on the surface of the infected macrophage in association with MHC II; the subsequent release of cytokines activates the macrophage and endows it with the ability to kill the organisms it has phagocytosed (Figure 12.16).

Examples of intracellular bacterial infections

Listeria

The organism *Listeria monocytogenes*, usually acquired by humans following the ingestion of contaminated foods such as unpasteurized dairy products, poses a particular risk to pregnant women due to its association with septic abortion. Following interaction of the bacterial cell surface molecule internalin A with E-cadherin on the epithelial cells, the organism passes through the epithelium and enters the bloodstream. Dissemination occurs to the spleen and liver where phagocytic internalization into macrophages occurs, and into hepatocytes via binding of another microbial surface molecule, internalin B, to the hepatocyte growth factor receptor. The actin-assembly-inducing protein ActA produced by *Listeria* facilitates its intercellular transmission. IFNγ secreted by NK and Th1 cells drives the macrophage activation required for the ultimate elimination of intracellular *Listeria* (Figure 12.17) The bactericidal action of neutrophils and the central role

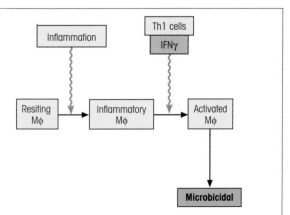

Figure 12.14. Stages in the activation of macrophages (Mφ) for microbicidal function.

Macrophages taken from sites of inflammation are considerably increased in size, acid hydrolase content, secretion of neutral proteases and phagocytic function. If we may give one example, the C3b receptors on resident resting Mφ are not freely mobile in the membrane and so cannot permit the "zippering" process required for phagocytosis (see p. 13); consequently, they bind but do not ingest C3b-coated red cells. Inflammatory Mφ, on the other hand, have C3 receptors that display considerable lateral mobility and the C3-opsonized erythrocytes are readily phagocytosed. In addition to the dramatic upregulation of intracellular killing mechanisms, striking changes in surface components accompany the activation that occurs in response to Th1 cytokines such as IFNγ.

of IL-12 also warrant our attention, as does the recruitment by the chemokine CCL2 (MCP-1) of dendritic cells producing TNF and nitric oxide. These or other populations of dendritic cells are thought to cross-prime CD8[+] T-cells with listeria antigens derived from infected macrophages. During primary infection, CD8 T-cells that are restricted to the nonclassical MHC molecule H2-M3 seem to play a particularly important role, whereas the classical class I restricted CD8 T-cells make a more profound contribution during secondary infection. Mutant mice lacking αβ and/or γδ T-cells reveal that these two cell types make comparable contributions to resistance against primary listeria infection, but that the αβ TCR set bears the major responsibility for conferring protective immunity. γδ T-cells control the local tissue response at the site of microbial replication and γδ knockout mutants develop huge abscesses when infected with *Listeria*.

Tuberculosis

Tuberculosis (TB) is on the rampage, aided by the emergence of multidrug-resistant strains of *Mycobacterium tuberculosis*. It is estimated that 1.7 million deaths worldwide resulted from TB in 2009, including 380 000 patients with AIDS who died of tuberculosis.

With respect to host defense mechanisms, as seen with listeria infection, murine macrophages activated by IFNγ can destroy intracellular mycobacteria, largely through the generation of toxic NO· radicals. *M. tuberculosis* within the macrophage can be engulfed by autophagy in these cells, with subsequent fusion to lysosomes containing a variety of microbicidal compounds. Some parasitized macrophages reach a stage at which they are too incapacitated to be stirred into action by T-cell messages, and here a somewhat ruthless

Figure 12.15. The role of the activated macrophage in the initiation and mediation of chronic inflammation with concomitant tissue repair, and in the killing of microbes and tumor cells.

It is possible that macrophages differentiate along distinct pathways to subserve these different functions. The electron micrograph shows a highly activated macrophage with many lysosomal structures that have been highlighted by the uptake of thorotrast; one (arrowed) is seen fusing with a phagosome containing the protozoan *Toxoplasma gondii*. (Courtesy of C. Jones.)

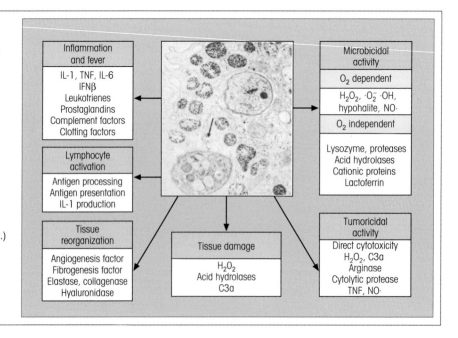

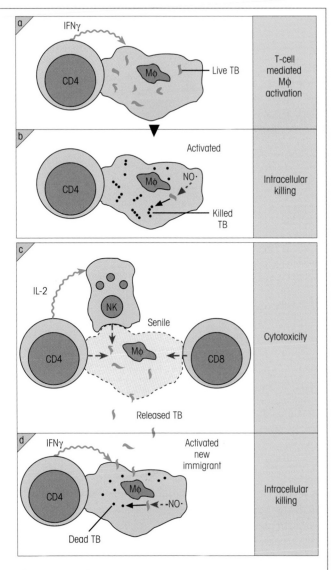

Figure 12.16. The "cytokine connection": nonspecific murine macrophage killing of intracellular bacteria triggered by a specific T-cell-mediated immunity reaction.

(a) Specific CD4 Th1 cell recognizes mycobacterial peptide associated with MHC class II and releases macrophage (Mϕ) activating IFNγ. (b) The activated Mϕ kills the intracellular TB, mainly through generation of toxic NO·. (c) A "senile" Mϕ, unable to destroy the intracellular bacteria, is killed by CD8 and CD4 cytotoxic cells and possibly by IL-2-activated NK cells. The Mϕ then releases live tubercle bacilli that are taken up and killed by newly recruited Mϕ susceptible to IFNγ activation (d). Human monocytes require activation by both IFNγ and IL-4 plus CD23-mediated signals for induction of iNO synthase and production of NO.

A vital role for both αβ and γδ T-cells in murine TB is indicated by an inability to control the infection in both TCR β-chain knockout mice (which lack an αβ TCR) and TCR δ-chain knockout mice (which lack a γδ TCR).

Inbred strains of mice differ dramatically in their susceptibility to infection by *Salmonella typhimurium, Leishmania donovani* and various mycobacteria. Resistance is associated with a T-cell-independent enhanced state of macrophage priming for bactericidal activity involving oxygen and nitrogen radicals. Moreover, macrophages from resistant strains have increased MHC class II expression and a higher respiratory burst, are more readily activated by IFNγ, and induce better stimulation of T-cells. By contrast, macrophages from susceptible strains tend to have suppressor effects on T-cell proliferation to mycobacterial antigens. The *M. tuberculosis*-infected macrophages secrete IL-6, which has the property of inhibiting IFNγ signaling in the surrounding macrophages. Susceptibility and resistance to *M. tuberculosis* in murine models depend upon a number of genes, including *SLC11A1* (solute carrier family 11 member 1, a proton-coupled divalent metal ion transporter previously called Nramp1) and genes in the *sst1* gene locus (susceptibility to tuberculosis 1, also involved in immunity to *Listeria monocytogenes* infection). A number of polymorphisms have been identified in the human *SLC11A1* gene and studies are ongoing to link individual polymorphisms to susceptibility.

Where the host has difficulty in effectively eliminating these organisms, the chronic CMI response to local antigen leads to the accumulation of densely packed macrophages that release angiogenic and fibrogenic factors and stimulate the formation of granulation tissue and ultimately fibrosis. The activated macrophages, probably under the stimulus of IL-4, transform to epithelioid cells and fuse to become giant cells. As suggested earlier, the resulting granuloma represents an attempt by the body to isolate a site of persistent infection.

The position is complicated in the human because IFNγ-stimulated human macrophages are unable to eliminate intracellular TB. Detection of the triacylated lipoprotein PAMP of *M. tuberculosis* by the TLR1/TLR2 heterodimer stimulates macrophage production of proinflammatory cytokines such as IL-1β, inducible NO synthase and expression of co-stimulatory molecules. Furthermore, the intracellular pattern recognition receptor NOD2 recognises the mycobacterial peptidoglycan muramyl dipeptide, again resulting in the production of proinflammatory cytokines. However, interference with the phagosome and a resistance to macrophage killing ensure the initial survival of the mycobacteria. Nonetheless, prolonged exposure of the macrophage to mycobacterial components leads to the induction of TNFα and subsequent macrophage cell death by both necrosis and apoptosis thereby depriving the mycobacteria of their safe haven.

The mycobacterial products Ag85B (a mycolyl transferase) and ESAT-6 (early secreted antigenic target-6) are potent inducers of IFNγ from human CD4⁺ T-cells. CD8⁺ T-cells can

strategy has evolved in which the host deploys cytotoxic CD8, and possibly CD4 and NK cells, to execute the helpless macrophage and release the live mycobacteria; these can now be taken up by newly immigrant phagocytic cells susceptible to activation by IFNγ and summarily disposed of (Figure 12.16).

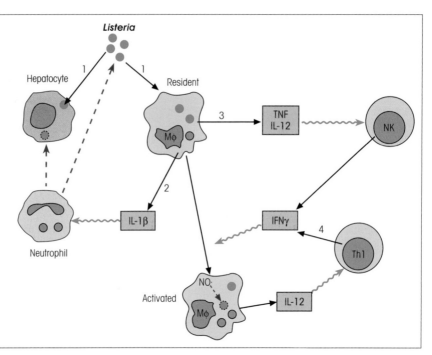

Figure 12.17. Macrophage activation in response to listeria infection.

(1) *Listeria* infects resident macrophages and hepatocytes; (2) the Mϕ release IL-1β, which activates neutrophils to destroy listeria bacilli by direct contact and are cytotoxic for infected hepatocytes; (3) the infected Mϕ release TNF and IL-12, which stimulate NK cells to secrete IFNγ, which in turn activates the macrophage to produce NO· and kill intracellular *Listeria*; IFNγ plus Mϕ-derived IL-12 recruit Th1 cells, which reinforce Mϕ activation through the production of IFNγ (4). (Based on an article by Rogers H.W., Tripps C.S. & Unanue E.R. (1995) *The Immunologist* **3**, 152.)

recognize mycobacterial peptide antigens presented by MHC class I. αβ T-cells have been described that proliferate in response to mycobacterial lipid-bearing antigens such as dide-hydroxymycobactins presented by host CD1a molecules and mycolic acid presented by CD1b. Although *in vitro* these cells can secrete IFNγ and TNFα and can be cytotoxic their function *in vivo* remains unclear. Regarding γδ T-cells, in the human those with a Vγ2Vδ2 TCR recognize protein antigens, isopentenyl pyrophosphates and prenyl pyrophosphates from *M. tuberculosis*, but again any possible protective role *in vivo* remains speculative.

Leprosy

Human leprosy presents as a spectrum ranging from the tuber-culoid form, with lesions containing small numbers of viable organisms, to the lepromatous form, characterized by an abundance of *Mycobacterium leprae* within the macrophages. CMI rather than humoral immunity is important for the control of the leprosy bacillus. Although the tuberculoid state is associated with good cell-mediated dermal hypersensitivity reactions and a bias towards Th1-type responses, these are still not good enough to eradicate the bacilli completely. In the lepromatous form, there is poor T-cell reactivity to whole bacilli and poor lepromin dermal responses, although there are numerous plasma cells that contribute to a high level of circulating antibody and indicate a more prominent Th2 activity. Leukocyte Ig-like receptor-A2 (LILRA2) expression is increased in lesions of lepromatous patients, causing a block in TLR-directed anti-microbial activity and a reduced production of proinflammatory IL-12, but enhanced secretion of immunosuppressive IL-10, by monocytes.

Immunity to viral infection

When outside of cells, viruses are surrounded by a protein coat; the capsid. In the case of enveloped viruses the capsid is enclosed by a lipid bilayer that, although derived from the host cell membrane, also incorporates viral proteins required for cell attachment. All viruses have to spend some of their life cycle inside host cells. They have no choice in this matter as they do not themselves possess all the components necessary to replicate their nucleic acid. During its extracellular existence the virus is susceptible to neutralization by antibodies able to block binding to receptors on the host cells, can be engulfed and destroyed by phagocytes, and can be damaged by the effects of complement (e.g. by opsonisation for phagocytosis or by lysis of enveloped viruses). However, like the intracellular bacteria discussed above, once inside the host cells the virus is effectively hidden from many host responses. Furthermore, many viruses cause latent infections in which the viral genome is in an inactive state inside host cells. Only upon re-activation will viral proteins be produced that can be processed for presentation by MHC class I molecules to CD8+ cytotoxic T-cells with subsequent destruction of the infected cell. This will deprive the virus of its habitat and any viruses released from the killed cell will become accessible to the combined effects of phagocytic cells, antibody and complement. Although this is a rather brutal approach in that it involves us killing our own cells, so long as it happens reasonably early on in the infection it is no big deal as we can usually regenerate the "missing" cells. However, during chronic infections with viruses the destruction of our own cells by cytotoxic T-cells can become so extensive that the immune response causes more damage than the virus itself, leading to immunopathology.

Viruses constitute a formidable enemy

HIV and influenza virus, among others, can quickly change their antigens by genetic mutation. Other viruses seem to come at us out of nowhere. Take the severe acute respiratory syndrome (SARS) caused by the SARS-associated coronavirus (SARS-CoV). This virus emerged as a human infection in Guangdong province in China in November 2002, almost certainly arising from one of the related coronaviruses found in a number of animal species. It spread rapidly to Hong Kong, and then on to Beijing, Hanoi and Singapore. Shortly afterwards it was brought into Toronto by an infected traveler. Fortunately the infection was swiftly brought under control by isolating infected individuals and tracing their contacts, and the chain of transmission was broken by July 2003. According to WHO figures, 8098 people became ill in 26 countries and 774 of these died. Hardly worth mentioning compared with the 7000 deaths per day from HIV infection, but nevertheless the brief SARS epidemic had a substantial economic effect, particularly in the Far East, and it is impossible to predict if and when there will be a future SARS outbreak.

Genetically controlled constitutional factors that render a host's cells nonpermissive (i.e. resistant to takeover of their replicative machinery by virus) play a dominant role in influencing the vulnerability of a given individual to infection. A group of proteins referred to as restriction factors provide a form of innate resistance to retroviruses via their ability to block the replication of some types of virus. Thus, the TRIM5α (*tri*partite *i*nteraction *m*otif 5α) protein targets the retroviral capsid in monkey cells and is responsible for the inability of HIV-1 to infect cells from most nonhuman primates. The APOBEC3 cytidine deaminases also act as restriction factors, in this case by hypermutating the retroviral genome.

Macrophages may readily take up viruses nonspecifically and kill them. However, in some instances, the macrophages allow replication and, if the virus is capable of producing cytopathic effects in vital organs, the infection may be lethal; with noncytopathic agents, such as lymphocytic choriomeningitis, Aleutian mink disease and equine infectious anemia viruses, a persistent infection may result. Viruses can avoid recognition by the host's immune system by latency or by sheltering in privileged sites, but they have also evolved a maliciously cunning series of evasive strategies.

Immunity can be evaded by antigenic changes

Influenza viruses change antigens by drift and shift

In the course of their constant duel with the immune system, viruses are continually changing the structure of their surface antigens. They do so by processes termed "antigenic drift" and "antigenic shift." For example, the surface of the influenza A virus contains a hemagglutinin (H), by which it adheres to cells prior to infection, and a neuraminidase (N), which releases newly formed virus from the surface sialic acid of the infected

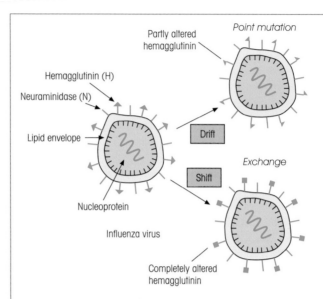

Figure 12.18. Antigenic drift and shift in influenza virus.

The changes in hemagglutinin structure caused by drift may be small enough to allow protection by immunity to earlier strains. This may not happen with radical changes in the antigen associated with antigenic shift and so new virus epidemics break out. There have been 32 documented influenza pandemics (widespread epidemics occurring throughout the population) since the first well-described pandemic of 1580. From 1900 onwards there have been four, associated with the emergence by antigenic shift of the Spanish flu in 1918 with the structure H1N1 (the official nomenclature assigns numbers to each hemagglutinin and neuraminidase major variant), Asian flu in 1957 (H2N2), Hong Kong flu in 1968 (H3N2) and "swine flu" in 2009 (another H1N1 variant); note that each new pandemic was due to a fundamental change in the hemagglutinin. The pandemic in 1918 killed an estimated 40 million people.

cell; of these, the hemagglutinin is the more important for the establishment of protective immunity. Minor changes in antigenicity of the hemagglutinin occur through point mutations in the viral genome (**drift**), but major changes (**shift**) arise through wholesale swapping of genetic material with reservoirs of different viruses in other animal hosts such as avian species (e.g. chickens, turkeys and ducks) and pigs (Figure 12.18). When alterations in the hemagglutinin are sufficient to render previous immunity ineffective, new influenza pandemics break out, as occurred in 1888, 1918, 1957 and 1968 following antigenic shifts in the influenza A virus. In 1997, the avian H5N1 virus infected humans in Hong Kong and is now in circulation across much of the globe and proving fatal in some cases. There has since been a number of other avian influenza viruses causing illness or occasionally death in humans, including H9N2 in Hong Kong in 1999 and 2003, H7N7 in The Netherlands in 2003 and H7N3 in Canada in 2004. In June 2009 the World Health Organisation declared the emergence of a worldwide pandemic due to a novel strain of H1N1 that had originated in swine. Fortunately the mortality rate associated with this virus was far lower than many had feared, although we may not be so lucky next time around.

Rhinovirus—the common cold virus

Mutated viruses can be favored by selection pressure from antibody. In fact, one current strategy for generating mutants in a given epitope is to grow the virus in tissue culture in the presence of a monoclonal antibody that reacts with that epitope; only mutants that do not bind the monoclonal will escape and grow out. This principle underlies the antigenic variation characteristic of the common cold rhinoviruses. The site on the virus for attachment to the viral receptor ICAM-1 on mucosal cells is a hydrophobic pocket lying on the floor of a canyon. Following binding, ICAM-1 catalyzes the penetration of the virus by forcing the viral capsid into an expanded open state with subsequent release of viral RNA. Antibodies produced in response to rhinovirus infection are often too large to penetrate the canyon, many of them reacting with the rim of the viral canyon. Mutations in the rim would thus enable the virus to escape from the host immune response without affecting the conserved site for binding to the target cell. However, some neutralizing monoclonal antibodies have been identified that contact a significant proportion of the canyon directly overlapping with the ICAM-1-binding site. Hydrophobic drugs have been synthesized that fit the rhinovirus canyon and cause a change in conformation that prevents binding to cells and, as host proteins have very different folds to those of the viral capsid molecule, the drugs have limited cytotoxicity. A more recent drug has been designed to slot into the substrate-binding site of the rhinovirus proteases 2A and 3C, so inhibiting their biological activity.

Mutation can produce nonfunctional T-cell epitopes

A number of infectious agents, including hepatitis B and C viruses, HIV and malaria, are capable of making mutations that prevent stimulation of cytotoxic T-cells. Such mutations modify residues that could contribute to peptides able to bind to MHC or be subsequently recognized by the TCR.

Some viruses interfere with antigen processing and/or presentation

Virtually every step in processing and presentation by MHC class I to cytotoxic T-cells can be sabotaged by one virus or another (Figure 12.19). Human cytomegalovirus (HCMV) is particularly adept at this, producing a whole gamut of proteins that interfere with antigen processing and presentation. The MHC class II pathway is not exempt from viral interference. HIV Nef affects vesicle traffic and endocytic processing involved in the generation of peptides, although the EIA protein of adenovirus interferes with IFNγ-mediated upregulation of MHC class II expression.

Viruses can interfere with immune effector mechanisms

Playing games with the host's humoral responses

Just as bacteria possess proteins capable of binding the Fc region of antibody (cf. p. 323), so certain viruses also possess such molecules. Herpes simplex virus (HSV) types 1 and 2, pseudorabies virus, varicella-zoster virus and murine cytomegalovirus all bear proteins that, by binding antibody "the wrong way round," may inhibit Fc-mediated effector functions.

As we saw for bacteria (cf. p. 318), viruses can block complement-mediated induction of the inflammatory response and thereby prevent viral killing. The vaccinia virus complement control protein (VCP) binds C3b and C4b, making both the classical and lectin $\overline{C4b2a}$ as well as the alternative $\overline{C3bBb}$ C3 convertases susceptible to factor I-mediated destruction. For its part, herpes simplex type 1 subverts the complement cascade by virtue of its surface glycoprotein C that binds C3b, interfering with its interaction with C5 and properdin.

Several viruses utilize complement receptors to gain entry into cells, especially as engagement of the complement receptor alone on a macrophage is a feeble activator of the respiratory burst. EBV infects B-cells by binding to the CR2 surface receptors, whereas flavivirus coated with iC3b enters through the CR3 receptors. Ominously, HIV coated with antibody and complement can be more virulent than unopsonized virus. Antibodies that mediate this effect are, for obvious reasons, referred to as "enhancing antibodies." Members of the regulators of complement activation (RCA) family are also used as cellular receptors for various viruses, such as CD46 (membrane cofactor protein) by measles virus and human herpes virus-6 (HHV-6), and CD55 (decay accelerating factor) by echoviruses and Coxsackieviruses.

Cell-mediated immunity can also be manipulated

Parainfluenza virus type 2 strongly inhibits Tc cell function by downregulating granzyme B expression (cf. p. 247). Viral homologs of host cytokines and their receptors act as immunosuppressants. The EBV protein BCRF1 (vIL-10) has an 84% homology to human IL-10 and helps the virus to escape the antiviral effects of IFNγ by downregulating Th1 cells. Poxviruses encode soluble homologs of both the IFNα/β receptor and the IFNγR, thereby competitively inhibiting the action of all three interferons. Human orthopoxvirus produces an IL-18 binding protein (IL-18BP) that inhibits IL-18-induced IFNγ production and NK responses. Herpesviruses and poxviruses possess several genes encoding chemokine-like and chemokine receptor-like proteins that can subvert the action of numerous chemokines. The list just goes on and on. Anti-IFN strategies are particularly abundant, with many viruses producing proteins able to block IFN-induced JAK/STAT pathway activation. A prime viral target is also the activation of the double-stranded RNA-dependent protein kinase (PKR) and other components of the cell involved in setting up an antiviral state following

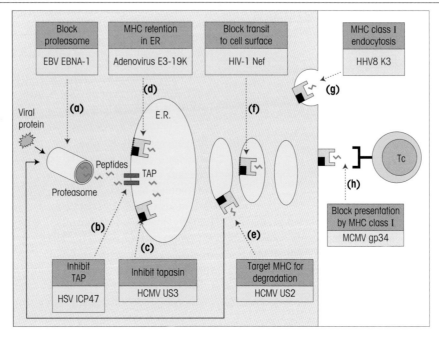

Figure 12.19. Viral interference with antigen processing and presentation by MHC class I.

Many viruses have evolved ways of avoiding detection by CD8+ cytotoxic T-cells, and here we provide just a few examples from among the many strategies that are employed. (a) The Epstein–Barr virus (EBV) nuclear antigen-1 (EBNA-1) contains glycine–alanine repeats that inhibit proteasome-mediated processing of viral proteins. (b) Peptide binding to TAP is inhibited by the infected cell protein 47 (ICP47) of herpes simplex virus (HSV). (c) Human cytomegalovirus (HCMV) produces a protein, US3, that inhibits tapasin, an essential component of the peptide-loading complex. (d) The E3-19K protein of adenovirus causes retention of MHC class I molecules in the endoplasmic reticulum (E.R.). (e) Redirection of the class I molecules to the cytosol for degradation by the proteasome is the very sneaky ploy of the HCMV US2 protein. (f) The Nef protein of HIV-1 causes retention of MHC class I molecules in the Golgi apparatus with subsequent targeting to lysosomes. (g) Even if it makes it to the cell surface, the MHC class molecule is not safe. The K3 protein of Kaposi's sarcoma-associated human herpesvirus 8 (HHV8) can remove it from the cell surface by a process involving endocytosis and ubiquitination. (h) The gp34 protein of murine CMV interferes with recognition of the peptide–MHC complex by the TCR on the CD8+ cytotoxic T-cell.

exposure to IFN. When the African swine fever virus (ASFV) infects macrophages, its A238L protein inhibits both NFκB and calcineurin-dependent cell activation pathways. The ASFV genome also encodes a homologue of the CD2 antigen (vCD2) that interferes with lymphocyte function.

Apoptosis of a cell could be considered bad news for a virus living very comfortably inside that cell. Therefore it is yet again not surprising that viruses have come up with ways of preventing apoptosis. Just a couple of examples: HHV8 produces a viral FLICE-inhibitory protein (vFLIP) that is a homolog of the prodomain of caspase 8 and thereby protects cells against apoptosis, whereas ASFV produces homologs of IAP and bcl2 in order to inhibit apoptosis. By contrast, some viral proteins including HIV-1 Vpr and HBV HBx are proapoptotic, in this case perhaps aiding dissemination of virus particles.

Protection by serum antibody

Antibodies can neutralize viruses by a variety of means. They may stereochemically inhibit combination with the receptor site on cells, thereby preventing penetration and subsequent intracellular multiplication, the protective effect of antibodies to influenza hemagglutinin providing a good example. Similarly, antibodies to the measles hemagglutinin prevent entry into the cell, and the spread of virus from cell to cell is stopped by antibodies to the fusion antigen. Antibody may destroy a free virus particle directly through activation of the classical complement pathway or produce aggregation, enhanced phagocytosis and subsequent intracellular death by the mechanisms already discussed. As far as any antibody-mediated effects are concerned, once infected the cells will need to rely upon ADCC (p. 48) as has been reported with herpes, vaccinia and mumps infection.

The most clear-cut protection by antibody is seen in diseases with long incubation times where the virus has to travel through the bloodstream before it reaches the tissue that it finally infects. For example, in poliomyelitis, the virus gains access to the body via the gastrointestinal tract and eventually passes through the circulation to reach the brain cells that become infected. Within the blood, the virus is neutralized by

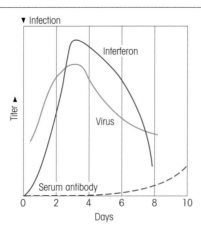

Figure 12.20. Appearance of interferon and serum antibody in relation to recovery from influenza virus infection of the lungs of mice.

(From Isaacs A. (1961) *New Scientist* **11**, 81.)

quite low levels of specific antibody, while the prolonged period before the virus infects the brain allows time for a secondary immune response in a primed host.

Local factors

With other viral diseases, such as influenza and the common cold, there is a short incubation time, related to the fact that the final target organ for the virus is the same as the portal of entry. There is little time for a primary antibody response to be mounted and in all likelihood the **rapid production of interferon** is the most significant mechanism used to counter the viral infection. Experimental studies certainly indicate that, after an early peak of interferon production, there is a rapid fall in the titer of live virus in the lungs of mice infected with influenza (Figure 12.20). Antibody, as assessed by the serum titer, seems to arrive on the scene much too late to be of value in aiding recovery. However, antibody levels may be elevated in the local fluids bathing the infected surfaces, e.g. nasal mucosa and lung, despite low serum titers, and it is the production of **antiviral antibody** (most prominently secretory IgA) by locally deployed immunologically primed cells that is of major importance for the **prevention of subsequent infection**. Unfortunately, in so far as the common cold is concerned, a subsequent infection is likely to involve an antigenically unrelated virus so that general immunity to colds is difficult to achieve.

Cell-mediated immunity gets to the intracellular virus

Antibodies are unable to access the cell cytosol. Therefore CMI is required for dealing with virus lurking inside infected host cells (Figure 12.21). The importance of CMI for recovery from viral infections is underlined by the inability of children with primary T-cell immunodeficiency to cope with such viruses,

whereas patients with Ig deficiency but intact CMI are not troubled in this way.

NK cells can kill virally infected targets

Early recognition and killing of a virally infected cell before replication occurs is of obvious benefit to the host. The importance of the NK cell in this role as an agent of preformed innate immunity can be gauged from observations on the exceedingly rare patients with complete absence of these cells who suffer recurrent life-threatening viral infections, including EBV, varicella and cytomegaloviruses (CMVs). The NK cell possesses two families of surface receptors. One, killer activating receptors, binds to carbohydrate and other structures expressed collectively by all cells; the other, killer inhibitory receptors, recognizes MHC class I molecules and overrules the signal from the activating receptor. Thus, NK cells survey tissues for the absence of self as indicated by aberrant or absent expression of MHC class I, which occurs in certain viral infections and on some tumor cells. The production of IFNα during viral infection not only protects surrounding cells but also activates NK cells.

Cytotoxic T-cells are crucial elements in immunity to viruses

T-lymphocytes from a sensitized host are directly cytotoxic to cells infected with viruses, the new MHC-associated peptide antigens on the target cell surface being recognized by specific αβ receptors on the cytotoxic T-lymphocytes (referred to as CTL or Tc). There is a quite surprising frequency of dual specificities in target cell recognition by virus-specific Tc clones, which can lyse uninfected allogeneic cells or targets expressing peptides with little homology from different regions of the same viral protein, from different proteins of the same virus, or even from different unrelated viruses. Thus activation by a second virus may help to maintain memory, and there may be a spontaneous immunity to an unrelated virus after initial infection with a cross-reacting strain. Downregulation of MHC class I poses no problems for those T-cells with a γδ T-cell receptor as these recognize native viral coat protein (e.g. herpes simplex virus glycoprotein) on the cell surface (Figure 12.21).

After a natural infection, both antibody and CTL are generated; subsequent protection is long-lived without reinfection, possibly being reinforced by bystander activation through cytokines released from other stimulated T-cells, or perhaps by random triggering with unrelated viruses based on the dual specificity described above. By contrast, injection of killed influenza produces antibodies but no Tc and protection is only short term.

Cytokines recruit effectors and provide a "cordon sanitaire"

Studies on the transfer of protection to influenza, lymphocytic choriomeningitis, vaccinia, ectromelia and CMV infections have indicated that CD8 rather than CD4 T-cells are the major

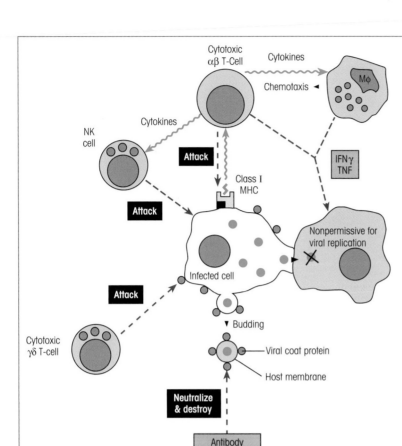

Figure 12.21. Control of infection by enveloped ("budding") viruses.

Free virus released by budding from the cell surface is neutralized by antibody. Specific cytotoxic T-cells kill virally infected targets directly and can release cytokines that attract macrophages (Mφ), prime contiguous cells to make them resistant to viral infection (IFNγ and TNF) and activate cytotoxic NK cells. NK cells can recognize a lack of MHC class I on the infected cell membrane in the case of viruses that cause a downregulation of class I expression, or partake in antibody-dependent cellular cytotoxicity (ADCC) if antibody to viral coat proteins is bound to the infected cell. Included in this group of budding viruses are: oncorna (= oncogenic RNA virus, e.g. murine leukemogenic), orthomyxo (influenza), paramyxo (mumps, measles), toga (dengue), rhabdo (rabies), arena (lymphocytic choriomeningitis), adeno, herpes (simplex, varicella zoster, cytomegalo, Epstein–Barr, Marek's disease), pox (vaccinia), papova (SV40, polyoma) and rubella viruses.

defensive force. The knee-jerk response would be to implicate cytotoxicity, but remember that CD8 cells also produce cytokines. This may well be crucial when viruses escape the cytotoxic mechanism and manage to sidle laterally into an adjacent cell. CMI can now play some new cards: if T-cells stimulated by viral antigen release cytokines such as IFNγ and macrophage or monocyte chemokines, the mononuclear phagocytes attracted to the site will be activated to secrete TNF, which will synergize with the IFNγ to render the cells nonpermissive for the replication of any virus acquired by intercellular transfer (Figure 12.21). In this way, the site of infection can be surrounded by a cordon of resistant cells. Like IFNα, IFNγ increases the nonspecific cytotoxicity of NK cells (see p. 26) for infected cells. This generation of "immune interferon" (IFNγ) and TNF in response to non-nucleic acid viral components provides a valuable back-up mechanism when dealing with viruses that are intrinsically poor stimulators of type I interferon (IFNα and IFNβ) synthesis.

Immunity to fungi

Opportunistic fungal infections often become established in immunocompromised hosts or when the normal commensal flora is upset by prolonged administration of broad-spectrum antibiotics. Phagocytosis, particularly following Th1-cell mediated activation of macrophages by IFN-γ and TNF, plays a major role in dealing with fungal infections. However, as already highlighted for certain bacteria, some fungi (e.g. *Histoplasma capsulatum*) are able to happily reside in macrophages. Reactive oxygen intermediates are fungicidal for most species by inducing protein modifications, damaging nucleic acid and causing lipid peroxidation. The fungal counterattack includes inhibition of the respiratory burst by catalase, mannitol and melanin. Following inhalation of *Aspergillus fumigatus* the alveolar macrophages phagocytose and destroy conidia (spores), although fungal proteases may help protect the spores from such activities. In the lungs the conidia can germinate into branching hyphae, which are probably dealt with by the release of oxidants and fungicidal granule contents from neutrophils.

NK cells have been shown to have constitutive antifungal activity against, for example, *Cryptococcus neoformans*, whereas such activity against this organism needs to be induced in CTL. In the case of *A. fumigatus* the adaptive immune response becomes activated following uptake of conidia and hyphae by local dendritic cells and subsequent presentation to T-cells in the draining lymph nodes. Fungal cell wall components can signal dendritic cells through a number of pattern recognition receptors (Figure 12.22), resulting in the release of IL-12, which drives a Th1 response. The role of antibody is complex and not always advantageous, although there are clear examples of protective effects such as the antibodies to *Candida albicans*

Figure 12.22. Pattern recognition receptor (PRR) mediated activation of immunity to fungi.

A number of different pathogen-associated molecular patterns present on fungal cell walls can activate both the innate and adaptive immune response through the canonical MyD88 pathway following their recognition by PRRs on the host cells. IL-1RI, interleukin-1 receptor type I; TLR, Toll-like receptor. (Modified from Romani L. (2004) *Nature Reviews Immunology* **4**, 1–23, with permission from the publishers.) *A. fumigatus*, *Aspergillus fumigatus*; *C. albicans*, *Candida albicans*.

heat-shock protein 90 (hsp90) that are protective against disseminated disease in patients with AIDS. Mannose-binding protein is able to agglutinate *Candida albicans* and subsequently activate the complement system.

The production of phospholipases, proteases and elastases by many fungi function as virulence factors. Dimorphic fungi such as *Blastomyces dermatitidis*, *Coccidioides immitis* and *Histoplasma capsulatum* transform from filamentous moulds to unicellular yeasts, although some species of *Candida*, including *Candida albicans*, can take on the form of yeasts, blastospores, pseudohyphae or hyphae depending on the site of the infection. The antigenic changes that accompany such morphological changes are presumed to act as virulence factors. Adhesins on the fungal surface also behave as virulence factors as their neutralization by antibody variable region fragments can block infection in an animal model of vaginal candidiasis.

Immunity to parasitic infections

The diverse organisms responsible for some of the major parasitic diseases are listed in Figure 12.23. The numbers affected are truly horrifying and the sum of misery these organisms engender is too large to comprehend. The consequences of parasitic infection could be, at one extreme, a lack of immune response leading to overwhelming superinfection, and, at the other, an exaggerated life-threatening immunopathological response. Like all infectious agents, a successful parasite must steer a course *between* these extremes, avoiding wholesale killing of the human host and yet at the same time escaping destruction by the immune system.

The host responses

A wide variety of defensive mechanisms are deployed by the host, but the rough generalization may be made that a humoral response develops when the organisms invade the bloodstream (malaria, trypanosomiasis), whereas parasites that grow within the tissues (e.g. cutaneous leishmaniasis) usually elicit CMI (Figure 12.24). Often, a chronically infected host will be resistant to reinfection with fresh organisms, a situation termed **concomitant immunity**. This is seen particularly in schistosomiasis but also in malaria. The resident and the infective forms must differ in some way yet to be pinpointed.

Humoral immunity

Antibodies of the right specificity present in adequate concentrations and affinity are reasonably effective in providing

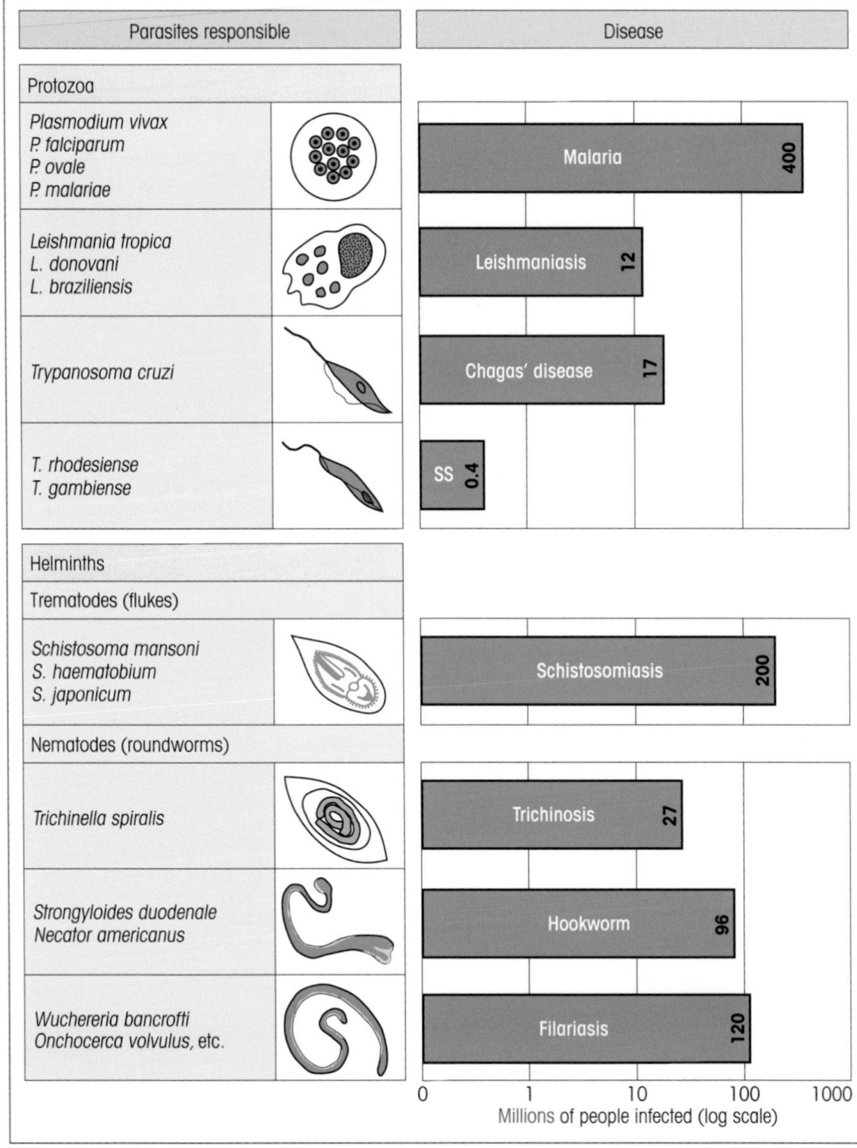

Figure 12.23. Some major parasites in humans and the sheer enormity of the numbers of people infected. SS, sleeping sickness.

(Data from World Health Organization, www.who.int)

protection against blood-borne parasites, such as *Trypanosoma brucei*, and the sporozoite and merozoite stages of malaria. Thus, individuals receiving IgG from solidly immune adults in malaria endemic areas are themselves temporarily protected against infection, the effector mechanisms being opsonization and phagocytosis, and complement-dependent lysis.

A marked feature of the immune reaction to helminthic infections, such as *Trichinella spiralis* in humans and *Nippostrongylus brasiliensis* in the rat, is the eosinophilia and the high level of IgE antibody produced. In humans, serum levels of IgE can rise from normal values of around 100 ng/ml to as high as 10 000 ng/ml. These changes have all the hallmarks of response to Th2-type cytokines (cf. p. 240) and it is notable that, in animals infected with helminths, injection of anti-IL-4 greatly reduces IgE production and anti-IL-5 suppresses the eosinophilia. IL-13 in the skin, which together with IL-4 is a switch factor for IgE production, seems to

play an important role in protection against schistosomes. Antigen-specific triggering of IgE-sensitized mast cells leads to exudation of serum proteins containing high concentrations of protective antibodies in all the major Ig classes and the release of eosinophil chemotactic factor. IgE can facilitate ADCC toward schistosomula, the early immature form of the schistosome, and this can be mediated by eosinophils, monocytes, macrophages and platelets. Schistosomula can also be killed by eosinophils using IgG for ADCC via binding through their FcγRII receptors to the IgG-coated organism (Figure 12.25); the major basic protein of the eosinophilic granules is released onto the parasite and brings about its destruction. There may also be a localized requirement for Th1 cells given that IFNγ in the liver has been shown to be important in immunity to schistosomes. Two further points are in order. The IgE-mediated reactions may be vital for recovery from infection, whereas the resistance in vaccinated

Figure 12.24. The relative importance of antibody and cell-mediated responses in protozoal infections.

Parasite	*Trypanosoma brucei*	*Plasmodium*	*Trypanosoma cruzi*	*Leishmania*
Habitat	Free in blood 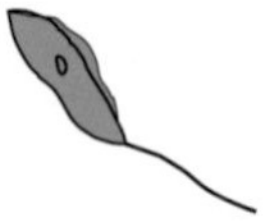	Inside erythrocyte or hepatocyte 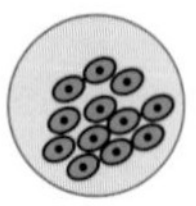	Inside macrophage 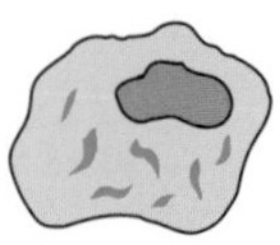	Inside macrophage 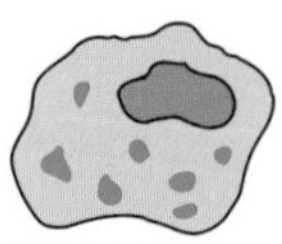
Antibody				
Importance	+ + + +	+ + +	+ +	+
Mechanism	Lysis with complement Opsonizes for phagocytosis	Blocks invasion Opsonizes for phagocytosis	Limits spread in acute infection	Limits spread
Means of evasion	Antigenic variation	Intracellular habitat Antigenic variation	Intracellular habitat	Intracellular habitat
Cell-mediated				
Importance	–	+	+ + + (Chronic phase)	+ + + +
Mechanism	–	Cytokine-mediated activation of macrophages for erythrocyte stage. CTL for liver stage	Macrophage activation by cytokines and killing by TNF, metabolites of O_2 and NO·. Role for cytotoxic T-cells	

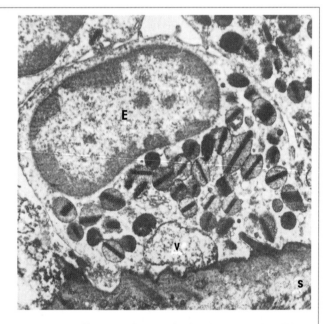

Figure 12.25. Electron micrograph showing an eosinophil (E) attached to the surface of a schistosomulum (S) in the presence of specific antibody.

The cell develops large vacuoles (V) that appear to release their contents on to the parasite (×16 500). (Courtesy of D.J. McLaren and C.D. Mackenzie.)

hosts may be more dependent upon preformed IgG and IgA antibodies.

Cell-mediated immunity

Just like certain bacteria and fungi, some parasites have adapted to life within the macrophage despite the possession by that cell of potent microbicidal mechanisms including NO·. Intracellular organisms, such as *Toxoplasma gondii*, *Trypanosoma cruzi* and *Leishmania* spp., use a variety of ploys to subvert the macrophage killing systems (see below) but again, as with for example mycobacterial infections, cytokine-producing T-cells are crucially important for the stimulation of macrophages to release their killing power and dispose of the unwanted intruders.

The balance of cytokines produced is of the utmost importance. Infection of mice with *Leishmania major* is instructive in this respect; the organism produces fatal disease in susceptible mice but other strains are resistant. This is partly controlled by alleles of the *SLC11A1* gene (cf. p. 327) but, as discussed earlier in Chapter 9, in susceptible mice there is excessive stimulation of Th2 cells producing IL-4 that do not help to eliminate the infection, whereas resistant strains are characterized by the expansion of Th1 cells that secrete IFNγ in response to antigen presented by macrophages harboring *living* protozoa. Combined therapy of susceptible strains with the leishmanicidal drug, Pentostam, plus IL-12, that recruits Th1 cells, provides promise that Th2 activities that exacerbate disease can be switched to protective Th1

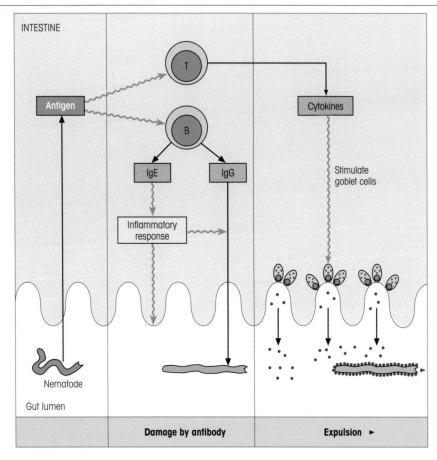

Figure 12.26. Expulsion of nematode worms from the gut.

The parasite is first damaged by IgG antibody passing into the gut lumen, perhaps as a consequence of IgE-mediated inflammation and possibly aided by accessory ADCC cells. Cytokines such as IL-4, IL-13 and TNF released by antigen-specific triggering of T-cells stimulate proliferation of goblet cells and secretion of mucus, which coat the damaged worm and facilitate its expulsion from the body by increased gut motility induced by mast cell mediators, such as leukotriene-D_4, and diarrhea resulting from inhibition of glucose-dependent sodium absorption by mast cell-derived histamine and PGE_2.

responses. Organisms such as malarial plasmodia, and incidentally rickettsiae and chlamydiae, that live in cells that are not professional phagocytes may be eliminated through activation of intracellular defense mechanisms. Of particular importance for protection, however, is the induction of IFNγ and CD8[+] T-cells. Interleukin-12 and nitric oxide are also required, and NK cells may play a subsidiary role by producing additional IFNγ. Direct cytotoxicity by CD8[+] T-cells has been observed against hepatic cells harboring malarial sporozoites. It is pertinent to note that, following the recognition of an association between HLA-B53 and protection against severe malaria, B53-restricted CTL reacting with a conserved nonamer from a liver stage-specific antigen were demonstrated in the peripheral blood of resistant individuals. A large case–control study of malaria in Gambian children showed that the protective B53 class I antigen is common in West African children but rare in other racial groups, lending further credence to the hypothesis that MHC polymorphism has evolved primarily through natural selection by infectious pathogens.

Eliminating worm infestations of the gut requires the combined forces of cellular and humoral immunity to expel the unwanted guest. One of the models studied is the response to *Nippostrongylus brasiliensis;* transfer studies in rats showed that, although antibody produces some damage to the worms, T-cells from *immune* donors are also required for vigorous expulsion, probably achieved through a combination of mast cell-mediated stimulation of intestinal motility and cytokine activation of the intestinal goblet cells. These secrete mucins that form a viscoelastic gel around the worm, so protecting the colonic and intestinal surfaces from invasion (Figure 12.26). Another model, this time of *Trichinella spiralis* infection in mice, reinforces the importance of activating the most appropriate T-cell cytokine responses. One strain, which expels adult worms rapidly, makes large amounts of IFNγ and IgG2a antibody, while, in contrast, more susceptible mice make miserly amounts of IFNγ and favor IgG1, IgA and IgE antibody classes. Clearly, the protective strategy varies with the infection.

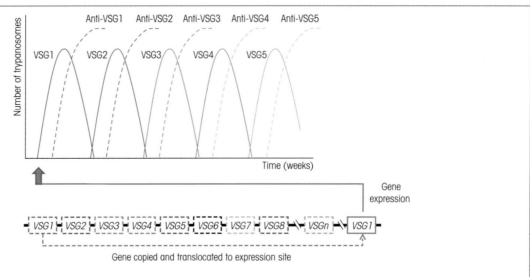

Figure 12.27. Antigenic variation during chronic trypanosome infection.

As antibody to the initial variant surface glycoprotein VSG1 is formed, the blood trypanosomes become coated prior to phagocytosis and are no longer infective, leaving a small number of viable parasites that have acquired a new antigenic constitution. This new variant (VSG2) now multiplies until it, too, is neutralized by the primary antibody response and is succeeded by variant VSG3. At any time, only one of the variant surface glycoproteins is expressed and covers the surface of the protozoan to the exclusion of all other antigens. Nearly 9% of the genome (approximately 1000 genes) is devoted to generation of VSGs. Switching occurs by insertion of a duplicate gene into a new genomic location in proximity to the promoter.

Evasive strategies by the parasite

Resistance to effector mechanisms

Some tricks to pre-empt the complement defenses are of interest. *T. cruzi* has elegantly created a DAF-like molecule (cf. p. 372) that accelerates the decay of C3b. The *Schistosoma mansoni* SCIP1 molecule (*schistosome C inhibitory protein 1*) is a surface-exposed form of the muscle protein paramyosin, which is able to bind C9 thereby inhibiting its polymerization and preventing formation of the membrane attack complex. The *Plasmodium falciparum erythrocyte membrane protein 1* (PfEMP1) is expressed on the surface of infected erythrocytes and can bind to CR1 (CD35) on other infected erythrocytes leading to rosette formation (clustering of the red cells), which may facilitate spread of the parasite with minimal exposure to the host immune system. In a similar fashion, malarial sporozoites shed their circumsporozoite antigen when it binds antibody, and *Trypanosoma brucei* releases its surface antigens into solution to act as decoy proteins (p. 318). In each case, these shedding and decoy systems are well suited to parasites or stages in the parasite life cycle that are only briefly in contact with the immune system.

Protozoal parasites that hide away from the effects of antibody by using the interior of a macrophage as a sanctuary block microbicidal mechanisms using similar methods to those deployed by intracellular bacteria (cf. p. 324). *Toxoplasma gondii* inhibits phagosome–lysosome fusion by lining up host cell mitochondria along the phagosome membrane. *Trypanosoma cruzi* escapes from the confines of the phagosome into the cytoplasm, while leishmania parasites are surrounded by a lipophosphoglycan that protects them from the oxidative burst by scavenging oxygen radicals. They also downregulate expression of MHC, CD80 and CD86 so diminishing T-cell stimulation.

Avoiding antigen recognition by the host

Some parasites **disguise** themselves to look like the host. This can be achieved by molecular mimicry as demonstrated by cross-reactivity between ascaris antigens and human collagen. Another way is to cover the surface with host protein. Schistosomes are very good at that; the adult worm takes up host red-cell glycoproteins, MHC molecules and IgG and lives happily in the mesenteric vessels of the host, despite the fact that the blood that bathes it contains antibodies that can prevent reinfection.

Another very crafty ruse, rather akin to moving the goalposts in football, is **antigenic variation**, in which the parasites escape from the cytocidal action of antibody on their cycling blood forms by the ingenious trick of altering their antigenic constitution. Figure 12.27 illustrates how the trypanosome continues to infect the host, even after fully protective antibodies appear, by switching to the expression of a new antigenic variant that these antibodies cannot recognise; as antibodies to the new antigens are synthesized, the parasite escapes again by changing to yet a further variant and so on. In this way, the parasite can remain in the bloodstream long enough to allow an opportunity for transmission by blood-sucking insects or blood-to-blood contact. The same phenomenon has been observed with *Plasmodium* spp. and this may explain why, in hyperendemic areas, children are subjected to repeated attacks of malaria for their first few years and are then solidly immune to further infection. Immunity must presumably be developed against all the antigenic variants before full protection can be attained, and indeed it is known that IgG from individuals with solid immunity can effectively terminate malaria infections in young children.

Deviation of the host immune response

Immunosuppression has been found in most of the parasite infections studied. During infection by trypanosomes, for example, there is polyclonal activation of both T- and B-cell responses that diverts the immune response away from specific antibody production. A secreted proline racemase (an enzyme that catalyses the interconversion of L- and D-forms of proline) from *T. cruzi* has been identified as a B-cell mitogen. Parasites may also manipulate T-cell subsets to their own advantage. Filariasis provides a case in point: it has been suggested that individuals with persistent microfilariae fail to mount presumably protective immediate hypersensitivity responses, including IgE and eosinophilia, as a result of active suppression of Th2 cells.

Epidemiological surveys accord with a protective role for IgE antibodies in schistosomiasis, but they also reveal a susceptible population producing IgM and IgG4 antibodies that can block ADCC dependent upon IgE. The ability of certain helminths to polyclonally activate IgE-producing B-cells is good for the parasite and correspondingly not so good for the host, as a high concentration of irrelevant IgE binding to a mast cell will crowd out the parasite-specific IgE molecules and diminish the possibility of triggering the mast cell by specific antigen to initiate a protective defensive reaction.

Transmissible spongiform encephalopathies

Variant Creutzfeldt–Jakob disease (vCJD) was first described in 1996 and, in common with sheep scrapie and bovine spongiform encephalopathy (BSE), is classed as a transmissible spongiform encephalopathy (TSE) caused by prions. The BSE prion, responsible for "mad cow disease," became adapted to humans after consumption of meat from cattle that had been fed with the remains of previously slaughtered livestock. This disease has caused much alarm, particularly at the epicenter of the infection in Great Britain, because of the unpredictable nature of the "epidemic." However, by late 2010 the number of deaths in the UK from vCJD stood at 170 and it may be that the huge number of fatalities that some mathematical models originally predicted will not actually occur.

In the TSE diseases the normal nonpathogenic cellular prion protein (PrP^c), of unknown function, becomes abnormally folded causing the generation of relatively protease-resistant pathogenic aggregates referred to as PrP^Sc (the "scrapie" protein). Unfortunately, the role of the immune system in prion diseases seems to be one of helping the disease rather than combating it. Infectivity usually replicates to high levels in lymphoid tissues before spreading to the central nervous system, with follicular dendritic cells (FDCs) in spleen, lymph node and Peyer's patches involved in this replication. This may be because FDCs naturally express high levels of PrP^c that then converts to PrP^Sc following exposure to the TSE agent. B-lymphocytes play a subsidiary role via their production of TNF and lymphotoxin, both cytokines being necessary for the formation of FDC networks in the secondary lymphoid tissues, the lymphotoxin being further required for the maintenance of the differentiated state in the FDCs. In addition to FDCs, macrophages and dendritic cells appear to be involved in the replication of PrP^Sc, thereby providing a reservoir of infectivity. Once they enter the CNS the infectious prions cause activation and proliferation of the microglial cells; the macrophages of the brain. Despite the fact that T-cells are seen to infiltrate the CNS, the available evidence from various knock-out mice suggest that once the prion pathology reaches the CNS further disease progression is independent of T- and B-cells, interferon, TNF, lymphotoxin, FcγRs, TLRs and complement.

Immunopathology

Where parasites persist chronically in the face of an immune response, the interaction with foreign antigen frequently produces tissue-damaging reactions. One example is the immune complex-induced nephrotic syndrome of Nigerian children associated with the quartan malaria that is caused by *Plasmodium malariae* and characteristically has a 72 hour chill and fever pattern related to the life cycle of the parasite. Increased levels of TNF are responsible for pulmonary changes in acute malaria, cerebral malaria in mice and severe wasting of cattle with trypanosomiasis. Another example is the liver damage resulting from IL-4-mediated granuloma formation around schistosome eggs (cf. Figure 15.28); one of the egg antigens directly induces IL-10 production in B-cells, thereby contributing to Th2 dominance. Remarkably, the hypersensitivity reaction helps the eggs to escape from the intestinal blood capillaries into the gut lumen to continue the cycle outside the body, an effect mediated by TNF.

Cross-reaction between parasite and self may give rise to autoimmunity, and this has been proposed as the basis for the cardiomyopathy in Chagas' disease. It is also pertinent that the nonspecific immunosuppression that is so widespread in parasitic diseases tends to increase susceptibility to bacterial and viral infections and, in this context, the association between Burkitt's lymphoma and malaria has been ascribed to an inadequate host response to the Epstein–Barr virus.

Immunity to infection involves a constant battle between the host defenses and the pathogen trying to evolve evasive strategies.

Inflammation revisited

- Inflammation is a major defensive reaction initiated by infection or tissue injury.
- The mediators released upregulate adhesion molecules on endothelial cells and leukocytes causing, first, rolling of leukocytes along the vessel wall and then passage across the blood vessel up the chemotactic gradient to the site of inflammation.
- IL-1, TNF and chemokines such as IL-8 are involved in maintaining the inflammatory process.
- Inflammation is controlled by complement regulatory proteins, PGE_2, TGFβ, glucocorticoids and IL-10.
- Inability to eliminate the initiating agent leads to a chronic inflammatory response dominated by macrophages often forming granulomas.

Extracellular bacteria susceptible to killing by phagocytosis and complement

- LPS is bound by LBP, which transfers the LPS to the CD14–TLR4 complex, thereby activating genes in the APC which encode proinflammatory cytokines.
- Bacteria try to avoid phagocytosis by surrounding themselves with capsules, secreting exotoxins that kill phagocytes or impede inflammatory reactions, deviating complement to inoffensive sites or by colonizing relatively inaccessible locations.
- Antibody combats these tricks by neutralizing the toxins, facilitating complement-mediated lesions on the bacterial surface, and overcoming the antiphagocytic nature of the capsules by opsonizing them with Ig and C3b.
- The secretory immune system protects the external mucosal surfaces. Secretory IgA inhibits adherence of bacteria and can opsonize them. IgE bound to mast cells can initiate the influx of protective IgG, complement and neutrophils.

Bacteria that grow in an intracellular habitat

- Intracellular bacteria such as tubercle and leprosy bacilli grow within macrophages. They defy killing mechanisms by blocking macrophage activation, neutralizing the pH in the phagosome, inhibiting lysosome fusion, and by escaping from the phagosome into the cytoplasm.
- They are killed by CMI: T-helpers release cytokines on contact with infected macrophages that powerfully activate the formation of nitric oxide (NO·), reactive oxygen intermediates (ROIs) and other microbicidal mechanisms.

Immunity to viral infection

- Viruses try to avoid the immune system by changes in the antigenicity of their surface antigens. Point mutations bring about antigenic drift, but radical changes leading to epidemics can result from wholesale swapping of genetic material with different viruses in other animal hosts (antigenic shift).
- Some viruses subvert the function of the complement system to their own advantage.
- Viruses can interfere with almost every step in the processing and presentation of antigen to T-cells.
- Antibody neutralizes free virus and is particularly effective when the virus has to travel through the bloodstream before reaching its final target.
- Where the target is the same as the portal of entry, e.g. the lungs, IFN is dominant in recovery from infection.
- Antibody is important in preventing reinfection.
- "Budding" viruses that can invade adjacent cells without becoming exposed to antibody are combated by CMI. Infected cells express a processed viral antigen peptide on their surface in association with MHC class I a short time after entry of the virus, and rapid killing of the cell by cytotoxic αβ T-cells prevents viral multiplication that depends upon the replicative machinery of the intact host cell. γδ Tc recognize native viral coat protein on the target cell surface. NK cells are also cytotoxic.
- T-cells and macrophages producing IFNγ and TNF bathe the adjacent cells and prevent them from becoming infected by lateral spread of virus.

Immunity to fungi

- Opportunistic fungal infections are common in immunosuppressed hosts.
- Phagocytosis plays a major role in dealing with fungi.
- CTL and NK cells exhibit anti-fungal activities.
- Antibody is not always advantageous, but does appear to help protect against systemic candida infections in patients with AIDS.

Immunity to parasitic infections

- Diseases involving *protozoal parasites* and *helminths* affect hundreds of millions of people. Antibodies are usually effective against the blood-borne forms. IgE production is increased in worm infestations and can lead to mast cell-mediated influx of Ig and eosinophils; schistosomes coated with IgG or IgE are killed by adherent eosinophils through extracellular mechanisms involving the release of cationic proteins and peroxidase.
- Organisms such as *Leishmania* spp., *Trypanosoma cruzi* and *Toxoplasma gondii* hide from antibodies inside macrophages, use the same strategies as intracellular parasitic bacteria to survive, and like

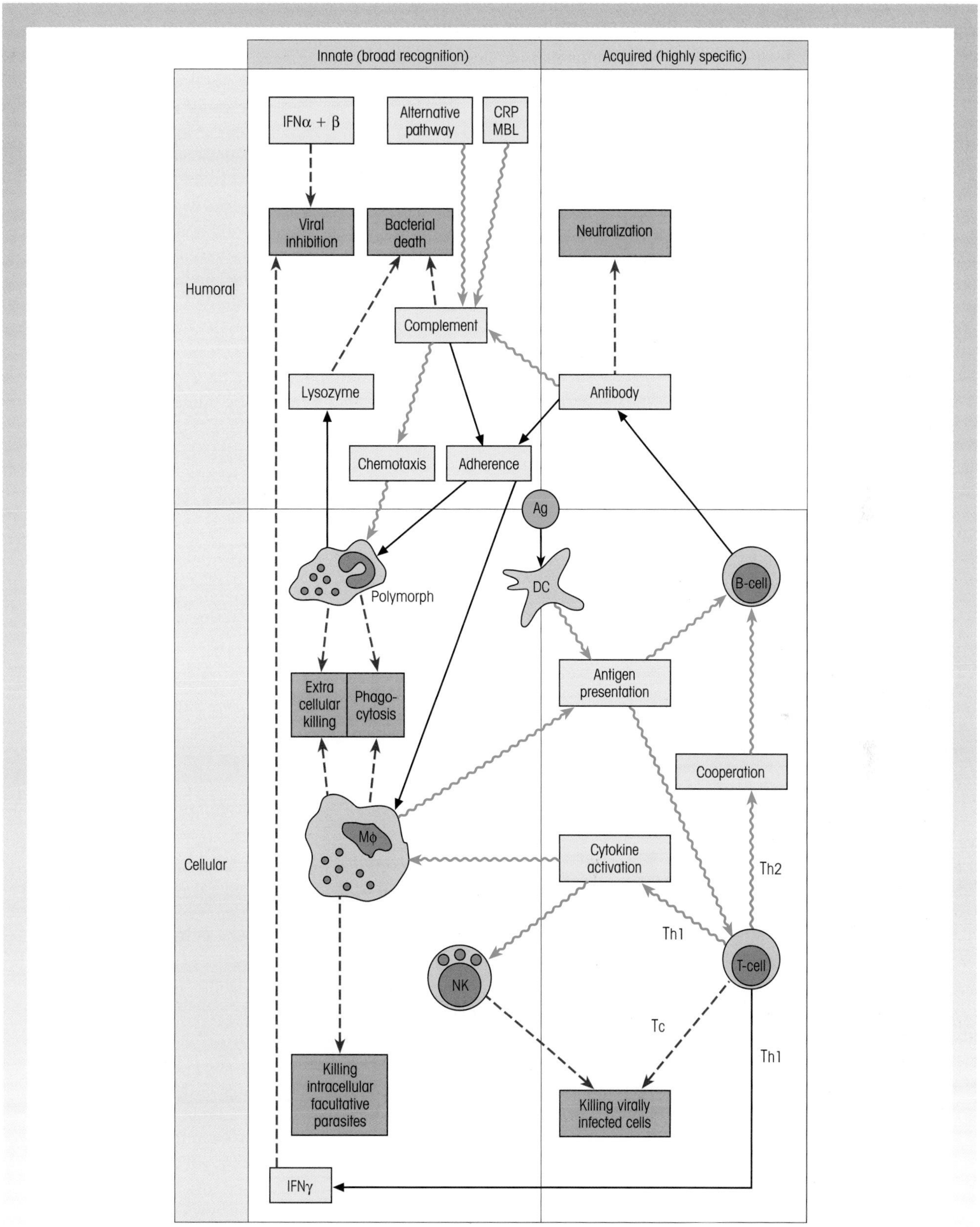

Figure 12.28. Simplified scheme to emphasize the interactions between innate and acquired immunity.

The dendritic cell that presents antigen to B-cells in the form of immune complexes is the follicular dendritic cell in germinal centers, whereas the MHC class II-positive interdigitating dendritic cell presents antigen to T-cells. CRP, C-reactive protein; MBL, mannose-binding lectin. (Developed from Playfair J.H.L. (1974) *British Medical Bulletin* **30**, 24.)

- them are killed when the macrophages are activated by Th1 cytokines produced during cell-mediated immune responses. NO· is an important killing agent.
- CD8 T-cells also have a protective role.
- Expulsion of intestinal worms usually depends on Th2 responses and requires the coordinated action of antibody, the release of mucin by cytokine-stimulated goblet cells and the production of intestinal contraction and diarrhea by mast cell mediators.
- Some parasites avoid recognition by disguising themselves as the host, either through molecular mimicry or by absorbing host proteins to their surface.
- Other organisms such as *Trypanosoma brucei* and various malarial species have the extraordinary ability to express on their surface a dominant antigen that is changed by genetic switch mechanisms to a different molecule as antibody is formed to the first variant.
- Most parasites also tend to nonspecifically suppress host responses.

- Chronic persistence of parasite antigen in the face of an immune response often produces tissue-damaging immunopathological reactions such as immune complex nephrotic syndrome, liver granulomas and autoimmune lesions of the heart. Generalized immunosuppression increases susceptibility to bacterial and viral infections.
- As the features of the response to infection are analysed, we see more clearly how the specific acquired response operates to amplify and enhance innate immune mechanisms; the interactions are summarized in Figure 12.28.

Prion diseases
- Scrapie, BSE and vCJD are transmissible spongiform encephalopathies caused by prions.
- Abnormally folded, protease-resistant forms of host prion protein (PrP) develop.
- FDCs in lymphoid tissues become infected prior to spread of the infectious agent to the CNS.

FURTHER READING

Alcami A., Hill A.B. & Koszinoski U.H. (2006) Viral interference with the host immune response. In *Topley & Wilson's Microbiology & Microbial Infections* 10th edn., pp. 617–644. Wiley-Blackwell, Oxford.

Berg D.E. & Kalia A. (2011) Pathogen evolution in adaptive landscapes. *Annual Review of Microbiology* **65**.

Black R.E., Cousens S., Johnson H.L. *et al.* (2010) Global, regional, and national causes of child mortality in 2008: a systematic analysis. *The Lancet* **375**, 1969–1987.

Blue C.E., Spiller O.B. & Blackbourn D.J. (2004) The relevance of complement to virus biology. *Virology* **319**, 176–184.

Flannagan R.S., Cosío G. & Grinstein S. (2009) Antimicrobial mechanisms of phagocytes and bacterial evasion strategies. *Nature Reviews Microbiology* **7**, 355–366.

Goering R. *et al.* (2007) Medical Microbiology, 4th edn. Mosby, London.

Hansen T.H. & Bouvier M. (2009) MHC class I antigen presentation: learning from viral evasion strategies. *Nature Reviews Immunology* **9**, 503–513.

Lambris J.D., Ricklin D. & Geisbrecht B.V. (2008) Complement evasion by human pathogens. *Nature Reviews Microbiology* **6**, 132–142.

Lewis D.B. (2006) Avian flu to human influenza. *Annual Review of Medicine* **57**, 139–154.

Lloyd-Smith J.O. *et al.* (2009) Epidemic dynamics at the human-animal interface. *Science* **326**, 1362–1367.

Papayannopoulos V. & Zychlinsky A. (2009) NETs: a new strategy for using old weapons. *Trends in Immunology* **30**, 513–521.

Romani L. (2004) Immunity to fungal infections. *Nature Reviews Immunology* **4**, 1–23.

Schmid-Hempel P. (2009) Immune defence, parasite evasion strategies and their relevance for 'macroscopic phenomena' such as virulence. *Philosophical Transactions of the Royal Society B* **364**, 85–98.

Templeton T.J. (2009) The varieties of gene amplification, diversification and hypervariability in the human malaria parasite, *Plasmodium falciparum*. *Molecular & Biochemical Parasitology* **166**, 109–116.

The following websites of the Centers for Disease Control and Prevention contain a large body of information: http://www.cdc.gov/DiseasesConditions/, Parasitic diseases: http://www.cdc.gov/parasites/

Now visit **www.roitt.com** to test yourself on this chapter.

CHAPTER 13
Vaccines

Key Topics

Just to Recap ...

The mechanisms by which we resist the onslaught of microbes have been discussed. These mechanisms include humoral, cellular and innate immunity. One of the great triumphs of medicine has been the ability to harness these mechanisms through vaccination to protect against a host of infectious diseases.

Introduction

The control of infection is approached from several directions. Improvements in public health—water supply, sewage systems, education in personal hygiene—prevent the spread of cholera and many other diseases. Antibiotics have had a major impact on bacterial diseases. Another strategy is to give the immune response a helping hand. This can be achieved by administering individual components of the immune response, such as defensins or antibodies, by using immunopotentiating agents such as cytokines, or more commonly by exposing the immune system to an antigen in order to stimulate the acquired immune response to generate memory—a procedure referred to as vaccination (see Milestone 13.1). Vaccines have traditionally been aimed at generating responses against infectious agents, but increasingly they are also being explored in areas such as malignancy.

Roitt's Essential Immunology, Twelfth Edition. Peter J. Delves, Seamus J. Martin, Dennis R. Burton, Ivan M. Roitt.
© 2011 Peter J. Delves, Seamus J. Martin, Dennis R. Burton, Ivan M. Roitt. Published 2011 by Blackwell Publishing Ltd.

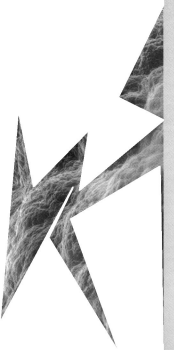

◉ Milestone 13.1—Vaccination

The notion that survivors of serious infectious disease seldom contract that infection again has been embedded in folklore for centuries. In an account of the terrible plague that afflicted Athens, Thucydides noted that, in the main, those nursing the sick were individuals who had already been infected and yet recovered from the plague. Deliberate attempts to ward off infections by inducing a minor form of the disease in otherwise healthy subjects were common in China in the Middle Ages. There, they developed the practice of inhaling a powder made from **smallpox** scabs as protection against any future infection. The Indians inoculated the scab material into small skin wounds, and this practice of **variolation** (Latin *varus*, a pustular facial disease) was introduced into Turkey where the inhabitants were determined to prevent the ravages of smallpox epidemics interfering with the lucrative sale of their gorgeous daughters to the harems of the wealthy.

The writer Voltaire, in 1773, tells us that the credit for spreading the practice of variolation to western Europe should be attributed to Lady Wortley Montague, a remarkably enterprising woman who was the wife of the English Ambassador to Constantinople in the time of George I. With little scruple, she inoculated her daughter with smallpox in the face of the protestations of her chaplain who felt that it could only succeed with infidels, not Christians. All went well however and the practice was taken up in England despite the hazardous nature of the procedure that had a case fatality of 0.5–2%. These dreadful risks were taken because, at that time, as Voltaire recorded "…three score persons in every hundred have the smallpox. Of these three score, twenty die of it in the most favorable season of life, and as many more wear the disagreeable remains of it on their faces so long as they live."

Edward Jenner (1749–1823) (Figure M13.1.1), a country physician in Gloucestershire, suggested to one of his patients that she might have smallpox, but she assured him that his diagnosis was impossible as she had already contracted cowpox through her chores as a milkmaid (folklore again!). This led Jenner to the series of experiments in which he showed that prior inoculation with cowpox, which was nonvirulent (i.e. nonpathogenic) in the human, protected against subsequent challenge with smallpox (cf. p. 351). His ideas initially met with violent opposition but were eventually accepted and he achieved world fame; learned societies

everywhere elected him to membership, although it is intriguing to note that the College of Physicians in London required him to pass an examination in classics and the Royal Society honored him with a Fellowship on the basis of his work on the nesting behavior of the cuckoo. In the end he inoculated thousands of people in the shed in the garden of his house in Berkeley, Gloucestershire, which now functions as a museum and venue for small symposia (rather fun to visit if you get the chance).

The next seminal development in vaccines came through the research of Louis Pasteur who had developed the germ theory of disease. A culture of chicken cholera bacillus, which had accidently been left on a bench during the warm summer months, lost much of its ability to cause disease; nonetheless, birds that had been inoculated with this old culture were resistant to fresh virulent cultures of the bacillus. This **attenuation** of **virulent** organisms was reproduced by Pasteur for anthrax and rabies using abnormal culture and passage conditions. Recognizing the relevance of Jenner's research for his own experiments, Pasteur called his treatment **vaccination**, a term that has stood the test of time.

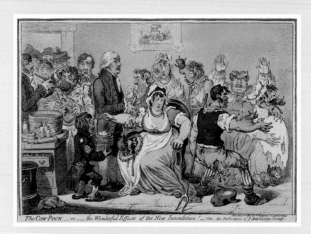

Figure M13.1.1. Edward Jenner among patients in the Smallpox and Inoculation Hospital at St Pancras, London.

Etching after J. Gillray, 1802. (Kindly supplied by the Wellcome Centre Medical Photographic Library, London.)

Passively acquired immunity

Passively administered antibody

Temporary protection against infection and clearance of toxins can be achieved by giving antibody isolated from the plasma of an individual having a high antibody titer to the pathogen or a hyperimmunized animal (Table 13.1 and Figure 13.1). Prior to the introduction of antibiotics, horse serum containing anti-tetanus or anti-diphtheria toxins was extensively employed prophylactically, but nowadays it is used less commonly because of the complication of serum sickness (a type III hypersensitivity)

and immediate (type I) hypersensitivity developing in response to the foreign protein. Furthermore, as the acquired antibodies are utilized by combination with antigen or are catabolized in the normal way, this protection is lost. The use of passive immunization is currently largely restricted to anti-venoms, in which an immediate therapeutic effect is required for a usually rare event such as a snake bite, and in prophylaxis for certain viral infections including cytomegalovirus (CMV) and rabies. However, with the emergence of antibiotic-resistant strains of bacteria, and concerns about possible bioterrorism, there is a renewed interest in passive immunization against infectious

Table 13.1. Examples of passive therapy against infection and toxins.

Condition	Source of antibody	Use
Tetanus infection	Human polyclonal	Antitoxin. Management of tetanus-prone wounds in patients where immunization is incomplete or uncertain
Botulism	Horse polyclonal	Antitoxin. Post-exposure prophylaxis of botulism
Snake bites (various)	Horse polyclonal	Antivenom. Treatment following venomous snake bite
Spider bites (various)	Horse polyclonal, rabbit polyclonal	Antivenom. Treatment following venomous spider bite
Paralysis tick bite	Dog polyclonal	Antivenom. Treatment following bite from paralysis tick
Stonefish sting	Horse polyclonal	Antivenom. Treatment following stonefish sting
Jellyfish sting	Sheep polyclonal	Antivenom. Treatment following venomous jellyfish sting
Hepatitis B infection	Human polyclonal	Antiviral. Prevention of infection in laboratory and other personnel accidentally inoculated with hepatitis B virus, and in infants of mothers infected during pregnancy or who are high-risk carriers
Rabies infection	Human polyclonal/monoclonal	Antiviral. Following bite from a possibly infected animal
Varicella-zoster virus infection	Human polyclonal	Antiviral. Seronegative individuals at increased risk of severe varicella (chickenpox)
Cytomegalovirus infection	Human polyclonal	Antiviral. Prophylaxis in immunosuppressed patients
Respiratory syncytial virus infection	Humanized mouse IgG1 monoclonal	Antiviral. Prevention of serious lower respiratory tract disease in high-risk children and infants

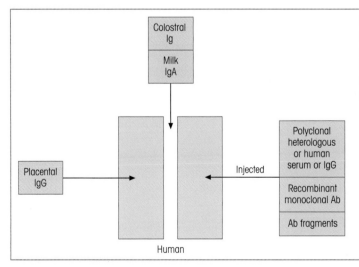

Figure 13.1. Passive immunization produced by: transplacental passage of IgG from mother to fetus, acquisition of IgA from mother's colostrum and milk by the infant, and injection of polyclonal antibodies, recombinant monoclonal antibodies, or antibody (Ab) fragments (Fab or scFv).

agents. Increasingly, it is likely that polyclonal antibody preparations will be replaced by human monoclonal antibodies or combinations of such antibodies. For instance, a humanized mouse monoclonal antibody (Synagis®, MedImmune) is in use to prevent disease due to respiratory syncytial virus (RSV) in babies and young infants. A cocktail of two human monoclonal antibodies against rabies virus is being developed for use as a post-exposure prophylactic following a bite or a scratch from a rabid animal such as a dog or a bat. In this case, there is a window of opportunity for intervention as the rabies virus needs to gain access to the CNS to cause disease and circulating antibody can prevent this. Passive antibody in rabies treatment is augmented with vaccination.

Maternally acquired antibody

In the first few months of life, while the baby's own lymphoid system is slowly getting under way, protection is afforded to the fetus by maternally derived IgG antibodies acquired by placental transfer and to the neonate by intestinal absorption of colostral immunoglobulins (Figure 13.1). The major immunoglobulin in milk is secretory IgA (SIgA) and this is not absorbed by the baby but remains in the intestine to protect the mucosal surfaces. In this respect it is quite striking that the SIgA antibodies are directed against bacterial and viral antigens often present in the intestine, and it is presumed that IgA-producing cells, responding to gut antigens, migrate and colonize breast tissue (as part of the mucosal immune system; see pp. 324–5), where the antibodies they produce appear in the milk. The case for mucosal vaccination of future mothers against selected infections is strong. It should also be noted that it has been argued that one of the most important functions of antibody is in the maternally acquired role. The hypothesis is that maternal antibody attenuates many infections allowing cellular immunity to mature under controlled conditions.

Intravenous immunoglobulin (IVIg)

Intravenous immunoglobulin (IVIg) is a preparation of IgG obtained by large-scale fractionation of plasma pooled from thousands of healthy blood donors. The preparations are given to individuals with immunodeficiencies associated with reduced or absent circulating antibody. IVIg is also of value in the treatment of a number of infection-associated conditions such as streptococcal toxic shock syndrome. IVIg also has efficacy in the treatment of several autoimmune and inflammatory diseases such as idiopathic thrombocytopenic purpura, chronic inflammatory demyelinating polyneuropathy and Guillain–Barré syndrome. The mechanism of action in these non-immunodeficient patients remains unclear, although recent evidence suggests IVIg probably modulates immune activity through sialic acids on the Ig molecule.

Adoptive transfer of cytotoxic T-cells

This is a labor-intensive operation and will be restricted to autologous cells or instances in which the donor shares an

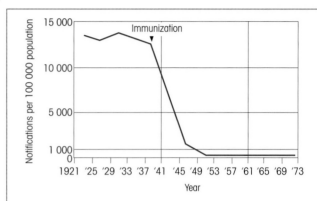

Figure 13.2. Notification of diphtheria in England and Wales per 100 000 population showing dramatic fall after immunization.

(Reproduced from Dick G. (1978) *Immunisation*. Update Books; with kind permission of the author and publishers.)

MHC class I allele. Adoptive transfer of autologous cytotoxic T-lymphocytes has been shown to be effective in enhancing EBV-specific immune responses and in reducing the viral load in patients with post-transplant lymphoproliferative disease.

Principles of vaccination

Herd immunity

In the case of tetanus, active immunization is of benefit to the individual but not to the community as it will not eliminate the organism that is found in the feces of domestic animals and persists in the soil as highly resistant spores. Where a disease depends on human transmission, immunity in just a proportion of the population can help the whole community if it leads to a fall in the reproduction rate (i.e. the number of further cases produced by each infected individual) to less than one; under these circumstances the disease will die out: witness, for example, the disappearance of diphtheria from communities in which around 75% of the children have been immunized (Figure 13.2). But this figure must be maintained; there is no room for complacency. In contrast, focal outbreaks of measles have occurred in communities that object to immunization on religious grounds, raising an important point for parents in general. Each individual must compare any perceived disadvantage associated with vaccination in relation to the increased risk of disease in their unprotected child.

How vaccines work

Vaccines are effective because of adaptive immunity and immune memory. Antibody memory exists in two compartments. First as pre-existing antibody in the blood and tissues ready to attack the pathogen without cellular triggering—this is probably the most powerful first line of defense against exposure to many pathogens. This antibody can be maintained at relatively high levels for many years, probably produced by long-lived plasma cells in the bone marrow, although this is not universally accepted. In a sense, the most crucial part of antibody "memory" might be equated with the long life of these plasma cells. However, the second form of the antibody memory component, memory B-cells, might also be crucial for vaccine-mediated protection in some cases. In this case, contact with pathogen stimulates B-cells to proliferate and differentiate to produce copious amounts of antibody. Equally, the contact of memory B-cells with pathogen might be important to boost plasma-cell numbers and serum-antibody concentrations for the next encounter with the pathogen. T-cell memory also exists in two compartments. Effector memory T-cells are found in peripheral tissues where they can respond immediately to pathogen-infected cell contact with effector activities. Central memory T-cells are found mainly in lymph nodes where they can respond to pathogen contact with expansion and differentiation to effectors. T-cell memory consists of both CD8$^+$ and CD4$^+$ T-cell responses. Clearly T cells responses are most pertinent to virus, parasite and intracellular bacterial infections.

The best correlate of protection for many current vaccines is antibody and it is likely that, in these cases, antibody is the most important mechanism of vaccine-induced resistance to disease. This is consistent with the notion that T-cells are the largest contribution to viral immunity during primary infection and antibodies during secondary infection (Figure 13.3). However, it is important to note that the mechanisms of vaccine protection may vary widely between different pathogens, different individuals, different doses of pathogen to which the individual is exposed and different routes of exposure.

In addition to an ability to engender effective immunity, a number of mundane but nonetheless crucial conditions must be satisfied for a vaccine to be considered successful (Table 13.2). The antigens must be readily available, and the preparation should be stable, cheap and certainly, safe, bearing in mind that the recipients are most often healthy children. Clearly, the first contact with antigen during vaccination should not be injurious and the maneuver is to avoid the pathogenic effects of infection, while maintaining protective immunogens.

The primary approaches to the generation of existing vaccines are shown in Figure 13.4. and these are now considered in turn.

Killed organisms as vaccines

The simplest way to destroy the ability of microbes to cause disease, yet maintain their antigenic constitution, is to prevent their replication by killing in an appropriate manner. Parasitic worms and, to a lesser extent, protozoa are extremely difficult to grow up in bulk to manufacture killed vaccines. This problem does not arise for many bacteria and viruses and, in these cases, the inactivated microorganisms have provided a number of safe antigens for immunization. Examples are influenza, cholera and inactivated poliomyelitis (Salk) vaccines (Figure 13.5). Care has to be taken to ensure that important protective antigens are not destroyed in the inactivation process.

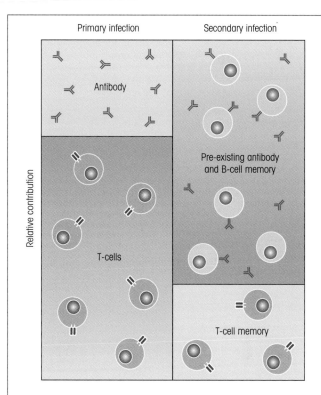

Figure 13.3. A schematic view of the relative contributions of humoral and cellular immunity during primary or secondary viral infection.

During primary viral infection, antiviral T-cell responses are critical for reducing viral replication in addition to contributing to the development of an effective antibody response. Primary T-cell-dependent antibody responses are mounted during the course of infection and take time to undergo immunoglobulin class-switching and somatic hypermutation to possibly provide assistance to virus specific T-cells in resolving the infection. Following recovery from primary infection (or vaccination), persisting virus-specific antibody represents the first line of defense against secondary infection. If secondary infection does occur, then circulating antibodies and presumably memory B-cells that proliferate and differentiate into antibody secreting cells will reduce virus dissemination and allow time for the development of an antiviral T-cell response. Memory B-cells are highly efficient at presenting specific antigen and therefore may also be involved with more rapid and efficient presentation to T-cells as well. Pre-existing T-cell memory will also play a role in protection against secondary infection. However, even if T-cell memory has declined or is lost, the long-term maintenance of antiviral antibody responses will suppress virus replication until a new virus-specific T-cell response is mounted from the naive repertoire. (Adapted from Amanna I.J. & Slifka M.K. (2009) *Antiviral Research* **84**, 119–130.)

Table 13.2. Factors required for a successful vaccine.

Factor	Requirements

Effectiveness	Must evoke protective levels of immunity:
	   at the appropriate site
	   of relevant nature (Ab, Tc, Th1, Th2)
	   of adequate duration

Availability	Readily cultured in bulk or accessible source of subunit
Stability	Stable under extreme climatic conditions, preferably not requiring refrigeration
Cheapness	What is cheap in the West may be expensive in developing countries but the Bill and Melinda Gates Foundation and governments help
Safety	Eliminate any pathogenicity

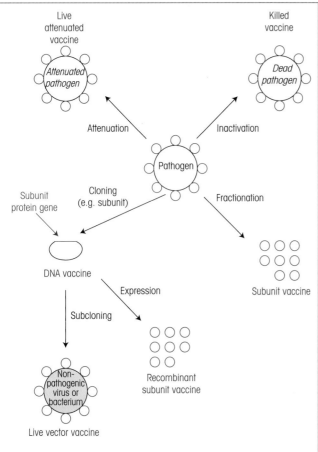

Figure 13.4. Classical vaccine approaches.

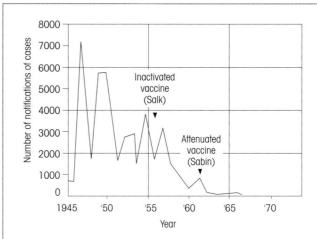

Figure 13.5. Notifications of paralytic poliomyelitis in England and Wales showing the beneficial effects of community immunization with killed and live vaccines.

(Reproduced from Dick G. (1978) *Immunisation*. Update Books; with kind permission of the author and publishers.)

Live attenuated organisms have many advantages as vaccines

The objective of attenuation is to produce a modified organism that mimics the natural behavior of the original microbe without causing significant disease. In many instances the immunity conferred by killed vaccines, even when given with adjuvant (see below), is often inferior to that resulting from infection with live organisms. This must be partly because the replication of the living microbes confronts the host with a **larger and more sustained dose of antigen** and that, with budding viruses, infected cells are required for the establishment of good **cytotoxic T-cell memory**. Another significant advantage of using live organisms is that the immune **response takes place largely at the site of the natural infection**. This is well illustrated by the nasopharyngeal IgA response to immunization with polio vaccine. In contrast with the ineffectiveness of parenteral injection of killed vaccine, intranasal administration evoked a good local antibody response; however, whereas this declined over a period of 2 months or so, per oral immunization with *live attenuated* virus established a persistently high IgA antibody level (Figure 13.6).

There is in fact a strong upsurge of interest in strategies for mucosal immunization. Remember, the mucosal immune system involves mucous membranes covering the aerodigestive

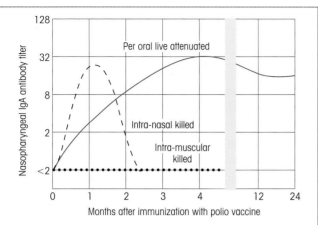

Figure 13.6. Local IgA response to polio vaccine.

Local secretory antibody synthesis is confined to the specific anatomical sites that have been directly stimulated by contact with antigen. (Data from Ogra P.L. *et al.* (1975). In Notkins A.L. (ed.) *Viral Immunology and Immunopathology*. Academic Press, New York, p. 67.)

and urogenital tracts as well as the conjunctiva, the ear and the ducts of all exocrine glands whose protection includes SIgA antibodies. Resident T-cells in these tissues produce large amounts of transforming growth factor-β (TGFβ), and the interleukins IL-10 and IL-4, which promote the B-cell switch to IgA, and note also that human intestinal epithelial cells themselves are major sources of TGFβ and IL-10.

Classical methods of attenuation

The objective of attenuation, that of producing an organism that causes only a very mild form of the natural disease, can be equally well attained if one can identify heterologous strains that are virulent for another species, but avirulent in humans. The best example of this was Jenner's seminal demonstration that cowpox would protect against smallpox. Subsequently, a truly remarkable global effort by the World Health Organization (WHO), combining extensive vaccination and selective epidemiological control methods, **completely eradicated smallpox as a human disease**—a wonderful achievement. Thus, although 300 million people are estimated to have died of smallpox in the twentieth century, no-one has died of the virus since 1978. Emboldened by this success, the WHO embarked upon a program to eradicate polio using attenuated polio vaccine to block transmission of the virus and, despite setbacks such as a temporary halt in vaccination in northern Nigeria following unfounded rumours regarding the safety of the vaccine, it is hoped that this goal will be achieved in the not too distant future. One can even follow the progress of this campaign on http://www.polioeradication.org.

Attenuation itself was originally achieved by empirical modification of the conditions under which an organism grows. Pasteur first achieved the production of live but non-

virulent forms of chicken cholera bacillus and anthrax (cf. Milestone 13.1) by such artifices as culture at higher temperatures and under anerobic conditions, and was able to confer immunity by infection with the attenuated organisms. A virulent strain of *Mycobacterium tuberculosis* became attenuated by chance in 1908 when Calmette and Guérin at the Institut Pasteur, Lille, France added bile to the culture medium in an attempt to achieve dispersed growth. After 13 years of culture in bile-containing medium, the strain remained attenuated and was used successfully to vaccinate children against tuberculosis. The same organism, bCG (bacille Calmette–Guérin), is widely used today in many countries for the immunization of infants and of tuberculin-negative children and adolescents. However, its efficacy varies widely from, for example, protection in 80% of vaccinated individuals in the UK, to a total lack of efficacy in Southern India. This variability is not fully understood, but is thought to be due to a number of factors including local differences in the antigenic composition of the vaccine and in the environmental mycobacterial strains, and differences in MHC alleles and other genetic factors in the various human populations. Attenuation by cold adaptation has been applied to influenza and other respiratory viruses; the organism can grow at the lower temperatures (32–34°C) of the upper respiratory tract, but fails to produce clinical disease because of its inability to replicate in the lower respiratory tract (37°C). An intranasal vaccine containing cold-adapted attenuated influenza virus strains was licensed for use in the USA in 2003.

Attenuation by recombinant DNA technology

It must be said that many of the classical methods of attenuation are somewhat empirical and the outcome is difficult to control or predict. With knowledge of the genetic makeup of these microorganisms, we can apply the molecular biologist's delicate scalpel to deliberately target the alterations that are needed for successful attenuation. Thus genetic recombination is being used to develop various attenuated strains of viruses, such as influenza, with not only a lower virulence for humans but also an increased multiplication rate in eggs (enabling newly endemic strains of influenza to be adapted for rapid vaccine production). Not surprisingly, strains of HIV-1, with vicious deletions of the regulatory genes, are being investigated as protective vaccines. The potential is clearly quite enormous.

The **tropism** of attenuated organisms for **the site** at which **natural infection** occurs is likely to be exploited dramatically in the near future to establish gut immunity to typhoid and cholera using attenuated forms of *Salmonella typhi* and *Vibrio cholerae* in which the virulence genes have been identified and modified by genetic engineering.

Microbial vectors as vaccines

An ingenious trick is to use a nonpathogenic virus as a Trojan horse for genes encoding proteins of a pathogen. Incorporation of such "foreign" genes into attenuated recombinant viral vectors, such as fowlpox and canarypox virus and the modified vaccinia Ankara (MVA) strain virus that infect mammalian hosts, but are unable to replicate effectively, provides a powerful vaccination strategy with many benefits. The genes may be derived from organisms that are difficult to grow or inherently dangerous, and the constructs themselves are replication deficient, non-integrating, stable and relatively easy to prepare. The proteins encoded by these genes are appropriately expressed *in vivo* with respect to glycosylation and secretion, and are processed for MHC presentation by the infected cells, thus effectively endowing the host with both humoral and cell-mediated immunity.

A wide variety of genes have been expressed in vaccinia virus vectors, and it has been demonstrated that the products of genes coding for viral envelope proteins, such as influenza virus hemagglutinin, vesicular stomatitis virus glycoprotein, HIV-1 gp120 and herpes simplex virus glycoprotein D, could be correctly processed. Hepatitis B surface antigen (HBsAg) was secreted from recombinant vaccinia virus-infected cells as the characteristic 22 nm particles (Figure 13.7). It is an impressive approach and chimpanzees have been protected against the clinical effects of hepatitis B virus, while mice that were inoculated with recombinant influenza hemagglutinin generated cytotoxic T-cells and were protected against influenza infection.

Attention has also been paid to bCG as a vehicle for antigens required to evoke CD4-mediated T-cell immunity. The

organism is avirulent, has a low frequency of serious complications, can be administered any time after birth, has strong adjuvant properties and gives long-lasting cell-mediated immunity after a single injection.

The ability of *Salmonella* to elicit **mucosal responses by oral immunization** has been exploited in the design of vectors that allow the expression of any protein antigen linked to *E. coli* enterotoxin, a powerful mucosal immunostimulant. There is an attractive possibility that the oral route of vaccination may be applicable not only for the establishment of gut mucosal immunity but also for providing systemic protection. For example, *Salmonella typhimurium* not only invades the mucosal lining of the gut, but also infects cells of the mononuclear phagocyte system throughout the body, thereby stimulating the production of humoral and secretory antibodies as well as CD4$^+$ and CD8$^+$ T cell-mediated immunity. As attenuated *Salmonella* can be made to express proteins from *Shigella*, cholera, malaria sporozoites and so on, it is entirely feasible to consider these as potential oral vaccines. *Salmonella* may also carry "foreign genes" within separate DNA plasmids and, after phagocytosis by antigen-presenting cells, the plasmids can be released from the phagosome into the cytosol if the plasmid bears a recombinant listeriolysin gene or the bacterium is a mutant whose cell walls disintegrate within the phagosome; the plasmid then moves to the nucleus where it is transcribed to produce the desired antigen. Quite strikingly, these attenuated organisms are very effective when inhaled and can elicit substantive mucosal and systemic immune responses comparable with those obtained by the parenteral route.

Constraints on the use of attenuated vaccines

Attenuated vaccines for poliomyelitis (Sabin), measles, mumps, rubella, varicella-zoster and yellow fever have gained general acceptance. However, with live viral vaccines there is a possibility that the nucleic acid might be incorporated into the host's genome or that there may be reversion to a virulent form. Reversion is less likely if the attenuated strains contain several mutations. Another disadvantage of attenuated strains is the difficulty and expense of maintaining appropriate cold-storage facilities, especially in out-of-the-way places. In diseases such as viral hepatitis, AIDS and cancer, the dangers associated with live vaccines are daunting. With most vaccines there is a very small, but still real, risk of developing complications and it cannot be emphasized too often that this **risk must be balanced against the expected chance of contracting the disease with its own complications**. Where this is minimal, some may prefer to avoid general vaccination and to rely upon a crash course backed up if necessary by passive immunization in the localities around isolated outbreaks of infectious disease.

It is important to recognize those children with immunodeficiency before injection of live organisms; a child with impaired T-cell reactivity can become overwhelmed by BCG and die. It is also inadvisable to give live vaccines to patients being treated with steroids, immunosuppressive drugs or

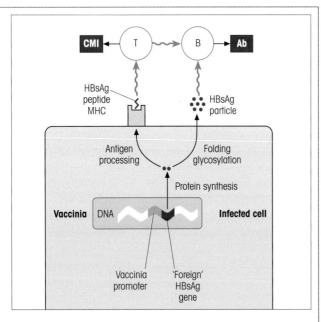

Figure 13.7. Hepatitis B surface antigen (HBsAg) vaccine using an attenuated vaccinia virus carrier.

The HBsAg protein is synthesized by the machinery of the host cell: some is secreted to form the HBsAg 22 nm particle that stimulates antibody (Ab) production, and some follows the antigen processing pathway to stimulate cell-mediated immunity (CMI) and T-helper activity.

radiotherapy or who have malignant conditions such as lymphoma and leukemia; pregnant mothers must also be included here because of the vulnerability of the fetus.

Use in a veterinary context

For veterinary use, of course, there is a little less concern about minor side-effects and excellent results have been obtained using existing vaccinia strains with rinderpest in cattle and rabies in foxes, for example. In the latter case, a recombinant vaccinia virus vaccine expressing the rabies surface glycoprotein was distributed with bait from the air and immunized approximately 80% of the foxes in that area. No cases of rabies were subsequently seen, but epidemiological considerations indicate that, with the higher fox density that this leads to, the higher the percentage that have to be made immune; thus, either one has to increase the efficacy of the vaccine, or culling of the animals must continue—an interesting consequence of interference with ecosystems. Less complicated is the use of such immunization to control local outbreaks of rabies in rare mammalian species, such as the African wild dog, which are threatened with extinction by the virus in certain game reserves.

Subunit vaccines

A whole pathogen usually contains many antigens that are not concerned in the protective response of the host but may give rise to problems by suppressing the response to protective antigens or by provoking hypersensitivity, as we saw in the last chapter. Vaccination with the isolated protective antigens may avoid these complications, and identification of these antigens then opens up the possibility of producing them synthetically in circumstances in which bulk growth of the organism is impractical or isolation of the individual components too expensive.

The use of purified components as bacterial vaccines

Bacterial exotoxins such as those produced by diphtheria and tetanus bacilli have long been used as immunogens. First, they must of course be detoxified and this may be achieved by formaldehyde treatment when this does not destroy the major immunogenic determinants (Figure 13.8). Immunization with the **toxoid** will, therefore, provoke the formation of protective antibodies, which neutralize the toxin by stereochemically blocking the active site, and encourage removal by phagocytic cells. The toxoid is generally given after adsorption to aluminum hydroxide, which acts as an adjuvant and produces higher antibody titers. In addition to their use as vaccines to generate a protective antibody response against tetanus and diphtheria, the toxoids are often conjugated to other proteins, peptides or polysaccharides to provide helper T-cell epitopes for these antigens. Nontoxic variants of the toxins themselves, such as the CRM197 variant of diphtheria toxin, can also be used to provide helper T-cell epitopes for antigens such as the *Haemophilus influenzae* type b (Hib) polysaccharide.

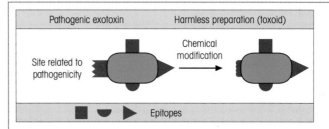

Figure 13.8. Modification of toxin to harmless toxoid without losing many of the antigenic determinants.

Thus, antibodies to the toxoid will react well with the original toxin.

The emphasis now is to move towards gene cloning of individual proteins once they have been identified immunologically and biochemically. In general, a protein subunit used in a vaccine should contain a sufficient number of T-cell epitopes to avoid HLA-related unresponsiveness within the immunized population. In order to maintain a pool of memory B-cells over a reasonable period of time, persistence of antigen on the follicular dendritic cells (DCs) in a form resistant to proteolytic degradation with retention of the native three-dimensional configuration is needed.

A viral subunit vaccine: hepatitis B virus (HBV)

In 1965, Baruch Blumberg first described an antigen in the blood of Australian aborigines associated with hepatitis. This "Australia antigen" was subsequently shown to be a particle formed from the surface antigen of hepatitis B virus. Initially antigen particles were isolated from the plasma of HBV carriers and inactivated and used as a vaccine. Later, the particles were prepared in yeast. The HBV subunit vaccine was a milestone in vaccinology as it was the first manufactured using recombinant DNA technology. One very interesting facet of this vaccine is that it was originally used for small at-risk groups exposed to blood products such as doctors and nurses. Later, it became very widely used including in the developing world. As HBV is associated with hepatic cancer and more than 300 million people are infected worldwide, the HBV vaccine represents the first to prevent cancer on a large scale.

Carbohydrate vaccines

The dense surface distribution of characteristic glycan structures on diverse pathogens and on malignant cells makes carbohydrates attractive antibody-based vaccine targets (Figure 13.9). However, the nature of glycans presents some severe problems in terms of the induction of protective antibodies. First, glycans tend to be poorly immunogenic. They should be coupled to a carrier protein to provide a source of CD4+ T-cell help. Second, anti-glycan antibodies typically have low affinities relative to anti-protein antibodies. They rely heavily on avidity effects to achieve binding at physiological concentrations. Third,

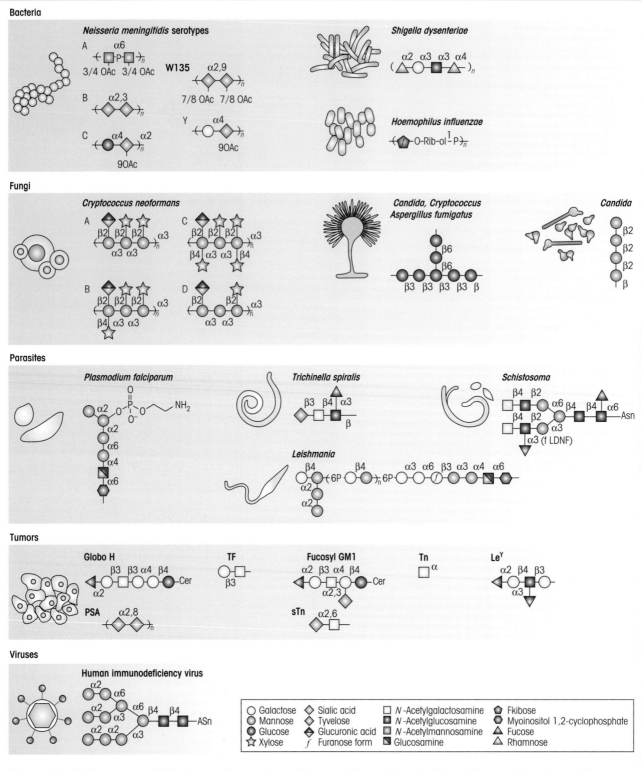

Figure 13.9. A diverse array of disease-causing agents and glycan antigens is targeted by existing and developmental carbohydrate vaccines.

Bacteria: capsular polysaccharide repeats associated with particular species (and serotypes). Fungi: common glucuronoxylomannan (GXM) motifs for serotypes A–D (*Cryptococcus*); β-glucan (*Candida*, *Cryptococcus* and *Aspergillus*); β-mannan (*Candida*). Parasites: synthetic glycosylphosphatidylinositol motif (*Plasmodium falciparum*); common tyvelose-containing antigen (*Trichinella*); LacdiNAc (LDN) and fucosylated LDN (LDNF) (*Schistosoma*); common lipophosphoglycan (*Leishmania*). Tumors: common glycan antigens associated with glycolipids (globohexaosylceramide (Globo H), fucosyl GM1, Lewis Y (Le^Y)) and glycoproteins (Thomsen–Friedenreich (TF), Le^Y, 2–6-α-*N*-acetylgalactosamine (Tn), sialyl Tn and polysialic acid (PSA)) found on various malignant tissues. Viruses: high mannose GlcNAc$_2$Man$_9$ (HIV). Mannose residues may be 6-*O*-acetylated on GXM motifs. (From Astronomo R.D. & Burton D.R. (2010) *Nature Reviews Drug Discovery* **9**, 308–324).

glycans are typically heterogeneous on target pathogens or cells and therefore the efficacy of any specific anti-glycan response is diluted. Nevertheless, glycoconjugates are increasingly being designed (Figure 13.10) as vaccine candidates. Licensed carbohydrate vaccines include those against *Haemophilus influenzae* type b (Hib), *Neisseria meningitidis*, *Salmonella typhi* and *Streptococcus pneumoniae*.

DNA vaccines

Teams working with J. Wolff and P. Felgner experimented with a new strategy for gene therapy that involved binding the negatively charged DNA to cationic lipids, which would themselves attach to the negatively charged surface of living cells and then presumably gain entry. The surprise was that controls injected with DNA without the lipids actually showed an *even higher uptake of DNA* and expression of the protein it encoded, so giving rise to the whole new technology of **DNA vaccination or genetic immunization**. As Wolff put it: "We tried it again and it worked. By the fourth or fifth time we knew we were onto something big. Even now I get a chill down my spine when I see it working." It was quickly appreciated that the injected DNA functions as a source of immunogen *in situ* and can induce strong immune responses, particularly cellular immune responses. The DNA used in this procedure is sometimes referred to as **naked DNA** to reflect the fact that the nucleic acid is stripped bare of its associated proteins.

The transcription unit composed of the cDNA gene with a poly A terminator is stitched in place in a DNA plasmid with a promoter such as that from cytomegalovirus and a CpG bacterial sequence as an adjuvant. It is usually injected into muscle where it can give prolonged expression of protein. The pivotal cell is the dendritic antigen-presenting cell that may be transfected directly, could endocytose soluble antigen secreted by the muscle cells into the interstitial spaces of the muscle, and could take up cells that have been killed or injured by the vaccine. The CpG immunostimulatory sequences engage Toll-like receptor 9 (TLR9) and thereby provoke the synthesis of IFNα and β, IL-12 and IL-18, which promote the formation of T helper (Th)1 cells; this in turn generates good cell-mediated immunity, helps the B-cell synthesis of certain antibody classes (e.g. IgG2a in the mouse) and induces good cytotoxic T-cell responses, presumably reflecting the cytosolic expression of the protein and its processing in the MHC class I pathway. Let's look at an example. It will be recalled that frequent point mutations (drift; p. 331) in the gene encoding influenza surface hemagglutinin give rise to substantial antigenic variation, whereas the major internal proteins, which elicit T-cell-mediated immunity responses, have been relatively conserved. On this line of reasoning, nucleoprotein DNA should give broad protection against other influenza strains and indeed it does (Figure 13.11). A combination of DNAs encoding the hemagglutinin (included only for statutory reasons) and nucleoprotein genes gave nonhuman primates and ferrets good protection against infection, and protected ferrets against challenge with an antigenically distinct epidemic human virus strain more effectively than the contemporary clinically licensed vaccine. Vaccination can also be achieved by coating the plasmids onto minute gold particles or cationic poly (lactide co-glycolide) (PLG) microparticles and shooting them into skin epidermal cells by the high-pressure "biolistic" helium gun, a technique that uses between 10- and 100-fold less plasmid DNA than the muscle injection.

To date, straightforward DNA vaccination has not been as successful in humans or nonhuman primates as in mice. Nevertheless the many potential advantages of the approach, including its simplicity and ease of quality control for example, mean that many efforts on improving DNA vaccination in humans are being explored. One is a "prime–boost" protocol. The persistent but low level of expression of the protein antigen by DNA vaccines establishes a pool of relatively high affinity memory B-cells that can readily be revealed by boosting with protein antigen (Figure 13.12). This has given rise to a prime–boost strategy in which these memory cells are expanded by boosting with a non-replicating viral vector, such as fowlpox virus or Ankara strain-modified vaccinia virus, bearing a gene encoding the antigen. Mice immunized in this fashion with influenza virus hemagglutinin produced satisfyingly high levels of IgG2a antibody and were protected against challenge with live virus. Remarkably, up to 30% of circulating CD8 T-cells were specific for the immunizing epitope as shown by MHC class I tetramer binding (cf. p. 176). A similar strategy with *Plasmodium berghei* produced high levels of peptide-specific CD8 T cells secreting IFNγ which protected against challenge by sporozoites. An ongoing HIV vaccine trial uses a DNA prime followed by an adenoviral boost, with both prime and boost encoding a number of HIV proteins.

Newer approaches to vaccine development

Conventional vaccines, which have been enormously successful against a range of pathogens, can be described as following a "simple mimicry" strategy going back to the work of Jenner and Pasteur. The essential strategy is to use attenuated or killed pathogens, with the occasional use of purified or recombinant subunits. These vaccines mostly target pathogens that have very little antigenic diversity and appear to be largely dependent on antibody-based protection. The conventional approach has tended to find much less success for a range of other pathogens, notably those showing considerable antigenic diversity or for which T-cell immunity may be of greater protective import (Figure 13.13). For example consider HIV. A live attenuated vaccine protects monkeys against challenge with the same strain of SIV (simian immunodeficiency virus, the monkey equivalent of HIV) but is far less effective against other strains of SIV. For a human vaccine against HIV to be effective clearly it should protect against the majority of circulating global viral strains. Killed and subunit vaccines against HIV/SIV tend to be ineffective because of the enormous variability and instability of the

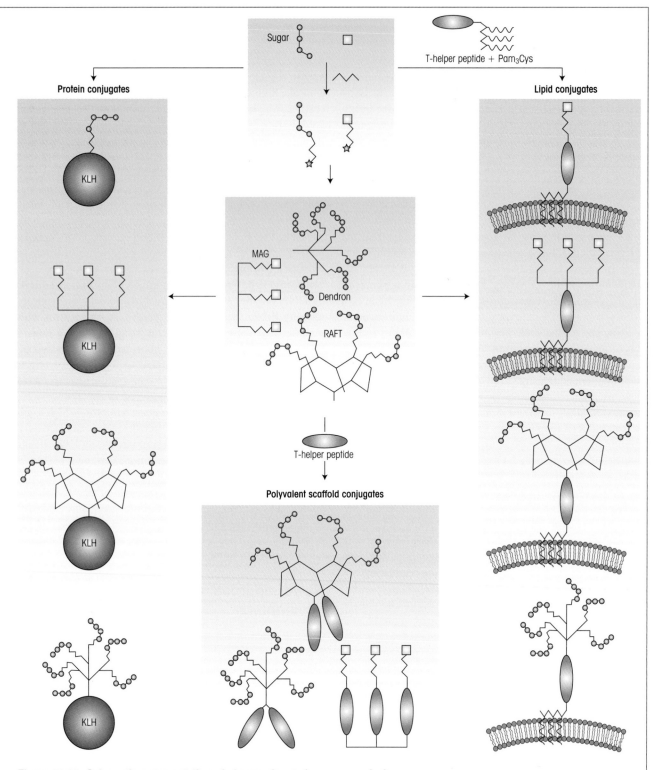

Figure 13.10. Schematic representation of glycoconjugate immunogen design.

Starting from activated glycans (star denotes activated group) from natural or synthetic sources, the production of three categories of glycoconjugate immunogens is shown: protein conjugates, lipid conjugates and polyvalent scaffold conjugates. The requirement for both polyvalent display and helper T-cell epitopes, crucial for achieving strong, long-lasting and class-switched antibody responses, are satisfied in each category. For protein conjugates, activated glycans are covalently attached to immunogenic protein carriers—for example, keyhole limpet hemocyanin (KLH)—which provide helper T-cell epitopes and enable polyvalent display. Lipid conjugates, made by covalent linkage of activated glycans to helper T-cell peptides attached to lipid moieties, allow polyvalency through formulation into lipid membranes. In addition, activated glycans may first be conjugated to synthetic polyvalent scaffolds—for example, dendron, multiple antigen glycopeptide (mAG) and regioselectively addressable functionalized template (RAFT)—which may then be used to make protein and lipid conjugates. Alternatively, polyvalent scaffold conjugates may be made through addition of helper T-cell peptides alone. Adjuvants (see later) are usually included in the final glycoconjugate vaccine formulations (for example, alum or QS-21). Note that tripalmitoyl-*S*-glyceryl-cysteinylserine (Pam$_3$Cys) has adjuvant properties. (From Astronomo R.D. & Burton D.R. (2010) *Nature Reviews Drug Discovery* **9**, 308–324.)

surface envelope proteins (see also chapter 14). Another highly problematical disease for vaccine development is tuberculosis; immunity to this intracellular pathogen is likely to involve T-cell rather than antibody-based protective activities.

In recent years, vaccine development has increasingly turned to the tools of modern molecular biology. For bacterial vaccines, the rise of genomics has been crucial. At least one complete sequence is now available for all of the major human pathogens. This has facilitated the development of "reverse vaccinology," championed by Rino Rappuoli and colleagues. The essential strategy identifies the complete repertoire of bacterial surface antigens, investigates the ability of antigens to elicit immunity in animal models and then designs a combination of antigens to be used in the vaccine. This elegant approach is illustrated in Figure 13.14 for the successful development of a vaccine to serogroup B *Neisseria meningitidis* (MenB), which is the most common cause of meningococcal disease in the developed world and had defined conventional vaccine approaches for decades.

Highly variable viruses such as HIV and hepatitis C virus (HCV) also provide severe vaccine development problems. Here one of the approaches being adopted can be described as reverse engineering or structural vaccinology. Thus broadly neutralizing antibodies capable of acting against a wide spectrum of global isolates as required by a vaccine have been described in natural infection and are being studied in terms of their interaction with surface envelope proteins. The notion is that the molecular information gained can be used to modify envelope proteins or to design novel immunogens that can be used as vaccines to elicit broadly neutralizing antibodies. This same concept might provide a universal influenza vaccine that would protect against most or all subtypes and stains of flu and obviate the need for annual immunizations. Immunodominance is one of the great problems in developing vaccines to highly variable pathogens i.e. the pathogen has evolved so that the strongest immune responses tend to be elicited to the most variable regions of the pathogen. A host of strategies are now being explored to try and focus B-cell and T-cell responses on to the most conserved epitopes.

Current vaccines

The established vaccines in current use and the schedules for their administration are set out in Tables 13.3 and 13.4. Regional differences in immunization schedules reflect not only different degrees of perceived risk of infection but also other local considerations. Children under 2 years of age make inadequate responses to the T-independent *H. influenzae* capsular polysaccharide, so they are now routinely immunized with the antigen conjugated with tetanus toxoid or the

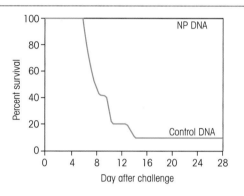

Figure 13.11. Protection from cross-strain influenza challenge after vaccination with nucleoprotein DNA.

Mice were immunized three times at 3-week intervals with 200 mg of nucleoprotein (NP) or vector (control) DNA and lethally challenged with a heterologous influenza strain 3 weeks after the last immunization. Survival of mice given NP DNA was significantly higher than in mice receiving vector ($p = 0.0005$). (Data kindly provided by Dr Margaret A. Liu and colleagues (1993) *DNA and Cell Biology* **12**, 777–783, and reproduced by permission of Mary Ann Liebert Inc.)

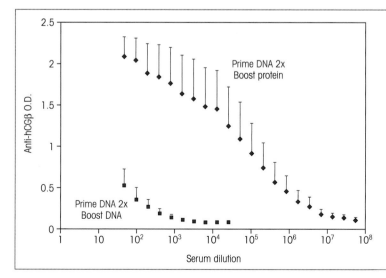

Figure 13.12. Induction of memory cells by DNA vaccine and boost of antibody production with the protein immunogen, human chorionic gonadotropin β-chain (hCG β).

Groups of five (C57BL/6 × BALB/c)F1 mice each received 50 mg of the hCG β DNA plasmid at weeks 0 and 2; one group received a further injection of the plasmid, while the other was boosted with 5 mg of the hCG β protein antigen in RIBI (cf. p. 365) adjuvant. Dilutions of serum were tested for antibodies to hCG β by indirect ELISA. Mean titers + SE are shown. (Data from Laylor R. *et al.* (1999) *Clinical and Experimental Immunology* **117**, 106.)

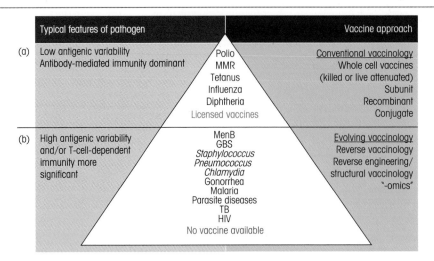

Typical features of pathogen		Vaccine approach
(a) Low antigenic variability Antibody-mediated immunity dominant	Polio MMR Tetanus Influenza Diphtheria Licensed vaccines	Conventional vaccinology Whole cell vaccines (killed or live attenuated) Subunit Recombinant Conjugate
(b) High antigenic variability and/or T-cell-dependent immunity more significant	MenB GBS Staphylococcus Pneumococcus Chlamydia Gonorrhea Malaria Parasite diseases TB HIV No vaccine available	Evolving vaccinology Reverse vaccinology Reverse engineering/ structural vaccinology "-omics"

Figure 13.13. Schematic view of conventional vaccinology and evolving vaccinology in the post-genome era.

(a) Most licensed vaccines target pathogens that have low antigenic variability and pathogens for which protection depends on antibody-mediated immunity. These vaccines have typically been developed using conventional vaccinology. (b) Several pathogens are shown for which no vaccine is available, due to either their high antigenic variability and/or the need to induce T-cell-dependent immunity to elicit protection. New approaches are being applied to vaccine development for these pathogens in the post-genome era. Vaccines/diseases shown in the figure are selected examples of each category and are not a complete list. TB, *Mycobacterium tuberculosis*; MMR, mumps, measles, rubella; MenB, meningitis B; GBS, group B *Streptococcus*. (Figure with permission from Rinuado C.D., Telford J.L., Rappuoli R. & Seib K.L. (2009) *Journal of Clinical Investigation* **9**, 2515–2525 and modified.)

Table 13.3. Current licensed vaccines for use in USA and/or Europe.

Vaccine	Antigenic component	Use
Bacterial infections (+ viral in some combinations)		
Anthrax	Alum adsorbed protective antigen (PA) from *Bacillus anthracis*	Individuals who handle infected animals or animal products. Laboratory staff working with *B. anthracis*
BCG	Bacillus Calmette-Guérin live attenuated strain of *Mycobacterium bovis*	Children and adolescents in geographical regions where the vaccine has been shown to be effective, including UK. Not routinely used in the USA
Cholera	Inactivated Vibrio cholerae together with recombinant B-subunit of the cholera toxin	Drinkable oral vaccine for travelers to endemic or epidemic areas
Diphtheria, tetanus, pertussis, poliomyelitis, hepatitis B	Alum-adsorbed diphtheria toxoid, tetanus toxoid, acellular pertussis, inactivated poliomyelitis virus and recombinant hepatitis B virus surface antigen	Routine immunization of children
Diphtheria, tetanus, pertussis, poliomyelitis, *Haemophilus influenzae* type b	Another pentavalent combination vaccine, including *Haemophilus influenzae* type b capsular polysaccharides conjugated to tetanus toxoid or to the CRM197 nontoxic variant of diphtheria toxin	Routine immunization of children

Table 13.3. (*Continued*)

Vaccine	Antigenic component	Use
Meningococcal group C	Four serotypes of meningococcus polysaccharide conjugated to diphtheria toxoid	Routine immunization of children in UK. As nearly all cases of childhood meningococcal disease in the UK are caused by groups B and C, the vaccine used for routine immunization contains only group C. A vaccine against meningococcal groups A, C, W-135 and Y is also available
Pneumococcal	Polysaccharide from either each of the 23 or from each of seven capsular types of pneumococcus, conjugated to diphtheria toxoid and adsorbed onto alum	Routine immunization of children (USA). Individuals at risk of pneumococcal infection, e.g. elderly, persons who have undergone splenectomy or with various chronic diseases (UK)
Typhoid fever	Vi polysaccharide antigen of *Salmonella typhi*	Travelers to countries with poor sanitation, laboratory workers handling specimens from suspected cases
Viral infections		
Hepatitis A	Alum-adsorbed inactivated hepatitis A virus	At risk individuals, e.g. laboratory staff working with the virus, patients with hemophilia, travelers to high-risk areas
Hepatitis B	Alum-adsorbed recombinant hepatitis B virussurface antigen (HBsAg)	Routine immunization of children (USA). Individuals at high risk of contracting hepatitis B (UK)
Influenza (inactivated)	Inactivated trivalent WHO recommended strains of influenza virus	Routine immunization of infants (USA). Individuals at high risk of complications from contracting influenza virus (UK)
Influenza (live attenuated)	Attenuated trivalent WHO recommended strains of influenza virus	Individuals aged 5–49 at high risk of complications from contracting influenza virus
Japanese encephalitis virus	Inactivated Japanese encephalitis virus	Individuals at risk of contracting Japanese encephalitis virus
Measles, Mumps and Rubella (MMR)	Live attenuated measles, mumps and rubella viruses	Routine immunization of children
Papillomavirus	Virus-like particles	Prophylaxis against human papillomavirus (HPV) infections including prevention of cervical cancer
Polio (Inactivated, Salk)	Inactivated poliovirus types 1, 2 & 3	Routine immunization of children. Protects against polio paralysis but does not prevent spread of wild polio virus (for which the oral polio vaccine [Sabin] containing live attenuated types 1, 2 & 3 virus is used)
Rabies	Inactivated rabies virus	At risk individuals
Rotavirus	Live attenuated virus	Oral, to prevent rotavirus-associated diarrhea and dehydration in infants
Tick-borne encephalitis	Inactivated tick-borne encephalitis virus	At risk individuals, e.g. working, walking or camping in infected areas
Varicella–zoster	Live attenuated varicella–zoster virus	Seronegative healthy children over 1 year old who come into close contact with individuals at high risk of severe varicella infections. Seronegative healthcare workers who come into direct contact with patients. A concentrated attenuated virus vaccine is used to prevent shingles in the elderly
Yellow fever	Live attenuated yellow fever virus	Those traveling or living in areas where infection is endemic, and laboratory staff who handle the virus or clinical samples from suspected cases

Vaccines separately containing the individual components of the polyvalent vaccines are also licensed.

Figure 13.14. MenB vaccine development.

Preclinical development was based on a reverse vaccinology approach, in which the genome sequence of the virulent meningitis B (MenB) strain MC58 was used to identify open reading frames (ORFs) predicted to encode proteins that were surface exposed (i.e. secreted [S] or located in the outer membrane [OM]), which were then expressed in *E. coli*, purified, and used to immunize mice. Antibodies generated in mice were then used to confirm surface exposure of the vaccine candidate by FACS and to identify proteins that induced bactericidal activity. This screening process resulted in identification of several novel vaccine candidates, including GNA 1870 (which is fHBP), GNA 1994 (which is NadA), GNA2132, GNA 1030, and GNA2091. The formulation for the comprehensive MenB vaccine consists of four components: fHBPGNA2091 and GNA2132–GNA1030 fusion proteins, NadA, and OMV from the New Zealand MeNZB vaccine strain. Clinical development using this formulation has shown in phase I and II trials that the vaccine is well tolerated and immunogenic. The vaccine induced bactericidal activity using human complement (hSBA) with titers greater than 1:4, which indicates the generation of antibodies able to kill the bacteria at a level that correlates with protection against the bacteria, in more than 90% of infants after the fourth dose. This vaccine entered phase III clinical trials in 2008. P, periplasm; IM, inner membrane; C, cytoplasm. (Figure with permission from Rinuado C.D., Telford J.L., Rappuoli R. & Seib K.L. (2009) *Journal of Clinical Investigation* **9**, 2515–2525.)

MenB vaccine development

Preclinical reverse vaccinology

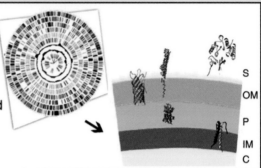

1998

2158 ORFs identified in the MenB MC58 genome

570 ORFs predicted to encode surface-expressed or secreted proteins

S
OM
P
IM
C

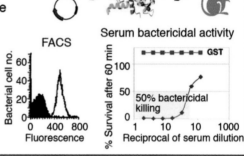

350 proteins expressed in *E. coli*, purified and used to immunize mice

91 novel surface-exposed proteins identified

28 novel proteins induced bactericidal antibodies

FACS

Serum bactericidal activity

GST

50% bactericidal killing

5 proteins selected for use in a four-component vaccine formulation

fHBP-GNA2091   GNA2132-GNA1030   NadA   OMV

Clinical

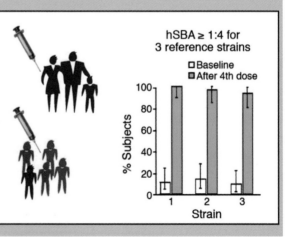

Phase I well tolerated, immunogenic

Phase II protective hSBA titers in > 90% of infants

2008 Phase III ongoing

hSBA ≥ 1:4 for 3 reference strains

☐ Baseline
☐ After 4th dose

Vaccine —

Table 13.4. Centers for Disease Control and Prevention (CDC)— recommended immunizations schedule for persons aged 0–6 years in the USA, 2008. Ranges are shown when there is flexibility in the immunization schedule e.g. for HepB, the first immunization is given at birth, the second at 1–2 months and the 3rd at 6–18 months. (http://www.cdc.gov/vaccines/recs/schedules/default.htm)

Vaccine ▼ / Age ▶	Birth	1 month	2 months	4 months	6 months	12 months	15 months	18 months	19–23 months	2–3 years	4–6 years
Hepatitis B	Hep B	Hep B			Hep B						
Rotavirus			Rota	Rota	Rota						
Diphtheria, tetanus, pertussis			DTaP	DTaP	DTaP		DTaP				DTaP
Haemophilus influenzae type b			Hib	Hib	*Hib*	Hib					
Pneumococcal			PCV	PCV	PCV	PCV				PPV	
Inactivated poliovirus			IPV	IPV		IPV					IPV
Influenza						Influenza (Yearly)					
Measles, mumps, rubella						MMR					MMR
Varicella						Varicella					Varicella
Hepatitis A						HepA (2 doses)				HepA Series	
Meningococcal										MCV4	

■ Range of recommended ages

■ Certain high-risk groups

CRM197 nontoxic variant of diphtheria toxin. The considerable morbidity and mortality associated with hepatitis B infection, its complex epidemiology and the difficulty in identifying high-risk individuals have led to routine vaccination in the USA from the time of birth. In the UK, BCG vaccination is routinely given. However, this is not the case in the USA, where the fact that vaccination leads to individuals becoming positive to the Mantoux skin test, thus resulting in an inability to use this test as a means of excluding tuberculosis during the investigation of suspected infection, is seen as too much of a disadvantage. Due to the constant antigenic drift and occasional antigen shift that occurs with the influenza virus, a new vaccine has to be produced each year for each hemisphere.

Vaccines under development

As with outer pharmaceutical agents, the development of vaccines comprises several stages. Successful pre-clinical studies in animal models are followed by phase I clinical trials in volunteers to initially evaluate safety and the immune response. If all goes well, phase II trials are then carried out in a small number of individuals to gain an indication of efficacy. If the phase II trial is successful, and the company and regulatory authorities decide to proceed, this is followed by a much larger (phase III) study to fully establish efficacy and safety, after which regulatory approval for distribution is given. Phase IV clinical trials finally establish efficacy and safety in large numbers of people. This whole process may take up to 20 years and cost in excess of $500 m.

There are many vaccines currently under development for diseases in which there is at present no vaccine available or where the vaccines that are available are left wanting (Table 13.5). **Tuberculosis** is a good example of the latter situation. The bacille Calmette–Guérin (bCG) vaccine has been in use for over 80 years but is only efficacious in protecting children and adolescents against disseminated and meningeal TB, and then only in some areas of the world, and is largely ineffective against pulmonary TB, which is the commonest form of the disease in adults. Indeed, TB remains a truly major problem in developing countries, and cases have also increased dramatically in Western countries. The alarmingly heightened susceptibility to TB in individuals with HIV/AIDS has led to TB in up to half of HIV-infected individuals, and worldwide multidrug-resistant strains are appearing. This has led to an urgent search for improved vaccine candidates.

Vaccines against parasitic diseases have proved particularly difficult to develop: malaria

A major advance in malaria control has been the finding that the impregnation of bed nets with the insecticide pyrethroid reduces *Plasmodium falciparum* deaths by 40%. However, with the emergence of drug-resistant strains of malaria parasites and reports of increasing mosquito resistance to insecticides, vaccines must be developed. The goal seems achievable as, although children are very susceptible, adults resident in highly endemic areas acquire a protective but non-sterilizing immunity possibly mediated by antibodies.

Malaria is a complex mosquito-borne parasitic disease (Figure 13.15). Traditionally, vaccines have targeted a single stage of the infectious cycle. These include the sporozoite,

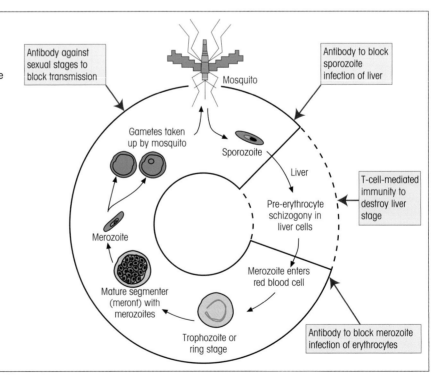

Figure 13.15. Vaccine targeting of the malaria life cycle.

Some of the most investigated potential stages of the cycle to be targeted by vaccine strategies are illustrated.

Antibody against sexual stages to block transmission

Antibody to block sporozoite infection of liver

Mosquito

Gametes taken up by mosquito

Sporozoite

Liver

Pre-erythrocyte schizogony in liver cells

T-cell-mediated immunity to destroy liver stage

Merozoite

Mature segmenter (meront) with merozoites

Merozoite enters red blood cell

Trophozoite or ring stage

Antibody to block merozoite infection of erythrocytes

Adjuvants in development for human vaccines		
Adjuvants	**Formulation**	**In pre-clinical or clinical trials**
Montanides	Water-in-oil emulsions	Malaria (Phase I), HIV, cancer (Phase I/II)
Saponins (QS-21)	Aqueous	Cancer (Phase II), herpes (Phase I), HIV (Phase I)
SAF	Oil-in-water emulsion conteining squalene, Tween™ 80, Pluronic™ L121	HIV (Phase I – Chiron)
AS03	Oil-in-water emulsion conteining α-tocopherol, squalene, Tween™ 80	Pandemic flu (GSK)
MTP-PtdEtn	Oil-in-water emulsion	HSV
Exotoxins	P. aeruginosa	P. aeruginosa, cystic fibrosis (AERUGEN – Crucell/Berna)
	E. coli heat-labile enterotoxin LT	ETEC (Phase II – Iornai Corp.)
ISCOMS	Phospholipids, cholesterol, QS-21	Influenza, HSV, HIV, HBV, malaria, cancer
TLR ligands		
MPL®-SE	Oil-in-water emulsion	Leishmania (Phase I/II – IDRI)
Synthetic Lipid A	Oil-in-water emulsion	Various indications (Avanti/IDRI)
MPL®-AF	Aqueous	Allergy (ATL); cancer (Biomira)
AS01	Liposomal	HIV (Phase I), malaria (ASO1, Phase III, GSK) cancer (Phase II/III, Biomira/MerckKGaA)
AS02	Oil-in-water emulsion containing MPL® and QS-21	HPV (Cervarix), HIV, tuberculosis, malaria (Phase III), herpes (GSK)
AS04	Alum + aqueous MPL®	HPV, HAV (GSK)
AS15	AS01 + CpG	Cancer therapy (GSK)
RC529	Aqueous	HBV, pneumovax
TLR-9	n/a	Cancer (ProMune – Coley/Pfizer)
(CpG)		HCV (ACTILON Coley)
TLR-9 ISS series	n/a	HIV, HBV, HSV, anthrax (VaxImmune Coley/GSK/Chiron) HBV (HEPLISAV, Phase III – Dynavax) Cancer (Phase II, Dynavax)
TLR-9 IMO series	n/a	Cancer (IMOxine, Phase I, Hybridon Inc.)
(YpG, CpR motif)	n/a	Cancer (IMO-2055, Phase II, Idera Pharm.) HIV (Remune, Phase I, Idera/IMNR)
TLR-9 agonist (MIDGE®)	n/a	Cancer (Phase I, Mologen AG)
TLR-7/8 (Imiquimod)	n/a	Melanoma (3M Pharmaceutical) HIV (prelinical), leishmaniasis
TLR-7/8 (Resiquimod)	n/a	HSV, HCV (Phase II – 3M Pharmaceuticals)

Table 13.5. Adjuvants in development for human vaccines. From Reed S.G. *et al.* (2008) *Trends in Immunology* **30**, 23–32.

Abbreviations: ETEC, enterotoxigenic *Escherichia coli*; HBV, hepatitis B virus; HCV, hepatitis C virus; HPV, human papillomavirus; HSV, herpes simplex virus.

which is the form with which the host is first infected after a mosquito bite, the liver stage of infection, the blood stage in which red blood cells become infected and the transmission stage in which gametes are taken up by the mosquito to complete the cycle. One of the problems faced by vaccine developers is the very considerate sequence variation apparent in malarial proteins.

In 2008, a candidate vaccine—RTS,S/AS01E (Glaxo-SmithKline, GSK)—was reported to have reduced the incidence of clinical malaria cases in trial of about 800 children aged 5–17 months in Kenya and Tanzania in a single malarial season by about a half. Thus there was only one episode of severe malaria in the vaccine group but eight episodes amongst seven children in the placebo group. This moderate success was hailed as a significant milestone along the road to an effective malaria vaccine as children in the age group of 0–5 years in sub-Saharan Africa are precisely the demographic most at risk from severe disease due to the parasite. The vaccine stimulates immune responses to the circumsporozoite protein (CSP) of *Plasmodium falciparum* in the liver stage of infection. The vaccine induces anti-CSP antibodies but no correlation was found between anti-CSP levels and protection from disease. The "AS01E" designator refers to the antigenic formulation used in the vaccine. The next stage in vaccine development is a phase III trial involving up to 16 000 African children across 7 countries. The trial was initiated in May 2009, the data will be made available to regulatory authorities in 2012 and the vaccine available for targeted use among children aged 5–17 months as early as 2013.

Despite the modest success of RTS,S/AS01E there is a strong argument made that the most effective vaccine is likely to target many antigens at different stages of the life-cycle of the parasite. For example, it has been noted that $CD8^+$ T-cells can provide sterile protection against liver-stage malaria parasites in mice. However, the number of antigen-specific $CD8^+$ T cells is very high suggesting that reliance on this mechanism alone might be unwise. Encouraging data has emerged on combining immune responses to liver and blood stages of the parasite, particularly using viral vectors that can induce both effective antibody and T-cell responses. In addition, data in humans and mice suggests that antibodies blocking transmission can be beneficial.

One of the most promising opportunities for malaria vaccine research relates to definition of the complete malaria genome that should help identify more vaccine targets as described above for "reverse vaccinology." Whole organism based malarial vaccines e.g. irradiated sporozoites are an alternative to recombinant vaccines that are being investigated.

Finally, it should be noted that, as with a number of viral infections, it is possible that T-cell-mediated immunity may contribute to malarial pathology. Infiltrating leukocytes have been observed in the brains of patients who have died of cerebral malaria and resistance to malarial disease has been correlated with a deficit in T-cell function in certain instances.

Vaccines for protection against bioterrorism

Biological warfare has a long and dark history. One early example occurred in 1346 when a group of Tartars catapulted plague-infected bodies and heads over the city walls of the Black Sea town of Kaffa in an attempt to re-capture the town from the Genovese. In 1763, the British were fighting Delaware Indians and, as a supposed gesture of "goodwill," donated smallpox-infected blankets to the Indians resulting in the death of many of the native tribes. Throughout the last century many countries throughout the world had biological weapons programs. Particularly alarming for citizens of the USA were the anthrax cases that occurred in late 2001 following exposure to mail items deliberately contaminated with anthrax spores and sent to news media offices in New York City and Boca Raton, Florida, and to two US Senators in Washington, DC. Aside from the anthrax (*Bacillus anthracis*), smallpox (variola) and plague (*Yersinia pestis*) mentioned above, many other infectious agents can potentially be used for bioterrorism including *Clostridium botulinum* toxin (botulism), *Francisella tularensis* (tularemia) and the Ebola, Marburg, Lassa and South American hemorrhagic fever viruses. Efforts are, therefore, underway to develop vaccines against these diseases in those cases in which effective vaccines are not currently available. Considerable success has been noted at the Vaccine Research Center of the National Institutes of Health in Bethesda, Maryland, USA in developing a vaccine that protects monkeys against lethal challenge with Ebola virus. The vaccine uses non-replicating adenovirus as a vector for the introduction of Ebola virus genes and expression of Ebola virus proteins in the animals prior to exposure to virus. Following the eradication of smallpox, routine vaccination against smallpox was discontinued. Concern that this agent could be used as a biological weapon has led to calls for the re-introduction of routine vaccination against smallpox. Currently only a small number of laboratory researchers, key healthcare workers and military personnel are vaccinated because it is felt that routine vaccination of the entire population would inevitably lead to a small number of vaccine-related deaths, a scenario accepted when a disease is endemic but not for a currently "extinct" disease. However, the vaccine is being stockpiled just in case. Incidentally, vaccination against smallpox would also protect against the related monkeypox virus.

Immunization against cancer

The realization that several different types of human cancer are closely associated with infectious agents suggests that vaccination against agents such as human papillomaviruses (cervical cancer), Epstein–Barr virus (Burkitt's and other lymphomas, nasopharyngeal carcinoma), *Helicobacter pylori* (stomach cancer), hepatitis B virus (liver cancer), HTLV-1 (adult T-cell leukemia) and human herpesvirus 8 (Kaposi's sarcoma) should lead to a substantial reduction in the incidence of such tumors. Cancer vaccines have also been developed against a number of tumor-associated antigens including carcinoembryonic antigen (colorectal cancer), immunoglobulin idiotypes (B-cell lymphoma), MAGE (melanoma), and so on. Results to date have been somewhat less than spectacular using tumor-associated self antigens but there is hope that strategies such as targeted activation of dendritic cells will lead to improved response rates.

Other applications for vaccines

A vaccine based on the human chorionic gonadotropin hormone, which is made by the preimplantation blastocyst and is essential for the establishment of early pregnancy, has undergone clinical trials as an immunological contraceptive. Vaccines are also being developed for the treatment of allergies and autoimmune diseases. These are generally aimed at re-setting the Th1/Th2 balance, activating regulatory T-cells, or re-establishing tolerance by clonal deletion or anergy. A vaccine for the treatment of addiction to tobacco consists of nicotine coupled to a bacteriophage Qb protein, which assembles into a complex of 180 protein monomers to form virus-like particles (VLPs). The vaccine has shown possible efficacy in a clinical trial in which there was a correlation between the levels of antibody induced against nicotine and continuous abstinence from smoking in some individuals. An anti-cocaine vaccine consisting of a derivate of cocaine conjugated to recombinant cholera toxin B with alum adjuvant is also undergoing clinical trials.

Adjuvants

For practical and economic reasons, prophylactic immunization should involve the minimum number of injections and the least amount of antigen. We have referred to the undoubted advantages of replicating attenuated organisms in this respect, but nonliving organisms, and especially purified products, frequently require an adjuvant that, by definition, is a substance incorporated into or injected simultaneously with antigen that potentiates the immune response (Latin *adjuvare*—to help).

Two types of action have been described for adjuvants; **immunostimulation** and **antigen delivery**. Immunostimulation results from the action of molecules to directly enhance immune responses. Immunostimulants include Toll-like receptor (TLR) agonists, cytokines and bacterial exotoxins. The explosion of understanding in innate immunity in the last decade has greatly increased the potential for the rational design of immunostimulants. The activation of DCs is particularly important here as this leads to increased antigen uptake, migration to lymph nodes and priming of CD4$^+$ T-cell help for B- and T-cell responses. Antigen delivery vehicles serve to optimally present antigens to the immune system by, at least in part, preventing dispersal of antigen and promoting slow release of antigen ("depot effects"). Such vehicles can deliver not only antigen but also immunostimulants more effectively. Examples include mineral salts such as alum, emulsions such as Freund's

adjuvant, liposomes and immune-stimulating complexes or ISCOMs. In reality many adjuvants combine to varying degrees the properties of immunostimulation and antigen delivery.

As stated above, conventional live attenuated vaccines typically do not require adjuvants, although responses sometimes can be enhanced by adjuvantation e.g. hepatitis A vaccination. However, the immunogenicity of proteins is typically relatively poor and the use of adjuvants is required. This is particularly the case if the protein is presented as a soluble monomeric form such as HIV gp120 as opposed to in a multimeric repeating particulate form like HBV surface antigen. The most widely used adjuvants in humans are based on gels formed by aluminium salts and are referred to collectively as **"alum" adjuvants**. Antigens are adsorbed on the aluminium particles and the appropriate adjuvant formulation selected based on immunogenicity. The activity of alum is ascribed to depot effects and immunostimulatory effects based on particle formation and induction of inflammation. Alum is used in several licensed vaccines, including hepatitis A, human papillomavirus (HPV), diphtheria–pertussis–tetanus (DPT), *Haemophilus influenze* b and inactivated polio.

Emulsions have been much used in vaccine research and are beginning to appear in human use. The classical adjuvant is Freund's, which is a water-in-oil emulsion. The complete form consists of a water-in-paraffin-oil emulsion plus inactivated mycobacteria; the incomplete form lacks the mycobacteria. The lifelong persistence of oil in the tissues and the occasional production of sterile abscesses mean this adjuvant (incomplete form, the complete form is even less suitable) is not used in human vaccines. The montanides are similar to incomplete Freund's but are biodegradable and have been used in HIV, malaria and cancer vaccine trials. Ribi, a commonly used formulation in experimental work, is a water-in-oil emulsion incorporating monophosphoryl lipid A (MPL) and mycobacterial trehalose dimycolate (TDM). MLA is a derivative of one of the most potent stimulators of antigen-presenting cells, namely lipid A from Gram-negative bacterial lipopolysaccharide (LPS). However, lipid A has many side effects although its derivative, MLA, is far less toxic. MF59 (Chiron—now Novartis) is an oil-in-water emulsion that has been safely used in millions of doses in an influenza vaccine in Europe. It effectively stimulates antibody and CD4$^+$ T-cell responses but not CD8$^+$ T-cell responses in humans and nonhuman primates. AS02 (GlaxoSmithKline) is an oil-in-water emulsion to which two immunostimulants, 3D-MPL and QS21 have been added. 3D-MPL is a derivative of MPL and QS21 is a saponin, originally derived from tree bark, that stimulates both antibody and cell-mediated immunity. Therefore AS02 is seen as a potentially powerful adjuvant for vaccines in which antibody and T-cell-mediated immunity may be important such as HIV or in which T-cell-mediated immunity is likely to be key such as TB.

Particulate antigens elicit much better immune responses than soluble proteins. ISCOMS or immune stimulating complexes take advantage of this by trapping antigens in cage-like structures with saponins. ISCOMATRIX (CSL) refines this basic concept. Synthetic oligonucleotides (deoxyribonucleotides) containing unmethylated CpG motifs (CpG ODN) are powerful immunostimulants acting through interaction with TLR9. Different families of CpG ODN can preferentially stimulate different cells—B-cells, NK cells, DCs, CD8$^+$ T-cells—involved in immune responses. Liposomes, virosomes and virus-like particles have the ability to present antigens in a multimeric form and can stimulate enhanced immune responses.

A number of pathogens gain entry to the body via mucosal surfaces and the induction of immune responses at these surfaces can be crucial in providing the best protection against disease. Many of the adjuvants described above can be used as mucosal adjuvants. However, there are also a number of molecules that are particularly effective as mucosal adjuvants, most notably cholera toxin (CT) and *E. coli* heat-stable enterotoxin (LT). Modified forms of the toxins and their subunits can powerfully stimulate mucosal responses through mechanisms that are not well understood.

Table 13.5 summarizes some of the adjuvants under development for use in human vaccines.

Passively acquired immunity

- Temporary protection against infection or clearance of toxins can be achieved with passively administered antibody preparations. Antisera from hyperimmunized animals and from immune humans are classically used in passive protection but increasingly human monoclonal antibodies are becoming available.
- Maternal antibody provides crucial protection to the newborn as its immune system matures.

Principles of vaccination

- Vaccines are effective because of humoral and cellular immune memory. Probably antibodies induced by vaccination are crucial in protecting against most bacteria and many viruses and parasites.
- Herd immunity is important in reducing disease incidence when transmission occurs between humans.

Killed organisms as vaccines

- Killed bacteria and viruses have been widely used as effective vaccines.

Live attenuated organisms

- The advantages include the larger antigen dose typically provided by a replicating organism, the tendency to elicit better cellular immunity and the generation of an immune response at the site of the natural infection.
- Nonpathogenic vectors such as adenovirus, attenuated fowlpox and modified vaccinia Ankara virus can serve as Trojan horses for genes from pathogenic organisms that are difficult to attenuate.
- BCG is a good vehicle for antigens requiring CD4 T-cell immunity and salmonella constructs may give oral and systemic immunity. Intranasal immunization is gaining popularity.
- The risk with live attenuated organisms is reversion to the virulent form and danger to immunocompromised individuals.

Subunit vaccines

- Whole organisms have a multiplicity of antigens, some of which are not protective, may induce hypersensitivity or might even be immunosuppressive.
- It makes particular sense in these cases to use purified components or those made recombinantly.
- Toxoids, inactivated toxins, are effective as vaccines in preventing illness due to some bacterial agents.
- The hepatitis B surface antigen particle is a classic example of an effective subunit viral vaccine.
- Many successful bacterial vaccines target glycans on the surface of the organism using glycoconjugate preparations.
- DNA encoding the proteins from a pathogen can be injected directly into muscle injected directly into muscle to generate the proteins *in situ* and produce immune responses. The advantages are stability, ease of production and cheapness. The method has not been as effective in humans as in mice but newer developments such as a DNA prime with a protein or vector boost are promising.

Newer approaches to vaccines

- The rise of genomics has been crucial in allowing a rational approach to the identification of many more bacterial vaccine targets. "Reverse vaccinology" has been successfully applied to the development of a MenB vaccine.
- Highly variable pathogens such as HIV and HCV present particular problems to vaccine design in that they require the elicitation of broadly protective immune responses. Here molecular approaches are being adopted to describe how broadly neutralizing antibodies interact with their targets and use the information to rationally design vaccine candidates.

Current vaccines

- Children in both the USA and UK are routinely immunized with diphtheria and tetanus toxoids and acellular pertussis (DTP triple vaccine), attenuated strains of measles, mumps and rubella (MMR), inactivated polio, and the capsular polysaccharide of *H. influenzae* type b (Hib) linked to a carrier.

■ Although in the UK and many other countries, BCG is given at 10–14 years of age, or for high-risk infants immediately after birth, it is not used routinely in the USA.

■ Vaccines against anthrax, Japanese encephalitis virus, hepatitis A, yellow fever, cholera and rabies, among others, are not given routinely but are available for travelers and high-risk groups.

Vaccines in development

■ A vaccine to malaria has been reported to significantly reduce the incidence of severe malarial disease in young children and intensive efforts are focused on follow-up. Many argue that a successful vaccine should target multiple antigens and multiple stages of the malarial life cycle.

■ A vaccine to HIV has reported possible success and efforts are focused on understanding possible correlates of any protection.

■ Vaccines are being developed for many pathogens including *Clostridium difficile*, dengue virus, herpes simplex virus and West Nile virus.

Adjuvants

■ Adjuvants generate enhanced longer-lived immune responses. They are generally not required for live attenuated vaccines but are crucial for protein subunit vaccines.

■ Adjuvants function by immunostimulation and antigen delivery or both.

■ Immunostimulation arises by the action of molecules such as TLR agonists, cytokines and bacterial exotoxins to directly enhance immune responses, particularly involving the dendritic cell (DC). Antigen delivery vehicles prevent antigen dispersal and promote slow release. They include mineral salts and emulsions.

■ Certain adjuvants such as cholera toxin are potent at stimulating mucosal responses, which may be most appropriate for certain pathogens infecting via mucosal surfaces.

FURTHER READING

Allen A. (2008) *Vaccine: the controversial story of medicine's greatest life saver.* W.W. Norton & Company, New York.

Amanna I.J., Messaoudi I. & Slifka M.K. (2008) Protective immunity following vaccination: how is it defined? *Human Vaccines* **4**, 316–319.

Amanna I.J. & Slifka M.K. (2009) Wanted, dead or alive: new viral vaccines. *Antiviral Research* **84**, 119–130.

Astronomo R.D. & Burton D.R. (2010) Carbohydrate vaccines: developing sweet solutions to sticky situations? *Nature Reviews Drug Discovery* **9**, 308–324.

Barrett A.D. & Beasley D.W. (2009) Development pathway for biodefense vaccines. *Vaccine* **27**, D2–D7.

Birkett A.J. (2010) PATH Malaria Vaccine Initiative (MVI): perspectives on the status of malaria vaccine development. *Human Vaccines* **6**, 139–145.

Casadevall A., Dadachova E. & Pirofski L.A. (2004) Passive antibody therapy for infectious diseases. *Nature Reviews Microbiology* **2**, 695–703.

Frazer I.H., Lowy D.R. & Schiller J.T. (2007) Prevention of cancer through immunization: prospects and challenges for the 21st century. *European Journal of Immunology* **37** (Suppl 1), S148–S155.

Haque A. & Good M.F. (2009) Malaria vaccine research: lessons from 2008/9. *Future Microbiology* **4**, 649–654.

Henderson D.A. (2009) *Smallpox—the death of a disease: the inside story of eradicating a worldwide killer.* Prometheus Books, New York.

Horimoto T. & Kawaoka Y. (2009) Designing vaccines for pandemic influenza. *Current Topics in Microbiology and Immunology* **333**, 165–176.

Offit P.A. (2007) *Vaccinated: one man's quest to defeat the world's deadliest diseases.* Smithsonian Books, New York.

Oldstone M.B. (2009) *Viruses, plagues, and history: past, present and future.* 2nd edn. Oxford University Press, Oxford.

Plotkin S.A. (2010) Correlates of protection induced by vaccination. *Clinical Vaccine and Immunology* **17**, 1055–1065.

Reed S.G., Bertholet S., Coler R.N. & Friede M. (2009) New horizons in adjuvants for vaccine development. *Trends in Immunology* **30**, 23–32.

Rinaudo C.D., Telford J.L., Rappuoli R. & Seib K.L. (2009) Vaccinology in the genome era. *Journal of Clinical Investigation* **119**, 2515–2525.

Sinden R.E. (2010) A biologist's perspective on malaria vaccine development. *Human Vaccines* **6**, 3–11.

Taylor K., Nguyen A. & Stéphenne J. (2009) The need for new vaccines. *Vaccine* **27**, G3–G8.

Virgin H.W. & Walker B.D. (2010) Immunology and the elusive AIDS vaccine. *Nature* **464**, 224–231.

Welsh R.M., Che J.W., Brehm M.A. & Selin L.K. (2010) Heterologous immunity between viruses. *Immunological Reviews* **235**, 244–266.

Now visit **www.roitt.com** to test yourself on this chapter.

CHAPTER 14
Immunodeficiency

Key Topics

Just to Recap ...

Pluripotent hematopoietic stem cells in the bone marrow can develop down either the myeloid or lymphoid pathway to differentiate into the various cell types that mediate the immune response. Migration of immune system cells from the blood circulation into the tissues involves cell adhesion molecules, chemotactic factors and complement components that regulate the inflammatory response. Upon entering the tissues the phagocytic cells of the innate response engulf and subsequently destroy pathogens using a plethora of microbicidal agents. Natural killer (NK) cells are involved in dealing with intracellular infections, a situation in which the pathogen is shielded from the effects of phagocytes and complement. Providing back-up to these innate responses is the acquired immune response that involves the antibody-producing B-cells together with helper, cytotoxic and regulatory T-cells. Although normally all the cells and molecules of the immune system interact effectively to fight infection there is always the possibility that one or more participants might fail, either due to inherited gene defects or due to damage caused by external factors.

Introduction

In accord with the dictum that "most things that can go wrong, do so," a multiplicity of immunodeficiency states in humans, which are **not secondary** to environmental factors, has been recognized. These "experiments of nature" provide valuable clues regarding the function of the defective factors concerned. We have earlier stressed the manner in which the interplay of complement,

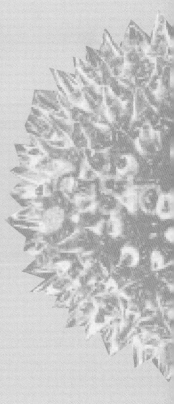

Roitt's Essential Immunology, Twelfth Edition. Peter J. Delves, Seamus J. Martin, Dennis R. Burton, Ivan M. Roitt.
© 2011 Peter J. Delves, Seamus J. Martin, Dennis R. Burton, Ivan M. Roitt. Published 2011 by Blackwell Publishing Ltd.

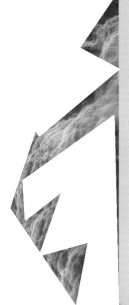

Introduction (*continued*)

antibody and phagocytic cells constitutes the basis of a tripartite defense mechanism against pyogenic (pus-forming) infections with bacteria that require prior opsonization before phagocytosis. It is not surprising, then, that deficiency in any one of these factors may predispose the individual to repeated infections of this type. Patients with T-cell deficiency of course present a markedly different pattern of infection, being susceptible to those intracellular bacteria, viruses and fungi that are normally eradicated by cell-mediated immunity (CMI).

The following sections deal first with some examples of these relatively uncommon genetically determined **primary immunodeficiency diseases (PIDs)**. We will then examine the various environmental factors, such as infection and malnutrition, that can be responsible for the much more prevalent **secondary immunodeficiencies.**

Deficiencies of innate immune mechanisms

Defective pattern recognition receptor signaling

Recognition of pathogen-associated molecular patterns is fundamental to the detection of microorganisms by cells of the innate response. Several gene defects have been described that result in impaired signaling through pattern recognition receptors. The MyD88 adaptor protein is required for signaling through a number of Toll-like receptors (TLRs), and patients with MyD88 deficiency suffer from severe life-threatening infections with pyogenic bacteria including pneumococci and *Salmonella*. The IL1R-associated kinase-4 (IRAK4) is involved in signaling through the IL-1 and IL-18 receptors and also through the TLR1/2 heterodimer, TLR2/6 heterodimer, TLR7 and TLR8. In IRAK4-deficient individuals it is Gram-positive pyogenic bacteria, including *Streptococcus pneumoniae* and *Staphylococcus aureus* that are most commonly seen. In response to engagement by their ligands, the intracellular TLRs (TLR3, -7, -8 and -9) interact with the ER-resident accessory molecule

UNC93B. Deficiencies in this protein are associated particularly with herpes simplex virus encephalitis.

Phagocytic cell defects (Table 14.1)

In **chronic granulomatous disease** the monocytes, macrophages and neutrophils fail to produce reactive oxygen intermediates due to a defect in the nicotinamide adenine dinucleotide phosphate (NADPH) oxidase system (cf. p. 13) normally activated by phagocytosis. The cytochrome b_{558} component of this system is composed of 91 and 22 kDa *phox* (*ph*agocyte *ox*idase) subunits and, in the X-linked form of the disease, there are mutations in the gene encoding the larger of these subunits (Figure 14.1). In the majority of cases, no cytochrome is produced, but one variant gp91 mutation permits the synthesis of low levels of the protein (Figure 14.2) and the condition can be improved by treatment with γ-interferon. Not unexpectedly, the knockout of gp91^{phox} provides a handy mouse model. The 30% of chronic granulomatous disease patients who inherit their disorder in an autosomal recessive

Table 14.1. Deficiencies of phagocytic cells.

Defective gene	Disorder	Typical infections
CD18 β-subunit	Leukocyte adhesion deficiency	Pyogenic bacteria
IFNγR1, IFNγR2, IL-12 p40, IL-12R/IL-23R shared β1 subunit or STAT1	Mendelian susceptibility to mycobacterial disease	Mycobacteria, *Salmonella*, viruses
IRAK4	IRAK4 deficiency	*Strep. pneumoniae, Staph. aureus*
LYST	Chediak-Higashi	*Staph. aureus, Strep. pyogenes*, pneumococci, *Aspergillus* spp., *Pseudomonas aeruginosa*
MEVF	Familial Mediterranean fever	None
MyD88	MyD88 deficiency	*Strep. pneumoniae, Staph. aureus, Pseudomonas aeruginosa*
p22phox, p40phox, p47phox, p67phox or gp91phox	Chronic granulomatous disease	*Staph. aureus, Aspergillus fumigatus, Candida albicans*
TNFRSFIA	TNF receptor-associated periodic syndrome	None
UNC93B	UNC93B deficiency	Herpes simplex virus

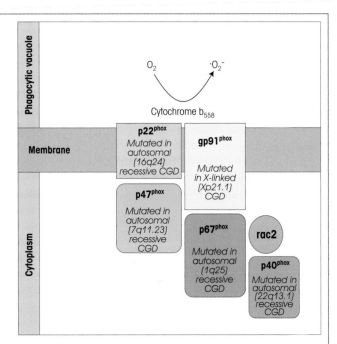

Figure 14.1. Mutations in NADPH oxidase components responsible for chronic granulomatous disease (CGD).

The cytochrome b_{558} found in the phagocyte membrane is composed of p22^{phox} and p91^{phox}. Upon cell activation the cytosolic proteins p47^{phox}, p67^{phox} and p40^{phox}, together with the small GTP-binding protein rac2, associate with cytochrome b_{558} to form the active NADPH oxidase complex, resulting in the generation of the superoxide anion (cf. Figure 1.16). Most patients with CGD have the X-linked form of the disease involving mutations in the gp91^{phox} gene. Mutations in the genes encoding other components of the NADPH oxidase are responsible for the autosomal forms of the disease.

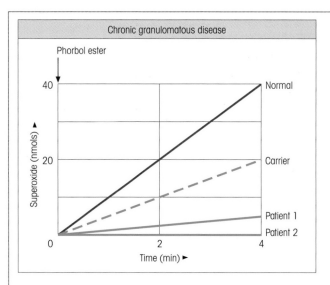

Figure 14.2. Defective respiratory burst in neutrophils of patients with chronic granulomatous disease.

The activation of the NADPH oxidase is measured by superoxide anion ($\cdot O_2^-$; cf. Figure 1.16) production following stimulation with phorbol myristate acetate. Patient 2 has a p91^{phox} mutation that prevents expression of the protein, whilst patient 1 has a different p91^{phox} mutation that results in very low but measurable levels. Many carriers of the X-linked disease express intermediate levels, as in the individual shown who is the mother of patient 2. (Data from Smith R.M. & Curnutte J.T. (1991) *Blood* **77**, 673.)

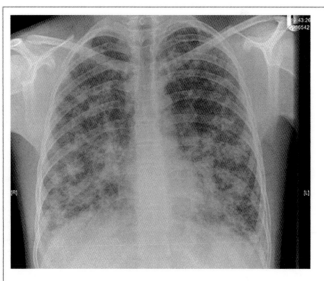

Figure 14.3. Fulminant pneumonitis in a patient with chronic granulomatous disease (CGD).

Chest radiograph of a 15-year-old boy with autosomal recessive CGD, showing bilateral dense infiltrates because of *Aspergillus fumigatus* and *Absidia corymbifera* pneumonitis. (From Slatter M.A. & Gennery A.R. (2008) *Clinical Experimental Immunology* **152**, 389–396. Courtesy of the Paediatric Immunology Unit, Newcastle General Hospital, UK.)

pattern express a defective form of the oxidase resulting from mutations in the smaller p22^{phox} cytochrome subunit or in the cytosolic p40^{phox}, p47^{phox} or p67^{phox} molecules (Figure 14.1).

Curiously, the range of infectious pathogens that trouble these patients is relatively restricted. The most common pathogen is *Staphylococcus aureus*, but certain Gram-negative bacilli and also fungi such as *Candida albicans* and *Aspergillus fumigatus* are frequently involved (Figure 14.3). The factors underlying this restriction are two-fold. First, many bacteria help to bring about their own destruction by generating H_2O_2 through their own metabolic processes, but if they are catalase positive, the peroxide is destroyed and the bacteria will survive. Thus neutrophils from these patients readily take up catalase-positive staphylococci in the presence of antibody and complement but fail to kill them intracellularly. Second, the organisms that are most virulent tend to be those that are highly resistant to the oxygen-independent microbicidal mechanisms of the phagocyte.

Lack of the CD18 β subunit of the β$_2$ integrins produces a **leukocyte adhesion deficiency** causing impaired neutrophil chemotaxis and recurrent bacterial infection. Emigration of monocytes, eosinophils and lymphocytes is unaffected as these can fall back on the alternative VCAM-1/VLA-4 β_1-integrin system. In **Chédiak–Higashi** disease and the "beige" murine counterpart, dysfunction of NK cells, cytotoxic T-cells and neutrophils is associated with defects in the *LYST* (**lys**osomal **t**rafficking) gene. Accumulation of giant intracytoplasmic granules occurs due to defective migration of the late endosomal/lysosomal compartment within the cell. The patients suffer from sometimes fatal pyogenic infections, particularly with *Staphylococcus aureus*. Most patients develop an "accelerated phase" of the disease in which there is unremitting T-cell proliferation, but this can potentially be brought under control by bone marrow transplantation.

Mendelian susceptibility to mycobacterial disease (MSMD) in humans involving BCG or nontuberculous mycobacteria can be traced to recessive mutations in five genes, two affecting the chains of the IFNγ receptor (IFNγR1 and IFNγR2) and, the others, the IL-12 p40 subunit, the IL-12R/IL-23R shared β1 subunit, and the signal transducer and activator of transcription-1 (STAT1) molecule. The latter is involved in signaling through a number of cytokine receptors including the interferon receptors. In addition to being particularly prone to mycobacterial infections, patients with MSMD also show increased susceptibility to other intracellular bacteria, particularly *Salmonella*, and to viruses. Because IL-12 drives the differentiation of the IFNγ-producing Th1 subset, collectively the genes involved in MSDM very nicely underline the role of IFNγ in mediating protection against intracellular infection.

There is a group of so-called **"autoinflammatory" disorders** characterized by apparently unprovoked inflammation. One such, *TNF receptor-associated periodic syndrome*

(TRAPS), presents with prolonged fever bouts and severe localized inflammation caused by dominantly inherited mutations in the *TNFRSFIA* gene encoding the p55 TNF receptor. Although the mechanisms resulting in persistent inflammation remain to be fully established, in some patients there may be impaired cleavage of the receptor ectodomain with diminished shedding of the potentially antagonistic soluble receptor. Indeed, it is salutary to note the beneficial effects of treatment with a recombinant p75 TNFR–Fcγ fusion protein (etanercept), or a monoclonal anti-TNF (infliximab) in some patients with TRAPS. Another hereditary periodic fever syndrome is **familial Mediterranean fever** due to mutations in the *MEFV* gene that encodes pyrin, an inflammatory regulator expressed predominantly in neutrophils and Th1 cytokine-activated monocytes.

Complement system deficiencies (Table 14.2)

Defects in control proteins

The importance of complement in defense against infections is emphasized by the occurrence of repeated life-threatening infection with pyogenic bacteria in patients lacking Factor I, the C3b inactivator. Because of this inability to destroy C3b, there is continual activation of the alternative pathway through the feedback loop, leading to very low C3 and Factor B levels with normal C1, C4 and C2.

Erythrocytes are bombarded daily with C3b generated through the formation of fluid phase alternative pathway C3 convertase from the spontaneous hydrolysis of the internal thiolester of C3. There are several regulatory components on the red cell surface to deal with this. The C3 convertase complex is dissociated by decay accelerating factor (DAF; CD55) and by CR1 complement receptors (not forgetting

Table 14.2. Deficiencies of complement pathways.

Defective gene	Disorder	Typical infections
C1q, C1r, C1s or *C4*	Predisposition to systemic lupus erythematosus	Usually none
C1 Inhibitor	Hereditary angioedema	Usually none
C2	Predisposition to systemic lupus erythematosus	Pyogenic bacteria, esp. pneumococci
C5, C6 or *C8*	Predisposition to systemic lupus erythematosus	*Neisseria gonorrhoeae*, *N. meningitidis*
C3 or *Factor H*	Age-related macular degeneration	Pyogenic bacteria
C7, C9, Factor D or *properdin*	–	*N. gonorrhoeae, N. meningitidis*
Factor 1	–	Pyogenic bacteria
MASP-2	–	*Strep. pneumoniae*
MBL	–	None
PIG-A	Paroxysmal nocturnal hemoglobinuria	Usually none

Factor H from the fluid phase; cf. p. 19), after which the C3b is dismembered by Factor I in concert with CR1, membrane cofactor protein (MCP) or Factor H (Figure 14.4). There are also two inhibitors of the membrane attack complex, homologous restriction factor (HRF) and the abundant protectin molecule (CD59) that, by binding to C8, prevent the unfolding of the first C9 molecule needed for membrane insertion. DAF,

HRF and protectin bind to the membrane through glycosyl phosphatidylinositol anchors. In a condition known as **paroxysmal nocturnal hemoglobinuria** (PNH), there is a defect in the ability to synthesize these anchors, caused by a mutation in the X-linked *PIG-A* gene that encodes the enzyme required for adding *N*-acetylglucosamine to phosphatidylinositol. In the absence of these complement regulators, lysis of the red cells occurs. The phenotype in which there are normal levels of these protective molecules is referred to as "type I." In the type II PNH disease phenotype, there is a defect in DAF, whereas in the more severe type III form protectin and HRF are also affected and susceptibility to spontaneous complement-mediated lysis is greatly increased (Figure 14.4). A monoclonal antibody to complement component C5, eculizumab, is effective in treating PNH by preventing C5 convertase-mediated cleavage and thus the generation of the membrane attack complex.

Factor H polymorphism, specifically the possession of a histidine rather than a tyrosine at residue 402, predisposes towards the development of **age-related macular degeneration,** as does the presence of a glycine rather than an arginine at position 102 in complement component C3. Quite why these polymorphisms are risk factors is currently unclear.

A defective gene for the C1 inhibitor is associated with **hereditary angioedema** and can lead to recurring episodes of acute circumscribed noninflammatory edema mediated by a vasoactive C2 fragment (Figure 14.5). The patients are heterozygotes (homozygotes have never been described) and synthesize small amounts of the inhibitor that can be raised to useful

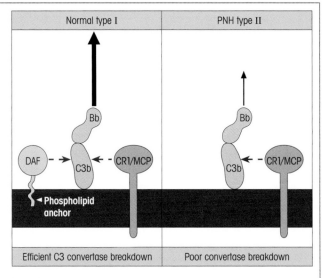
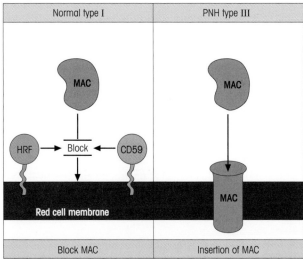

Figure 14.4. Paroxysmal nocturnal hemoglobinuria (PNH).

A mutation in the *PIG-A* gene, which encodes α-1,6-*N*-acetyl-glucosaminyltransferase, results in an inability to synthesize the glycosyl phosphatidylinositol anchors, deprives the red cell membrane of complement control proteins and renders the cell susceptible to complement-mediated lysis. Type II is associated with a DAF defect and the more severe type III with additional CD59 (protectin) and HRF deficiency. DAF, decay accelerating factor; CR1, complement receptor type 1; MCP, membrane cofactor protein; HRF, homologous restriction factor; MAC, membrane attack complex.

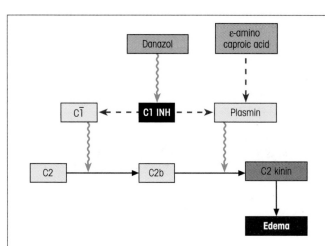

Figure 14.5. C1 inhibitor deficiency and angioedema.

C1 inhibitor stoichiometrically inhibits C1, plasmin, kallikrein and activated Hageman factor and deficiency leads to formation of the vasoactive C2 kinin by the mechanism shown. The synthesis of C1 inhibitor can be boosted by methyltestosterone or preferably the less masculinizing synthetic steroid, danazol; alternatively, attacks can be controlled by giving ε-aminocaproic acid to inhibit the plasmin.

levels by administration of the synthetic anabolic steroid danazol or, in critical cases, of the purified inhibitor itself. ε-Aminocaproic acid, which blocks the plasmin-induced liberation of the C2 kinin, provides an alternative treatment.

Deficiency in components of the complement pathways

Deficiencies in C1q, C1r, C1s, C2, C4, C5, C6 and C8 can all predispose to the development of immune-complex-mediated autoimmune diseases such as systemic lupus erythematosus (SLE, cf. p. 495), perhaps due to a decreased ability to mount an adequate host response to infection with a putative etiologic agent or, in the case of the earlier components, more probably to eliminate antigen–antibody complexes effectively (cf. p. 410). Bearing in mind the focus of the autoimmune response in SLE on the molecular constituents of the blebs appearing on the surface of apoptotic cells (cf. p. 496), the importance of C1q in binding to and clearing these apoptotic bodies becomes paramount. So it is that C1q-deficient mice develop high titer antinuclear antibodies and die with severe glomerulonephritis.

Patients who are deficient in either C7 or C9 exhibit increased susceptibility to disseminated *Neisseria gonorrhoeae* and *N. meningitidis*. Such infections are also characteristic of deficiencies in the alternative pathway components factor D and properdin. Interestingly, the inability to produce a membrane attack complex involving complement components C5b–9 does not have a substantial effect on the incidence of other types of infection. Adequate protection must be largely afforded by opsonization of microorganisms with antibody and/or the C3b, C4b and iC3b complement components for subsequent phagocytosis, and the immune adherence mechanism whereby organisms coated with these early complement components become bound to the CR1 complement receptor on erythrocytes and are then taken to the liver or spleen for destruction. C3 deficiency, whilst very rare, will affect all three pathways of complement activation and is associated with recurrent pyogenic infections.

Mutations that lead to reduced levels of mannose-binding lectin (MBL) are fairly common but this does not lead to a detectable increase in infections in most cases. Presumably complement activation by other mammalian lectins such as ficolin, or indeed by the antibody-mediated classical pathway, compensates for the absence of the MBL-mediated pathway. However, other individuals with a MBL-associated serine protease-2 (MASP-2) deficiency due to a mutation that renders the enzyme non-functional exhibit increased pyogenic infections by organisms such as *Streptococcus pneumoniae*.

Primary B-cell deficiency (Table 14.3)

Agammaglobulinemia due to early B-cell maturation failure

X-linked agammaglobulinemia (XLA) is one of several immunodeficient syndromes that have been mapped to the X chromosome (Figure 14.6). The defect occurs at the pre-B-cell stage and the production of immunoglobulin in affected males is grossly depressed, there being few lymphoid follicles or plasma cells in lymph node biopsies. Mutations occur in the Bruton's tyrosine kinase (*Btk*) gene, as is also seen in *xid* mice. The children are subject to repeated infection by pyogenic bacteria—*Staphylococcus aureus*, *Streptococcus pyogenes* and *S. pneumoniae*, *Neisseria meningitidis*, *Haemophilus influenzae*—and by a protozoan, *Pneumocystis jirovecii*, which produces a strange form of pneumonia. Cell-mediated immune responses are normal and viral infections are readily brought under control.

Mutations in either the μ heavy chain or the λ₅ chain, which together form the surrogate IgM receptor on pre-B-cells (cf. p. 300), result in a phenotype similar to that seen in XLA with arrest at the pro-B stage. The implication would be that *Btk* provides the signal for pro- to pre-B differentiation through this pre-B-cell receptor complex. Other mutations that cause a similar phenotype include those in the genes for the Igα (CD79a) signal transducing protein and for the BLNK

Table 14.3. Deficiencies affecting B-lymphocytes.

Defective gene	Disorder	Typical infections
BAFFR, CD19, ICOS or *TACI*	Common variable immunodeficiency	*S. pneumoniae, H. influenzae, Mycoplasma* spp.
Btk	X-linked agammaglobulinemia	*S. aureus, S. pyogenes, S. pneumoniae, N. meningitidis, H. influenzae, Pneumocystis jirovecii*
Ig Cμ, λ5, Igα or *BLNK*	—	*S. aureus, S. pyogenes, S. pneumoniae, N. meningitidis, H. influenzae, Pneumocystis jirovecii*
Unknown	Selective IgA deficiency	Mostly asymptomatic, sometimes bronchopulmonary infections

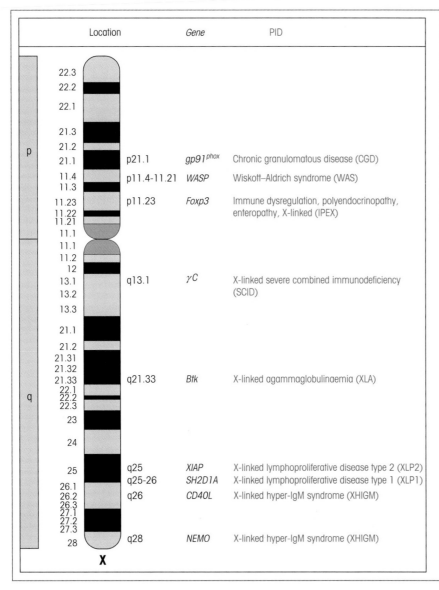

Figure 14.6. Loci of the major X-linked immunodeficiency syndromes.

Males are more likely to be affected by X-linked recessive genes because, unlike the situation with females when there are two X chromosomes, homozygosity is not needed. In some cases the precise location of the relevant gene is still to be ascertained. A number of other rare X-linked immunodeficiencies have also been described. Some of the primary immunodeficiency diseases (PIDs) listed (e.g. CGD, SCID, HIGM) can also be due to defective genes on other chromosomes.

B-cell *link*er protein that is again required for the transition from pro-B to pre-B-cells.

Deficiencies affecting particular antibody isotypes

The most common of all the primary immunodeficiencies is **selective IgA deficiency**, which affects both circulating IgA and the secretory dimeric form and can also broaden to include the IgG2 isotype. In some patients there is a complete absence of IgA whereas others have low levels of these antibodies. The majority of patients with selective IgA deficiency are asymptomatic. **Common variable immunodeficiency** (CVID), in which there is low IgG and IgA and/or IgM, often occurs within the same family as patients with selective IgA deficiency, and individual family members sometimes gradually convert from one disease to the other. The gene defects for both these PIDs in most patients have yet to be fully defined but a small

number of CVID patients have mutations in the B-cell surface BAFF receptor, TAC1 or CD19 molecules, or in the T-cell surface molecule ICOS. All these molecules are involved in lymphocyte activation, perhaps going some way to explain the increased incidence of autoimmune disease seen in patients with CVID, an association also seen in individuals with selective IgA deficiency. Patients with these antibody deficiencies can be protected against recurrent pyogenic infections with intravenous or subcutaneous injections of pooled human immunoglobulin.

Transient hypogammaglobulinemia is seen in early life

A degree of immunoglobulin deficiency occurs naturally in human infants as the maternal IgG level wanes (p. 303), and may become a serious problem in very premature babies. A more protracted **transient hypogammaglobulinemia of infancy**, characterized by recurrent respiratory infections, is associated with low IgG levels that often return to normal by 4 years of age. There is a deficiency in the number of circulating lymphocytes and in their ability to generate help for Ig production by B-cells activated by pokeweed mitogen, but this becomes normal as the disease resolves spontaneously.

Primary T-cell deficiency (Table 14.4)

Patients with no T-cells or poor T-cell function are vulnerable to opportunistic infections and, as B-cell function is to a large extent T-dependent, T-cell deficiency also impacts negatively on humoral immunity. Dysfunctional T-cells often permit the emergence of allergies, lymphoid malignancies and autoimmune syndromes, the latter presumably arising from inefficient

negative selection in the thymus or the failure to generate appropriate regulatory cells.

Defective thymic development

The **DiGeorge syndrome**, in which mutations in the TBX1 transcription factor involved in embryonic development are present, is characterized by a failure of the thymus to develop properly from the third and fourth pharyngeal pouches (DiGeorge syndrome children also lack parathyroids and have severe cardiovascular abnormalities). Consequently, hematopoietic stem cells cannot differentiate to become T-lymphocytes and the "thymus-dependent" areas in lymphoid tissue are sparsely populated; in contrast, lymphoid follicles are seen but even these are poorly developed. Cell-mediated immune responses are undetectable and, although the infants can deal

Table 14.4. Deficiencies affecting T-lymphocytes.

Defective gene	Disorder	Typical infections
AIRE	Autoimmune polyendocrine syndrome-1	*Candida albicans*
ATM	Ataxia telangiectasia	Bronchopulmonary
CIITA	MHC class II deficiency	Bronchopulmonary
CD3γ	CD3γ deficiency	Bacteria and viruses
CD40L, CD40, AID, NEMO or UNG	Hyper-IgM syndrome	*Pneumocystis jirovecii*, *Toxoplasma*, *Cryptosporidium parvum*
FAS or FASL	Autoimmune lymphoproliferative syndrome	None
Foxp3	Immune dysregulation, polyendocrinopathy, enteropathy, X-linked (IPEX)	None
γC, RAG-1, RAG-2, artemis, ADA or IL-7R α chain	Omenn syndrome	Broad (viral, bacterial, fungal) including *Pneumocystis jirovecii* and *S. aureus* sepsis
NBS1	Nijmegen breakage syndrome	Bronchopulmonary
PNP	PNP deficiency	Broad (viral, bacterial, fungal)
SH2DIA	X-linked lymphoproliferative disease type 1	Epstein–Barr virus
STAT3	Hyper-IgE syndrome	Extracellular bacteria, staphylococci, *Aspergillus* spp., *C. albicans*
TAP-1, TAP-2 or tapasin	MHC class I deficiency	Brochopulmonary
TBX1	DiGeorge syndrome	Multiple
WASP	Wiskott–Aldrich syndrome	Encapsulated extracellular bacteria
XIAP	X-linked lymphoproliferative disease type 2	Epstein–Barr virus
ZAP70	ZAP70 deficiency	Broad (viral, bacterial, fungal)

with common bacterial infections, they may be overwhelmed by live attenuated vaccines such as measles or bacille Calmette–Guérin (BCG) if given by mistake. Antibodies can be elicited, but the response is subnormal, reflecting the need for the cooperative involvement of T-cells. (The similarity of this condition to neonatal thymectomy and of B-cell deficiency to neonatal bursectomy in the chicken should not go unmentioned.) Treatment by grafting neonatal thymus leads to restoration of immunocompetence, but some matching between the MHC on the nonlymphocytic thymus cells and peripheral cells is essential for the proper functioning of the T-lymphocytes (p. 122). Complete absence of the thymus is pretty rare and more often one is dealing with partial DiGeorge syndrome in which the T-cells may rise from 6% at birth to around 30% of the total circulating lymphocytes by the end of the first year (compared with 60–70% in normal 1-year olds); antibody responses are adequate.

Arrest of early T-cell differentiation

Mutation of the gene encoding the purine degradation enzyme, **purine nucleoside phosphorylase**, results in the accumulation of the metabolite deoxy-GTP, which is toxic to T-cell precursors through its ability to inhibit ribonucleotide reductase, an enzyme required for DNA synthesis. Targeting of the T-cell lineage by this deficiency could well be linked to a relatively low level of 5′-nucleotidase. Some T-cells "leak through" but they give inadequate protection against infection and the disease is usually fatal unless a hematopoietic stem cell transplant life-line is offered. In addition to recurrent infections, patients usually suffer from neurologic dysfunction and autoimmunity.

Quite a few different genes, including for RAG-1, RAG-2, Artemis, IL-7 receptor α chain, adenosine deaminase, and the γC shared interleukin receptor chain, have been linked to the development of **Omenn syndrome.** As we shall see very shortly mutations of these genes are also responsible for severe combined immunodeficiency (SCID), but in Omenn syndrome the particular mutations involved are "leaky" and result in a less devastating phenotype. For example, the mutations in RAG allow some T-cells to sneak through because VDJ recombination is not completely abolished. Patients often exhibit eosinophilia and raised IgE, and sometimes have autoimmune disease affecting the skin and gut.

MHC class II deficiency (sometimes referred to as "bare lymphocyte syndrome") is associated with recurrent bronchopulmonary infections and chronic diarrhea occurring within the first year of life, with death from overwhelming viral infections at a mean age of 4 years unless these affected infants are successfully treated with a hematopoietic stem cell transplant. The condition arises from mutations affecting any of several transcription factors controlling the expression of class II genes, for example the *class II trans*activator (CIITA). Feeble expression of class II molecules on thymic epithelial cells grossly impedes the positive selection of CD4 T-helpers, and those that do leak

through will not be encouraged by the lack of class II on antigen-presenting cells. Note also that rare patients with mutations in the *TAP-1, TAP-2* or *tapasin* genes have MHC class I deficiency.

Deficiencies leading to dysfunctional T-cell–B-cell collaboration

Cell-mediated immunity (CMI) is depressed in immunodeficient patients with thrombocytopenia and eczema (**Wiskott–Aldrich syndrome**) or with **ataxia telangiectasia.** The *Wiskott–Aldrich syndrome protein* (**WASP**) plays a critical role in linking signal transduction pathways and the actin-based cytoskeleton by clustering physically with actin through the GTPase Cdc42 and the Arp2/3 (*actin-related protein*) complex that regulates actin polymerization. Mutations in the *WASP* gene on the X chromosome thus adversely affect T-cell motility, phagocyte chemotaxis, dendritic cell (DC) trafficking and the polarization of the T-cell cytoskeleton towards the B-cells during T-cell–B-cell collaboration. Poor cell-mediated immunity and impaired antibody production in affected boys are hardly surprising consequences. **Ataxia telangiectasia,** a chromosomal breakage syndrome, is an autosomal recessive disorder of childhood characterized by progressive cerebellar ataxia with degeneration of Purkinje cells, a hypersensitivity to X-rays and an unduly high incidence of cancer. The *ataxia telangiectasia mutated* (*ATM*) gene encodes the Atm protein kinase, a member of the phosphatidylinositol 3-kinase family involved in regulating cell cycle and DNA double-stranded break repair. Furthermore, the Atm kinase is required for hematopoietic stem cell self-renewal by inhibiting oxidative stress in these cells. Another disease characterized by immune dysfunction, radiation sensitivity and increased incidence of cancer is the **Nijmegen breakage syndrome** in which there is a mutation in the *NBS1* gene encoding nibrin, a component of the double-stranded DNA break repair complex that becomes phosphorylated by Atm. Both Atm and nibrin are required for efficient class switch recombination in B-cells.

It is exciting to see the molecular basis of diseases being unraveled and an excellent example of Nature yielding its secrets has been provided by studies on the **hyper-IgM syndrome**, a rare disorder characterized by recurrent bacterial infections, very low levels or absence of IgG, IgA and IgE and normal to raised concentrations of serum IgM and IgD. Most patients have an X-linked form of the disease involving point mutations and deletions in the T-cell CD40L (CD154). These mutations largely map to the part of the molecule involved in the interaction with B-cell CD40 (cf. p. 221), thereby rendering the T-cells incapable of transmitting the signals needed for Ig class switching in B-cells. Less commonly, mutation of the X-linked *NEMO* gene (NFκB essential modifier, alternatively known as IKKγ), or the autosomal *CD40*, activation-induced cytidine deaminase (*AID*) or uracil-DNA glycosylase (*UNG*) genes are responsible. In these cases it is the B-cells, rather than the helper T-cell, that are defective.

The most common genetic cause of **hyper-IgE syndrome** (HIES) is a mutation in the *STAT3* gene. In addition to elevated IgE levels there are decreased numbers of Th17 cells. The HIES phenotype also includes several distinctive anatomical features such as hyperextensible joints and a failure or delay in shedding primary teeth so that patients have two sets of teeth.

Rare cases of T-cell functional deficiency arise from mutation in the γ chain of the CD3 complex, in which patients have normal levels of circulating T-cells but with a reduced expression of T-cell receptors on their cell surface, and ZAP-70 kinase mutations that result in reduced numbers of CD8⁺ T-cells.

Some immunodeficiencies can rather paradoxically cause an overactive immune response

We have already mentioned that excessive production of certain classes of antibody (IgM or IgE, for example) can result from particular gene defects. It is now also clear that "immunodeficiency" affecting regulatory or tolerance mechanisms will result in an undesirable enhancement of particular types of immune response. Thus, given the critical role of Foxp3 in the induction of regulatory T-cells, it will come as no surprise to hear that loss-of-function mutations in the *Foxp3* gene have a profound effect, being responsible for the **IPEX** (*i*mmune dysregulation, *p*olyendocrinopathy, *e*nteropathy, *X*-linked) syndrome in which unregulated T-cell activity leads to multisystemic and often fatal autoimmune disease. The somewhat less severe clinical condition **autoimmune polyendocrine syndrome-1** (APS-1, sometimes referred to as APECED—*a*utoimmune *p*olyendocrinopathy with *c*andidiasis and *e*ctodermal *d*ystrophy)—is due to mutations in the *AIRE* gene leading to inadequate central tolerance of T-cells. In contrast APS-2 is genetically much more complex and, like the vast majority of autoimmune diseases (see Chapter 18), is not caused by a single gene defect.

Defects in either Fas (CD95) or Fas ligand (CD95L) lead to **autoimmune lymphoproliferative syndrome** (ALPS) in which there is defective lymphocyte apoptosis resulting in increased numbers of CD4⁻CD8⁻ (double negative) T-cells and the development of autoimmune disease.

Combined immunodeficiency

In the primary T-cell deficiencies described above there are at least some mature T-cells present, albeit functionally defective. However, in **severe combined immunodeficiency disease** (SCID) there is normally an absolute failure in T-cell development and therefore SCID represents the most severe form of primary immunodeficiency, affecting one child in approximately every 80 000 live births. These infants exhibit profound defects in cellular and humoral immunity and without medical intervention death occurs within the first year of life due to severe and recurrent opportunistic infections. Prolonged diarrhea resulting from gastrointestinal infections and pneumonia due to *Pneumocystis jirovecii* are common; *Candida albicans* grows vigorously in the mouth or on the skin. If vaccinated with attenuated organisms these immunocompromised infants usually die of progressive infection.

Several different gene defects can be responsible for the development of SCID

Mutations in several different genes can cause SCID, which involves a block in T-cell development together with a direct or indirect B-cell deficiency. In some cases NK cells also fail to develop (Figure 14.7).

Cytokine signaling pathway defects

Approximately 40% of patients with SCID have mutations in the **common γ (γc) chain** of the receptors for interleukins IL-2, -4, -7, -9, -15 and -21. Of these, IL-7R is the most crucial for lymphocyte differentiation, and mutations in the **IL-7R α**

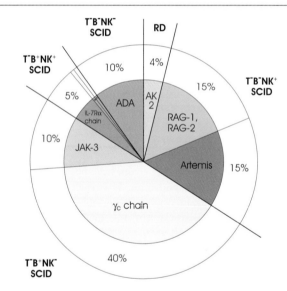

Figure 14.7. Genetic defects responsible for severe combined immunodeficiency (SCID).

The SCID phenotype is dependent upon the particular gene defect that is responsible. For example, in the 15% of SCID cases caused by mutation of the *Artemis* gene there is a complete lack of both T- and B-cells but NK cells are present (i.e. T⁻B⁻NK⁺ SCID) whereas in the 10% of cases due to ADA gene defects NK cells are also lacking (T⁻B⁻NK⁻SCID). Mutations in CD3δ, CD3ε, CD3ζ or CD45, (*) or the actin-regulator coronin-1A (†) each account for <1% of SCID cases. Mutations in the AK2 gene give rise to reticular dysgenesis (RD). There may be a few rare cases of SCID in which other gene mutations are responsible.

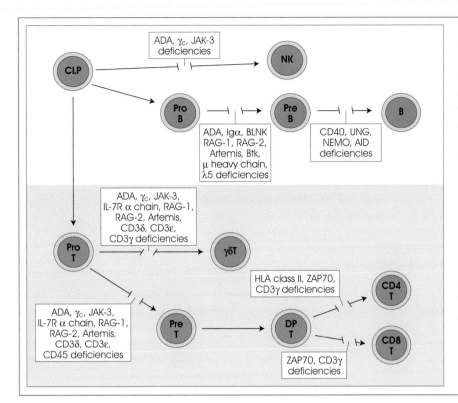

Figure 14.8. Blocks in lymphoid cell development result in immunodeficiency.

The site and nature of the mutation will determine the extent to which the function of the gene product is compromised. Thus, although homozygous inheritance of the mutated gene will often lead to an absolute block in development of the relevant lymphocyte populations, some mutations only cause a partial block in development. Furthermore, even some loss of function mutations will only partially abrogate lymphocyte differentiation. This is the case with CD3 γ chain and HLA class II deficiencies where the consequences are usually less severe than in many other immunodeficiencies. ADA, adenosine deaminase; AID, activation-induced cytidine deaminase; CLP, common lymphoid progenitor; DP, double positive; RAG, recombination-activating gene..

chain, or in **JAK-3** which transduces the γ_c signal, also result in SCID (Figure 14.8).

SCID can arise from grossly deficient VDJ recombination

Unlike the sneak through of immunocompetent T-cells that accompanies the partial *RAG* deficiency in Omenn syndrome, grossly dysfunctional mutations in the recombinase enzymes, which catalyze the introduction of the double-stranded breaks permitting subsequent recombination of the *V, D* and *J* segments of the immunoglobulin and T-cell receptor gene loci, prevent the emergence of any mature lymphocytes (Figure 14.8). Failure of the VDJ recombination mechanism is also a feature of the radiosensitive cells from those SCID patients with a defective *Artemis* gene. Artemis is an essential component of the DNA-dependent protein kinase complex that realigns and repairs the free coding ends created by the RAG enzymes.

Other causes of SCID

Ten percent of SCID patients have a genetic deficiency of the purine degradation enzyme, adenosine deaminase (ADA), which results in the accumulation of the metabolite, dATP, which is toxic to early lymphoid progenitor cells (Figure 14.8). If either the CD3 δ or ε chain of the T-cell receptor complex is mutated there is a block in T-cell development, in marked contrast to the CD3 γ chain deficiency mentioned previously which does not prevent T-cell differentiation but does result in

defective T-cell activation. Mutations of the CD45 protein tyrosine phosphatase can also give rise to SCID in very rare instances. **Reticular dysgenesis**, in which there are mutations in the mitochondrial adenylate kinase-2 (*AK2*) gene, is a rapidly fatal variant of SCID associated with a block in the differentiation of both myeloid and lymphoid cell precursors.

Combined immunodeficiency resulting from inherited defective control of lymphocyte function

X-linked lymphoproliferative disease (XLP), or Duncan's syndrome, is a progressive immunodeficiency disorder characterized by fever, pharyngitis, lymphadenopathy and dysgammaglobulinemia (i.e. a selective deficiency of one or more, but not all, the classes of antibody). Patients are particularly vulnerable to Epstein–Barr virus (EBV) infection. Mutations occur in the *SH2DIA* gene encoding SAP (*s*ignaling lymphocytic *a*ctivation molecule (SLAM)-*a*ssociated *p*rotein), which binds to SLAM through its SH2 domain. As triggering of SLAM leads to strong induction of IFNγ in T-cells and acts on B-cells to enhance proliferation and increase susceptibility to apoptosis, mutations in SAP that adversely affect the activation of SLAM will weaken the immune response, especially with regard to EBV infection in which viral replication in B-cells is heavily controlled by host T-cells.

Diagnosis of immunodeficiencies

Defects in immunoglobulins can be assessed by quantitative estimations; levels of 2 g/l arbitrarily define the practical lower limit of normal. The humoral immune response can be examined by first screening the serum for natural antibodies (A and B isohemagglutinins, heteroantibody to sheep erythrocytes, bactericidins against *E. coli*) and then attempting to induce active immunization with diphtheria, tetanus, pertussis and killed poliomyelitis—but no live vaccines. CD19, CD20 and CD22 are the main markers used to enumerate B-cells by immunofluorescence.

Patients with T-cell deficiency will be hypo- or unreactive in skin tests to such antigens as tuberculin, *Candida* and mumps. Active skin sensitization with dinitrochlorobenzene may be undertaken. The reactivity of peripheral blood mononuclear cells to the phytohemagglutinin mitogen is a good indicator of T-lymphocyte reactivity as is also the one-way mixed lymphocyte reaction (see Chapter 16). Enumeration of T-cells is most readily achieved by flow cytometry using CD3, CD4 and CD8 monoclonal antibodies.

In vitro tests for complement and for the bactericidal and other functions of neutrophils are available, while the reduction of nitroblue tetrazolium (NBT) or the stimulation of superoxide production provides a measure of the oxidative enzymes associated with active phagocytosis.

Treatment of primary immunodeficiencies

Early intervention with antibiotics and antifungals is of immediate importance, with the option of long-term low-dose prophylactic antimicrobials to prevent reinfection and subsequent complications such as hearing loss following otitis media (infection of the middle ear).

Replacing the missing components

As already mentioned above, if a suitable matched donor is available then bone marrow, peripheral blood or cord blood hematopoietic stem cell transplantation is the treatment of choice and has led to reconstitution of immune responses in patients with various primary immunodeficiencies including SCID, leukocyte adhesion deficiency, Chédiak–Higashi disease and Wiskott–Aldrich syndrome. In patients with ADA⁻SCID for whom no matched donor is available, the missing enzyme can be replaced by weekly intramuscular injections of bovine ADA conjugated to polyethylene glycol, the latter phenomenally improves the biological half-life of ADA from a few minutes for the free enzyme to 48–72 hours for the conjugate.

Deficiencies affecting humoral responses can to some extent be compensated for by intravenous immunoglobulin (IVIg) given every 3–4 weeks. Where innate responses are compromised, cytokine therapy can be helpful, for example by stimulating the defective phagocytes in chronic granulomatous disease by injections of interferon gamma.

Gene therapy

The ideal treatment in which a matched transplant is not available is correction of the gene defect. The first gene therapy trials for primary immunodeficiencies were initiated over 20 years ago and there has been a steady improvement in this approach, with some setbacks along the way. The majority of patients treated by this procedure have been those with ADA⁻SCID in which the normal gene for ADA is inserted into a retroviral vector that is then used to introduce the functional gene into the patient's own CD34⁺ hematopoietic stem cells (Figure 14.9). More recently this approach has been extended to the replacement of the defective γ_c cytokine receptor gene in patients with this form of SCID, although in this case more caution is required as some of these patients have developed leukemia following treatment. However, in both types of SCID the gene therapy approach has led to a sustained clinical benefit with restoration of immune responses to common pathogens. A small number of patients with the X-linked form of chronic granulomatous disease have been treated with a functional *gp91^{phox}* gene with encouraging results. Future progress will depend upon improvements in vector design to enhance the efficiency and safety of the gene transfer, and a more precise targeting of the gene integration sites. The use of self-inactivating lentiviral vectors (lentiviruses, which include HIV, are a subfamily of retroviruses) incorporating tissue-specific promoters has been proposed, although their efficacy and safety remain to be established.

Secondary immunodeficiency

Immune responsiveness can be depressed nonspecifically by many factors. CMI in particular may be impaired in a state of malnutrition, even of the degree which may be encountered in urban areas of the more affluent regions of the world. Iron deficiency is particularly important in this respect, as are zinc and selenium deficiencies.

Viral infections are not infrequently immunosuppressive, and the profound fall in cell-mediated immunity that accompanies **measles infection** has been attributed to specific suppression of IL-12 production by viral cross-linking of monocyte surface CD46 (membrane cofactor protein; cf. p. 373). The most notorious immunosuppressive virus, human immunodeficiency virus (HIV), will be elaborated upon in the next section. In lepromatous leprosy and malarial infection there is evidence for a constraint on immune responsiveness imposed by distortion of the normal lymphoid traffic pathways and, additionally, in the latter instance, macrophage function appears to be aberrant. Skewing of the balance between Th1 and Th2 cells as a result of infection may also depress the subset most appropriate for immune protection.

Many therapeutic agents, such as X-rays, cytotoxic drugs and corticosteroids, can have dire effects on the immune system. **B-lymphoproliferative disorders**, such as chronic lymphocytic leukemia, myeloma and Waldenstrom's macroglobulinemia, are associated with varying degrees of hypogammaglobulinemia and impaired antibody responses. Their common infections with pyogenic bacteria contrast with the situation in Hodgkin's disease in which the patients display all the hallmarks of defective CMI—susceptibility to tubercle bacillus, *Brucella*, *Cryptococcus* and herpes zoster virus.

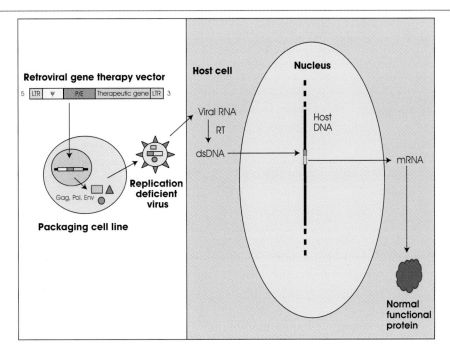

Figure 14.9. Gene therapy.

In a typical retroviral vector the Gag (core protein), Pol (reverse transcriptase [RT]) and Env (viral envelope) genes are replaced with the therapeutic gene, together with appropriate promoter (P) and enhancer (E) regulatory sequences. The 5′ and 3′ long terminal repeats (LTR) include sequences involved in gene integration, and the ψ (psi) sequence directs packaging of the viral nucleic acid. The retroviral vector containing the therapeutic gene is transfected into a packaging cell line that contains previously integrated genes encoding the essential Gag, Pol and Env proteins. The virus particles that are produced by this cell line will lack the genes for these proteins and therefore cannot go on to produce further infectious particles following delivery of the therapeutic gene to the host hematopoietic stem cells. In the patient's cells the viral RNA is reverse transcribed into double-stranded DNA that subsequently integrates into the host chromosomal DNA. The therapeutic gene can then be transcribed into mRNA for production of a functional form of the previously defective protein.

Acquired immunodeficiency syndrome (AIDS)

Acquired immunodeficiency syndrome (AIDS) is a devastating illness that had killed more than 25 million people by the end of 2008. According to the 2008 UNAIDS report, approximately 35 million people are currently living with human immunodeficiency virus (HIV), the agent responsible for AIDS (Figure 14.10). There were approaching 3 million new infections in 2008 alone. The epicentre of the plague is sub-Saharan Africa with nearly two-thirds of worldwide HIV infections and an adult infection rate estimated at about 5%. As of the end of 2008, 14 million children in sub-Saharan Africa had been orphaned because of AIDS. Increasingly, HIV/AIDS has a female face; females over 16 years of age account for nearly 50% of all people living with HIV or AIDS (closer to 60% in sub-Saharan Africa) and their rate of infection is increasing. The other key demographic is young people 15–24 years old, who account for about one-third of all infected individuals.

The first reported case of AIDS was in 1981. The syndrome was characterized by a predisposition to opportunistic infec-tions, i.e. those easily warded off by a normally functioning immune system; the incidence of an aggressive form of Kaposi's sarcoma or B-cell lymphoma; and the concurrent depletion of CD4+ T-cells. It was suspected that AIDS was caused by a previously unknown virus as it spread through contact with bodily fluids, and in 1983, HIV-1 was isolated and identified. There are in fact two closely related HIVs, HIV-1 and the less virulent HIV-2, which differ both in origin and sequence. The majority of AIDS cases are caused by HIV-1. HIV-2 is found predominantly in West Africa.

Both HIV-1 and HIV-2 have their origins in nonhuman primates. Based on sequence similarities (Figure 14.11) with simian immunodeficiency viruses (SIVs), HIV is likely the evolutionary product of closely related SIVs that crossed from their nonhuman primate hosts into humans in the early to mid part of the twentieth century. The closest relative of HIV-1 is SIVcpz, the natural host of which is the chimpanzee, *Pan troglodytes*. HIV-2 is more closely related to SIVsmm from the sooty mangabey, *Cercocebus atys*. Phylogenetic mapping and sequence analyses indicate several independent zoonoses of SIV_{cpz} and SIV_{smm} within the past century. The leading hypothesis is that SIV_{cpz} and SIV_{smm} were transmitted to

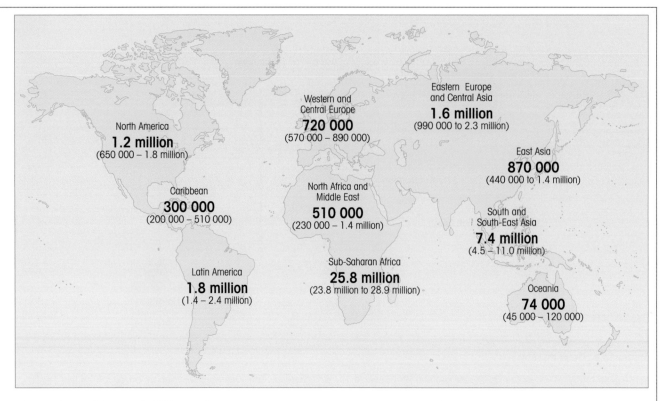

Figure 14.10. Adults and children estimated to be living with HIV as of the end of 2008 across the regions of the world.

It is estimated that a total of 33.4 (31.1–35.8) million individuals are infected (from the UNAIDS website, http://www.unaids.org).

Figure 14.11. Evolution of AIDS viruses.

Two evolutionary trees are shown in which the scale bar indicates 10% protein sequence divergence. (a) Tree showing the origins of primate lentiviruses. SIV strains have a suffix indicating their species of origin, e.g. SIV$_{cpzUS}$ is SIV from a chimpanzee in captivity in the USA. The distinct origins of HIV-1 and HIV-2 (shown in red) are apparent. This tree was derived using Pol protein sequences. (b) Tree showing the relationship between HIV-1 groups and clades and SIV$_{cpz}$. This tree was derived from Env protein sequences. (Kindly provided by Paul Sharp; after Sharp P.M. (2002) *Cell* **108**, 305–312.)

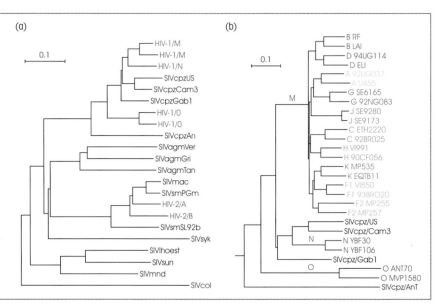

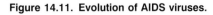

humans through cutaneous or mucosal membrane exposure to infected animal blood. This scenario is consistent with regular direct exposure of hunters in the bushmeat trade to primate blood.

Based on viral sequences, HIV-1 is categorized into four groups: M (main), O (outlier), N (non-M, non-O) and P (a recently discovered virus likely transmitted to humans from gorillas) each representing separate zoonoses (Figure 14.11). HIV-2 is similarly categorized into eight groups, A through H. HIV-1 from group M has spread throughout the world and is further subcategorized into clades A through K, which predominate in different geographical regions. The other three groups, N, O and P, are mainly confined to Gabon, Cameroon and neighboring countries in West Africa.

The evolution of the different group M clades most probably occurred within the human population following one cross-species transmission event. The discovery of an HIV-1 isolate from 1959 that appears to be an ancestor of clades B and D is consistent with this viewpoint. Furthermore, the recent discovery of a second isolate from 1960 that is highly divergent from the 1959 isolate shows that the virus had already undergone substantial diversification 50 years ago. The oldest common ancestor of group M has been estimated to date to the early part of the twentieth century, suggesting that HIV-1 has been infecting humans longer than originally thought, unnoticed clinically among populations in West Central Africa. The early spread of AIDS may have resulted from various economic, social and behavioral factors (e.g. use of nonsterilized needles for parenteral injections and vaccinations) that facilitated virus transmission.

HIV does not usually cause AIDS immediately and controversy still remains as to precisely how the virus damages the immune system and whether all HIV-1 infected individuals will necessarily develop disease. Great strides have been made since the identification of HIV but much remains a puzzle and a cure or a vaccine are elusive.

 ## The clinical course of disease: from infection to AIDS

Initial infection generally occurs by exposure to bodily fluids from an infected individual. HIV is found as free virus particles and infected cells in semen, vaginal fluid and mother's milk. Currently, the most common route of transmission worldwide is through sexual intercourse. The use of contaminated needles for intravenous drug delivery and the use of blood or blood products for therapeutic purposes are also common means of infection with HIV. Screening the blood supply for HIV has virtually eliminated transmission via the inadvertent administration of infected human blood in developed countries. Another important route of transmission is from infected mothers to their children. Mothers can pass HIV to their child either during birth or by breastfeeding. In Africa, the perinatal transmission rate is around 25%. The chance of perinatal transmission can be significantly reduced if the mother is undergoing antiretroviral therapy.

Two to 8 weeks after infection (Figure 14.12), 80% of individuals experience acute viremia. Symptoms are reminiscent of a bout of influenza and include a high spiking fever, sore throat, headaches and swollen lymph nodes. This is referred to as the acute retroviral syndrome, the symptoms of which usually subside spontaneously in 1–4 weeks. During this acute phase, there is an explosion of viral replication, particularly in CD4$^+$ T-cells in the gut, and a corresponding marked decline in circulating CD4$^+$ T-cells. At this time, most individuals also launch a strong HIV-specific CD8$^+$ T-cell response (Figure 14.12) that kills infected cells, followed by the production of HIV-specific antibodies (seroconversion). CD8$^+$ T-cells are thought to be important for controlling primary viremia.

Virus levels spike, then fall as CD4$^+$ T-cell counts rebound but to levels still below normal (800 cells/ml compared with 1200 cells/ml). The baseline level of virus persisting in the blood after the symptoms of acute viremia subside (the "set point") is currently the best indicator for an individual's prognosis.

Following primary infection, a period of clinical latency (no or few symptoms) follows during which time HIV continues to replicate while CD4$^+$ T-cells gradually decline in function and number. There are several mechanisms proposed to contribute to the depletion of CD4$^+$ T-cells during HIV infection. First, there are the direct cytopathic effects of the virus on its host T-cell. Second, infected cells have an increased susceptibility to the induction of apoptosis. Third, "bystander" effects can lead to the demise of uninfected cells by exposure to viral products or molecules leading to immune activation. Finally, there is the elimination of infected CD4$^+$ T-cells by CD8$^+$ T-cells that recognize viral peptides displayed by MHC class I.

The great majority of HIV-infected individuals will, over the course of years, progress to AIDS. The asymptomatic period typically lasts somewhere between 2 and 15 years; however, the number of functional CD4$^+$ T-cells eventually drops below a threshold (about 400 cells/ml) and opportunistic infections begin to appear. Once the CD4$^+$ T-cell count has dropped below 200 cells/ml, the individual is classified as having AIDS.

In the earlier stages of HIV-1 disease, typical opportunistic microbes to evade the impaired cellular immune system are oral *Candida* species and *Mycobacterium tuberculosis*, which manifest as oral thrush and tuberculosis respectively. Later, patients often suffer from shingles due to the activation of latent varicella zoster virus from a previous case of chickenpox. Also common is the development of EBV-induced B-cell lymphomas and Kaposi's sarcoma, a cancer of endothelial cells, likely due to the effects of cytokines secreted in response to both the existing HIV infection and a herpes virus (HHV-8) found in these tumors. Hepatitis C/HIV co-infection is also common and disease progression due to hepatitis C is accelerated. Pneumonia caused by the fungus *Pneumocystis jirovecii* is a frequent occurrence in patients and was often fatal prior to the introduction of effective antifungal therapy. In the final stages of AIDS, the prominent pathogens causing infection are *Mycobacterium avium* and cytomegalovirus. Respiratory infections are the major cause of death for AIDS sufferers. Although the above-mentioned infections and cancers are typical, not all AIDS patients will develop these illnesses and a number of other tumors and infections, though less prominent, are still of note.

The time of progression from HIV infection to AIDS varies greatly due to genetic variations in virus and/or host. For example, some viruses are naturally attenuated and are associated with slower disease progression. The HLA type of the host can be important. Homozygosity of HLA class I is linked to faster progression, probably due to a less diverse T-cell response to the infection. Certain HLA types are associated

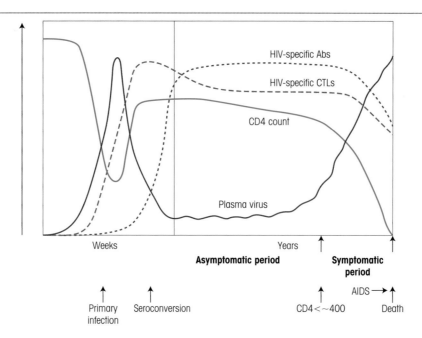

Figure 14.12. The typical course of HIV infection.

Primary infection is characterized by a rapid rise in plasma virus and a rapid decline in circulating CD4+ T-cells. The plasma virus levels peak and decline to a low roughly constant level ("the set point"), which is predictive of the time of progression to disease. The CD4+ T-cell count recovers somewhat but to a lower level than prior to infection. The HIV-specific CD8+ T-cell response is activated as virus peaks and is probably important in controlling primary infection. The HIV-specific antibody response takes somewhat longer to initiate and results in seroconversion. The neutralizing antibody response is yet slower to initiate (see Figure 14.17). Clinical latency follows primary infection for a period of the order of a decade. No symptoms are apparent but depletion of CD4+ T-cells in lymphoid tissues continues. Eventually, CD4+ T-cell depletion is so pronounced that resistance to opportunistic infections begins to wane, leading ultimately to a complete collapse of a functioning immune system and death. Drug intervention can take plasma viral loads below the level of detection and prevent CD4+ T-cell depletion.

with different prognoses: HLA-B57 and HLA-B27 are associated with slower progression while HLA-B35 is associated with more rapid progression. There are also individuals who are highly resistant to HIV infection because they have a mutation in the chemokine receptor CCR5, which serves as a coreceptor for HIV, as discussed later.

Two small groups of people are of particular interest to researchers due to their ability to remain disease free after exposure to HIV. The first group, long-term nonprogressors, are clearly infected with virus but control virus replication at low levels and have not progressed to disease. Within this group, some individuals have barely detectable virus and are referred to as elite controllers. The second group, highly exposed seronegative individuals, have been repeatedly exposed to HIV yet remain disease free and have no detectable virus. Intriguingly, some members of this latter group appear to possess HIV-specific CD8+ T-cells suggesting previous exposure to the virus or at least to noninfectious viral antigens. Whether the immune response seen in these individuals is responsible for clearing an HIV infection is unclear. Nonetheless, these individuals are the focus of much interest for vaccine design and development. We will now review key aspects of the virus itself including its cellular tropism, genome and life cycle.

HIV-1 genome

HIV-1 is a retrovirus, which means that it has an RNA genome but that replication passes through DNA with the involvement of the enzyme reverse transcriptase. It belongs to a group of retroviruses called the lentiviruses, from the Latin *lentus* meaning "slow", because of the slow course of disease associated with infection by these viruses. The HIV-1 genome is composed of approximately 9 kb of RNA, which consists of nine different genes encoding 15 proteins. Two copies of the single-stranded genome are packaged in the virus particle along with additional enzymes and accessory proteins. Three of the reading frames encode Gag (group specific antigen), Pol (polymerase) and Env (envelope) polyproteins, which are proteolytically cleaved into individual structural proteins and enzymes (Figure 14.13). Gag is cleaved into four structural proteins, MA (matrix), CA (capsid), NC (nucleocapsid) and p6, while Env is cleaved into two, SU (surface gp120) and TM (transmembrane gp41). Pol cleavage produces the enzymes PR (protease), RT (reverse transcriptase) and IN (integrase), which are encapsulated in the virus particle. Several accessory proteins are also encoded, three of which—Vif, Vpr and Nef—are packaged inside the virus particle. The remaining accessory proteins are Tat, Rev and Vpu. The functions of the 15 HIV proteins

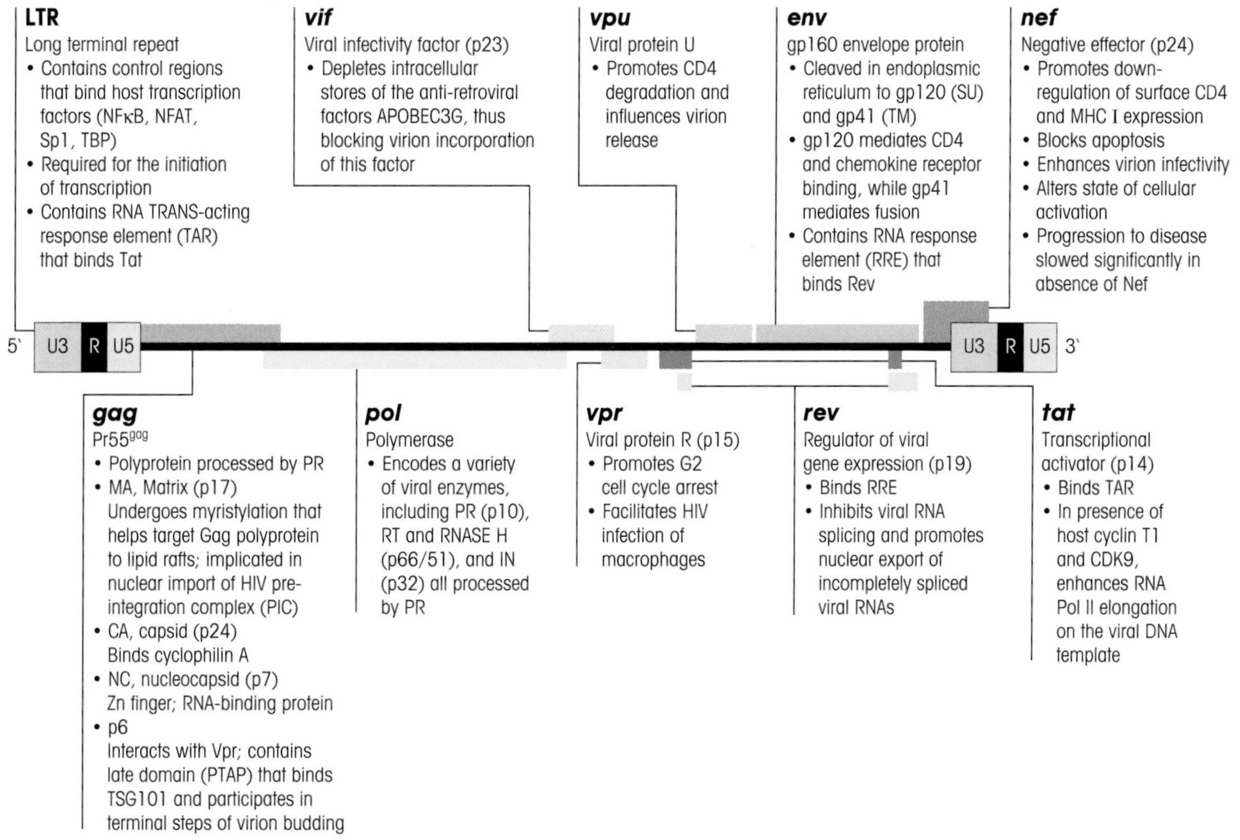

Figure 14.13. The HIV-1 genome.

The organization of the genome is shown and the functions of the gene products summarized. (Kindly provided by Warner Greene; after Greene W.C. & Peterlin B.M. (2002) *Nature Medicine* **8**, 673–680.)

are summarized in Figure 14.13 and discussed in relation to the HIV life cycle below.

The life cycle of HIV-1

Viral entry

Initial virus–cell attachment is believed to be mediated primarily through nonspecific interactions between the envelope spikes that decorate the surface of the virus and target T-cell surface molecules. The envelope spike is a trimer of heterodimers composed of noncovalently associated surface glycoprotein (gp120) and transmembrane glycoprotein (gp41) subunits. The sugar moieties and positively charged patches on gp120 probably mediate binding to cell surface lectins and negatively charged heparan sulfate proteoglycans, respectively.

The first receptor-specific binding event occurs when gp120 on the viral envelope spike engages CD4 on the target T-cell surface (Figure 14.14). HIV-1 specifically infects cells expressing CD4, including T-lymphocytes, macrophages and dendritic cells. CD4 binds with high affinity to a recessed cavity of gp120 as revealed by a structure of gp120 in complex with CD4. This binding event triggers multiple conformational changes in gp120 that expose and form the coreceptor

binding site. The coreceptor is most often the chemokine receptor CCR5 or CXCR4. These receptors normally function in chemoattraction, in which immune cells move along gradients of chemokine molecules to sites of inflammation. HIV-1s are often grouped by their coreceptor usage. R5 viruses use CCR5, X4 viruses use CXCR4 and dual tropic R5X4 viruses use both CCR5 and CXCR4. R5 viruses only require low levels of CD4 expressed on the surface of target T-cells, whereas X4 viruses require higher levels. Thus, differential expression of CD4 and coreceptors makes different T-cell types (or subtypes) more susceptible to infection by either X4 or R5 viruses: X4 viruses infect naive CD4$^+$ T-cells and mature DCs while the preferred *in vivo* targets of R5 viruses include immature dendritic cells, macrophages and activated effector or memory CD4$^+$ T-cells. Initially, R5 variants were labeled as "macrophage-tropic" when variants were classified based on the cell lines in which they could grow *in vitro* and likewise, X4 viruses were labeled as "lymphocyte-tropic." These former designations for HIV variants are misleading, as R5 viruses do infect lymphocytes, and therefore the designations were changed to reflect coreceptor usage.

Coreceptor binding induces conformational changes in the transmembrane glycoprotein, gp41, that result in the exposure

Figure 14.14. Steps in the HIV replication cycle (courtesy of NIAID).

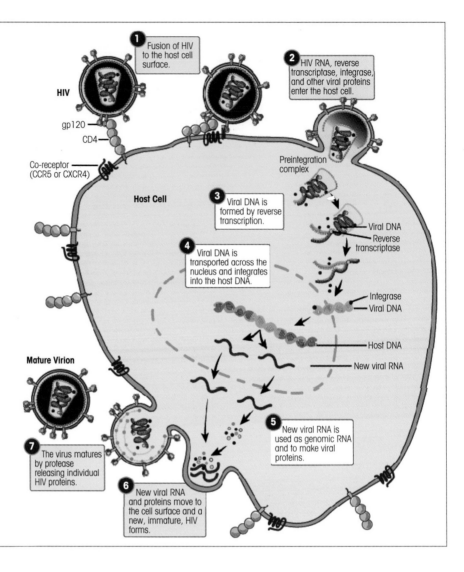

of the highly hydrophobic N-terminal fusion peptide of gp41, previously buried in the spike structure. The fusion peptide inserts into the host T-cell membrane like a harpoon, both destabilizing the target T-cell membrane and generating an extended α-helical gp41 fusion intermediate, designated the "pre-hairpin intermediate." This intermediate is unstable and readily collapses back onto itself forming a six-helix bundle, or "hairpin," comprising three internal α-helices arranged antiparallel to three external α-helices. The only high-resolution structure of gp41 available to date is of gp41 in this putative postfusion form. The collapse of gp41 into this extremely stable six-helical bundle is thought to provide the thermodynamic driving force for fusion. Six-helical bundles are a common structural motif among other viral and cellular fusion proteins; other viruses having surface proteins with structural similarities to gp41 include influenza virus, SARS and Ebola virus. Although it is not well understood how six-helical bundle formation enables the merging of cellular and viral membranes, if bundle formation is prevented using peptide analogs that compete for the occupancy of the external α-helices,

fusion is also abrogated. One such peptide has been developed into an HIV drug, the first of a class of drugs referred to as viral entry inhibitors.

Fusion is a highly cooperative process that occurs on a time scale of minutes and has been proposed to require the interaction of one to several spikes with corresponding receptors and coreceptors to be an efficient process.

Following fusion, the virus particle has lost its enveloped exterior, and the viral core, or reverse transcription complex, remains. This complex is composed of two viral RNAs, RT, IN, tRNA^{Lys}, matrix (p17), nucleocapsid (p7), capsid protein (p24) and Vpr.

Reverse transcription and integration

En route to the nucleus, RT uses the two single-stranded RNA molecules enclosed within the viral core as a template to convert the viral genome into a double-stranded cDNA copy of the viral genome. RT has no proofreading mechanism and introduces approximately one mutation per genome per reverse transcription. RNase H degrades the RNA template as the minus strand DNA is synthesized and DNA polymerase catalyzes the generation of a double-stranded viral cDNA genome.

Upon reverse transcription, the complex contains essentially the same factors as before, except that the RNA genome has been replaced with a newly synthesized cDNA genome. This complex is referred to as the preintegration complex, which translocates to the nucleus, possibly via actin filaments and microtubules by a mechanism only partially understood, given the large size of the complex.

Integration of the viral cDNA genome into the host T-cell genome is mediated by integrase and the actions of several host proteins (Figure 14.14). It requires the viral LTR sequence and is preferentially targeted to areas of active transcription. Integration can lead to latent or transcriptionally active viral cDNA referred to as a provirus. Active provirus serves as the template for viral replication and transcription. Latency explains the inability of viral therapies employed to date to eliminate virus completely from infected individuals and is the great challenge to a complete cure for HIV. The number of latently infected cells in an infected individual is very small, of the order of 10^5–10^6.

Replication

Replication of the virus commences postintegration with the production of nascent viral transcripts by cellular RNA polymerases (Figure 14.14). Transcription is regulated by proteins that bind within the LTR sequences, which flank the genome of the virus. For example, activation of T-cells results in the expression of transcription factor NFκB. NFκB binds to several promoters including those within the 5′-LTR.

Production of the viral proteins is biphasic. During the early phase (also called the Rev-independent phase), the viral transcripts are completely processed (i.e. all internal splice sites are utilized), polyadenylated and exported to the cytoplasm as all other cellular transcripts. Translation of these transcripts results in three gene products: Tat, Rev and Nef. Like other viruses, HIV-1 makes full use of a single template and therefore, in order for the other genes to be expressed, alternative splicing patterns are utilized (four different 5′-splice sites, eight different 3′-splice sites); however, this cannot occur until a critical threshold of Rev is achieved in the nucleus. A nuclear localization signal in the N-terminus of Rev guides it back to the nucleus post-translation with the help of cellular factor importin β. This arginine-rich domain also serves as a binding site for an RNA target, the Rev response element (RRE), which is located within the env intron of all incompletely spliced mRNAs. Splicing of HIV transcripts by cellular splicing factors is an inefficient process, and this allows time for Rev to bind the RRE. Rev cooperatively multimerizes (up to 12 additional Rev monomers) along the RNA and this Rev–RRE complex associates with exportin/Crm-1 via a nuclear export signal in the C-terminus of Rev. This allows for efficient transport of the partially spliced or unspliced transcripts from the nucleus to the cytoplasm before the splicing factors are able to process the transcripts.

These actions by Rev permit the second phase of gene expression to commence and the partially spliced and unspliced mRNAs are translated into Env, Vif, Vpr and Vpu and Gag and Gag–Pol, respectively. This is a crucial adaptation on the part of the virus as transcripts with introns are normally retained and degraded if they cannot be processed. Without Rev, HIV-1 is not able to transport its genetic material (containing multiple introns) to the cytoplasm where newly synthesized virus particles assemble; indeed, in experiments in which Rev is removed from the genome, the resulting virus clones are replication incompetent.

Tat and Nef are also crucial in HIV replication. In the absence of Tat, transcription begins but the polymerase fails to elongate efficiently along the viral genome. Tat binds to a well defined structure on the RNA, recruits positive elongation factors and promotes the rate of viral replication. Nef acts differently to Tat and Rev; it does not bind directly to viral RNA but rather acts upon the environment of the infected cell to favor replication. The activities of Nef include the ability to affect signaling cascades, downregulate CD4 expression at the infected cell surface and promote the generation of more infectious virions as well as virus dissemination. In addition by downregulating MHC class I molecules from the cell surface, Nef impairs immunological responses to HIV and inhibits apoptosis, thereby prolonging the life of the infected cell and increasing viral replication.

The number of mechanisms by which HIV promotes its own reproduction is staggering. It reflects the rapid turnover and inherent infidelity in HIV replication. The virus has sampled a huge number of different protein–protein and protein–nucleic acid interactions in its dance with humans and selection pressure has brought forth those interactions that favor virus survival and expansion. This is evolution on a time scale far shorter than normally experienced.

Virus assembly, budding and maturation

New virus particle assembly occurs at the plasma membrane of the infected cell (Figure 14.4). One of the viral proteins translated in the cytosol during the late phase of gene expression is the Gag precursor protein p55. p55 traffics to the plasma membrane or late endosomes and attaches to lipid bilayer where Env glycoproteins are attached via the transmembrane anchor of gp41. Assembly is dependent on the cellular protein HP68 that binds p55 and promotes the formation of an immature viral core. Other structural viral proteins assemble at the cell membrane with two copies of the viral RNA genome, RT, protease and integrase to be packaged into an immature virus particle. One of the key structural proteins present is p6, which connects the virus core to components of the endosomal sorting complex at sites of budding in the plasma membrane and late endosomes. Just before budding, other host factors including cytoplasmic viral restriction factors such as APOBEC3G can be incorporated into the virion. Coincident with budding of the immature virion from the plasma membrane, proteolytic processing of capsid occurs, generating the mature viral particle.

APOBEC3G is an interesting molecule that can restrict viral replication by cysteine deamination of DNA and resultant loss of functionality of viral genomes. The HIV-1 protein vif binds to APOBEC3G and by targeting it for professional degradation reduces its incorporation into virions. APOBEC3G is expressed in primary cells such as lymphocytes and macrophages and, as a consequence, Vif is essential for viral replication in these cells.

Another important HIV-1 restriction factor is TRIM5α, which is responsible for the resistance of primate cells to diverse retrovirus infection. It targets the capsid protein and blocks an early step of retroviral infection prior to reverse transcription. Finally, tetherin is a molecule that can suppress virus release from infected cells—its action can be counteracted by the HIV-1 protein Vpu.

In closing, it is important to note that much propagation of infection in HIV-1 *in vivo* probably occurs by cell-to-cell spread of virus rather than by free virus particles. Env proteins on the infected cell surface engage receptors on neighboring target T-cells, but HIV-1 transfer still requires viral budding. It appears that HIV-1 particles transfer directionally through sites of contact between infected and uninfected T-cells in an arrangement that has been termed the virological synapse with similarities to the immunological synapse found between T-cells and DCs. Nef promotes the formation of such synapses between infected macrophages and T-cells.

Vaginal transmission of HIV and the early stages of infection

Most HIV infections are now acquired through heterosexual transmission, most frequently by women through vaginal intercourse. There has therefore been an increased focus on understanding how vaginal transmission takes place and how one might intervene to prevent transmission. The SIV/monkey model has been very useful in this area (Figure 14.15). It appears that the virus struggles against the odds in the early phases of infection, but once it gains a foothold, circumstances rapidly change in favor of the virus to the point that progression to disease is virtually inevitable without drug intervention.

The first problem the virus encounters is the mucosal barrier. If this barrier is damaged, e.g. by ulcerative genital diseases, bacterial vaginosis or after the use of some microbicides such as nonoxynol-9, then transmission rates are increased. If the barrier is largely intact, then very few viruses will make it across, probably via small breaks or by transport on DCs. DCs express C-type lectins, such as DC-SIGN and DC-SIGNR, which bind high mannose glycans displayed on the surface of gp120, thereby capturing virions that may be internalized into a low-pH, nonlysosomal compartment, where they remain infectious. Once across the barrier, free virus infects target T-cells such as CD4$^+$ T-cells, macrophages and DCs in the lamina propria. Infectious virus inside DCs can enter resting and activated CD4$^+$ T-cells via DC–T-cell conjugates as bursts of viral replication are observed at DC–T-cell synapses. In addition, HIV-1 Nef-induced upregulation of DC-SIGN and β-chemokines in DCs may promote lymphocyte clustering and viral spread. Other studies suggest that Nef may also alter the physiological characteristics of infected macrophages so as to enhance conditions for viral dissemination.

Nevertheless, at this point in time, there is only a small founder population of infected cells, which must spread infection to the relatively few in number and spatially dispersed susceptible cells in the mucosa. Infection is still fragile and probably susceptible to intervention at this time. Then sometime between a day and a week, the virus finds its way to lymphoid tissue, a rich source of activated CD4$^+$ T-cells. Now conditions favor the virus as access is provided to large numbers of closely packed target T-cells leading to an extremely rapid rise in virus production to give peak viral loads in plasma. One very important lymphoid tissue compartment is the lamina propria of the gut where massive killing of CD4$^+$ memory T-cells occurs either via direct killing or via apoptosis. The counter-attack by the host's immune system has been described as "too little, too late."

HIV-1 therapy

Great advances have been made in recent years in the containment of HIV replication in infected individuals and the slowing down or blocking of the progression to AIDS. Many new drugs are available. Many steps in the virus life cycle are potential targets for drugs, including: (i) entry; (ii) fusion; (iii) reverse transcription; (iv) integration; (v) transcription/transactivation; (vi) assembly; and (vii) maturation.

Currently, five classes of drugs targeting four steps are in clinical use. The first antiretroviral class to become available was the nucleoside/nucleotide reverse transcription inhibitors. These nucleoside/nucleotide analogs are incorporated into the growing strand of viral DNA leading to chain termination and the production of noninfectious virus. Reverse transcription can also be inhibited by a second class of drugs, the non-nucleoside/nucleotide reverse transcription inhibitors, which bind allosterically to a site distant from the substrate-binding site. Viral protease inhibitors inhibit cleavage of the gag and pol polyproteins. The first fusion inhibitor, enfuvirtide, was approved by the Federal Food and Drug Administration (FDA) in the USA in 2003, and is a peptide that binds to gp41 to inhibit fusion. The first integrase inhibitor was approved in the USA in 2007.

A major problem in HIV therapy is the development of drug resistance. The error-prone nature of reverse transcription, the large viral load and the rapid rate of virus replication in many infected individuals means that they typically harbor a very large number of HIV variants. Administration of drugs may select for a variant that has resistance. Drug resistance against many protease inhibitors and some of the more potent

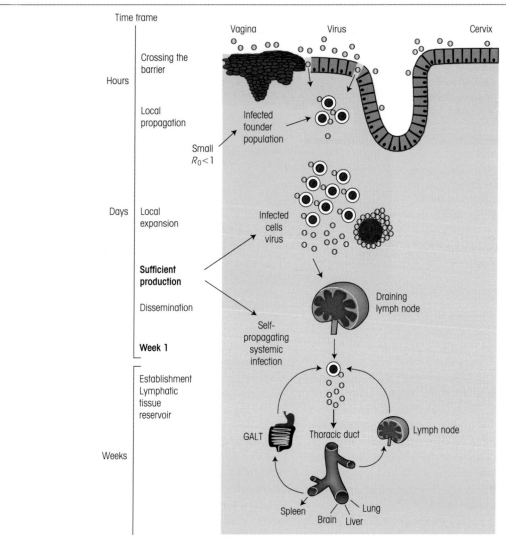

Figure 14.15. Time frame, sites and major events in vaginal transmission of HIV/SIV.

The SIV rhesus macaque animal model provides a window through which to view early infection. Within hours, virus in the inoculum may gain access through breaks in the mucosal epithelial barrier to susceptible target cells. The small focal infected founder population is initially composed mainly of infected resting CD4 T-cells. The founder population expands locally in these "resting" and in activated CD4 T-cells. Local expansion is necessary to disseminate infection to the draining lymph node and subsequently through the bloodstream to establish a self-propagating infection in secondary lymphoid organs. Crossing the barrier, small founder populations (with the associated risk that the basic reproductive rate, R_0, will fall below one), and local expansion are vulnerabilities for the virus in week 1 of infection. These vulnerabilities create opportunities for prevention of infection. Microbicides and vaccines that could reduce the size of the founder populations of infected cells might abort infection at the point of entry or prevent the efficient viral seeding of distant sites required for the establishment of a systemic infection. In humans, HIV-1 infection is first clinically manifest in the time frame of weeks and hence the need for the animal model to view sexual mucosal transmission and the earlier stages of infection. (Kindly provided by Ashley Haase; after Haase A.T. (2010) *Nature* 464, 217–223.)

nucleoside analogs can develop within a few days as a single mutation in the target enzyme confers resistance to many of these drugs. Resistance to other antiretrovirals, such as zidovudine (AZT), requires multiple mutations (three or four for AZT) and correspondingly longer to develop. Due to the relatively rapid development of resistance to all HIV drugs used singly, successful suppression of HIV currently necessitates combination therapy. Antiretroviral therapy (ART) typically involves the administration of a combination of drugs operating by different mechanisms.

ART has proven very effective in the management of viral levels in infected individuals. During the first 2 weeks of treatment, plasma virus loads decrease very rapidly reflecting the inhibition of virus production from infected cells and the rapid clearance of free virus from the circulation (half-life about 30 min). The results indicate that the half-life of productively

Figure 14.16. Model for neutralization of HIV by antibody.

Viral entry is mediated by the interaction of envelope spikes on the virus surface with CD4 and CCR5 on the target cell surface. The antibody molecule (Ab) has a molecular volume approaching that of a spike. Therefore the attachment of an antibody molecule to a spike is expected to show strong steric interference with virus attachment and/or fusion. (After Poignard *et al.* (2001) *Annual Review of Immunology*, **19**, 253–274; and Schief *et al.* (2010) *Current Opinion in HIV and AIDS* **4**, 431–440).)

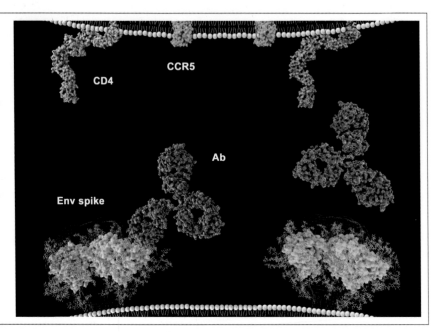

infected cells is about 2 days. At the end of 2 weeks, viral plasma levels have decreased by more than 95%, signifying a nearly complete loss of productively infected CD4$^+$ T-cells. There is a concomitant rise in CD4$^+$ T-cell counts in the peripheral blood as HIV replication and infection is controlled. This rise has been attributed to three mechanisms: redistribution of CD4$^+$ memory cells from lymphoid tissues into the circulation; reduction in the abnormal levels of immune activation associated with reduced CD8$^+$ T-cell killing of infected cells; and the emergence of new naive T-cells from the thymus.

After the initial rapid and almost complete clearance of free virus, a second slow phase of viral decay reflects the very slow decay of virus production in longer-lived reservoirs, such as in DCs and macrophages, from latently infected memory CD4$^+$ T-cells that have been activated. A third phase has been postulated, which is even slower, resulting from reactivation of integrated provirus in memory T-cells and other long-lived reservoirs of infection. Follicular DCs store virus in the form of immune complexes, making them potential long-term sources of infectious virus. These latent reservoirs may persist for years and are resistant to current HIV drug therapy.

HIV-1 vaccines

Most epidemiologists agree that the most efficient means to control the HIV-1 pandemic would be an effective vaccine. Unfortunately, the development of such a vaccine faces some major hurdles intimately associated with features of the virus. These include the variability of the virus, the nature of the envelope spikes of the virus and the ability of the virus to integrate into host chromosomes and become latent.

Most viral vaccines appear to be effective because they mimic natural infection and elicit neutralizing antibody responses. Long-lived plasma cells in the bone marrow secrete neutralizing antibodies that are present in serum and can act immediately to inactivate virus particles (Figure 14.16). Indeed, the likelihood that a vaccine will be effective is often assessed by looking at serum neutralizing antibody levels. Additionally on contact with virus, vaccine-induced memory B-cells are stimulated to secrete neutralizing antibodies. Studies in monkeys show that neutralizing antibodies can protect against HIV. If neutralizing antibodies are administered systemically and then the monkeys challenged with a hybrid human (HIV)/monkey (SIV) virus, they show no signs of infection, i.e. they exhibit sterilizing immunity. However, there is a requirement that the neutralizing antibodies elicited by vaccination be active against a wide spectrum of different HIV variants (so-called broadly neutralizing antibodies). Such antibodies are known to exist but the design of immunogens to elicit them has not yet been achieved. Indeed, natural HIV infection elicits relatively weak broadly neutralizing antibody responses, highlighting the difficulties of finding an appropriate immunogen. Natural infection tends to elicit type-specific neutralizing antibodies (Figure 14.17). When these antibodies reach a critical threshold, a resistant virus emerges. Eventually, a neutralizing antibody response to this virus develops and a new resistant virus emerges and so on. Apparently the virus always stays one step ahead of the neutralizing antibody response.

For the reasons outlined above, it appears that it will be challenging to design an HIV vaccine that will provide sterilizing immunity through elicitation of broadly neutralizing antibodies. In fact, most current vaccines effective against other viruses are not thought to provide sterilizing immunity. Rather they elicit sufficient serum titers of neutralizing antibody to blunt infection, which is then contained by cellular or innate immunity and overt symptoms are avoided. In other words, vaccination protects against disease rather than infection.

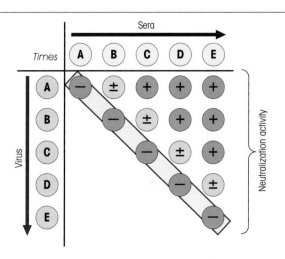

Figure 14.17. Evolution of the neutralizing antibody response in HIV infection.

A–E refer to virus and sera from time points A–E during the course of infection of an individual. Serum taken at time point A has no significant neutralizing activity against virus isolated from the plasma of the infected individual at time point A. Serum taken at time point B has some weak activity. Serum taken at time point C and points thereafter clearly neutralizes virus from time point A. Once the serum neutralizing antibody concentration has reached a certain threshold following exposure to a given predominant virus variant, selection pressure is exerted such that a new neutralization-resistant variant emerges from the huge pool of variants present in the infected individual. A neutralizing antibody response develops to this new variant and the cycle is repeated. (Courtesy of Doug Richman; after Richman D.D. *et al.* (2003) *Proceedings of the National Academy of Sciences of the USA* **100**, 4144–4149.)

Studies in animal models have shown that protection against disease for a number of viruses can be achieved by eliciting a cellular immune response through vaccination. In the absence of effective methods to elicit broadly neutralizing antibodies, much HIV vaccine research has targeted cellular immune responses. The primary rationale has been that if potent T-cellular immune responses can be elicited in vaccinees, the response may reduce the damage to CD4+ T-cells following primary infection and lower the viral set point. As

viral set point has been correlated with time of progression to AIDS, this would provide direct benefit to vaccinees. Furthermore, reduction of average plasma viral loads in vaccinated individuals should reduce transmission rates since transmission correlates with plasma viral load. Thus, vaccination should provide benefit to the population at large. Finally, reducing the damage to CD4+ T-cells in primary infection may help to maintain immunity against many pathogens over a long period.

Most studies on so-called "T-cell vaccines" have been carried out in monkeys. The results have been mixed. The best CD8+ T-cell responses, at least in terms of ELISPOT measurements, have been achieved using recombinant viral vectors to express HIV/SIV gene products. In particular, adenovirus vectors, either alone or in combination with other vectors or DNA vaccination, have elicited significant T-cellular responses. These responses have shown some protection in some monkey models but not in others.

Four larger-scale human HIV vaccine trials have been carried out. Two trials reporting in 2003 were based on recombinant monomeric gp120 and could be described as "antibody vaccines" in that they were expected to elicit primarily antibody responses. However the responses did not neutralize typical HIV isolates and the vaccines showed no efficacy. A trial reporting in 2007 was based on an adenovirus vector encoding HIV internal proteins gag, pol and nef and was described as a "T-cell vaccine." The vaccine showed no efficacy. Initially, it was thought that the vaccine had enhanced infection rates but detailed studies have brought this interpretation into question. The most recent trial reporting in 2009 was based on a canarypox vector encoding HIV gag, pro and env with boosting by env (recombinant gp120). This has been described as an "antibody and T-cell vaccine." The trial described possible modest efficacy close to the limits of statistical significance that appeared to have very short duration. Intensive efforts are ongoing to see if any correlate of protection in this trial can be identified.

Overall, it is clear that the development of an HIV vaccine is one of the major challenges facing modern medicine. Many believe that success will require the development of immunogens that can elicit both potent broadly neutralizing antibody and cellular immune responses.

Primary immunodeficiency diseases (PIDs)
- Primary immunodeficiencies are much less common than secondary, occur as a result of a gene defect, and can affect almost any component of the immune response.
- They are characterized by opportunistic infections.
- Several X-linked mutations produce PIDs in males.
- PIDs illuminate the importance of individual components of the immune system in combating particular infectious agents.

- Treatment includes prophylactic antibiotics, intravenous Ig, bone marrow transplantation and, potentially, gene therapy.

PIDs affecting innate responses
- Mutations in the genes encoding pattern recognition receptors or their associated adaptor and signaling molecules will particularly affect innate responses.
- Phagocytic cell or complement defects result in infection with bacteria that would normally

be disposed of by opsonization and phagocytosis.

■ Where there is an inability to produce the membrane attack complex there is only a very limited spectrum of increased infections, mainly with *Neisseria* spp.

■ Defects in complement components are associated with age-related macular degeneration or systemic lupus erythematosus.

■ A mutation in any one of several genes involved in the IFNγ response leads to increased susceptibility to mycobacterial infections.

■ Mutations that influence TNF pathways can lead to conditions in which inflammation occurs in the absence of a stimulus.

B-cell primary immunodeficiencies

■ Selective IgA deficiency is the most common PID but affected individuals are often symptomless.

■ In X-linked agammaglobulinemia all classes of antibodies are absent or only present at extremely low concentrations due to a defect in the Bruton's tyrosine kinase resulting in maturation arrest at the pre-B-cell stage.

■ Common variable immunodeficiency is associated with low IgG and IgA and/or IgM.

T-cell primary immunodeficiencies

■ Patients with T-cell deficiencies are susceptible to intracellular bacteria, viruses and fungi.

■ A lack of functional T-cells will impair B-cell responses.

■ In complete DiGeorge syndrome the absence of a thymus leads to an inability to produce T-cells, although in most cases there is only a partial defect.

■ Mutations affecting the enzyme purine nucleoside phosphorylase lead to the accumulation of toxic metabolites that particularly affect T-cells.

■ The genes linked to Omenn syndrome are similar to those responsible for SCID but the site of the actual mutation is different and does not have quite such a profound effect.

■ An absence of either MHC class I or class II molecules will result in the inability of T-cells to undergo positive selection in the thymus.

■ A number of gene defects, including those associated with Wiskott–Aldrich syndrome and with hyper-IgM syndrome, adversely affect the ability of T-cells to interact with B-lymphocytes.

■ Mutations in genes required for regulatory T-cell activity result in autoimmune conditions.

Severe combined immunodeficiency

■ Null mutations in a number of different genes, including γC, ADA, RAG-1, RAG-2, JAK-3, Artemis and the IL-7R α chain, can result in SCID.

■ There is a complete block in the development of T-cells, and thus complete lack of help for B-cells. Depending on the particular gene defect, B-cells and/or NK cells may also be absent.

■ Most cases of gene therapy for PIDs have attempted to insert a normal gene for ADA or γC.

Secondary immunodeficiency

■ Immunodeficiency may arise as a secondary consequence of malnutrition, lymphoproliferative disorders, agents such as X-rays and cytotoxic drugs, and viral infections.

Acquired immunodeficiency syndrome (AIDS)

■ AIDS results from infection with the lentiviruses HIV-1 or HIV-2, with HIV-1 being much more prevalent worldwide.

■ HIV-1 infects CD4$^+$ cells, including CD4$^+$ T-cells, macrophages and dendritic cells.

■ Depletion of CD4$^+$ T-cells, dramatically in primary infection particularly in the gut and then more slowly over a period of years during clinical latency, leads to damage to the immune system, which renders an individual susceptible to opportunistic pathogens (AIDS).

■ HIV-1 is a retrovirus, which gains entry to cells by interaction of envelope spikes with CD4 and the chemokine receptors, CCR5 or CXCR4. The RNA genome is reverse transcribed and the resulting viral cDNA integrated into host T-cell chromosomes.

■ Integrated proviral DNA can remain latent in cells for very long times, posing enormous problems for complete elimination of the virus from an individual and therefore hampering a complete cure for HIV-1 infection.

■ Proviral DNA can be transcribed to generate new viral particles with the aid of several viral accessory proteins, which act to aid viral replication and/or adapt the host T-cell machinery to virus production.

■ A major hallmark of HIV is the enormous diversity of the virus, present even in a single infected individual, because of the inherent errors involved in transcribing from an RNA genome, the rapid turnover of the virus and the high viral burden typically carried by the individual.

■ Viral diversity and latency present major challenges to drug therapy but nevertheless drug design has been highly successful and combination drug regimes can hold the virus in check for many years, if not indefinitely.

■ Vaccine design has also struggled with viral diversity and no immunogens that elicit broadly

neutralizing antibodies or sufficiently potent T-cell responses to significantly contain challenge with a wide diversity of HIVs have yet been designed, although efforts are intense and there are promising leads.

FURTHER READING

Arhel N. & Kirchhoff F. (2010) Host proteins involved in HIV infection: new therapeutic targets. *Biochimica et Biophysica Acta* **1802**, 313–321.

Austen K.F., Burakoff S.J., Rosen F.S. & Strom T.B. (eds) (2001) *Therapeutic Immunology*, 2nd edn. Blackwell Science, Oxford.

Bonilla F.A. & Geha R.S. (2006) Update on primary immunodeficiency diseases. *Journal of Allergy and Clinical Immunology* **117** (2 suppl), S435–441.

Broder S. (2010) The development of antiretroviral therapy and its impact on the HIV-1/AIDS pandemic. *Antiviral Research* **85**, 1–18.

Buckley R.H. (2002) Primary immunodeficiency diseases: dissectors of the immune system. *Immunological Reviews* **185**, 206–219.

Conley M.E. *et al.* (2009) Primary B cell immunodeficiencies: comparisons and contrasts. *Annual Review of Immunology* **27**, 199–227.

Greene W.C. & Peterlin B.M. (2002) Charting HIV's remarkable voyage through the cell: basic science as a passport to future therapy. *Nature Medicine* **8**, 673–680.

Haase A.T. (2010) Targeting early infection to prevent HIV-1 mucosal transmission. *Nature* **464**, 217–223.

Klasse P.J., Shattock R. & Moore J.P. (2008) Antiretroviral drug-based microbicides to prevent HIV-1 sexual transmission. *Annual Review of Medicine* **59**, 455–471.

Kohn D.B. (2010) Update on gene therapy for immunodeficiencies. *Clinical Immunology* **135**, 247–254.

Malim M.H. & Emerman M. (2008) HIV-1 accessory proteins—ensuring viral survival in a hostile environment. *Cell Host & Microbe* **3**, 388–398.

McMichael A.J., Borrow P., Tomaras G.D., Goonetilleke N. & Haynes B.F. (2010) The immune response during acute HIV-1 infection: clues for vaccine development. *Nature Reviews Immunology* **10**, 11–23.

Notarangelo L.D. *et al.* (2009) Primary immunodeficiencies: 2009 update. International Union of Immunological Societies Expert Committee on Primary Immunodeficiencies, *Journal of Allergy and Clinical Immunology* **124**, 1161–1178.

Ochs H.D., Smith C.I.E. & Puck J.M. (eds.) (2007) *Primary Immunodeficiency Diseases—A Molecular and Genetic Approach*. 2nd edn. Oxford University Press, Oxford.

Richman D.D., Margolis D.M., Delaney M., Greene W.C., Hazuda D. & Pomerantz R.J. (2009) The challenge of finding a cure for HIV infection. *Science* **323**, 1304–1307.

Sharp P.M. & Hahn B.H. (2008) AIDS: prehistory of HIV-1. *Nature* **455**, 605–606.

Simonte S.J. & Cunningham-Rundles C. (2003) Update on primary immunodeficiency: defects of lymphocytes. *Clinical Immunology* **109**, 109–118.

Tilton J.C. & Doms R.W. (2010) Entry inhibitors in the treatment of HIV-1 infection. *Antiviral Research* **85**, 91–100.

Turvey S.E., Bonilla F.A. & Junker A.K. (2009) Primary immunodeficiency diseases: a practical guide for clinicians. *Postgraduate Medical Journal* **85**, 660–666.

van de Vosse E., van Dissel J.T. & Ottenhoff T.H. (2009) Genetic deficiencies of innate immune signalling in human infectious disease. *The Lancet Infectious Diseases* **9**, 688–698.

Virgin H.W. & Walker B.D. (2010) Immunology and the elusive AIDS vaccine. *Nature* **464**, 224–231.

Walker L.M. & Burton D.R. (2010) Rational antibody-based HIV-1 vaccine design: current approaches and future directions. *Current Opinion in Immunology* **22**, 358–366.

 Now visit **www.roitt.com** to test yourself on this chapter.

CHAPTER 15
Allergy and other hypersensitivities

Key Topics

Just to Recap ...

Infections are dealt with by appropriate immune responses that detect foreign antigens. In the case of adaptive responses there is a necessity for clonal proliferation of lymphocytes in order to generate sufficient numbers of antigen-specific cells. Antibody of a class appropriate to clear the infection is produced and binds to the surface of the pathogen. The formation of IgM- or IgG-containing immune complexes triggers the activation of the classical complement pathway. IgG and complement components opsonise microorganisms for subsequent phagocytosis. In the case of parasitic infections, Th2-derived IL-4 and IL-13 encourage IgE production by B-cells. Intracellular pathogens are dealt with by NK cells, cytotoxic T-cells and by Th1 cells producing macrophage activating factors such as IFNγ.

Introduction

In **allergy** the immune response extends beyond its usual boundary of recognizing only foreign pathogens to also encompass what should be innocuous environmental antigens. This is a form of **hypersensitivity**, overzealous immunity that can also take the form of reactivity to antigens from the same or different species. Such responses lead to tissue damage, **immunopathology**, if the antigen is present in relatively large amounts or if the acquired immune response is at a heightened level. It should be emphasized that the mechanisms underlying hypersensitivity reactions are the same as those normally employed by the body in combating infection. The various hypersensitivity states were originally classified into types I–IV by Gell and Coombs and this classification remains broadly useful. However, it is often the case that in a particular disease state more than one of these types coexist.

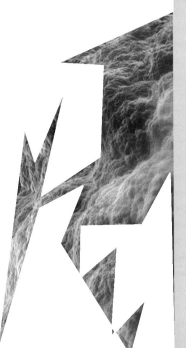

Roitt's Essential Immunology, Twelfth Edition. Peter J. Delves, Seamus J. Martin, Dennis R. Burton, Ivan M. Roitt.
© 2011 Peter J. Delves, Seamus J. Martin, Dennis R. Burton, Ivan M. Roitt. Published 2011 by Blackwell Publishing Ltd.

⚲ Milestone 15.1—The Discovery of Anaphylaxis

Hypersensitive reactions in some individuals to normally innocuous environmental agents have been observed from time immemorial. Scientific interest in such reactions was aroused by the observations of Charles Richet and Paul Portier. During a South Sea cruise on Prince Albert of Monaco's yacht, the Prince, presumably smarting from an encounter with *Physalia* (the jellyfish known as the Portugese man-of-war with very nasty tentacles), suggested that toxin production by the jellyfish might be of interest. Let Richet and Portier take up the story in their own words (1902):

"On board the Prince's yacht, experiments were carried out proving that an aqueous glycerin extract of the filaments of *Physalia* is extremely toxic to ducks and rabbits. On returning to France, I could not obtain *Physalia* and decided to study comparatively the tentacles of *Actiniaria* (sea anemone). While endeavouring to determine the toxic dose (of extracts), we soon discovered that some days must elapse before fixing it; for several dogs did not die until the fourth or fifth day after

administration or even later. We kept those that had been given insufficient to kill, in order to carry out a second investigation upon these when they had recovered. At this point an unforeseen event occurred. The dogs that had recovered were intensely sensitive and died a few minutes after the administration of small doses. The most typical experiment, the one in which the result was indisputable, was carried out on a particularly healthy dog. It was given at first 0.1 ml of the glycerin extract without becoming ill: 22 days later, as it was in perfect health, I gave it a second injection of the same amount. In a few seconds it was extremely ill; breathing became distressful; it could scarcely drag itself along, lay on its side, was seized with diarrhea, vomited blood and died in 25 minutes."

The development of sensitivity to relatively harmless substances was termed by these authors **anaphylaxis**, in contrast to **prophylaxis**.

Anaphylactic hypersensitivity (type I)

The phenomenon of anaphylaxis

The earliest accounts of inappropriate responses to foreign antigens relate to **anaphylaxis** (Milestone 15.1). The phenomenon can be readily reproduced in guinea-pigs that, like humans, are a highly susceptible species. A single injection of 1 mg of an antigen such as egg albumin into a guinea-pig has no obvious effect. Repeat the injection 2–3 weeks later and the sensitized animal reacts very dramatically with the symptoms of generalized anaphylaxis; almost immediately, the guinea-pig begins to wheeze and within a few minutes dies from asphyxia. Examination shows intense constriction of the bronchioles and bronchi and generally there is: (i) contraction of smooth muscle; and (ii) dilatation of capillaries. Similar reactions occur in human subjects highly allergic to insect stings, pollens, foods, drugs such as penicillin, or other agents that have the potential to cause life-threatening anaphylactic responses. In many instances only a timely injection of epinephrine, which rapidly reverses the action of histamine on smooth muscle contraction and capillary dilatation, can prevent death. Individuals known to be at risk are given self administration preloaded epinephrine syringes.

Sir Henry Dale recognized that histamine mimics the systemic changes of anaphylaxis and, furthermore, that exposure of the uterus from a sensitized guinea-pig to antigen induces an immediate contraction associated with an explosive degranulation of mast cells (see Figure 1.20) responsible for the release of histamine and a number of other mediators (see Figure 1.21).

Anaphylaxis is triggered by clustering of IgE receptors on mast cells through cross-linking

In rodents two main types of **mast cell** have been recognized, those in the intestinal mucosa and those in the peritoneum and other connective tissue sites. They differ in a number of respects, for example in the type of protease and proteoglycan in their granules, and in their ability to proliferate and differentiate in response to stimulation by interleukin 3 (IL-3) (Table 15.1). The two types have common precursors and are interconvertible depending upon the environmental conditions, with the mucosal MC_t (*t*ryptase) phenotype favored by IL-3 and connective tissue MC_{tc} (both *t*ryptase and *c*hymase) being promoted by relatively high levels of stem cell factor (c-kit ligand). In humans most mast cells in the intestinal mucosa and lung alveoli are tryptase-only positive, whereas those in skin, intestinal submucosa and other connective tissues are tryptase, chymase and carboxypeptidase positive. A third, less frequent, population is chymase-only positive and is found in the nasal mucosa and intestinal submucosa.

Mast cells, and their circulating counterpart the basophil, abundantly display the FcεRI high-affinity (K_a 10^{10} M^{-1}) receptor for IgE (cf. Table 3.2). The receptor is also expressed, albeit at considerably lower levels, on Langerhans' cells, dendritic cells, monocytes, macrophages, neutrophils, eosinophils, platelets and the intestinal epithelium. On basophils and mast cells the receptor is a tetramer consisting of an α chain, a tetraspan β chain and two disulfide-linked γ chains, whereas on other cell types, where the receptor is involved in antigen presentation rather than triggering degranulation, the β chain is absent and therefore the receptor is a trimer. The α chain possesses

Table 15.1. Comparison of the two main types of mast cell.

Characteristics	Mucosal mast cell	Connective tissue mast cell
General		
Abbreviation*	MC$_t$	MC$_{tc}$
Distribution	Gut & lung	Most tissues**
Differentiation favored by	IL-3	Stem cell factor
T-cell dependence	+	–
High affinity Fcε receptor	2×10^5/cell	3×10^4/cell
Granules		
Alcian blue and Safranin staining	Blue & brown	Blue
Ultrastructure	Scrolls	Gratings/lattices
Protease	Tryptase	Tryptase & chymase
Proteoglycan	Chondroitin sulfate	Heparin
Degranulation		
Histamine release	+	++
LTC$_4$:PGD$_2$ release	25:1	1:40
Blocked by disodium cromoglycate/theophylline	–	+

*Based on protease in granules.
**Predominate in normal skin and intestinal submucosa.

two external Ig-type domains responsible for binding the Cε3 region of IgE (Figure 15.1), whereas the γ chains and β chain each contain a cytoplasmic *i*mmunoreceptor *t*yrosine-based *a*ctivation *m*otif (ITAM) for cell signaling. In the absence of bound IgE the level of FcεRI drops substantially. However, in its presence there is upregulation of the receptor on mast cells and, because the γ chain is shared with the mast cell FcγRIIIA, a consequent competitive downregulation of the Fc receptor for IgG. Anaphylaxis is mediated by the reaction of the allergen with the IgE antibodies held on the surface of the mast cell, cross-linking of these antibodies triggering mediator release (Figure 15.2). The critical event is aggregation of the receptors by cross-linking as clearly shown by the ability of divalent antibodies reacting directly with the receptor to trigger the mast cell.

Aggregation of the FcεRI α chains activates the Lyn and Fyn protein tyrosine kinases associated with the β chains and, if the aggregates persist, this leads to transphosphorylation of the β and γ chains of other FcεRI receptors within the cluster and recruitment of the Syk kinase (Figure 15.3). The subsequent series of phosphorylation-induced activation steps ultimately leads to mast cell degranulation with release of preformed mediators and the synthesis of arachidonic acid metabolites formed by the cyclo-oxygenase and lipoxygenase pathways (cf. Figure 1.21). To recapitulate, the preformed mediators released from the granules include histamine,

heparin, tryptase, chymase, carboxypeptidase, eosinophil, neutrophil and monocyte chemotactic factors, platelet activating factor and serotonin. By contrast, leukotrienes LTB$_4$, LTC$_4$ and LTD$_4$, the prostaglandin PGD$_2$ and thromboxanes are all newly synthesized. The Th2-type cytokines IL-4, IL-5, IL-6, IL-9, IL-10, IL-13, as well as IL-1, IL-3, IL-8, IL-11, *g*ranulocyte–*m*acrophage *c*olony-*s*timulating *f*actor (GM-CSF), TNF (tumor necrosis factor), CCL2 (*m*onocyte *c*hemotactic *p*rotein-1, MCP-1), CCL5 (RANTES) and CCL11 (eotaxin), are all also released. Under normal circumstances, these mediators help to orchestrate the development of a defensive acute inflammatory reaction (and in this context let us not forget that complement fragments C3a and C5a can also trigger mast cells through complement receptors). When there is a massive release of these mediators under abnormal conditions, as in atopic disease, their bronchoconstrictive and vasodilatory effects predominate and become distinctly threatening.

Atopic allergy

The allergy march

Food allergy, eczema (atopic dermatitis), **hayfever** (seasonal allergic conjunctivitis and rhinitis) and **asthma** often occur in the same individual. Indeed in many individuals allergies develop in an ordered sequence that has been referred to as the "allergy march" (Figure 15.4). Thus gastrointestinal and

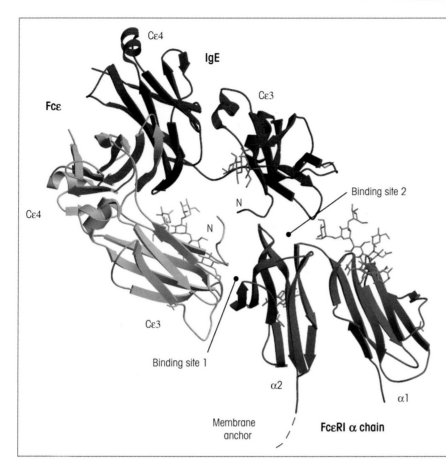

Figure 15.1. The structural basis of the binding of IgE to the high-affinity mast cell receptor FcεRI.

Side view of the complex with the two Fc chains in yellow and red and the FcεRI α chain in blue; carbohydrate residues are shown as sticks. The two Cε3 domains of the heavy chain dimer of IgE bind asymmetrically to two distinct interaction sites on the α chain of the receptor. The β-turn loop on one Cε3 binds along one side of the α2 domain, while surface loops plus the Cε2–Cε3 linker region on the other Cε3 interact with the top of the α1–α2 interface. The 1:1 stoichiometry of this asymmetric binding precludes the linkage of one IgE to two receptor molecules and ensures that triggering due to α–α aggregation only occurs through multivalent binding to surface IgE (see Figure 15.2). (Photograph kindly provided by Ted Jardetzky and reproduced by permission of the Nature Publishing Group.)

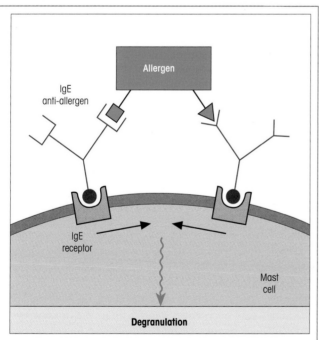

Figure 15.2. Clustering of IgE receptors

Cross-linking of FcεRI by binding of multivalent allergen to IgE sensitizing the mast cell leads to degranulation. Note that the two antibodies are against different epitopes on the same allergen, and therefore will need to be represented on the mast cell surface at a reasonably high frequency in order for efficient cross-linking to occur.

cutaneous allergies developing early in life can be followed later on by asthma and hayfever.

Clinical responses to extrinsic allergens

It has been claimed that in westernized countries up to 30% of adults and 45% of children may suffer to a greater or lesser degree with allergies involving localized IgE-mediated reactions to allergens such as grass pollens, animal danders, the feces from mites in house dust (Figure 15.5) and so on. Even if these are overestimates, it is clear that allergies affect a large number of people and that they are on the increase. A large number of allergens have now been cloned and expressed (Table 15.2), several of which turn out to be enzymes. For example, Der p 1 is a cysteine protease that increases the permeability of the bronchial mucosa, thereby facilitating its own passage along with other allergens across the epithelium and allowing access to and sensitization of cells of the immune system. The CD23 low affinity receptor for IgE (FcεRII) on B-cells downregulates IgE synthesis upon antigen-mediated cross-linking of the bound IgE. However, Der p 1 proteolytically cleaves CD23 and thereby reduces its negative impact on IgE synthesis. Furthermore, Der p 1 also cleaves CD25 (the IL-2 receptor α chain) on T-cells and thus limits the activation of Th1 cells, biasing the immune response to Th2-dependent

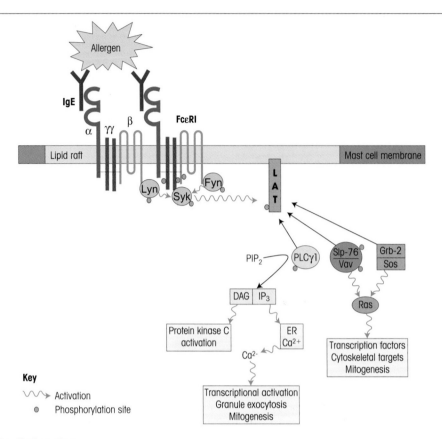

Figure 15.3. Mast cell triggering.

Simplified scheme of some of the signaling events through the high affinity IgE receptor, FcεRI. Aggregation of the FcεRI α chains in lipid rafts through cross-linking of bound IgE by multivalent antigen (allergen) leads to ITAMs in the β and γ chains of the receptor interacting with the Lyn, Syk and Fyn protein tyrosine kinases. Phosphorylation of Syk leads to its activation and it in turn phosphorylates and activates the membrane adaptor LAT1 and LAT2 (NTAL) proteins that recruit phospholipase Cγ1 (PLCγ1) and adaptor molecules concerned in the activation of GTPase/kinase cascades. Activation of PLCγ1 generates diacylglycerol (DAG) that targets protein kinase C, while inositol 1,4,5-triphosphate (IP₃) elevates cytoplasmic Ca²⁺ by depleting the ER stores. The raised calcium concentration activates transcriptional factors and causes granule exocytosis. The Grb-2/Sos and Slp-76/Vav complexes associate with the LAT1 adaptor, and Grb-2/Sos additionally with LAT2, and trigger the Ras GTPase-induced serial kinase cascade leading to the activation of transcription factors and rearrangements of the actin cytoskeleton. (Figure essentially designed by Helen Turner, based on the article by Turner H. & Kinet J.-P. (1999) *Nature* (Supplement on Allergy and Asthma) **402**, B24.)

IgE production. Short cuts to allergen purification can be achieved by screening cDNA expression libraries with IgE. This was a godsend for the purification of the allergen from the venom of the Australian jumper ant, *Myrmecia pilosula;* just think of trying to accumulate ants by the kilogram to isolate the allergen using conventional protein fractionation.

The local anaphylactic reaction to injection of antigen into the skin of atopic patients is manifest as a weal and flare (Figure 15.6), which is maximal at 30 minutes or so and resolves within about an hour; it may be succeeded by a late phase response involving eosinophil infiltrates that peak at around 5 hours. Contact of the allergen with cell-bound IgE in the bronchial tree, the nasal mucosa and the conjunctival tissues releases mediators of anaphylaxis and produces the symptoms of **asthma** or **allergic rhinitis and conjunctivitis** (hay fever) as the case may be. A proportion of the patients who experience late phase responses after bronchial challenge with allergen eventually develop chronic **asthma**. Three hundred million individuals worldwide suffer from asthma and it costs over US$6 billion a year to treat in the USA alone. Indeed, according to the World Health Organization, the worldwide economic costs associated with asthma are estimated to exceed those of tuberculosis and HIV/AIDS combined. Asthma can be associated with agents encountered in the workplace, and is then described as **occupational asthma**. Allergens here include toluene diisocyanate in spray paints, colophony fumes

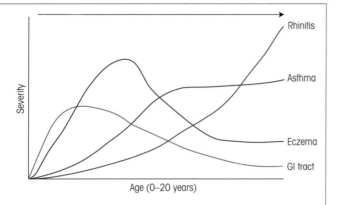

Figure 15.4. The allergy march.

In many children there is a temporal progression in the development of allergies. (Modified with kind permission from a figure produced by Ulrich Wahn for the World Allergy Organization (http://www.worldallergy.org)).

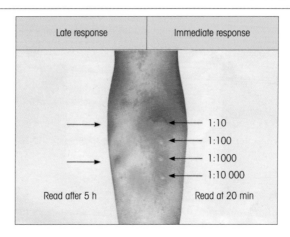

Figure 15.6. Atopic allergy.

Skin prick tests with grass pollen allergen in a patient with typical summer hay fever. Skin tests were performed 5 hours (left) and 20 minutes (right) before the photograph was taken. The tests on the right show a typical titration of a type I immediate weal and flare reaction. The late phase skin reaction (left) can be clearly seen at 5 hours, especially where a large immediate response has preceded it. Figures for allergen dilution are given.

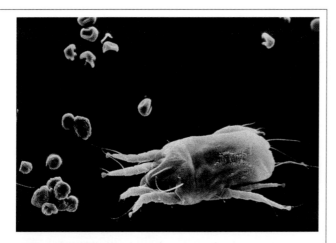

Figure 15.5. House dust mite—a major cause of allergic disease. The electron micrograph shows the rather nasty looking mite graced by the name *Dermatophagoides pteronyssinus* and fecal pellets on the bottom left. A typical double bed can contain up to 200 million mites, each mite producing approximately 20 fecal pellets/day and each pellet containing 0.2 ng of proteolytically active Der p 1 allergen. The biconcave pollen grains (top left) shown for comparison indicate the size of particle that can become airborne and reach the lungs. The mite itself is much too large for that. (Reproduced by courtesy of E. Tovey.)

Bronchial biopsy and lavage of asthmatic patients reveal an unequivocal involvement of **mast cells and eosinophils** as the major mediator-secreting effector cells, while T-cells provide the microenvironment required to sustain the chronic inflammatory response, which is an essential feature of the histopathology (Figure 15.7). The resulting variable airflow obstruction and bronchial hyper-responsiveness are the cardinal clinical and physiological features of the disease.

The atopic trait can also manifest itself as an **atopic dermatitis** (eczema) (Figure 15.8), with house dust mite, domestic cats and German cockroaches often proving to be the environmental offenders. Recalling the inflammation in asthma, skin patch tests with Der p 1 in these eczema patients produce an infiltrate of eosinophils, T-cells, mast cells and basophils. The number of individuals affected is comparable to the number affected by asthma. The beneficial effect of the calcineurin inhibitors cyclosporine and, more recently, topical tacrolimus in patients with eczema highlights the important role of T-cells in the pathogenesis of this disease.

Awareness of IgE sensitization to **food allergens** in the gut has increased dramatically. Contact with allergens such as those present in cows' milk, eggs, nuts and shellfish before mucosal protective mechanisms, especially IgA, are reasonably established leads to an increase in the incidence of atopy in the newborn (Figure 15.4). Although, overall, children who are breastfed have a lower incidence of allergies, sensitization to dietary allergens can also occur in early infancy through breastfeeding, with antigen passing into the mother's milk.

from solders used in the electronics industry and danders (particles of old skin on animal hair) encountered by animal handlers. Although the majority of asthma patients have **extrinsic asthma** associated with **atopy** (from the Greek *atopos,* meaning "out of place"), i.e. the genetic predisposition to synthesize inappropriate levels of IgE specific for external allergens, some patients are nonatopic and therefore are said to have **intrinsic or idiopathic asthma**.

Table 15.2. Some examples of allergens.

Category	Origin	Allergens	Example
Insect	House dust mite (*Dermatophagoides pteronyssinus*) feces	Der p 1–Der p 14	Der p 1: cysteine protease
	Honeybee (*Apis mellifera*) venom	Api m 1–7	Api m 1: phospholipase A$_2$
	German cockroach (*Blattella germanica*)	Bla g 1–6	Bla g 2: aspartic protease
Companion animals	Cat (*Felis domesticus*)	Fel d 1–7	Fel d 4: lipocalin
	Dog (*Canis domesticus*)	Can f 1–4	Can f 3: albumin
Trees	Birch (*Betula verrucosa*)	Bet v 1–7	Bet v7: cyclophilin
	Hazel (*Corylus avellana*)	Cor a 1–11	Cor a 8: lipid transfer protein
Grasses and plants	Timothy grass (*Phleum pretense*)	Phl p 1–13	Phl p 13: polygalacturonase
	Perennial ryegrass (*Lolium perenne*)	Lol p 1–11	Lol p 11: trypsin inhibitor
	Short ragweed (*Ambrosia artemisiifolia*)	Amb a 1–7	Amb a 5: neurophysin
Molds	*Aspergillus fumigatus*	Asp f 1–23	Asp f 12: heat shock protein p90
	Cladosporium herbarum	Cla h 1–12	Cla h 3: aldehyde dehydrogenase
Foods	Peanut	Ara h 1–8	Ara h 1: vicilin
	Cows' milk (*Bos domesticus*)	Bos d 1–8	Bos d 4: α-lactalbumin
	Chickens' eggs (*Gallus domesticus*)	Gal d 1–5	Gal d 2: ovalbumin
Drugs	Penicillin	–	Amoxicillin
	Fluoroquinolone	–	Ciprofloxacin
Occupational allergens	Toluene diisocyanate	–	–
	Latex (derived from the rubber tree, *Hevea brasiliensis*)	Hev b 1–13	Hev b 1: elongation factor

For a complete list see International Union of Immunological Societies Allergen Nomenclature Sub-Committee http://www.allergen.org

One could argue that breastfeeding mothers should limit their intake of common allergens. Allergy to peanuts is seen in approximately 1% of children and, as with other allergens, reactions are sometimes life threatening or even occasionally fatal. Food additives such as sulfiting agents can also cause adverse reactions. Contact of the food with specific IgE on mast cells in the gastrointestinal tract may produce local reactions resulting in abdominal pain, cramps, diarrhea and vomiting, or may allow the allergen to enter the body by causing a change in gut permeability through mediator release; the allergen may complex with antibodies and cause distal lesions by depositing in the joints, for example, or it may diffuse freely to other sensitized sites, such as the skin (Figure 15.8) or lungs, where it will cause a further local anaphylactic reaction. Thus eating strawberries may produce **urticarial reactions** (**hives**, raised areas of itchy skin) and egg may precipitate an asthmatic attack in appropriately sensitized individuals. The role of the sensitized gut in acting as a "gate" to allow entry of allergens is strongly suggested by experiments in which oral sodium cromoglycate, a mast cell stabilizer, prevented subsequent asthma after ingestion of the provoking food (Figure 15.9).

Anaphylactic drug allergy is manifest in the dramatic responses to drugs such as **penicillin**, which haptenate body proteins by covalent coupling to induce IgE synthesis. In the case of penicillin, the β-lactam ring links to the ε-amino of lysine to form the penicilloyl determinant. The fine specificity of the IgE antibodies permits discrimination between closely similar drugs, such that some patients may be allergic to amoxicillin but tolerate benzylpenicillin, which differs by only very minor modifications of the side chains.

Pathological mechanisms in asthma

We should now look in more depth at those events that generate the chronicity of asthma. Remember that there is an *early phase* bronchial response to inhaled antigen essentially involving mast cell mediators, and an inflammatory *late phase* dominated by eosinophils. **Both phases are IgE-dependent** as shown by their marked attenuation in asthmatics treated with the humanized monoclonal anti-IgE antibody Omalizumab, which reduces IgE to almost undetectable levels. Activated mast cells produce IL-11, which contributes towards the development of the asthma-associated structural changes

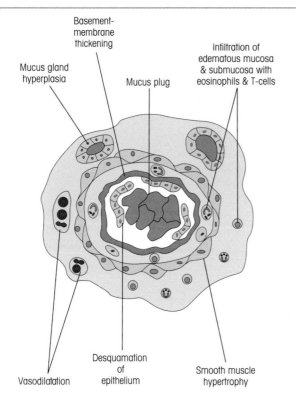

Figure 15.7. Pathological changes in asthma.

Diagram of cross-section of an airway in severe asthma.

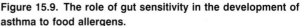

Figure 15.9. The role of gut sensitivity in the development of asthma to food allergens.

A patient challenged by feeding with egg developed asthma within hours, as shown here by the depressed lung function test of measuring peak air flow; the symptoms at the end-organ stage were counteracted by the β-adrenoreceptor agonist, isoprenaline. However, oral sodium cromoglycate (SCG), which prevents antigen-specific mast cell triggering, also prevented the onset of asthma after oral challenge with egg. Note that SCG taken orally has no effect on the response of an asthmatic to inhaled allergen. (From Brostoff J. (1986), In Brostoff J. & Challacombe S.J. (eds) *Food Allergy*, p. 441. Baillière Tindall, London, reproduced with permission.)

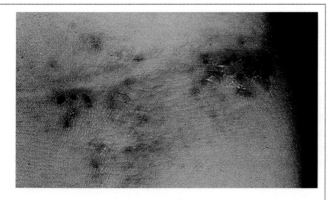

Figure 15.8. An atopic eczema reaction on the back of a knee of a child allergic to rice and eggs.

(Kindly provided by J. Brostoff.)

referred to as **airway remodeling**; thickening of the airway walls, and increases in the adventitia (the outermost connective tissue), submucosal tissue and smooth muscle. The mast cells also contribute to eosinophil recruitment by secretion of tryptase, which can activate coagulation Factor II receptor-like 1 (F2RL1, protease-activated receptor-2 [PAR-2]) on the surface of endothelial and epithelial cells, fibroblasts and smooth muscle. Activation of the receptor leads to TNF, IL-1 and IL-4 production, promoting the expression of the vascular endothelial adhesion molecules VCAM-1, ICAM-1 and P-selectin, which recruit eosinophils and basophils. An important trigger of the late phase reaction is the **activation of alveolar macrophages** through the interaction of allergen with IgE bound to the low affinity FcεRII leading to a significant increase in the production of TNF and IL-1β. These cytokines stimulate the release of the powerful **eosinophil chemoattractants** CCL5 (RANTES), CCL11 (eotaxin), and CCL12 (MCP5) (cf. p. 232) from bronchial epithelial cells and fibroblasts. Note also that CCL5 and CCL11 can contribute directly to local inflammation by IgE-independent degranulation of basophils.

A new player now enters the field: primed T-cells traffic into the inflamed site under the influence of CCL11. The GATA-3 transcription factor, c-maf and the presence of prostaglandin E_2 all promote **Th2 development**, and responses are heavily skewed towards this particular T-cell subset in **asthma** (Figure 15.10). Encounter with allergen-derived peptides on antigen-presenting cells will promote the synthesis of IL-4, -5 and -13. IL-4 stimulates further CCL11 release, while IL-5 upregulates chemokine receptors on eosinophils, maintains their survival through an inhibitory effect on natural apoptosis and is involved in their longer term recruitment from bone marrow. Th17 cells are also present and promote

Figure 15.10. Th2 dominance in atopic allergy.

Shown by cytokine profiles of antigen-specific CD4 T-cell clones from (a) patients with type I atopic allergy and (b) subjects with type IV contact sensitivity, compared with normal controls. Each point represents the value for an individual clone. Archetypal Th1 clones have high IFNγ and IL-2 and low IL-4 and IL-5; Th2 clones show the converse. The high level of IL-4 drives the switch to IgE production by B-cells and further promotes the Th2 bias. (Data from Kapsenberg M.L., Wierenga E.A., Bos J.D. & Jansen H.M. (1991) *Immunology Today* **12**, 392.)

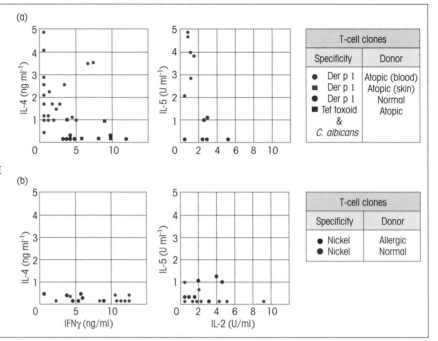

both neutrophil and macrophage inflammatory responses in the lung.

Things now look bad for the bronchial tissues and a multitude of factors contribute to allergen-induced airway dysfunction: (i) a virtual soup of bronchoconstrictors, the leukotrienes being especially important, bathe the smooth muscle cells; (ii) edema of the airway wall; (iii) altered neural regulation of airway tone through binding of eosinophil major basic protein (MBP) to M2 autoreceptors on the nerve endings with increased release of acetylcholine; (iv) airway epithelial cell desquamation due to the toxic action of MBP, there being a strong correlation between the number of desquamated cells in bronchoalveolar lavage fluid and the concentration of MBP; (v) mucus hypersecretion due to IL-13 and, to a lesser extent, IL-4, leukotrienes and platelet activating factor acting on submucosal glands and their controlling neural elements; and finally (vi) a repair-type response involving the production of fibroblast growth factor, TGFβ and platelet-derived growth factor, the laying down of collagen, scar and fibrous tissue and hypertrophy of smooth muscle, leading to an exaggerated narrowing of the airways in response to a variety of environmental stimuli (Figure 15.7). The wide range of cytokines and mediators produced by lung epithelial and endothelial cells, fibroblasts and smooth muscle cells may account for the persistence of airway inflammation and the permanent structural changes in chronic disease sufferers, even in the absence or apparent absence of ongoing exposure to inhalant allergens to which subjects are sensitized, a state where conventional immunotherapy might not be expected to be beneficial.

Unlike atopic asthmatics, **intrinsic asthmatics** have negative skin tests to common aeroallergens, no clinical or family history of allergy, normal levels of serum IgE and no detectable specific IgE antibodies to common allergens. Nonetheless, they resemble the atopics in important respects: bronchial biopsies show enhanced expression of IL-4, IL-13, CCL5 and CCL11, and of the mRNA for the ε heavy chain, suggestive of local IgE synthesis. Is there a role for virus-specific IgE or for IgE autoantibodies to the FcεRI?

The inflammatory infiltrate in **atopic dermatitis** resembles that in asthma and includes mast cells, basophils, eosinophils and T-cells. Epidermal dendritic cells express FcεRI, and incoming allergens are taken up as allergen–IgE complexes and passed to the MHC class II processing pathway for presentation to Th2 cells. CC chemokines produced by keratinocytes and fibroblasts preferentially attract eosinophils and the skin-homing CLA+ memory Th2-cells. The latter comprise 80–90% of the T-cells in the infiltrate and account for the specific response to the offending allergen.

Etiological factors in the development of atopic allergy

There is a strong familial predisposition to the development of atopic allergy (Figure 15.11) suggestive of genetic factors. Indeed, it is clear that the development of atopic allergy depends upon complex multiple genetic interactions with various environmental factors. Age, sex, infection history, nutritional status and allergen exposure all play a role. One obvious factor is the overall ability to synthesize the IgE isotype—the higher the level of IgE in the blood, the greater the likelihood of becoming atopic (Figure 15.11). Genetic studies have provided evidence that many different genes

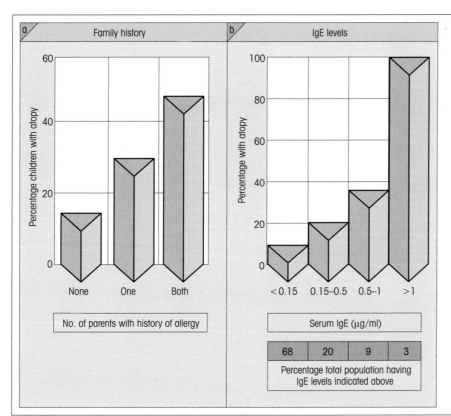

Figure 15.11. Risk factors in allergy

(a) Family history; (b) IgE levels—the higher the serum IgE concentration, the greater the chance of developing atopy.

contribute to susceptibility to develop asthma (Figure 15.12) although no one single gene is a particularly strong predisposing factor on its own. One interesting association, however, is with polymorphisms in a number of pattern recognition receptors (PRR). What relevance might this have for atopic disease? Well, the PRR-mediated recognition of pathogens by dendritic cells is important in developing the correct balance between Th1 and Th2 responses. Current thinking goes along the following lines. At the time of birth the neonatal immune system is skewed towards Th2-type responses, but in the face of a hostile microbial environment there is a shift towards Th1 responses. This shift extends to inhaled allergens, and is sometimes referred to as immune deviation. However, in the absence of repeated infections with common pathogens (due to a "cleaner" environment and widespread early use of antibiotics) the immune system maintains a Th2 phenotype, which will favor the secretion of IL-4 (promoting IgE production) and IL-5 (promoting eosinophilia). This idea forms the basis of the hygiene hypothesis put forward to explain the rise in allergies seen in highly developed countries, and even more tellingly in countries that *become* highly developed, such as the former East Germany where levels of atopic allergy started to catch up with those in West Germany following re-unification. The overall picture relating to economic development is, however, complex—let us not forget that a finger has been pointed at environmental pollutants such as diesel exhaust particles as cofactors for asthma attacks.

Recently there has also been a great deal of interest in trying to understand the role of the barrier function of the epithelium in allergic responses. Compromise of the normally tight junctions between the epithelial cells, perhaps caused by chemical or physical pollutants or by infection, will clearly lead to increased access of both pathogens and allergens. Yet another piece of the jigsaw relates to the role of regulatory T-cells (Tregs) in atopic disease. Evidence is accumulating that indicates a deficit of these cells in patients with allergy, with both naturally-occuring CD4+CD25+Foxp3+ Tregs and inducible Tregs being implicated. The Tregs may themselves be influenced by interactions with distinct dendritic cell subsets. And where do Th17 cells fit into all of this? Watch this space, as they say.

Clinical tests for allergy

Sensitivity is normally assessed by the response to intradermal challenge with antigen. The release of histamine and other mediators rapidly produces a **weal and erythema** (see Figure 15.6), maximal within 30 minutes and then subsiding. These immediate weal and flare reactions may be followed by a late phase reaction (see Figure 15.6), which sometimes lasts for 24 hours, redolent of those seen following challenge of the bronchi and nasal mucosa of allergic subjects and similarly characterized by dense infiltration with eosinophils and T-cells.

The correlation between skin prick test responses and the **radioallergosorbent test** (RAST, see p. 167) for

Figure 15.12. Gene products that influence susceptibility to asthma.

Multiple genes have been implicated that act at various stages in the type I hypersensitivity response. ADAM33, disintegrin and metalloprotein domain-containing protein 33; DPP10, dipeptidyl peptidase 10; NPSR1, neuropeptide S receptor 1; PCDH1, protocadherin-1; PTGDR, prostaglandin D_2 receptor; TIM1, T-cell, immunoglobulin and mucin domain-containing protein 1. (Modified from Cookson W. & Moffatt M. (2004) *New England Journal of Medicine* **351**, 1794–1796, with permission from the publishers.)

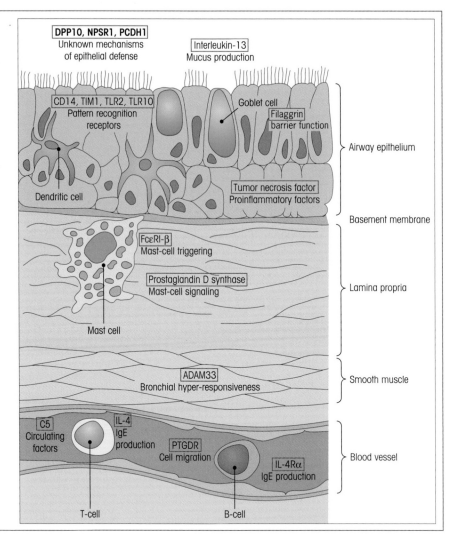

allergen-specific serum IgE is fairly good. In some instances, intranasal challenge with allergen may provoke a response even when both of these tests are negative, probably as a result of local synthesis of IgE antibodies.

The presence of proteins secreted from mast cells or eosinophils in the serum or urine could provide important surrogate markers of disease and might predict exacerbations.

Therapy

If one considers the sequence of reactions from initial exposure to allergen right through to the production of atopic disease, it can be seen that several points in the chain provide legitimate targets for therapy (Figure 15.13).

Allergen avoidance. Avoidance of contact with *potential* allergens is often impractical, although, to give one example, feeding cows' milk to infants at too early an age is discouraged. After sensitization, avoidance where possible is obviously worthwhile, but the reluctance of some parents to dispose of the family cat to stop little Algernon's wheezing is sometimes quite surprising.

Modulation of the immunological response. Desensitization by repeated **subcutaneous injection** of small amounts of allergen can lead to worthwhile improvement in individuals subject to insect venom anaphylaxis or hay fever. **Sublingual allergen immunotherapy** (SLIT) is less time consuming for the patient and carries less risk of severe systemic reactions than subcutaneous administration; but this has to be balanced against the fact that it is sometimes not quite as effective as injection immunotherapy. The purpose of allergen hyposensitization therapy was originally to boost the synthesis of IgG "blocking" antibodies, whose function was to divert the allergen from contact with tissue-bound IgE. While this may well be a contributory factor, downregulation of IgE synthesis by engagement of the FcγRIIB receptor (cf. p. 264) on B-cells by allergen-specific IgG linked to allergen molecules bound to surface IgE receptors also seems likely (cf. p. 264; see Chapter 10 on IgG regulation of Ab production). Additionally, T-lymphocyte cooperation is important for IgE synthesis and eosinophil-mediated pathogenesis, and therefore the beneficial effects of antigen injection may also be mediated through induction of anergic or regulatory T-cells and a switch from Th2 to Th1 cytokine production.

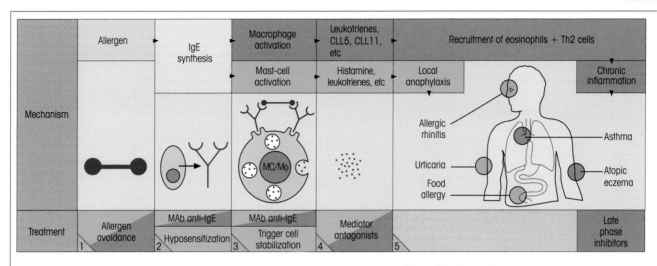

Figure 15.13. Atopic allergies and their treatment: sites of local responses and possible therapies.

Events and treatments relating to local anaphylaxis are in green and to chronic inflammation in red. MAb, monoclonal antibody.

Injection of heat-killed *Mycobacterium vaccae* induces IL-10 and TGFβ secretion by regulatory T-cells with a resultant decrease in Th2 activity. Inhibition of the Th2-associated transcription factor GATA-3 using PPAR (peroxisome proliferator-activated receptor) agonists, or stimulating Th1-associated T-bet expression with CpG motifs, may provide future therapeutic options for promoting Th1 rather than Th2 responses. The administration of tolerizing or antagonist peptide epitopes represents another possible therapeutic modality. Fortunately, most patients respond to a remarkably limited number of T-cell epitopes on any given allergen, and so it may not be necessary to tailor the therapeutic peptide to each individual. Clinical trials of immunotherapy with Fel d 1-derived peptides from cat allergen have resulted in a decrease of both early and late-phase reactions. A case can be made for future prophylactic hyposensitization of children with two asthmatic parents given that such youngsters have an approximately 50% probability of developing the disease.

Blocking the action of IgE. We have already mentioned the humanized monoclonal **Omalizumab** directed against the FcεRI-binding Cε3 domain of IgE (cf. p. 396), which provides an exciting new therapy for severe forms of asthma. It reduces the circulating IgE levels almost to vanishing point by direct neutralization, and as a secondary effect this decreases the IgE-dependent expression of the FcεRI receptor on mast cells. Thus there are far fewer receptors on the mast cell to bind IgE, and virtually no IgE to be bound anyway. It is not surprising therefore that this antibody successfully completed phase II clinical trials and was subsequently approved by the FDA for use in those adults and adolescents with moderate or severe persistent atopic asthma whose symptoms are inadequately controlled with inhaled corticosteroids.

Stabilization of the triggering cells. Much relief has been obtained with agents such as inhalant **isoprenaline** and

sodium cromoglycate (cromolyn sodium), which render mast cells resistant to triggering. Sodium cromoglycate blocks chloride channel activity and maintains cells in a normal resting physiological state, which probably accounts for its inhibitory effects on a wide range of cellular functions, such as mast cell degranulation, eosinophil and neutrophil chemotaxis and mediator release, and reflex bronchoconstriction. Some or all of these effects are responsible for its anti-asthmatic actions.

The triggering of macrophages through allergen interaction with surface-bound IgE is clearly a major initiating factor for late reactions, as discussed above, and resistance to this stimulus can be very effectively achieved with corticosteroids. Unquestionably, **inhaled corticosteroids** have revolutionized the treatment of asthma. Their principal action is to suppress the transcription of multiple inflammatory genes, including in the present context those encoding several cytokines.

Mediator antagonism. **Histamine H₁-receptor antagonists** have for long proved helpful in the symptomatic treatment of atopic disease. Newer drugs of this class such as **loratadine** and **fexofenadine** are effective in rhinitis and in reducing the itch in atopic dermatitis, although they have little benefit in asthma. **Cetirizine** additionally has useful effects on eosinophil recruitment in the late phase reaction. Short-acting selective **β₂-agonists** such as Ventolin, the active ingredient of which is **albuterol** (salbutamol), are inhaled to alleviate mild-to-moderate symptoms of asthma. Such β-adrenergic receptor agonist drugs increase cAMP levels leading to relaxation of bronchial smooth muscle and inhibition of mast cell degranulation. An important advance has been the introduction of **long-acting β₂-agonists** such as **salmeterol** and **formoterol,** which protect against bronchoconstriction for over 12 hours. Potent **leukotriene receptor antagonists** such as **pranlukast** also block constrictor challenges and show striking efficacy in certain patients, particularly aspirin-sensitive asthmatics.

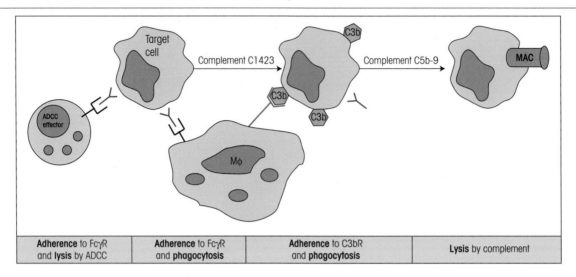

Figure 15.14. Antibody-dependent cytotoxic hypersensitivity (type II).

Antibodies directed against cell surface antigens cause cell death not only by complement-dependent lysis using the C5b–C9 membrane attack complex (MAC) but also by Fcγ and C3b adherence reactions leading to phagocytosis, or through nonphagocytic extracellular killing by **antibody-dependent cellular cytotoxicity (ADCC)**. Human monocytes and IFNγ-activated neutrophils kill Ab-coated tumor cells using their FcγRI receptors; NK cells kill targets through FcγRIII receptors.

Theophylline was introduced for the treatment of asthma over 60 years ago and, as a **phosphodiesterase (PDE) inhibitor**, it increases intracellular cAMP, thereby causing bronchodilatation. Generally good news for the patient, although concern over some of its side effects mean that it is often only used when other treatment options prove ineffective.

Attacking chronic inflammation. Certain drugs impede atopic disease at more than one stage. **Cetirizine** is a case in point with its dual effects on the histamine receptor and on eosinophil recruitment. **Corticosteroids** seem to do almost everything; apart from their role in stabilizing macrophages, they solidly inhibit the activation and proliferation of Th2 cells, which are the dominant underlying driving force in chronic asthma, and may call a halt to the development of irreversible narrowing of the airways. So it is that inhaled steroids (e.g. budesonide, mometasone furoate, fluticasone propionate) with high anti-inflammatory potency but minimal side-effects due to hepatic metabolism, provide first-line therapy for most chronic asthmatics, with supplementation by long-acting β_2-agonists.

Antibody-dependent cytotoxic hypersensitivity (type II)

Where an antigen is present on the surface of a cell, combination with antibody will encourage the demise of that cell by promoting contact with phagocytes by **opsonic adherence** to Fcγ receptors and, often, to C3b receptors following activation of complement by the classical pathway. Cell death may also occur through activation of the full complement system up to C8 and C9 producing **direct membrane damage** (Figure 15.14), although this will have to overcome the protective effect of cell surface complement regulatory proteins.

A quite distinct cytotoxic mechanism, **antibody-dependent cellular cytotoxicity (ADCC)**, occurs when target cells coated with antibody are killed through an extracellular nonphagocytic process involving leukocytes that bind to the target by their specific Fc receptors, e.g. FcγR in the case of IgG (Figure 15.14). ADCC can be mediated by a number of different types of leukocyte including NK cells (see p. 26), monocytes, neutrophils and eosinophils. Although readily observed as a phenomenon *in vitro*, e.g. schistosomules coated with either IgG or IgE can be killed by eosinophils (cf. Figure 12.25), whether ADCC plays a role *in vivo* remains a tricky question. Functionally this extracellular cytotoxic mechanism would be expected to be of significance where the target is too large for ingestion by phagocytosis, e.g. large parasites and solid tumors. It could also act as a back-up system for T-cell mediated killing.

Type II reactions between members of the same species (alloimmune)

Transfusion reactions

Of the many different polymorphic constituents of the human red cell membrane, **ABO blood groups** form the dominant system. The antigenic groups A and B are derived from H substance (Figure 15.15) by the action of glycosyltransferases encoded by *A* or *B* genes, respectively. Individuals with both genes (group AB) have the two antigens on their red cells, while those lacking these genes (group O) synthesize H substance

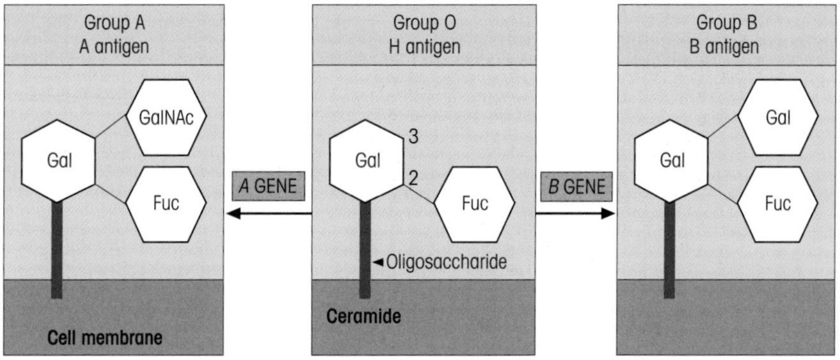

Figure 15.15. The ABO system.

The allelic genes A and B code for transferases that add either *N*-acetylgalactosamine (GalNAc) or galactose (Gal), respectively, to H substance. The oligosaccharide is anchored to the cell membrane by coupling to a sphingomyelin called ceramide.

Eighty-five percent of the population secrete blood group substances in the saliva, where the oligosaccharides are present as soluble polypeptide conjugates formed under the action of a secretor (*se*) gene. Fuc, fucose.

Table 15.3. ABO blood groups and serum antibodies.

Blood group (phenotype)	Genotype	Antigen	Serum antibody
A	AA,AO	A	ANTI-B
B	BB,BO	B	ANTI-A
AB	AB	A and B	NONE
O	OO	H	ANTI-A ANTI-B

only. Antibodies to A or B occur spontaneously when the antigen is absent from the red cell surface; thus a person of blood group A will possess anti-B and so on. These **isohemagglutinins** are usually IgM and probably belong to the class of "natural antibodies"; they would be boosted through contact with antigens of the gut flora that are structurally similar to the blood group carbohydrates, so that the antibodies formed cross-react with the appropriate red cell type. If an individual is blood group A, she/he would be tolerant to antigens closely similar to A and would only form cross-reacting antibodies capable of agglutinating B red cells; similarly an O individual would make anti-A and anti-B (Table 15.3). On transfusion, mismatched red cells will be coated by the isohemagglutinins, which will cause severe complement-mediated intravascular hemolysis.

Clinical refractoriness to platelet transfusions is frequently due to HLA alloimmunization, but one can usually circumvent this problem by depleting the platelets of leukocytes.

Rhesus incompatibility

The **rhesus (Rh) blood groups** form the other major antigenic system, the RhD antigen being of the most consequence for

isoimmune reactions. A mother with an RhD –ve blood group (i.e. *dd* genotype) can readily be sensitized by red cells from a baby carrying RhD antigens (*DD* or *Dd* genotype). This occurs most often at the birth of the first child when a placental bleed can release a large number of the baby's erythrocytes into the mother. The antibodies formed are predominantly of the IgG class and, unlike the IgM anti-A and anti-B mentioned above for the ABO blood group system, are therefore able to cross the placenta in any subsequent pregnancy. Reaction with the D-antigen on the fetal red cells leads to their destruction through opsonic adherence, giving hemolytic disease of the newborn (Figure 15.16a and b).

These anti-D antibodies fail to agglutinate RhD +ve red cells *in vitro* ("incomplete antibodies") because the low density of antigenic sites does not allow sufficient antibody bridges to be formed between the negatively charged erythrocytes to overcome the electrostatic repulsive forces. Erythrocytes coated with anti-D can be made to agglutinate by addition of an anti-immunoglobulin serum (Coombs' reagent; Figure 15.17).

If a mother has natural isohemagglutinins that can react with any fetal erythrocytes reaching her circulation, sensitization to the D-antigens is less likely due to "deviation" of the red cells away from the antigen-sensitive cells. For example, a

Figure 15.16. Hemolytic disease of the newborn due to rhesus incompatibility.

(a) RhD +ve red cells from the first baby sensitize the RhD –ve mother. (b) The mother's IgG anti-D crosses the placenta and coats the erythrocytes of the second RhD +ve baby causing type II hypersensitivity hemolytic disease.
(c) IgG anti-D given prophylactically during the first pregnancy and birth removes the baby's red cells through phagocytosis and prevents sensitization of the mother.

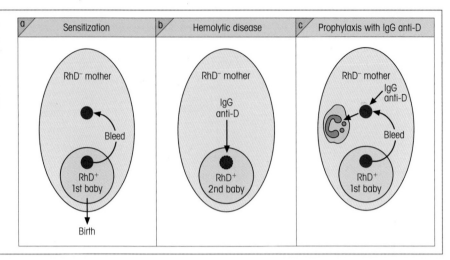

Figure 15.17. The Coombs' test for antibody-coated red cells.

This test is used for detecting rhesus antibodies and in the diagnosis of autoimmune hemolytic anemia. (Photographs courtesy of A. Cooke.)

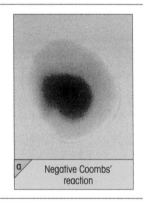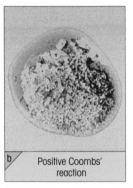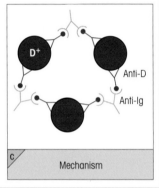

group O RhD –ve mother with a group A RhD +ve baby would destroy any fetal erythrocytes with her anti-A before they could immunize to produce anti-D. In an extension of this principle, **RhD –ve mothers are treated prophylactically with IgG anti-D at 28 weeks and 34 weeks gestation and then again at the time of birth if the baby is RhD +ve** (Figure 15.16c). This greatly reduces the risk of sensitization—another success for immunology.

Another disease resulting from transplacental passage of maternal antibodies is **neonatal alloimmune thrombocytopenia**. The fall in platelet numbers is greatly ameliorated by i.v. injections of pooled human IgG (IVIg). The efficacy of Fcγ fragments and of anti-FcγR suggests that this works by blockade of the Fcγ receptors.

Organ transplants

Allografts can evoke humoral antibodies in the host directed against surface transplantation antigens. These may be directly cytotoxic or cause adherence of phagocytic cells or attack by ADCC. The antibodies may also lead to platelet adherence when they bind antigens on the surface of the vascular endothe-

lium (Figure 16.6, p. 427). Hyperacute rejection is mediated by preformed antibodies in the graft recipient.

Autoimmune type II hypersensitivity reactions

Autoantibodies to the patient's own red cells are produced in **autoimmune hemolytic anemia**. They react at 37°C with epitopes on antigens of the rhesus complex distinct from those that incite transfusion reactions. Erythrocytes coated with these antibodies have a shortened half-life, largely through their adherence to splenic macrophages. Similar mechanisms account for the anemia in patients with cold hemagglutinin disease who have monoclonal anti-I after infection with *Mycoplasma pneumoniae,* and in some cases of paroxysmal cold hemoglobinuria associated with the actively lytic Donath–Landsteiner antibodies specific for blood group P. These antibodies are primarily of IgM isotype and only react at temperatures well below 37°C. IgG autoantibodies against platelet surface glycoproteins are responsible for the depletion of platelets in **idiopathic thrombocytopenic purpura**; primarily through Fcγ receptor-mediated clearance by tissue macrophages in spleen and liver.

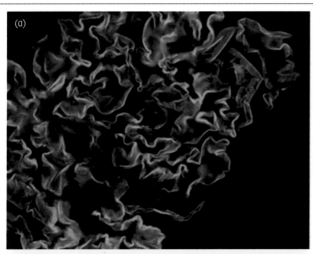

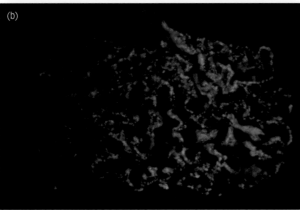

Figure 15.18. Glomerulonephritis.

(a) In Goodpasture's syndrome due to a type II hypersensitivity with linear deposition of antibody to glomerular basement membrane, here visualized by staining the human kidney biopsy with a fluorescent anti-IgG; and in contrast to (b) in systemic lupus erythematosus (SLE, cf. p. 495) where a type III hypersensitivity is associated with deposition of antigen–antibody complexes, which can be seen as discrete masses lining the glomerular basement membrane following immunofluorescent staining with anti-IgG. Similar patterns to these are obtained with a fluorescent anti-C3. (Courtesy of S. Thiru.)

Patients with Hashimoto's thyroiditis have autoantibodies that, in the presence of complement, are directly cytotoxic for isolated human thyroid cells in culture. In Goodpasture's syndrome, autoantibodies recognize type IV collagen in kidney glomerular basement membrane. These antibodies, together with complement components, bind to the basement membranes where the action of the full complement system leads to serious damage (Figure 15.18a). One could also include the stripping of acetylcholine receptors from the muscle endplate by autoantibodies in myasthenia gravis as a further example of type II hypersensitivity.

Type II drug reactions

Drugs can become coupled to body components and thereby undergo conversion from a hapten to a full immunogen that may elicit an immune response in some individuals. If IgE antibodies are produced, anaphylactic reactions can result. In some circumstances, particularly with topically applied ointments, cell-mediated hypersensitivity may be induced. In other cases where coupling to serum proteins occurs, the possibility of type III immune complex-mediated reactions may arise. In the present context, we are concerned with those instances in which the drug appears to form an antigenic complex with the surface of circulating blood cells and evokes the production of antibodies that are cytotoxic for the cell–drug complex. When the drug is withdrawn, the sensitivity is no longer evident. Examples of this mechanism occur in the **hemolytic anemia** sometimes associated with continued administration of chlorpromazine or phenacetin, in the **agranulocytosis** associated with the taking of amidopyrine or of quinidine, and the now classic situation of **thrombocytopenic purpura**, which may be produced by sedormid, a sedative of yesteryear. In the latter case, freshly drawn serum from the patient will lyse platelets in the presence, but not in the absence, of sedormid; inactivation of complement by preheating the serum at 56°C for 30 minutes abrogates this effect.

Immune complex-mediated hypersensitivity (type III)

The body may be exposed to an excess of antigen over a protracted period in a number of circumstances: persistent infection, autoimmunity to self-components and repeated contact with environmental agents. The union of such antigens and antibodies to form a complex within the body may well give rise to acute inflammatory reactions through a variety of mechanisms (Figure 15.19). For a start, intravascular complexes can aggregate platelets with two consequences: they provide a source of vasoactive amines and may also form microthrombi that can lead to local ischemia (Figure 15.19a). Immune complexes can also stimulate macrophages, through their Fcγ receptors, to generate the release of proinflammatory cytokines IL-1 and TNF, reactive oxygen intermediates and nitric oxide (Figure 15.19b). Complexes that are insoluble often cannot be digested after phagocytosis by macrophages and so provide a persistent activating stimulus. If complement is fixed, the C5a chemotactic factor will be generated leading to an influx of neutrophils (Figure 15.19c), which begin the phagocytosis of the immune complexes; this in turn results in the extracellular release of the neutrophil granule contents, particularly when the complex is deposited on a basement membrane and cannot be phagocytosed (so-called "frustrated phagocytosis"). The proteolytic enzymes (including neutral proteases and collagenase), kinin-forming enzymes, polycationic proteins and reactive oxygen and nitrogen intermediates that are released will of course damage local tissues and intensify the inflammatory

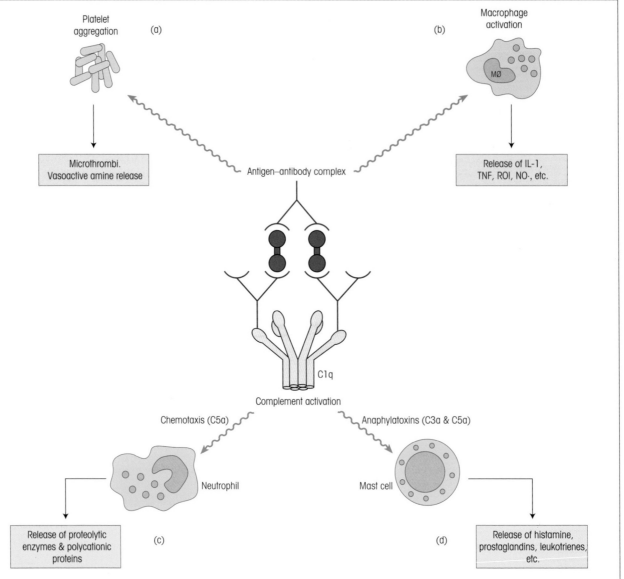

Figure 15.19. Immune complex-mediated (type III) hypersensitivity—underlying pathogenic mechanisms. ROI, reactive oxygen intermediates; NO, nitric oxide.

responses. The anaphylatoxins C3a and C5a produced following complement activation will cause release of mast cell mediators resulting in vascular permeability changes (Figure 15.19d). Further havoc may be mediated by reactive lysis in which activated C5, C6 and C7 becomes adventitiously attached to the surface of nearby cells and subsequently binds C8 and C9. Given all these potential consequences of immune complex formation the need for the system of inhibitors present in the body should be absolutely clear.

The outcome of the formation of immune complexes *in vivo* depends not only on the absolute amounts of antigen and antibody, which determine the intensity of the reaction, but also on their *relative* proportions, which govern the nature of the complexes (cf. Figure 6.24, p. 164) and hence their distribution within the body. Between **antibody excess** and **mild antigen excess**, the complexes are rapidly precipitated and tend to be localized to the site of introduction of antigen, whereas in **moderate** to **gross antigen excess**, soluble complexes are formed.

Covalent attachment of C3b prevents the Fc–Fc interactions required to form large insoluble aggregates, and these small complexes bind to CR1 complement receptors on the human erythrocyte and are transported to fixed macrophages in the liver and spleen where they are safely inactivated. This is an important role of the erythrocyte, a cell often unfairly ignored in discussion of the immune system. If there are defects in this process, for example deficiencies in classical pathway components, or perhaps if the system is overloaded, then

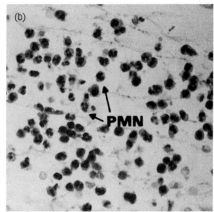
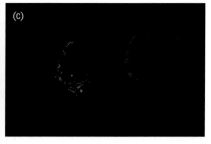

Figure 15.20. Histology of acute inflammatory reaction in polyarteritis nodosa associated with immune complex formation with hepatitis B surface antigen (HBsAg).

(a) A vessel showing thrombus (Thr) formation and fibrinoid necrosis (FN) is surrounded by a mixed inflammatory infiltrate, largely neutrophils. (b) High-power view of acute inflammatory response in loose connective tissue of patient with polyarteritis nodosa—polymorphonuclear neutrophils (PMN) are prominent. (c) Immunofluorescence studies of immune complexes in the renal artery of a patient with chronic hepatitis B infection stained with fluoresceinated antihepatitis B antigen (left) and rhodaminated anti-IgM (right). The presence of both antigen and antibody in the intima and media of the arterial wall indicates the deposition of the complexes at this site. IgG and C3 deposits are also detectable with the same distribution. ((a) and (b) provided by courtesy of N. Woolf; (c) kindly provided by A. Nowoslowski.)

widespread disease involving deposition of complexes in the kidneys, joints, skin and choroid plexus (networks of capillaries in the walls of the ventricles in the brain) may result.

Inflammatory lesions due to locally formed complexes

The Arthus reaction

Maurice Arthus found that injection of soluble antigen intradermally into hyperimmunized rabbits with high levels of precipitating antibody produced an erythematous and edematous reaction reaching a peak at 3–8 hours that then usually resolved. The lesion was characterized by an intense infiltration with neutrophils (cf. Figure 15.20a and b). The injected antigen precipitates with antibody often within the venule, too fast for the classical complement system to prevent it; subsequently, the complex is able to bind complement and, using fluorescent reagents, antigen, immunoglobulin and complement components can all be demonstrated in this lesion, as illustrated by the inflammatory response to deposits of immune complexes containing hepatitis B surface antigen in a patient with periarteritis nodosa (Figure 15.20c). Anaphylatoxin production, mast cell degranulation, macrophage activation, platelet aggregation and influx of neutrophils all make their contribution. The Arthus reaction can be attenuated by depletion of neutrophils by nitrogen mustard or of complement by anti-C5a; soluble forms of the complement regulatory proteins CD46 (membrane cofactor protein) and CD55 (delay accelerating factor) are also inhibitory.

Reactions to inhaled antigens

Intrapulmonary Arthus-type reactions to exogenous inhaled antigen are responsible for a number of hypersensitivity disorders. The severe respiratory difficulties associated with **farmer's lung** occur within 6–8 hours of exposure to the dust from mouldy hay. The patients are found to be sensitized to thermophilic actinomycetes that grow in the mouldy hay, and extracts of these organisms give precipitin reactions with the subject's serum and Arthus reactions on intradermal injection. Inhalation of bacterial spores in dust from the hay introduces antigen into the lungs and an immune complex-mediated hypersensitivity reaction occurs. Similar situations arise in pigeon-fancier's disease, where the antigen is probably serum protein present in the dust from dried feces, and in many other quaintly named cases of **extrinsic allergic alveolitis** resulting from continual inhalation of organic particles, e.g. cheese washer's disease (*Penicillium casei* spores), furrier's lung (fox fur proteins) and maple bark stripper's disease (spores of *Cryptostroma*). Evidence that an immediate anaphylactic type I response may sometimes be of importance for the initiation of an Arthus reaction comes from the study of patients with allergic bronchopulmonary aspergillosis who have high levels of IgE and precipitating IgG antibodies to *Aspergillus* species.

Reactions to internal antigens

Type III reactions are often provoked by the local release of antigen from infectious organisms within the body; for example, living filarial worms, such as *Wuchereria bancrofti,* are

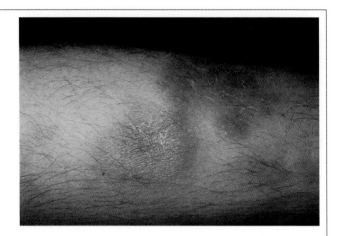

Figure 15.21. Erythema nodosum leprosum, forearm.

The patient has lepromatous leprosy with superimposed erythema nodosum leprosum. These acutely inflamed nodules were extremely tender and the patient was pyrexial. (Photograph kindly provided by G. Levene.)

relatively harmless, but the dead parasite found in lymphatic vessels initiates an inflammatory reaction thought to be responsible for the obstruction of lymph flow and the ensuing, rather monstrous, elephantiasis. Microbial cell death following chemotherapy may cause an abrupt release of microbial antigens and in individuals with high antibody levels produce quite dramatic immune complex-mediated reactions, such as **erythema nodosum leprosum** in the skin of dapsone-treated lepromatous leprosy patients (Figure 15.21) and the Jarisch–Herxheimer reaction in syphilitics on penicillin.

An interesting variant of the Arthus reaction is seen in rheumatoid arthritis where complexes are formed locally in the joint due to the production of self-associating IgG anti-IgG by synovial plasma cells (cf. p. 496).

Complexes could also be generated at a local site by a quite different mechanism involving nonspecific adherence of an antigen to tissue structures followed by the binding of soluble antibody—in other words, the antigen becomes fixed in the tissue *before* not *after* combining with antibody. Although it is not clear to what extent this mechanism operates in patients with immune complex disease, let us describe the experimental observation on which it is based. After injection with bacterial endotoxin, mice release DNA into their circulation that binds specifically to the collagen in the basement membrane of the glomerular capillaries; the endotoxin also polyclonally activates B-cells making anti-DNA that gives rise to antigen–antibody complexes in the kidney.

Disease resulting from circulating complexes

Immune complex glomerulonephritis

The deposition of complexes is a dynamic affair and longlasting disease is only seen when the antigen is persistent, as in chronic infections and autoimmune diseases. In the glomeruli, the **smallest complexes reach the epithelial side** but progressively **larger complexes are retained in or on the endothelial side of the glomerular basement membrane** (Figure 15.22). They build up as "lumpy" granules staining for antigen, immunoglobulin and complement (C3) by immunofluorescence (Figure 15.18b), and appear as large amorphous masses in the electron microscope (cf. Figure 18.18). The inflammatory process damages the basement membrane through engagement of the complexes with effector cells bearing Fcγ receptors, as revealed by the absence of glomerulonephritis despite immune complex deposition in the kidneys of FcγR-knockout New Zealand (B × W) F1 hybrids (a murine model of human systemic lupus erythematosus, SLE; p. 495). Proteinuria results from the leakage of serum proteins through the damaged membrane and serum albumin, being small, appears in the urine (Figure 15.23, lane 3).

Many cases of glomerulonephritis are associated with circulating complexes, and biopsies give a fluorescent staining pattern similar to that of Figure 15.18b, which depicts DNA/anti-DNA/complement deposits in the kidney of a patient with SLE (cf. p. 496). Well known is the disease that can follow infection with certain strains of so-called "nephritogenic" streptococci and the nephrotic syndrome associated with malaria, where complexes with antigens of the infecting organism have been implicated. Immune complex nephritis can arise in the course of chronic viral infections; as seen in individuals co-infected with HIV and hepatitis C virus.

Deposition of immune complexes at other sites

The choroid plexuses in the brain are a major filtration site and therefore also favored for immune complex deposition. This factor could account for the frequency of central nervous system disorders in SLE. Neurologically affected patients tend to have depressed complement component C4 in the cerebrospinal fluid (CSF) and, at postmortem, SLE patients with neurologic disturbances and high-titer anti-DNA were shown to have scattered deposits of immunoglobulin and DNA in the choroid plexus. Subacute sclerosing panencephalitis is associated with a high CSF to serum ratio of measles antibody, and deposits containing Ig and measles Ag may be found in neural tissue.

Vasculitic skin rashes are also characteristic of both systemic and discoid lupus erythematosus (Figure 15.24), and biopsies of the lesions reveal amorphous deposits of Ig and C3 at the basement membrane of the dermo-epidermal junction (cf. Figure 18.19).

Another example of immune complex hypersensitivity is the hemorrhagic shock syndrome found in South-East Asia during a second infection with dengue virus. There are four types of virus, and antibodies to one type produced during a first infection may not neutralize a second strain but rather facilitate its entry into, and replication within, human monocytes by attachment of the complex to Fc receptors. The

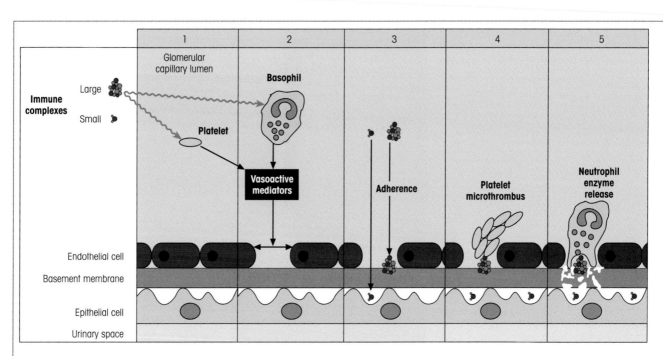

Figure 15.22. Deposition of immune complexes in the kidney glomerulus.

(1) Complexes induce release of vasoactive mediators from basophils and platelets that cause (2) separation of endothelial cells. (3) Attachment of larger complexes to exposed basement membrane, with smaller complexes passing through to the epithelial side. (4) Complexes induce platelet aggregation. (5) Chemotactically attracted neutrophils release granule contents in "frustrated phagocytosis" to damage basement membrane and cause leakage of serum proteins. Complex deposition is favored in the glomerular capillary because it is a major filtration site and has a high hydrodynamic pressure. Deposition is greatly reduced in animals depleted of platelets or treated with vasoactive amine antagonists.

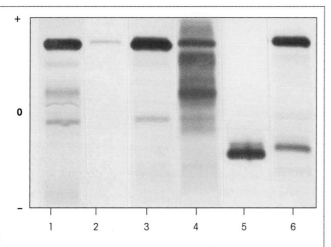

Figure 15.23. Proteinuria demonstrated by electrophoresis.

Lane 1: Normal serum as reference. The major band nearest to the cathode is albumin. Lane 2: Normal urine showing a trace of albumin. Lane 3: Glomerular proteinuria showing a major albumin component. Lane 4: Proteinuria resulting from tubular damage with a totally different electrophoretic pattern. Lane 5: Bence Jones proteinuria representing excreted paraprotein light chains. Lane 6: Bence Jones proteinuria with a trace of the intact paraprotein. Some of the samples have been concentrated. (Electropherograms kindly supplied by T. Heys.)

enhanced production of virus leads to immune complex formation and a massive intravascular activation of the classical complement pathway. In some instances drugs such as penicillin become antigenic after conjugation with body proteins and form complexes that mediate hypersensitivity reactions.

It should be said that persistence of circulating complexes does not invariably lead to type III hypersensitivity (e.g. in many cancer patients and in individuals with idiotype–anti-idiotype reactions). Perhaps in these cases the complexes lack the ability to initiate the changes required for complex deposition, but some hold the view that complexes detected in the serum may sometimes be artifacts released from their *in vivo* attachment to the erythrocyte CR1 receptors by the action of factor I during processing of the blood.

Treatment

The avoidance of exogenous inhaled antigens inducing type III reactions is obvious. Elimination of microorganisms associated with immune complex disease by chemotherapy may provoke a further reaction due to copious release of antigen. Suppression of the accessory factors thought to be necessary for the deposition of complexes would seem logical. Sodium cromoglycate, heparin and salicylates are often used, the latter being an effective platelet stabilizer as well as a potent anti-inflammatory

Figure 15.24. Vasculitic skin rashes due to immune complex deposition.

(a) Facial appearance in systemic lupus erythematosus (SLE). Lesions of recent onset are symmetrical, red and edematous. They are often most pronounced on the areas of the face that receive most light exposure, i.e. the upper cheeks and bridge of the nose, and the prominences of the forehead. (b) Vasculitic lesions in SLE. Small purpuric macules are seen.

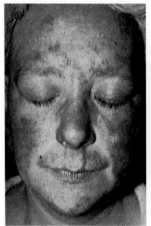
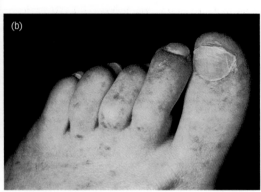

Figure 15.25. Cell-mediated (type IV) hypersensitivity reactions.

(a) Mantoux test showing cell-mediated hypersensitivity reaction to tuberculin, characterized by induration and erythema. (b) Chronic type IV inflammatory lesion in tuberculous lung showing caseous necrosis (CN), epithelioid cells (E), giant cells (G) and mononuclear inflammatory cells (M). (c) Diagrammatic representation of a granuloma with central caseous ("cheesy") necrosis. (d) Type IV contact hypersensitivity reaction to nickel caused by the clasp of a necklace. ((a) Kindly provided by J. Brostoff and (b) by R. Barnetson; (d) reproduced from the British Society for Immunology teaching materials with permission of the Society and the Dermatology Department, London Hospital.)

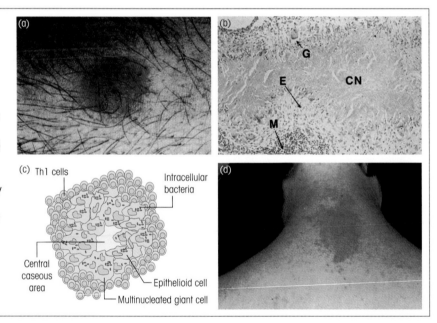

agent. Corticosteroids are particularly powerful inhibitors of inflammation and are immunosuppressive. In many cases, particularly those involving autoimmunity, conventional immunosuppressive agents may be justified.

Cell-mediated (delayed-type) hypersensitivity (type IV)

Delayed-type hypersensitivity (DTH) is encountered in many allergic reactions to infectious agents, in the contact dermatitis resulting from sensitization to certain simple chemicals and in transplant rejection. Perhaps the best known example is the **Mantoux reaction** obtained by injection of tuberculin into the skin of an individual in whom previous infection with the mycobacterium had induced a state of cell-mediated immunity

(CMI). The reaction is characterized by erythema and induration (Figure 15.25a), which appears only after several hours (hence the term "delayed") and reaches a maximum at 24–48 hours, thereafter subsiding. Histologically, the earliest phase of the reaction is seen as a perivascular cuffing with mononuclear cells followed by a more extensive exudation of mono- and polymorphonuclear cells. The latter soon migrate out of the lesion leaving behind a predominantly mononuclear cell infiltrate consisting of lymphocytes and cells of the monocyte–macrophage series (Figure 15.25b). This contrasts with the essentially "neutrophil" character of the Arthus reaction (Figure 15.20b).

Comparable reactions to soluble proteins are obtained when sensitization is induced by incorporation of the antigen into complete Freund's adjuvant (see p. 365). In some, but not

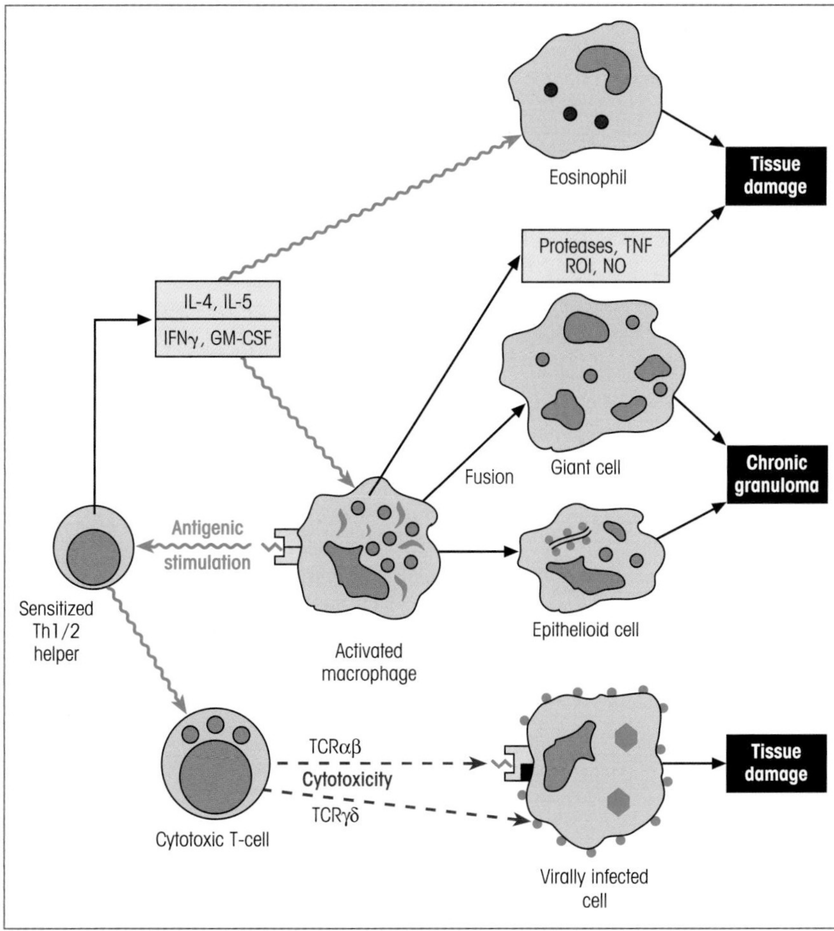

Figure 15.26. The cellular basis of type IV hypersensitivity.

Th1 cells will activate macrophages and cytotoxic T-cells, whereas Th2 cells will recruit eosinophils. ROI, reactive oxygen intermediates; NO, nitric oxide.

all cases, if animals are primed with antigen alone or in incomplete Freund's adjuvant (which lacks the mycobacteria present in the complete adjuvant), the delayed hypersensitivity state is of shorter duration and the dermal response more transient. This is known as "Jones–Mote" sensitivity but has more recently been termed **cutaneous basophil hypersensitivity** on account of the high proportion of basophils infiltrating the skin lesion.

The cellular basis of type IV hypersensitivity

Unlike the other forms of hypersensitivity that we have discussed, delayed-type reactivity cannot be transferred from a sensitized to a nonsensitized individual with serum antibody; T-lymphocytes are required. It cannot be stressed too often that the hypersensitivity lesion results from an exaggerated interaction between antigen and the *normal* cell-mediated immune mechanisms (cf. p. 237). Following earlier priming, memory T-cells recognize the antigen peptide together with MHC class II molecules on an antigen-presenting cell and are activated to undergo proliferation. The stimulated T-cells release a number of cytokines that mediate the ensuing hypersensitivity response, particularly by attracting and activating macrophages if they belong to the Th1 subset, or eosinophils if they are Th2. Helper

T-cells also assist Tc precursors to become killer cells that can cause damage to virally infected target cells (Figure 15.26), the CD8 TCRαβ cytotoxic cells being activated by recognition of MHC class I complexes with processed viral proteins and TCRγδ killers operating through binding to native viral proteins on the surface of the infected cells. It is also thought that Th17 cells play a role. Thus, IL-17 knockout mice have impaired DTH responses, and IL-17 is secreted by cutaneous lymphocyte antigen (CLA)+ nickel-specific T-cell clones from patients allergic to this allergen. Cytokines released by Th1 and Th17 cells cause the activation of NK cells that then release proinflammatory cytokines and exert killing activity by inducing apoptosis in keratinocytes. IL-17 is known to synergise with IFNγ in upregulating ICAM-1 expression and chemokine production by human keratinocytes, which may hasten their demise.

Tissue damage produced by type IV reactions

Infections

The development of a state of cell-mediated hypersensitivity to bacterial products is probably responsible for the lesions, such as the cavitation, caseation and general toxemia, seen in human tuberculosis and the granulomatous skin lesions found in patients with the borderline form of leprosy. When the battle between the replicating bacteria and the body defenses fails to be resolved in favor of the host, persisting antigen provokes a chronic local delayed hypersensitivity reaction. Continual release of cytokines from sensitized T-lymphocytes leads to the accumulation of large numbers of macrophages, many of which give rise to arrays of epithelioid cells (macrophages that morphologically resemble epithelial cells), while others fuse to form multinucleated giant cells. Macrophages presenting peptides derived from bacterial antigens using their surface MHC class I molecules may become targets for cytotoxic T-cells and be destroyed. Further tissue damage will occur as a result of indiscriminate cytotoxicity by cytokine-activated macrophages. Morphologically, this combination of cell types with proliferating lymphocytes and fibroblasts associated with areas of fibrosis and necrosis is termed a **chronic granuloma** and represents an attempt by the body to wall off a site of persistent infection (Figures 15.25b,c and 15.26). It should be noted that granulomas can also arise from the persistence of indigestible antigen–antibody complexes or inorganic materials, such as talc, within macrophages, although nonimmunological granulomas may be distinguished by the absence of lymphocytes.

The skin rashes in measles and the lesions associated with herpes simplex infection may be largely attributed to delayed-type reactions with extensive Tc-mediated damage to virally infected cells. By the same token, specific cytotoxic T-cells can cause extensive destruction of liver cells infected with hepatitis B virus. Cell-mediated hypersensitivity has also been demonstrated in the fungal diseases candidiasis, dermatomycosis, coccidioidomycosis and histoplasmosis, and in the parasitic disease leishmaniasis.

Crohn's disease and ulcerative colitis are the two main forms of **inflammatory bowel disease** (IBD) and are distinct entities, although both probably result from dysregulated mucosal immune responses to microbial antigens in the gut. **Crohn's disease** is characterized by transmural granulomatous inflammation involving the entire bowel wall from mucosa to serosa, and the development of fibrosis, microperforations and fistulas. Inflammation can occur throughout the gastrointestinal tract. By contrast, in **ulcerative colitis** there is a more superficial inflammation that is confined to the colon and rectum. Mutations in the *NOD2* gene, encoding a cytoplasmic pattern recognition receptor for the muramyl dipeptide of bacterial cell wall peptidoglycan, are strongly associated with susceptibility to Crohn's disease. IBD can be induced in severe combined immunodeficient (SCID) mice by the transfer of CD45RB^{hi} (naive) CD4 T-cells, but the colitis that develops can be cured by the subsequent transfer of CD4$^+$, CD25$^+$, CD45RB^{lo} regulatory T-cells. The aggressor cells belong to the IL-12-driven Th1 population producing TNF and IFNγ, which are highly toxic for enterocytes, whereas the regulators secrete the suppressor cytokines TGFβ and IL-10. Monoclonal anti-TNF is a very effective therapy; probiotic treatment with lactobacilli and *Streptococcus salivarius* would appear to main-

tain remission in severe colitis, is less draconian and is easier on the budget (remember the friendly yoghurt adverts). Clinical trials to establish the efficacy of such treatments in large cohorts of patients are underway.

Experimental colitis induced in SJL/J mice by administration of oxazolone presents as a relatively superficial inflammation resembling human ulcerative colitis. It is initially mediated by IL-4-producing Th2 cells but rapidly superceded by an atypical Th2 response involving IL-13-producing NKT cells. The inflamed tissue in patients with ulcerative colitis has also been shown to contain increased numbers of IL-13-producing nonclassical NKT cells (unlike most NKT cells, these do not bear an invariant TCR) which have the potential to be cytotoxic for human epithelial cells.

Sarcoidosis

Sarcoidosis is a disease of unknown etiology affecting lymphoid tissue and involving the formation of chronic granulomas. A chronic inflammatory Th1 response to an infectious, environmental or autoantigen is thought to be responsible. Increased numbers of activated B-cells and hypergammaglobulinemia are often present. Evidence for atypical mycobacteria has been obtained, but delayed-type hypersensitivity is depressed and the patients are anergic on skin testing with tuberculin, perhaps due to the presence of increased numbers of regulatory T-cells in those patients with active disease. Patients develop a granulomatous reaction a few weeks after intradermal injection of spleen extract from another sarcoid patient—the **Kveim reaction**.

Contact dermatitis

The epidermal route of inoculation tends to favor the development of a Th1 response through processing by class II-rich dendritic Langerhans' cells (cf. Figure 2.7f), which migrate to the lymph nodes and present antigen to T-lymphocytes. Thus, delayed-type reactions in the skin are often produced by foreign low molecular weight materials capable of binding to peptides within the groove of MHC molecules on the surface of Langerhans' cells, to form new antigens. The reactions are characterized by a mononuclear cell infiltrate peaking at 12–15 hours, accompanied by edema of the epidermis with microvesicle formation (Figure 15.27). There is a most unusual twist to this story, however, possibly because the inciting reagent is a reactive hapten. The late mononuclear reaction is entirely dependent upon very early events (1–2 hours) mediated by hapten-specific IgM produced by B-1 cells that, together with complement, activates local vessels to permit T-cell recruitment. Contact hypersensitivity can occur in people who become sensitized while working with chemicals, such as picryl chloride and chromates, or who repeatedly come into contact with the substance urushiol from the poison ivy plant. *p*-Phenylene diamine in certain hair dyes, neomycin in topically applied ointments, and nickel salts formed from articles such as nickel jewellery clasps (Figure 15.25d) can provoke similar

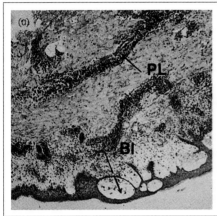
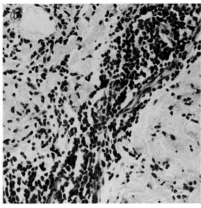

Figure 15.27. Contact sensitivity.

(a) Perivascular lymphocytic infiltrates (PL) and blister (Bl) formation characterize a contact sensitivity reaction of the skin. (b) High-power view to show the lymphocytic nature of the infiltrate in a contact hypersensitivity reaction. (Photographs kindly provided by N. Woolf.)

reactions. T-cell clones specific for nickel salts isolated from the latter group produce a Th1-type profile of cytokines (IFNγ, IL-2) on antigen stimulation (Figure 15.10b). Invariant NKT cells producing both the "Th1" cytokine IFNγ and the "Th2" cytokine IL-4 are also present in the skin infiltrate of patients with contact dermatitis.

Other examples

Excessive responses by Th2 cells can damage tissues through activation of eosinophils (Figure 15.26). As recounted earlier, T-cells synthesizing IL-5 are largely responsible for the sustained influx of eosinophils in asthma and atopic dermatitis (cf. p. 401). Th2 cells also account for the liver pathology in schistosomiasis that has been attributed to a reaction against soluble enzymes derived from the eggs that lodge in the capillaries (Figure 15.28).

It has been suggested that the relatively mixed Th1–Th2 DTH response induced by bites from blood-feeding insects such as sand flies (*Phlebotomus papatasi*) might represent an adaptation of the insect to direct the host immune response to its own advantage. Thus, it was shown that the increased blood flow associated with the DTH sites allowed sand flies to feed twice as fast relative to feeding from normal skin sites.

The contribution of DTH reactions to allograft rejection is covered in Chapter 16, whereas the potential role of Tc cells for the control of cancer cells is discussed in Chapter 17. In certain organ-specific autoimmune diseases, such as type I diabetes, cell-mediated hypersensitivity reactions undoubtedly provide the major engine for tissue destruction.

The intestinal inflammation in **celiac disease**, an HLA-DQ2/8-associated enteropathy, is precipitated by exposure to dietary wheat gliadin. The disorder involves what is probably a genetically related increased mucosal activity of transglutaminase (the main target antigen of anti-endomysium autoantibodies; cf. p. 495). This enzyme deamidates the glutamine residues in gliadin and creates a new T-cell epitope that binds efficiently to DQ2 and is recognized by IFNγ-secreting intraepithelial CD4$^+$ Th1-cells. Local production of IL-15 also

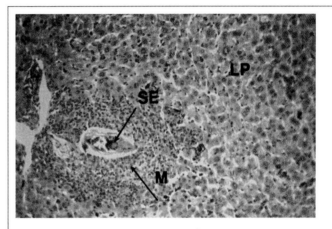

Figure 15.28. Th2-mediated response to schistosome egg.

Th2-type hypersensitivity lesion of inflammatory cells (M) around a schistosome egg (SE) within the liver parenchyma (LP). (Photograph by courtesy of M. Doenhoff.)

plays a role by increasing expression of nonclassical MHC class I molecules such as MICA on epithelial cells and receptors for these such as NKG2D on intraepithelial CD8$^+$ αβ T-cells, γδ T-cells and NK cells, leading to cytotoxic killing of the epithelial cells.

Psoriasis involves marked proliferation of epidermal keratinocytes and accelerated incomplete epidermal differentiation. For reasons that are not understood, in around 10% of patients the skin manifestations are associated with psoriatic arthritis involving joint inflammation and destruction. The skin inflammation involves neutrophils and both CD4 and CD8 T-cells that are CD45RO$^+$ indicating that they are antigen experienced. The release of IFNγ induces epidermal hyperplasia and, together with TNF, increases the expression of ICAM-1 on epidermal keratinocytes, thereby facilitating the adhesion of T-cells. Experiments in a skin xenograft model of psoriasis involving the transplantation of human skin onto severe combined immunodeficient (SCID) mice have identified that the activated form of the *s*ignal *t*ransducer and *a*ctivator of *t*ranscription *3* (STAT3) cell signaling molecule localizes to the nucleus of epidermal keratinocytes following the transfer of CD4 but not CD8 T-cells, indicating a central role for STAT3 signaling in the interactions between activated CD4 cells and keratinocytes. Biological agents that are effective in the treatment of psoriasis include etanercept (TNF receptor-IgG fusion protein) and the monoclonal antibodies adalimumab (human anti-TNF), infliximab (chimeric anti-TNF) and ustekinumab (human anti-IL-12 and IL-23). Efalizumab, a humanized IgG1 monoclonal antibody against CD11a (LFA-1), is also effective but has been withdrawn due to safety concerns. Recently IL-22 production by Th17 cells has been shown to mediate keratinocyte proliferation and epidermal cell hyperplasia, providing yet another potential therapeutic target.

An addition to the original classification— stimulatory hypersensitivity ("type V")

Although Gell and Coombs only categorized four types of hypersensitivity reaction, a fifth type (type V) is sometimes added. This is where antibody to a cell surface receptor acts as an agonist leading to stimulation of the cell. When thyroid-stimulating hormone (TSH) binds to its receptor on the thyroid epithelial cells, adenylyl cyclase is activated, and the cAMP "second messenger" is generated to stimulate thyroid hormone production. Once sufficient levels of the hormones are produced a negative feedback loop shuts off the production of TSH. The **thyroid-stimulating antibody** present in patients with Graves' disease (cf. p. 493) is an autoantibody against the TSH receptor and mimics the effect of TSH, except in this case there is continuous secretion of the autoantibody by plasma cells that provides a constant stimulation of the thyroid leading to hyperthyroidism. Agonistic autoantibodies that stimulate the angiotensin II AT1 receptor have been described in patients with preeclampsia and with hypertension.

"Innate" hypersensitivity reactions

Many infections provoke a **"toxic shock syndrome"** characterized by hypotension (low blood pressure), hypoxia (shortage of oxygen), oliguria (decreased urine output) and microvascular abnormalities and mediated by elements of the innate immune system independently of the operation of acquired immune responses.

Septicemia associated with **Gram-negative bacteria** results in excessive release of TNF, IL-1 and IL-6 through stimulation of macrophages and endothelial cells by the lipopolysaccharide (LPS) endotoxin. Normally this would enhance host defenses, aiding the recruitment of phagocytes by promoting adherence to endothelium, priming neutrophils for subsequent release of reactive oxygen intermediates, inducing febrile responses (immune responses improve steadily from 33 to 44°C), and so on. Unfortunately, the excess of circulating LPS, and the cytokines released in response to its presence, lead to unwanted

pathophysiology at distant sites. This occurs in, for example, the **adult respiratory distress syndrome** brought about by an overwhelming invasion of the lung by neutrophils. There is a prolonged pathologically high concentration of nitric oxide but, additionally, LPS can activate the alternative complement pathway, and this may be linked to its ability to induce the release of thromboxane A_2 and prostaglandin from platelets leading to **disseminated intravascular coagulation**.

Whereas the major culprit in Gram-negative sepsis is LPS, **Gram-positive organisms** possess a variety of components that act on host defense elements to initiate septic shock. Thus adherence of *Staphylococcus aureus* to macrophages induces TNF synthesis, and peptidoglycan-mediated aggregation of platelets by the same organism leads to disseminated intravascular coagulation. The staphylococcal and streptococcal enterotoxins induce toxic shock syndrome by quite different means. By functioning as **superantigens** (cf. p. 136), they react directly with particular T-cell receptor families and give rise to massive cytokine release, including TNF and macrophage migration inhibitory factor (MIF), which is detected in high concentrations in the plasma of patients with septic shock. Various treatments are under investigation. Pentoxifylline blocks TNF production by macrophages. Experimental models of septic shock can be blocked by anti-MIF and by a peptide derived from the natural sequence 150–161 of staphylococcal enterotoxin B, which is part of a domain crucial for T-cell activation.

The reader's attention has already been drawn to both the **tumor necrosis factor receptor-associated periodic syndrome** (TRAPS) (p. 372) and to **paroxysmal nocturnal hemoglobinuria** (p. 373) in the previous chapter. Undue C3 consumption is associated with mesangiocapillary glomerulonephritis and partial lipodystrophy (degeneration of adipose tissue) in patients with the so-called **C3 nephritic factor**, an IgG autoantibody capable of activating the alternative pathway by combining with and stabilizing the C3bBb convertase.

In patients with **idiopathic pulmonary fibrosis** there is a defective response to tissue damage in the lung with an imbalance between wound repair and fibrinolysis. TGFβ and TNF production by epithelial cells and macrophages cause fibroblasts to proliferate and overproduce extracellular matrix. Anti-inflammatory agents have not generally proved of benefit in this disease, indeed there is some indication that IFNγ may have some therapeutic potential by acting as an anti-fibrotic agent.

The neuropathological hallmarks of **Alzheimer's disease** are extracellular plaques and intracellular neurofibrillary tangles. The senile plaques contain 4 kDa β-amyloid hydrophobic peptides derived from β-*a*myloid *p*recursor *p*rotein (APP). Normally APP is cleaved by an α-secretase into soluble products that cannot form the Alzheimer's β-amyloid fragment. However, in individuals with this neurodegenerative disease the pathogenic 4 kDa peptides are produced following sequential proteolytic processing of APP by β-secretase (BACE, β-site *A*PP *c*leavage *e*nzyme) and γ-secretase (composed of presenilin-1 and -2). Aggregated β-amyloid peptides produced by this pathway are thought to trigger apoptosis in neurons. The APOE4 variant of the gene encoding apolipoprotein E, a cholesterol transporter, is the only established susceptibility gene, although other genes are also thought to be involved. Following the observation that individuals treated with high doses of nonsteroidal anti-inflammatory drugs (NSAIDs) for conditions such as rheumatoid arthritis appear to have a reduced likelihood of developing Alzheimer's disease, clinical trials are underway to test the ability of these immunomodulatory agents to delay or prevent the onset of Alzheimer's disease.

■ Excessive stimulation of the normal effector mechanisms of the immune system can lead to tissue damage and we speak of hypersensitivity reactions, several types of which can be distinguished.

Anaphylactic hypersensitivity (type I)
■ Anaphylaxis involves contraction of smooth muscle and dilatation of capillaries.
■ This depends upon the reaction of antigen with specific IgE antibody bound through its Fc to the mast cell high affinity receptor FcεRI.
■ Cross-linking and clustering of the IgE receptors activates the Lyn protein tyrosine kinase, recruits other kinases and leads to release from the granules of mediators including histamine, leukotrienes and platelet activating factor, plus eosinophil and neutrophil chemotactic factors and numerous other cytokines.

Atopic allergy
■ Atopy stems from an excessive IgE response to extrinsic antigens (allergens) that leads to local anaphylactic reactions at sites of contact with allergen.
■ Hay fever and extrinsic asthma represent the most common atopic allergic disorders resulting from exposure to inhaled allergens. Atopic dermatitis is also extremely common.
■ Whereas the immediate reaction to extrinsic allergen (maximum at 30 minutes) is due to mast cell triggering, a late phase reaction peaking at 5 hours, involving eosinophil infiltration, is initiated by the activation of alveolar and other macrophages through surface-bound IgE; secreted TNF and IL-1β now act upon epithelial cells and fibroblasts to release powerful eosinophil chemoattractants such as CCL5 and CCL11.
■ In asthma, serious prolongation of the response to allergen is caused by Th2 cells that sustain the recruitment of tissue-damaging eosinophils through the release of IL-5. The soup of powerful bronchoconstrictors, the injurious effect of eosinophil major basic protein and the mucus hypersecretion stimulated by IL-13 and IL-4, all contribute to the airway damage characteristic of chronic asthma.
■ Many food allergies involve type I hypersensitivity.
■ Genetic factors include linkage to the propensity to make the IgE isotype and to genes encoding a number of pattern-recognition receptors.
■ Exposure to Th1-stimulating infections may strongly influence the "immunostat" setting of the tendency to either Th1 or Th2 responses, the latter increasing the risk of allergy through promotion of IgE synthesis and eosinophil recruitment.
■ The offending antigen is identified by intradermal prick tests, giving immediate weal and erythema reactions, by provocation testing and by RAST.
■ Where possible, allergen avoidance is the best treatment.
■ A monoclonal antibody directed to the receptor-binding domain of IgE dramatically reduces IgE levels and synthesis, and decreases mast cell responsiveness.
■ Symptomatic treatment involves the use of long-acting β2-agonists and leukotriene antagonists. Sodium cromoglycate blocks chloride channel activity thereby stabilizing mast cells and inhibiting bronchoconstriction. Theophylline is a phosphodiesterase inhibitor that raises intracellular cAMP, causing bronchodilatation.
■ Chronic asthma is dominated by activated Th2 cells and is treated with inhaled steroids that display a wide range of anti-inflammatory actions, including the ability to block the production of mediators by stimulated macrophages or Th2 cells. These are supplemented where necessary by long-acting β2-agonists.
■ Courses of antigen injection or sublingual administration can desensitize by the formation of blocking or regulatory IgG antibodies, or through T-cell regulation. T-cell epitope peptides may be manipulated to modulate the atopic state.

Antibody-dependent cytotoxic hypersensitivity (type II)
■ This involves the death of cells bearing antibody attached to a surface antigen.

- The cells may be taken up by phagocytic cells to which they adhere through their coating of IgG or C3b, lysed by complement or killed by ADCC effectors.
- Examples are: transfusion reactions, hemolytic disease of the newborn through rhesus incompatibility, antibody-mediated graft destruction, autoimmune reactions directed against the formed elements of the blood and kidney glomerular basement membranes, and hypersensitivity resulting from the coating of erythrocytes or platelets by a drug.

Complex-mediated hypersensitivity (type III)

- This results from the effects of antigen–antibody complexes through: (i) activation of complement resulting in mast cell degranulation and the attraction of neutrophils, which release tissue-damaging mediators on contact with the complex; (ii) stimulation of macrophages to release proinflammatory cytokines; and (iii) aggregation of platelets to cause microthrombi and vasoactive amine release.
- Where circulating antibody levels are high, the antigen is precipitated near the site of entry into the body. The reaction in the skin is characterized by neutrophil infiltration, edema and erythema maximal at 3–8 hours (Arthus reaction).
- Examples are farmer's lung, pigeon-fancier's disease and pulmonary aspergillosis where inhaled antigens provoke high antibody levels, reactions to an abrupt increase in antigen caused by microbial cell death during chemotherapy for leprosy or syphilis, polyarteritis nodosa linked to complexes with hepatitis B virus and an element of the synovial lesion in rheumatoid arthritis.
- In relative *antigen excess*, soluble complexes are formed that are removed by binding to the CR1 C3b receptors on red cells. If this system is overloaded or if the classical complement components are deficient, the complexes circulate in the free state and are deposited under circumstances of increased vascular permeability at certain preferred sites: the kidney glomerulus, the joints, the skin and the choroid plexus.
- Examples are: glomerulonephritis associated with systemic lupus erythematosus (SLE) or infections with streptococci, malaria and co-infection with HIV and hepatitis C virus; neurological disturbances in SLE and subacute sclerosing panencephalitis; and hemorrhagic shock in dengue viral infection.

Cell-mediated or delayed-type hypersensitivity (type IV)

- This is based upon the interaction of antigen with primed T-cells and represents tissue damage resulting from inappropriate cell-mediated immunity reactions.
- Cytokines, including IFNγ, are released that activate macrophages and account for the events that occur in a typical delayed hypersensitivity response such as the Mantoux reaction to tuberculin, that is, the delayed appearance of an indurated and erythematous reaction that reaches a maximum at 24–48 hours and is characterized histologically by infiltration with mononuclear phagocytes and lymphocytes.
- Continuing provocation of delayed hypersensitivity by persisting antigen leads to formation of chronic granulomas.
- Th2-type cells producing IL-5 can also produce tissue damage through their ability to recruit eosinophils.
- CD8 T-cells are activated by class I MHC antigens to become directly cytotoxic to target cells bearing the appropriate antigen.
- IL-22 production by Th17 cells in patients with psoriasis results in keratinocyte proliferation and epidermal cell hyperplasia.
- Examples are: tissue damage occurring in bacterial (tuberculosis, leprosy), viral (measles, herpes), fungal (candidiasis, histoplasmosis) and parasitic (leishmaniasis, schistosomiasis) infections, contact dermatitis from exposure to chromates and poison ivy, insect bites and psoriasis. Inflammatory bowel disease can result from Th1-type (Crohn's disease) or "Th2-like" NKT (ulcerative colitis) reactions to intestinal bacteria. Celiac disease is an aberrant response to wheat gliadin.

Stimulatory hypersensitivity (type V)

- The antibody reacts with a key surface component such as a hormone receptor and "switches on" the cell.
- An example is the hyperthyroidism in Graves' disease due to a stimulatory anti-TSHR autoantibody. Features of these five types of acquired hypersensitivity are compared in Table 15.4.

"Innate" hypersensitivity reactions

- Some infections provoke a "toxic shock syndrome" involving excessive release of TNF, IL-1 and IL-6 and activation of the alternative complement pathway.

Table 15.4. Comparison of types of hypersensitivity involving acquired responses.

		Anaphylactic (I)	Cytotoxic (II)	Complex-mediated (III)	Cell-mediated (IV)	Stimulatory (V)
Antibody mediating reaction		Homocytotropic Ab Mast-cell binding	Humoral Ab ±CF*	Humoral Ab ±CF*	None (T-cell mediated)	Humoral Ab Non-CF*
Antigen		Usually exogenous (e.g. grass pollen)	Cell surface	Extracellular	Associated with MHC on macrophage or target cell	Cell surface
Response to intradermal antigen:	Max. reaction	30 min (+late reaction)	—	3–8 h	24–48 h	—
	Appearance	Weal and flare	—	Erythema and edema	Erythema and induration	—
	Histology	Degranulated mast cells; edema; (late reaction cellular including eosinophils)	—	Acute inflammatory reaction; predominant neutrophils	Perivascular inflammation: polymorphs migrate out leaving predominantly mononuclear cells	—
Transfer sensitivity to normal subject		← Serum antibody	Serum antibody	↑	Lymphoid cells	Serum antibody
Examples:		Atopic allergy, e.g. hay fever	Hemolytic disease of newborn (Rh)	Immune complex glomerulonephritis Farmer's lung	Mantoux reaction to TB Granulomatous reaction to TB Contact sensitivity	Graves' disease

*CF, complement fixation.

- Acute respiratory distress syndrome associated with Gram-negative bacteria is primarily due to the lipopolysaccharide (LPS) endotoxin provoking a massive invasion of the lung by neutrophils.
- Gram-positive organisms cause release of TNF and macrophage migration inhibitory factor (MIF) through

direct action on macrophages and stimulation of selected T-cell families by the enterotoxin superantigens.
- Aberration of innate mechanisms may underlie idiopathic pulmonary fibrosis and contribute to the β-amyloid plaques in Alzheimer's disease.

FURTHER READING

Alcorn J.F., Crowe C.R. & Kolls J.K. (2010) T$_H$17 cells in asthma and COPD. *Annual Review of Physiology* **72**, 495–516.

Broide D.H. (2009) Immunomodulation of allergic disease. *Annual Review of Medicine* **60**, 279–291.

Chapel H., Haeney M., Misbah S. & Snowden N. (2006) *Essentials of Clinical Immunology*, 5th edn. Blackwell Publishing, Oxford.

Frew A.J. (2008) Sublingual immunotherapy. *New England Journal of Medicine* **358**, 2259–2264.

Holgate S.T., Church M.K. & Lichtenstein L.M. (2006) *Allergy*, 3rd edn. Mosby, London.

Medoff B.D., Thomas S.Y. & Luster A.D. (2008) T cell trafficking in allergic asthma: the ins and outs. *Annual Review of Immunology* **26**, 205–232.

Meyer E.H., DeKruyff R.H., & Umetsu D.T. (2008) T cells and NKT cells in the pathogenesis of asthma. *Annual Review of Medicine* **59**, 281–292.

Palomares O. *et al.* (2010) Role of T regulatory cells in immune regulation of allergic diseases. *European Journal of Immunology* **40**, 1232–1240.

Rothenberg M.E. & Hogon S.P. (2006) The eosinophil. *Annual Review of Immunology* **24**, 147–174.

Sicherer S.H. & Sampson H.A. (2009) Food allergy: recent advances in pathophysiology and treatment. *Annual Review of Medicine* **60**, 261–277.

Valenta R. *et al.* (2010) From allergen genes to allergy vaccines. *Annual Review of Immunology* **28**, 211–241.

 Now visit **www.roitt.com** to test yourself on this chapter.

CHAPTER 16
Transplantation

Key Topics

Just to Recap ...

Whilst the cells of the innate response, and the B-lymphocytes of the adaptive response recognize intact antigen, T-lymphocytes recognize processed antigens in the form of peptides presented by cell surface MHC molecules. At the population level there is an incredible diversity of MHC genes that is thought to have evolved in response to pathogen diversity. The V(D)J recombination mechanisms associated with antibodies and T-cell receptors have the potential to generate responses again virtually any foreign antigen, including allogeneic MHC molecules.

Introduction

The replacement of diseased organs by a transplant of healthy tissue has long been an objective in medicine but has been frustrated to no mean degree by the uncooperative attempts by the body to reject grafts from other individuals. Unfortunately a relatively high percentage of T-cells have T-cell receptors specific for "allo-MHC," i.e. the MHC variants of other individuals. Antibodies can also be produced against nonself antigens on transplanted tissues or organs. These constraints necessitate both tissue type matching and immunosuppression in most cases of transplantation from genetically nonidentical individuals.

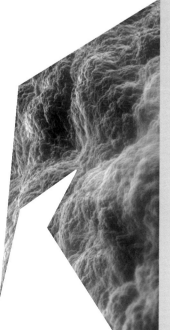

Roitt's Essential Immunology, Twelfth Edition. Peter J. Delves, Seamus J. Martin, Dennis R. Burton, Ivan M. Roitt.
© 2011 Peter J. Delves, Seamus J. Martin, Dennis R. Burton, Ivan M. Roitt. Published 2011 by Blackwell Publishing Ltd.

Types of graft

We first need to define the terms used for transplants between individuals and species:

- *Autograft*—tissue grafted back on to the original donor.
- *Isograft*—graft between **syngeneic** individuals (i.e. of identical genetic constitution) such as identical twins or mice of the same pure inbred strain.
- *Allograft*—graft between **allogeneic** individuals (i.e. members of the same species but different genetic constitution), e.g. human to human and one mouse strain to another.
- *Xenograft*—graft between **xenogeneic** individuals (i.e. of different species), e.g. pig to human.

Most cases of clinical transplantation involve allografts, although there is now a serious interest in the use of grafts from other species. The most common allografting procedure is blood transfusion where the unfortunate consequences of mismatching include hemolysis (lysis of red cells), intravascular coagulation, chills and nausea. However, such events are rare because infused blood would of course normally have been cross-matched for the ABO and rhesus (Rh) blood groups.

Considerable attention has been paid to the rejection of solid grafts such as skin and the sequence of events is worth describing. In mice, for example, the skin allograft settles down and becomes vascularized within a few days. Between 3 and 9 days the circulation gradually diminishes and there is increasing infiltration of the graft bed with lymphocytes and monocytes. Necrosis begins to be visible macroscopically and within a day or so the graft is sloughed completely (Figure M16.1.1). **Rejection is an immunological phenomenon**, showing both memory and specificity (Milestone 16.1). Furthermore, the recipient of T-cells from a donor who has already rejected a graft will give accelerated rejection of a further graft of the same type (Figure 16.1), showing that the lymphoid cells are primed and retain memory of the first contact with graft antigens.

Genetic control of transplantation antigens

The specificity of the antigens involved in graft rejection is under genetic control. Genetically identical individuals, such as mice of a pure strain or monozygotic twins, have identical transplantation antigens and grafts can be freely exchanged between them. The mendelian segregation of the genes controlling these antigens has been revealed by interbreeding experi-

---

♀ Milestone 16.1—The Immunological Basis of Graft Rejection

The field of transplantation owes a tremendous debt to Sir Peter Medawar, the outstanding scientist who kick-started and inspired its development. Even at the turn of the twentieth century it was an accepted paradigm that grafts between unrelated members of a species would be unceremoniously rejected after a brief initial period of acceptance (Figure M16.1.1). That there was an underlying genetic basis for rejection became apparent from Padgett's observations in Kansas City in 1932 that skin allografts between family members tended to survive for longer than those between

unrelated individuals and J.B. Brown's critical demonstration in St. Louis in 1937 that monozygotic (i.e. genetically identical) twins accepted skin grafts from each other. However, it was not until Medawar's research in the early part of the Second World War, motivated by the need to treat aircrew with appalling burns, that rejection was laid at immunology's door. He showed that a second graft from a given donor was rejected more rapidly and more vigorously than the first and, further, that an unrelated graft was rejected with the kinetics of a first set reaction (Figure M16.1.2). This **second set rejection**

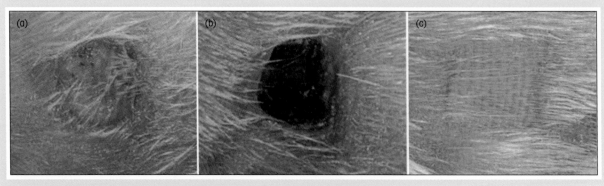

Figure M16.1.1. Appearance of skin grafts in mice.

(a) Graft undergoing rejection; (b) complete rejection (scab); and, for comparison, (c) a completely healed skin graft without evidence of rejection. (Reproduced from McFarland H.I. &

Rosenberg A.S. *Current Protocols in Immunology*. Unit Number: UNIT 4.4. DOI: 10.1002/0471142735.im0404s84).

📍 Milestone 16.1—*Continued*

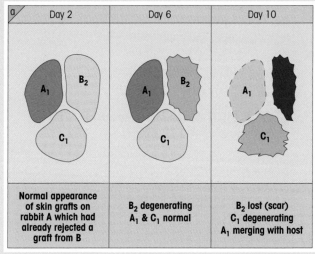

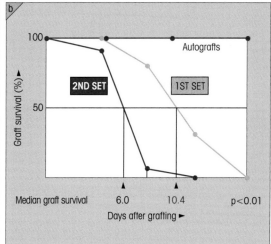

Figure M16.1.2. Memory and specificity in skin allograft rejection in rabbits.

(a) Skin autografts and allografts from two unrelated donors B and C are applied to rabbit A that has already rejected a first graft from B (B_1). While the autograft A remains intact, graft C_1 seen for the *first* time undergoes first set rejection, whereas a *second* graft from B (B_2) is sloughed off very rapidly.

(b) Median survival times of first and second set skin allografts showing faster second set rejection with a median 50% graft survival of 6 days compared with 10 days for a first set rejection. (From Medawar P.B. (1944) *Journal of Anatomy* **78**, 176.)

is characterized by **memory** and **specificity** and thereby bears the hallmarks of an immunological response. This was later confirmed by transferring the ability to express a second set reaction with lymphocytes.

The message was clear: to achieve successful transplantation of tissues and organs in the human, it would be necessary to overcome this immunogenetic barrier. Limited success was obtained by Murray at the Peter Bent Brigham Hospital (Boston) and Hamburger in Paris, who grafted kidneys between dizygotic twins using sublethal X-irradiation. The key breakthrough came when Schwartz and Damashek's report on the immunosuppressive effects of the antimitotic drug 6-mercaptopurine was applied independently by Calne

and Zukowski in 1960 to the prolongation of renal allografts in dogs. This finding was followed very rapidly by Murray's successful grafting in 1962 of an unrelated cadaveric kidney under the immunosuppressive umbrella of azathioprine, the more effective derivative of 6-mercaptopurine devised by Hutchings and Elion.

This story is studded with Nobel Prize winners and readers of a historical bent will gain further insight into the development of this field and the minds of the scientists who gave medicine this wonderful prize in Hakim N.S. and Papalois V. (eds.) (2003) *History of Organ and Cell Transplantation*, Imperial College Press, London and in Brent L. (1996) *A History of Transplantation Immunology*, Academic Press, London.

ments between mice of different pure strains. As these mice breed true within a given strain and always accept grafts from each other, they must be homozygous for the "transplantation" genes. Consider two such strains A and B with allelic genes differing at one locus. In each case paternal and maternal genes will be identical and they will have a genetic constitution of, say, A/A and B/B respectively. Crossing strains A and B gives a first familial generation (F1) of constitution A/B. Now, all F1 mice accept grafts from either parent showing that they are immunologically tolerant to both A and B due to the fact that the transplantation antigens from each parent are codominantly expressed (see Figure 4.26). By intercrossing

the F1 generation, one would expect an average distribution of genotypes for the F2s as shown in Figure 16.2; only one in four would have no A genes and would therefore reject an A graft because of lack of tolerance, and one in four would reject B grafts for the same reason. Thus, for each locus, three out of four of the F2 generation will accept parental strain grafts.

In the mouse around 40 such loci have been established but, as we have seen earlier, the complex set of loci termed H-2 (HLA in the human) predominates in the sense that it controls the "strong" transplantation antigens that provoke intense allograft reactions. We have looked at the structure (cf.

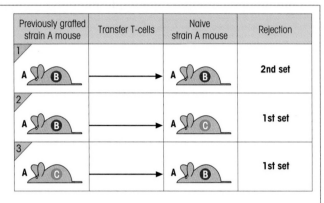

Figure 16.1. Graft rejection induces memory that is specific and can be transferred by T-cells.

In experiment 1, an A strain recipient of T-cells from another A strain mouse, which had previously rejected a graft from strain B, will give accelerated (i.e. 2nd set) rejection of a B graft. This occurs even though the mouse that has received the graft has not itself previously been grafted. Experiments 2 and 3 show the specificity of the phenomenon with respect to the genetically unrelated third party strain C.

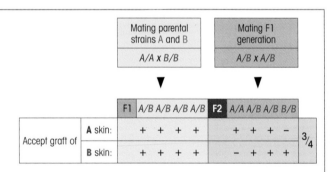

Figure 16.2. Inheritance of genes controlling transplantation antigens.

A represents a gene expressing the A antigen and *B* the corresponding allelic gene at the same genetic locus. The pure strains are homozygous for *A/A* and *B/B* respectively. As the genes are codominant, an animal with *A/B* genome will express both antigens, become tolerant to them and therefore accept grafts from either A or B donors. The illustration shows that, for each gene controlling a transplantation antigen specificity, three-quarters of the F2 generation will accept a graft of parental skin. For *n* genes the fraction is $(3/4)^n$. If F1 *A/B* animals are back-crossed with an *A/A* parent, half the progeny will be *A/A* and half *A/B;* only the latter will accept B grafts.

Figure 4.17) and biology of this **major histocompatibility complex (MHC)** in some detail in previous chapters (see Milestone 4.2, p. 100). Given the mendelian segregation and codominant expression of these genes, it should be evident that in outbred populations siblings have a 1:4 chance of identity

with respect to MHC. The non-H-2 or "minor" transplantation antigens, such as the male H-Y, are recognized by T-cells as processed peptides in association with the MHC molecules. One should not be misled by the term "minor" into thinking that these antigens cannot give rise to serious rejection problems; they do, albeit more slowly than the MHC.

Some other consequences of MHC incompatibility

Class II MHC differences produce a mixed lymphocyte reaction (MLR)

When peripheral blood mononuclear cells (PBMCs) from individuals of different class II haplotype are cultured together, lymphocyte activation and proliferation occurs (MLR), the T-cells of each population reacting against MHC class II determinants on the surface of the cells of the other population. The responding cells are predominantly CD4+ T-cells and are stimulated by the class II determinants present mostly on B-cells, macrophages and especially dendritic cells. Thus, the MLR is inhibited by antisera to class II determinants on the stimulator cells.

The graft-versus-host (GVH) reaction

When competent T-cells are transferred from a donor to a recipient who is incapable of rejecting them, the grafted cells survive and have time to recognize the host antigens and react immunologically against them. Instead of the normal transplantation reaction of host against graft, we have the reverse, a graft-versus-host (GVH) reaction. In the young rodent there can be inhibition of growth (runting), spleen enlargement and hemolytic anemia (due to the production of red cell antibodies). In the human, fever, anemia, weight loss, rash, diarrhea and splenomegaly are observed, with cytokines, especially tumor necrosis factor (TNF), being major mediators of pathology. The "stronger" the transplantation antigen difference, the more severe the reaction. Where donor and recipient differ at HLA or H-2 loci, the consequences can be fatal, although it should be noted that reactions to dominant minor transplantation antigens, or combinations of them, may be equally difficult to control.

Two possible situations leading to GVH reactions are illustrated in Figure 16.3. In humans this may arise in immunologically compromised subjects receiving hematopoietic stem cell grafts, e.g. for severe combined immunodeficiency (see p. 378) or as a form of cancer therapy. Competent T-cells in blood or present in grafted organs given to immunosuppressed patients may also mediate g.v.h. reactions.

Mechanisms of graft rejection

Various immune system components can mediate an attack upon the foreign organ or tissue and thereby contribute towards **hyperacute**, **acute** or **chronic** rejection (Table 16.1).

Table 16.1. The various types of graft rejection.

Graft rejection	Time course	Cause	Characteristics
Hyperacute	Minutes	Pre-existing antibodies due to either blood group incompatibility or presensitization to class I MHC through blood transfusion	Antibodies bind to blood vessel endothelium in the graft, resulting in complement activation, neutrophil recruitment, platelet aggregation and blood clotting
Acute	Several days	Activation of lymphocytes	Cytotoxic T-cells attack the donor cells expressing foreign MHC. Helper T-cells and B-cells collaborate in production of antibodies to alloantigens
Chronic	Months to years	Multiple immune mechanisms or recurrence of the original disease	Mechanisms not fully understood. Can involve lymphocytes, phagocytes, antibody and complement

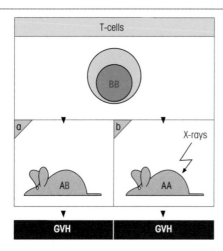

Figure 16.3. Graft-versus-host reaction.

When competent T-cells are inoculated into a host incapable of reacting against them, the grafted cells are free to react against the antigens on the host's cells that they recognize as foreign. The ensuing reaction may be fatal. Two of several possible situations are illustrated: (a) the hybrid AB receives cells from one parent (BB) that are tolerated but react against the A antigen on host cells; (b) an X-irradiated AA recipient restored immunologically with BB cells cannot react against the graft and a graft-versus-host (GVH) reaction will result.

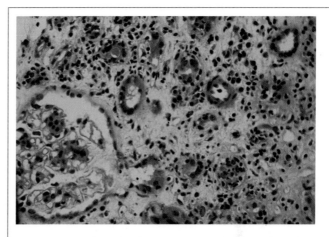

Figure 16.4. Acute rejection of human renal allograft showing dense cellular infiltration of interstitium by mononuclear cells. (Photograph courtesy of M. Thompson and A. Dorling.)

Lymphocytes can mediate rejection

A primary role of lymphocytes in first set rejection is consistent with the histology of the early reaction showing infiltration by mononuclear cells with very few polymorphonuclear cells or plasma cells (Figure 16.4). The dramatic effect of neonatal thymectomy on prolonging skin transplants, and the long survival of grafts in children with thymic deficiencies, implicate the T-cells in these reactions. In the chicken, allograft rejection and GVH reactivity are influenced by neonatal thymectomy but not bursectomy. More direct evidence has come from *in vitro* studies showing that T-cells taken from mice rejecting an allograft could kill target cells bearing the graft antigens *in vitro*. Although CD8 cytotoxic T-cells play a major role in allograft rejection, a number of murine models have indicated that in the absence of CD4 T-cells allografts can be accepted indefinitely. Indeed, rejection can be mediated by CD4 T-cells in the absence of CD8 T-cells, perhaps because the CD4 cells sometimes have cytotoxic potential for class II targets. However, in intact animals, cytokine secretion from CD4 T-cells will recruit and activate CD8 T-cells, B-cells, NKT cells and macrophages that all have the potential to contribute to the rejection process. Furthermore, γ-interferon (IFNγ) upregulates MHC expression on the target graft cell, so increasing its vulnerability to CD8 cytotoxic cells.

Recognition of allogeneic MHC by the recipient's T-cells

Remember, we defined the MHC by its ability to provoke the most powerful rejection of grafts between members of the same species. This intensity of MHC mismatched rejection is a consequence of the **very high frequency of alloreactive T-cells** (i.e. cells that react with allografts) **present in normal individuals.** Whereas merely a fraction of a percent of the normal T-cell population is specific for a given single peptide, upwards of 10% of T-cells react with alloantigens. Two main pathways of recognition have been described. In the **direct pathway** large numbers of recipient alloreactive T-cells recognize **allo- (i.e. graft) MHC** on the surface of donor cells, whereas in the **indirect pathway** a smaller number of recipient T-cells recognize peptides derived from **allo-MHC** (and allo-minor transplantation antigens) presented by self MHC molecules on the recipient's own antigen-presenting cells (Figure 16.5a and c). A third, **semi-direct**, pathway has also been proposed, in which intact MHC molecules are acquired from the donor cells by the dendritic cells of the recipient (Figure 16.5b).

Allogeneic MHC differs from the recipient essentially in the groove residues that contact processed peptide, but much less so in the more conserved helical regions that are recognized by the TCR. Having a different groove structure, the allo-MHC will be able to bind a number of peptides derived from proteins common to donor and host that might be unable to fit the groove in the host MHC and therefore fail to induce self-tolerance. Thus the host T-cells that recognize allo-MHC plus common peptides will not have been eliminated, and will be available to react with the large number of different peptides binding to the allo-groove of the donor antigen-presenting cells (APCs) that migrate to the secondary lymphoid tissue of the graft recipient. In some cases, the polymorphic residues may lie within the regions of the MHC helices that contact TCR directly and, by chance, a proportion of the T-cell repertoire cross-reacts and binds to the donor MHC with high affinity. Attachment of the T-cell to the APC will be particularly strong

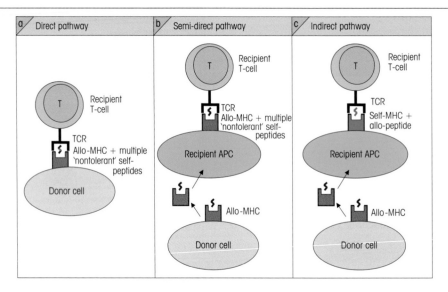

Figure 16.5. Recognition of graft antigens by alloreactive T-cells.

(a) **Direct pathway.** T-cell receptors (TCR) on the recipient's T-cells directly recognize allogeneic MHC (brown) on the surface of donor antigen-presenting cells. Polymorphic differences between MHC allotypes largely affect peptide binding rather than TCR contact by the donor MHC. Under these circumstances, the donor allogeneic MHC molecule will be seen as similar to "self" MHC by the recipient's T-cells but, unlike the self-MHC, the donor MHC groove on graft antigen-presenting cells will bind large numbers of processed peptides common to graft and recipient to which the responder host T-cells have not been rendered tolerant and that can therefore provoke a reaction in up to 10% of these host T-cells. This provides the intensity of the allograft response. This explanation for the high frequency of alloreactive T-cells is given further credibility by the isolation of individual T-cell clones that react with self- and allo-MHC, each binding a different peptide sequence. Direct recognition of donor MHC by recipient T-cells can also occur if the limited polymorphism in the α-helix adventitiously allows binding of TCRs to the allo-MHC independently of the associated peptide. Multiple bonds of this nature between the APC and T-cell may give rise to a strong enough interaction to permit T-cell activation. (b) **Semi-direct pathway.** It has been proposed that recipient dendritic cells may acquire intact MHC molecules from donor cells and then show these intact MHC molecules to the recipient's T-cells. Again, "nontolerant" peptides derived from antigens common to donor and recipient are presented. (c) **Indirect pathway.** The recipient's APCs (antigen-presenting cells) process donor MHC (brown) and donor minor histocompatibility molecules and, just as they would any protein molecule, then present the generated allogeneic peptides (brown) using their own, i.e. self, MHC (green). The initially small population of T-cells that are stimulated by the indirect pathway will expand with time.

as the TCRs will bind to all the donor MHC molecules on the APC, whereas in the case of normal MHC–peptide recognition, only a small proportion of the MHC grooves will be filled by the specific peptide in question. These direct pathways of immunization by the allograft MHC that are usually initiated by the most powerful APC, the dendritic cell, dominate the early sensitization events, as this acute phase of rejection (see below) can be blocked by antibodies to the allo-MHC class II.

However, with time, as the donor APCs in the graft are replaced by recipient cells, another rejection mechanism based on an indirect pathway of sensitization involving the presentation of processed **allogeneic peptides** by **host MHC** (Figure 16.5c) becomes possible. Although T-cells recognizing peptides derived from polymorphic graft proteins would be expected to be present in low frequency comparable to that observed with any foreign antigen, a graft that has been in place for an extended period will have the time to expand this small population significantly so that later rejection may depend progressively on this indirect pathway. In these circumstances, antirecipient MHC class II can now be shown to prolong renal allografts in rats.

The role of antibody

Allogeneic cells can be destroyed by antibody-mediated cytotoxic (type II hypersensitivity) reactions (p. 406). Consideration of the different ways in which kidney allografts can be rejected illustrates the contribution of antibody to the rejection process.

Hyperacute rejection occurs within minutes of transplantation and is the result of pre-existing anti-donor antibodies in the recipient binding to blood vessel endothelium in the donated kidney. The antibodies activate the classical pathway of complement and initiate the blood clotting cascade. The blood vessels become blocked with aggregated platelets, and neutrophils are also rapidly recruited as a result of the complement activation.

Acute rejection is characterized by dense cellular infiltration (Figure 16.4) and rupture of peritubular capillaries. CD8+ cytotoxic T-cells attack the graft cells whose MHC antigen expression has been upregulated by γ-interferon. CD4+ T-cells are also present, including cells of the Th17 phenotype. Upregulated expression of the CD80 and CD86 co-stimulatory molecules occurs on tubular epithelial cells thereby promoting activation of these cell-mediated responses, further aided by the local production of a number of chemokines. Although some T-cells may become sensitized within the graft itself, antigen presentation by dendritic cells of both donor and recipient origin occurs predominantly in the draining lymph nodes Acute humoral rejection involving anti-donor MHC contributes to acute rejection episodes in around 25% of kidney transplant patients. Binding of graft-specific antibody leads to the deposition of substantial amounts of complement component C4d in the peritubular capillaries. Immunoglobulin deposits on the vessel walls induce platelet aggregation in the glomerular capillaries leading to acute renal shutdown (Figure

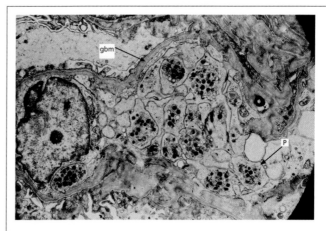

Figure 16.6. Acute late rejection of human renal allograft showing platelet aggregation in a glomerular capillary induced by deposition of antibody on the vessel wall.

Electron micrograph. gbm, glomerular basement membrane; P, platelet. (Photograph courtesy of K. Porter.)

16.6). The possibility of damage to antibody-coated cells through antibody-dependent cellular cytotoxicity must also be considered.

Chronic rejection involves glomerular and tubular fibrosis and is often associated with subendothelial deposits of immunoglobulin and C4d in the glomerular and peritubular capillaries. This may sometimes be an expression of an ongoing immune complex disorder (causing the renal pathology that originally resulted in the necessity to replace a damaged kidney) or possibly of complex formation with soluble antigens derived from the grafted kidney.

The complexity of the action and interaction of cellular and humoral factors in graft rejection is therefore considerable and an attempt to summarize the postulated mechanisms involved is presented in Figure 16.7.

There are also circumstances when antibodies may actually protect a graft from destruction, a phenomenon termed enhancement.

The prevention of graft rejection

Matching tissue types on graft donor and recipient

Given the fact that demand for transplantation far outstrips the supply of available organs (Figure 16.8) it is essential to maximize the chances that the graft will be immunologically accepted by the recipient. As MHC differences provoke the most vicious rejection of grafts, a prodigious amount of effort has gone into defining these antigen specificities, in an attempt to minimize rejection by matching graft and recipient in much the same way that individuals are cross-matched for blood transfusions (incidentally, the ABO group provides strong transplantation antigens).

Figure 16.7. Mechanisms of target cell destruction.

(a) Direct killing by Tc cells and indirect tissue damage through release of cytokines such as IFNγ and TNF from Th1-cells. (b) Direct killing by NK cells (see p. 26) enhanced by interferon. (c) Attack by antibody-dependent cellular cytotoxicity (d) Phagocytosis of target coated with antibody (heightened by bound C3b). (e) Sticking of platelets to antibody bound to the surface of graft vascular endothelium leading to formation of microthrombi. (f) Complement-mediated cytotoxicity. (g) Macrophages activated nonspecifically by agents such as IFNγ and possibly C3b can be cytotoxic for graft cells, perhaps through extracellular action of TNF and $\cdot O_2^-$ radicals generated at the cell surface (see p. 13). IFN, interferon; Mφ, macrophage; NK, natural killer cell; P, polymorphonuclear leukocyte; TNF, tumor necrosis factor.

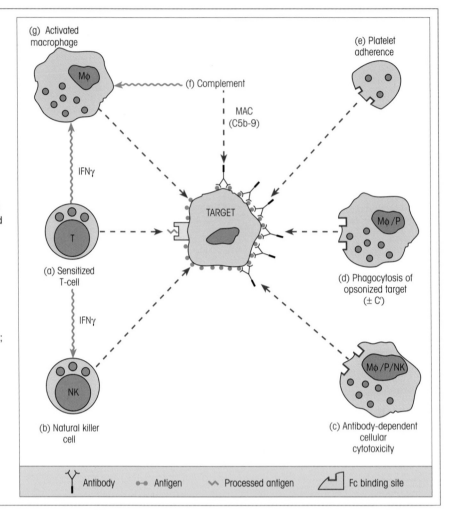

Figure 16.8. The unmet demand for kidney transplants.

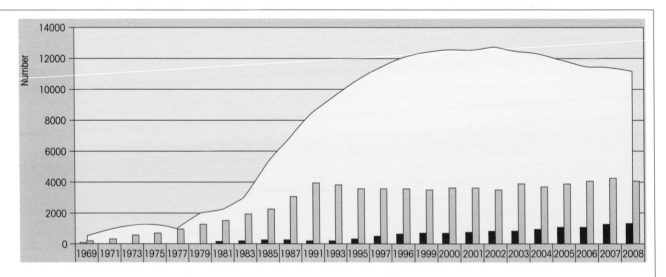

Dynamics of the Eurotransplant kidney transplant waiting list and transplants between 1969 and 2008. The curved line indicates the number of patients awaiting a kidney transplant, and underneath the far fewer number of transplants that have taken place is shown by the histogram, with deceased donor transplants indicated by the orange bars and living donor transplants by the black bars.

HLA tissue typing

HLA alleles are defined by their gene sequences and individuals can be typed by the *polymerase chain reaction* (PCR) using discriminating pairs of primers. Molecules encoded by the class II *HLA-DP, -DQ* and *-DR* loci provoke CD4 T-cell responses, whereas *HLA-A, -B* and *-C* gene products are targets for alloreactive CD8 T-cells.

The polymorphism of the human HLA system

With so many alleles at each locus and several loci in each individual (Figure 16.9), it will readily be appreciated that this gives rise to an exceptional degree of polymorphism. This is of

great potential value to the species, as the need for T-cells to recognize their own individual specificities provides a defense against microbial molecular mimicry in which a whole species might be put at risk by its inability to recognize as foreign an organism that generates MHC–peptide complexes similar to self. It is also possible that in some way the existence of a high degree of polymorphism helps to maintain the diversity of antigenic recognition within the lymphoid system of a given species and also ensures heterozygosity (hybrid vigor).

The value of matching tissue types

Improvements in surgical techniques and the use of drugs such as cyclosporine have diminished the effects of mismatching

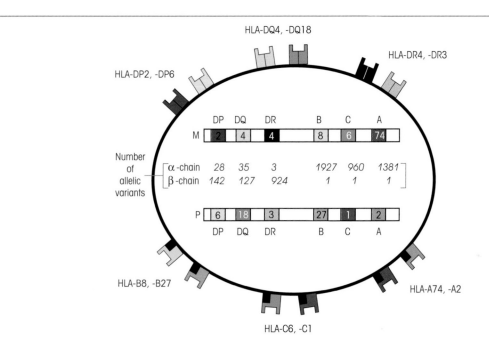

Figure 16.9. Polymorphic HLA specificities and their inheritance.

As there are several possible alleles at each locus, the probability of a random pair of subjects from the general population having identical HLA specificities is very low. Indeed, the class I and II MHC genes are the most polymorphic in the genome and the number of different allelic variants based upon nucleotide sequences assigned as of October 2010 are indicated by the numbers in italics in the center of the figure (data from http://www.anthonynolan.org.uk/HIG). In the example given the individual expresses the particular α- and β-chain alleles at the DP loci (see Figure 4.22) on the maternal (M) chromosome that specify HLA-DP2, and has inherited those for HLA-DP6 on the paternal (P) chromosome, and so on. These genes are codominantly expressed and therefore cells can express up to six different alleles of the main class I molecules and, on their professional antigen-presenting cells, additionally up to at least six different class II molecules. The fact that there are usually two DRβ genes inherited on both copies of chromosome 6, and the

potential for *trans* pairing as well as *cis* pairing of some class II α and β-chains, further increases the HLA diversity in the individual. Conversely, homozygosity at any of the loci will reduce the number of variants. Note that not all polymorphisms in nucleotide sequence will result in a polymorphism at the protein level, and furthermore that not all polymorphisms in the polypeptide chain will affect binding of antigenic peptides or T-cell receptors to the MHC molecule and therefore impact upon transplant rejection. The MHC class I molecules all employ the same β-chain, β_2-microglobulin, that is nonpolymorphic, encoded outside of the MHC, and does not form part of the peptide-binding groove. There is a 1:4 chance that two siblings will be MHC identical because each group of specificities on a single chromosome forms a haplotype that will usually be inherited *en bloc*, giving four possible combinations of paternal and maternal chromosomes. Parent and offspring can only be identical (1:2 chance) if the mother and father have one haplotype in common.

HLA specificities on solid graft survival but, nevertheless, most transplanters favor a reasonable degree of matching (see Figure 16.18). Tissue typing can be carried out using serological methods that employ panels of antibodies each specific for a different HLA allele, and which enable the detection of the HLA variants on the cell surface of leukocytes. These techniques are increasingly being replaced by molecular genetics techniques, such as the use of sequence-specific oligonucleotide primers, to determine the variants. HLA-DR matching is the most critical, followed by HLA-B and then HLA-A. In fact, it is only these three loci that are usually typed, although recent studies have suggested that typing of HLA-C might also be advantageous in optimizing the success of some transplants. Mismatches at HLA-DQ are thought to generally be less important, and those at the HLA–DP loci appear to have minimal consequences. In addition to typing recipients and potential donors, cross-matching is carried out to ensure the absence of pre-existing antibodies to donor antigens in the proposed recipient. Hematopoietic stem cell grafts, including bone marrow grafts, require a very high degree of compatibility because of the increased potential for graft-versus-host disease in addition to host-versus-graft reactions; the greater accuracy of DNA typing methods and the inclusion of HLA-DQ typing can be most helpful in this respect.

Because of the many thousands of different HLA phenotypes possible (Figure 16.9), it is usual to work with a large pool of potential recipients on a continental basis (e.g. Eurotransplant), so that when graft material becomes available the best possible match can be made. The position will be improved when the pool of available organs can be increased through the development of long-term tissue storage banks, but techniques are not good enough for this at present, except in the case of hematopoietic stem cells that can be kept viable even after freezing and thawing. With a paired organ such as the kidney, living donors may be used; siblings provide the best chance of a good match. However, the use of living donors poses difficult ethical problems and organs are most commonly obtained from brain dead donors in which there has been a loss of all brain function including that of the brain stem that controls respiration.

There is active interest in the possibility of using animal organs (see below) or mechanical substitutes, while some are even trying to prevent the disease in the first place!

Agents producing general immunosuppression

Graft rejection can be held at bay by the use of agents that nonspecifically interfere with the induction or expression of the immune response (Figure 16.10). Because these agents are nonspecific, patients on immunosuppressive therapy tend to be susceptible to infections; they are also more prone to develop lymphoreticular cancers, particularly those of viral etiology.

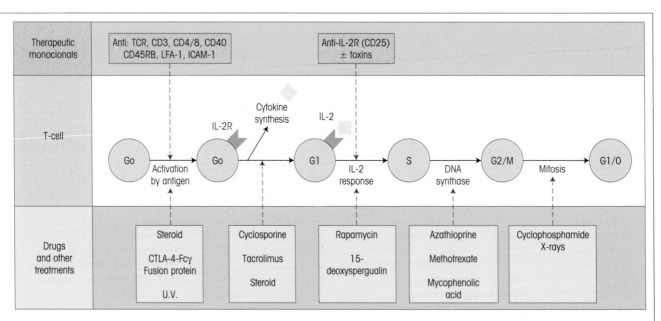

Figure 16.10. Immunosuppressive agents used to control graft rejection.

Mycophenolate mofetil is a powerful immunosuppressant that, when metabolized into the purine analog mycophenolic acid, inhibits proliferation but also suppresses expression of CD25, -71, -154 (CD40L) and CD28. Another potent drug is 15-deoxyspergualin (DSG), which interferes with lymphocyte function by binding to heat shock protein and thereby inhibiting NFκB translocation to the nucleus. Simultaneous treatment with agents acting at sequential stages in development of the rejection response would be expected to lead to strong synergy and this is clearly seen with cyclosporine and rapamycin.

Targeting lymphoid populations

Anti-CD3 monoclonals are in widespread use as anti-T-cell reagents to reverse acute graft rejection. Originally the mouse monoclonal antibody OKT3 was used and, although shown to have a beneficial effect, its efficacy was to some extent compromised by its immunogenicity in the human host. Furthermore, it possesses a mitogenic activity responsible for triggering a severe cytokine release syndrome involving "flu-like" symptoms. These problems are circumvented by the use of engineered antibodies (see p. 146). The otelixizumab (ChAglyCD3) antibody is a humanized nonmitogenic version of a rat monoclonal antibody in which position 297 in the heavy chain has been mutated to prevent glycosylation and consequently binding to Fc receptors and to complement. Teplizumab, a humanized OKT3γ1 Ala–Ala antibody in which leucines were replaced with alanines at positions 234 and 235 to eliminate FcγR binding, is also nonmitogenic and efficacious.

The IL-2 receptor α chain (CD25), expressed by activated but not resting T-cells, represents another exploitable target. Daclizumab is a humanized monoclonal anti-IL-2Rα, and basiliximab a chimeric (mouse V region, human C region) antibody of similar specificity. They are of particular benefit in the prevention of acute kidney transplant rejection when used in combination with cyclosporine plus corticosteroids.

Yet another effective biologic is belatacept, a fusion protein of the extracellular domain of CTLA-4 with human IgG1 Fc in which two amino acid replacements in CTLA-4 provide an increased ability to block the activity of the CD80/CD86 co-stimulatory molecules required for T-cell activation. In phase II clinical trials this drug was shown to be as effective as cyclosporine but with less damaging effects on the kidney.

Immunosuppressive drugs

The development of an immunological response requires the active proliferation of a relatively small number of antigen-sensitive lymphocytes to give a population of sensitized cells large enough to be effective. Many of the immunosuppressive drugs now employed were first used in cancer chemotherapy because of their toxicity to dividing cells. Aside from the complications of blanket immunosuppression mentioned above, these antimitotic drugs are especially toxic for cells of the bone marrow and small intestine and must therefore be used with great care.

A commonly used drug in this field is **azathioprine**, which inhibits nucleic acid synthesis and has a preferential effect on T-cell-mediated reactions. Another drug, **methotrexate**, through its action as a folic acid antagonist also inhibits synthesis of nucleic acid. The N-mustard derivative **cyclophosphamide** attacks DNA by alkylation and cross-linking, so preventing correct duplication during cell division. These agents appear to exert their damaging effects on cells during mitosis and, for this reason, are most powerful when administered after presentation of antigen at a time when the antigen-sensitive cells are dividing. An exciting group of fungal metabolites dramatically improved graft survival in human transplantation and are also of benefit in the therapy of immunological disorders through their ability to target T-cells. **Cyclosporine** (Sandimmune, or its microemulsion version Neoral, which exhibits increased bioavailability) is a neutral hydrophobic 11 amino acid cyclical peptide generated by the fungus *Beauvaria nivea*. It selectively blocks the transcription of IL-2 in activated T-cells. Resting cells that carry the vital memory for immunity to microbial infections are spared and there is little toxicity for dividing cells in gut and bone marrow. The drug also directly affects dendritic cells, inhibiting a number of their functions including antigen processing, production of TNF and IL-12, expression of chemokine receptors and cell migration. Cyclosporine is firmly established as a first-line therapy in the prophylaxis and treatment of transplant rejection; Figure 16.11 gives an example of its use in kidney transplantation. Another T-cell-specific immunosuppressive drug, **tacrolimus** (FK506), contains a macrolide ring structure and although originally also found in a fungus is isolated from the bacterium *Streptomyces tsukubaensis*. Like cyclosporine, it blocks various T-cell and dendritic cell activities. **Rapamycin** (sirolimus), a product of *Streptomyces hygroscopicus*, is also a macrolide but in contrast to tacrolimus acts to block signals induced by combination of IL-2 with its receptor.

Regarding the molecular details of the mode of action of these drugs, cyclosporine complexes with cyclophilin A, a member of the **immunophilin** family, whilst tacrolimus complexes with another immunophilin family member, *FK-b*inding protein (FKBP) (Figure 16.12). These complexes then interact with and inhibit the calcium- and calmodulin-dependent phosphatase, calcineurin, which activates the NFAT (*n*uclear *f*actor of *a*ctivated *T*-cells) transcription factor for IL-2 in activated T-cells. Although rapamycin also binds to FKBP, the complex has a quite different activity and inhibits the TOR

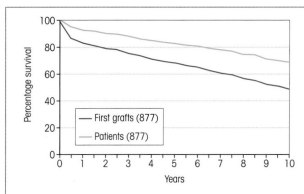

Figure 16.11. Actuarial survival of primary cadaveric kidney grafts in 877 patients treated at the Oxford Transplant Centre with triple therapy of cyclosporine, azathioprine and prednisolone.

(Data kindly provided by Peter J. Morris.)

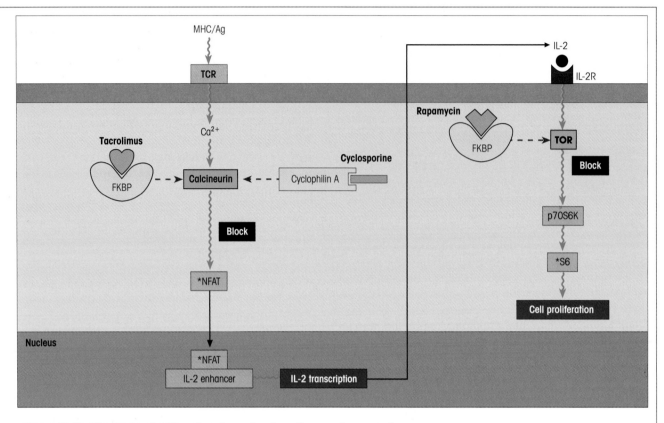

Figure 16.12. The mode of action of cyclosporine, tacrolimus and rapamycin.

The complexes of cyclosporine with cyclophilin A and of tacrolimus with FKBP (*FK*506 [tacrolimus]-*b*inding *p*rotein) bind to and inactivate the phosphatase calcineurin responsible for activating the *n*uclear *f*actor of *a*ctivated *T*-cells (NFAT)

transcription factor for IL-2 synthesis. The rapamycin–FKBP complex inhibits the TOR (*t*arget *of* *r*apamycin) kinase and thereby blocks the activation of p70 S6 kinase by transduced IL-2 signals, thus inhibiting cell proliferation.

(*t*arget *of* *r*apamycin) serine/threonine kinase. The immunosuppressive activity of rapamycin is at least partially explained by the fact that TOR plays a central role in transducing proliferative signals, such as those through the IL-2 receptor. In addition to its role in transplantation, cyclosporine is used in a wide range of disorders where T-cell-mediated hypersensitivity reactions are suspected. Indeed, the benefits of cyclosporine in diseases such as rheumatoid arthritis, psoriasis, idiopathic nephrotic syndrome, type 1 diabetes, Behçet's syndrome, active Crohn's disease, aplastic anemia and severe corticosteroid-dependent asthma have been interpreted to suggest or confirm a pathogenic role for the immune system. Inhibition of keratinocyte proliferation by cyclosporine may contribute to the favorable outcome seen in patients with psoriasis who are treated with this drug. A rapid onset of benefit, and of relapse when treatment is stopped, are common features of cyclosporine therapy. There are, of course, side effects, the most significant being nephrotoxicity. It has to be used at doses below those causing renal fibrosis due to stimulation of TGFβ production by several cell types.

Tacrolimus is greatly superior to cyclosporine on a molar basis *in vitro* but is not substantially more effective. Because they act at different stages in the activation of the T-cell (Figure 16.10), cyclosporine and rapamycin show an impressive degree of synergy that allows the two drugs to be used together at considerably lower dose levels with correspondingly less likelihood of side effects. Steroids such as prednisolone intervene at many points in the immune response, affecting lymphocyte recirculation and the generation of cytotoxic effector cells, for example; in addition, their outstanding anti-inflammatory potency rests on features such as inhibition of neutrophil adherence to vascular endothelium in an inflammatory area and suppression of monocyte/macrophage functions such as microbicidal activity and response to cytokines. Corticosteroids form complexes with intracellular receptors that then bind to regulatory genes and block transcription of TNF, IFNγ, IL-1, -2, -3, -6 and MHC class II, i.e. they block expression of cytokines from both lymphocytes and macrophages, whereas cyclosporine has its main action on the former.

Inducing tolerance to graft antigens

If the disadvantages of blanket immunosuppression are to be avoided, we must aim at knocking out only the reactivity of the host to the antigens of the graft, leaving the remainder of the immunological apparatus intact—in other words, the induction of **antigen-specific tolerance**.

It turns out that hematopoietic cells represent an excellent source of tolerogenic alloantigens, and the production of stable mixed chimerism by such cells engrafted from bone marrow is proving to be a potent means of inducing robust specific transplantation tolerance to solid organs across major MHC mismatches. However, successful allogeneic bone marrow transplantation in immunocompetent adults normally requires cytoablative treatment of recipients with irradiation or cyto-

toxic drugs and this has tended to restrict its use to malignant conditions. A most encouraging study in mice showed the feasibility of inducing long-lasting tolerance not only to bone marrow cells but also to fully MHC-mismatched skin grafts in naive recipients receiving high-dose bone marrow transplantation and **co-stimulatory blockade** by single injections of monoclonal anti-CD154 (CD40L) plus a CTLA-4–Ig fusion protein (Figure 16.13). A persistent hematopoietic macrochimerism is achieved with a significant proportion of donor-type lymphocytes in the thymus indicating intrathymic deletion of donor-reactive T-cells.

While this protocol permits long-term engraftment of bone marrow and solid organs, it seems that direct blockade with just anti-CD154 and CTLA-4–Ig is sufficient to induce tolerance to solid organ grafts. Stimulation of alloreactive T-cells by

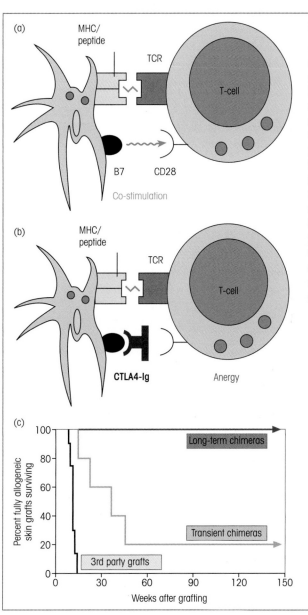

Figure 16.13. Co-stimulatory blockade.

(a) T-cell activation requires co-stimulatory signals, in particular engagement of CD28 on the T-cell surface by the B7 molecules (CD80 and CD86) on the surface of the antigen-presenting cell. (b) CTLA-4 binds to CD80/86 with higher affinity than CD28 and therefore the soluble CTLA-4-Ig fusion protein is able to block these co-stimulatory signals, resulting in T-cell anergy. Similarly, a monoclonal antibody to CD40L on the T-cell would block co-stimulatory signals normally provided by CD40 on the antigen-presenting cell. (c) Induction of tolerance and macrochimerism by fully allogeneic bone marrow transplantation plus co-stimulatory blockade. B6 mice received bone marrow cells from the fully allogeneic B10.A strain with injections of anti-CD154 (CD40L) and the CTLA-4–Ig fusion protein that blocks CD80/CD86–CD28 interactions. Eight mice showing long-term persistence of multilineage donor cells (macrochimerism) were fully tolerant to B10.A skin grafts. Five mice with transient chimerism showed moderate prolongation of skin graft survival relative to unrelated third party grafts. (Data taken from Wekerle T. *et al.* (2000) *Nature Medicine* **6**, 464, with permission.)

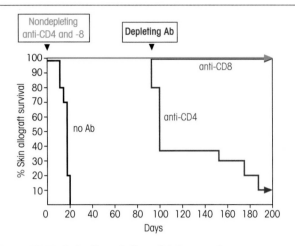

Figure 16.14. Induction of allograft tolerance by nondepleting anti-CD4 plus anti-CD8.

Tolerance to skin grafts from donors with multiple minor transplantation antigen mismatches was achieved by concurrent injection of IgG2a monoclonal antibodies to CD4 and CD8 that do not induce cell depletion (green arrow). The maintenance of tolerance depends upon the continued presence of antigen, which enables the unresponsive cells to interact with newly arising immunocompetent cells on the surface of the same antigen-presenting cells and render them unresponsive through an infectious tolerance mechanism (cf. Figures 11.8 and 18.31). Loss of tolerance on depletion of CD4 but not CD8 cells (red arrows) shows that active tolerance is maintained by the CD4 subset. Indeed, tolerance can be transferred by CD4⁺CD25⁺ T-regulatory cells. (Figure synthesized from data kindly provided by S.P. Cobbold and H. Waldmann.)

the graft in the presence of co-stimulatory blockade leads to apoptosis, a process promoted by rapamycin that improves the tolerant state. Bcl-x$_L$ (cf. Figure 10.4, p. 266) prevents both T-cell apoptosis and tolerance induction by this treatment revealing the importance of apoptotic T-cell deletion for the establishment of antigen-specific unresponsiveness. In a further twist to the tale, the apoptotic T-cells "reach from beyond the grave" by producing IL-10, so that their phagocytosis along with antigen leads to the presentation of the antigen in a tolerogenic form that maintains tolerance through the production of immunoregulatory cells.

Despite the role of the *mature* dendritic cell as the champion stimulator of resting T-cells, the dendritic cell *precursors* may present antigen in the absence of B7 co-stimulators and, by mechanisms echoing those described above in the co-stimulatory blockade experiments, would appear to have a powerful potential for tolerance induction. This concept is of particular relevance to the specific unresponsiveness generated by grafts of liver that, being a hematopoietic organ, continually exports large numbers of these immature dendritic cells.

Nondepleting anti-CD4 and anti-CD8 monoclonals, by depriving T-cells of fully activating signals, can render them

anergic when they engage antigen through their specific receptors. These anergic cells can induce unresponsiveness in newly recruited T-cells ("infectious tolerance," p. 296) and so establish specific and indefinite acceptance of mouse skin grafts across class I or multiple minor transplantation antigen barriers (Figure 16.14). It should be noted that skin allografts provide the most difficult challenge for tolerance induction, and transplants of organs such as the heart, which are less fastidious than skin, require less aggressive immunotherapy.

Given the wide variety of different peptide epitopes presented by the graft MHC, full-frontal attack on the alloreactive T-cells by administration of tolerogenic peptides represents quite a challenge, and the strategy of using co-stimulatory blockade with the antigens being provided by the graft itself looks to be a more promising route.

Is xenografting a practical proposition?

Because the supply of donor human organs for transplantation lags seriously behind the demand, a widespread interest in the feasibility of using animal organs is emerging. Pigs are more favored than primates as donors both on the grounds of ethical acceptability and the hazards of zoonoses. Indeed, pig heart valves have been successfully used for decades on millions of patients in valve replacement procedures. However, in this case the valves have greatly reduced immunogenicity due to prior treatment with glutaraldehyde. This fixation procedure cannot be used where an entire functioning heart or other organ is to be transplanted. The first hurdle to be overcome in these cases is therefore the **hyperacute rejection** that occurs due to xenoreactive natural antibodies in the host. The sugar structure galactose α-1,3-galactose is absent in humans, apes and Old World monkeys due to a mutation in the gene encoding α-1,3-galactosyltransferase in these species. They are therefore not immunologically tolerant to this nonself sugar structure. Furthermore, they have pre-existing antibodies to the Gal α-1,3-Gal epitope, which is present on many common bacteria and expressed abundantly on the xenogeneic pig vascular endothelium. The natural antibodies bind to the endothelium and activate complement in the absence of regulators of the human complement system, such as decay accelerating factor, CD59 and MCP (cf. Figure 14.4), precipitating the hyperacute rejection phenomenon. Novel genetic engineering strategies for the solution of this problem are outlined in Figure 16.15.

The next crisis is **acute vascular rejection** occurring within 6 days as *de novo* antibody production is elicited in response to the xenoantigens on donor epithelium. Interleukin-12 and IFNγ inhibit acute vascular rejection of xenografts and, over the long term, IFNγ may protect the graft by promoting the formation of NO· which prevents constriction of blood vessels. A limited degree of success has been achieved using baboons as recipients of hearts or kidneys from α-1,3-galactosyltransferase knockout pigs, although fairly hefty immunosuppressive regimens were employed together with, in the case of the kidney

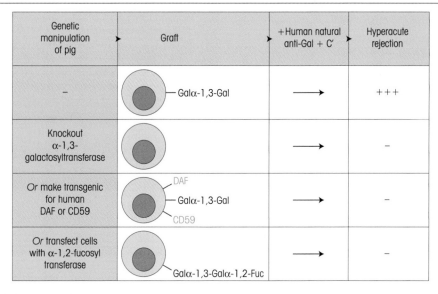

Genetic manipulation of pig	Graft	+Human natural anti-Gal + C′	Hyperacute rejection
–	Galα-1,3-Gal	⟶	+++
Knockout α-1,3-galactosyltransferase		⟶	–
Or make transgenic for human DAF or CD59	DAF — Galα-1,3-Gal — CD59	⟶	–
Or transfect cells with α-1,2-fucosyl transferase	Galα-1,3-Galα-1,2-Fuc	⟶	–

Figure 16.15. Strategies for avoiding complement-mediated hyperacute rejection of a xenograft caused by reaction of natural antigalactose antibodies with Galα-1,3-Gal on the surface of the pig graft cells.

Heart or kidney xenografts from α-1,3-galactosyltransferase knockout pigs can function for reasonable periods of time in baboons, as can hearts from transgenic pigs expressing the human complement regulatory proteins decay accelerating factor (DAF) or CD59. Transfection of pig cells with α-1,2- fucosyltransferase leads to the "covering up" of the Galα-1,3-Gal structure with a terminal fucose, thus preventing the binding of the antigalactose. Other strategies involve transfection with genes encoding an α-galactosidase or intracellular recombinant scFv reacting with α-1,3-galactosyltransferase.

grafts, cotransplantation of thymic tissue with the aim of inducing tolerance in the recipient.

Even when the immunological problems are overcome, it remains to be seen whether the xenograft will be compatible with human life over a prolonged period. There is also concern over the presence of porcine endogenous retroviruses (PERVs), which are related to viruses associated with leukemias in a number of species. Given that the PERV-A receptors PAR-1 and PAR-2 are widely distributed in human tissues such concerns are warranted, although it is unclear if infection of human cells with such viruses would have detrimental consequences.

Stem cell therapy

The ideal transplant is one created **entirely from cells of the recipient**, i.e. an autograft, which would eliminate the need for immunosuppression. It is possible to isolate stem cells from various adult organs including bone marrow. By way of an example, human bone marrow-derived multipotent stem cells have been shown to induce therapeutic neovascularization and cardiomyogenesis in a rat model of myocardial infarction. Recent advances in cell nuclear replacement have also opened up the possibility of therapeutic cloning using embryonic stem cells (Figure 16.16). Knowledge is steadily accumulating concerning the various growth factors required to guide relatively undifferentiated stem cells into the desired mature form,

for example pancreatic, nerve or liver cells for regenerative therapy, or erythrocytes for transfusion.

An exciting development came a few years back from the cloning of "Dolly" the sheep, the first cloned animal produced from a cell taken from an adult animal. Such reproductive cloning has led to concerns that cloned human embryos could be re-implanted and used in attempts to produce cloned humans. However, in therapeutic cloning the embryo is only allowed to grow for a few days in order to provide a source of stem cells for subsequent differentiation and expansion in vitro. A major step in this direction was the announcement in 2005 that a team at the University of Newcastle in the UK had succeeded in their attempts to clone a human blastocyst. More recently several groups have been able to genetically reprogramme adult tissue cells by introducing genes encoding a number of transcription factors in order to generate what are referred to as induced pluripotent stem cells. These powerful technologies have the potential to eventually revolutionize the treatment of paralysis and neurodegenerative conditions such as Parkinson's and Alzheimer's diseases using transfer of stem cell-derived neuronal cells. Stem cell therapy is also being very actively explored for the treatment of heart disease, diabetes, visual impairment and many other afflictions. The potential to grow stem cells on a matrix in order to engineer tissues or even whole organs provides further opportunities to circumvent the problem of allograft rejection (Figure 16.17). The first

Figure 16.16. Cell nuclear replacement for therapeutic cloning.

The nucleus of an egg is replaced with the nucleus from a body cell, such as a mammary gland cell or skin cell. The egg is then stimulated electrically or with chemicals to initiate cell division. Following its development into an embryo the stem cells can be isolated and are then driven to develop into the desired cell type by culture with appropriate growth and differentiation factors.

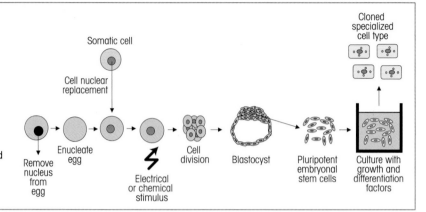

Figure 16.17. Production of autologous grafts by tissue engineering.

Undifferentiated cells are obtained directly from the patient either as adult stem cells or by cell nuclear replacement into enucleated oocytes. They are cultured in a biodegradable matrix with appropriate growth factors to provide a tissue populated with differentiated cells that can function as an autologous graft.

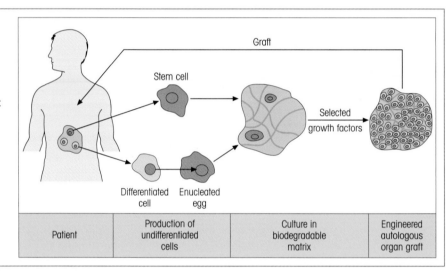

successful transplant of an engineered tissue was reported in 2008 in which a trachea grown from the recipient's own stem cells was given to a patient with collapsed airways following a severe *M. tuberculosis* infection.

Clinical experience in grafting

Privileged sites

Corneal grafts survive without the need for immunosuppression. Because they are avascular they tend not to sensitize the recipient. This privileged protection is boosted by the local production of immunosuppressive factors such as TGFβ, IL-1Ra, limited expression of MHC and the strategic presence of FasL which can induce apoptosis in infiltrating lymphocytes. Nonetheless, they do become cloudy if the individual has been *presensitized*. Grafts of **cartilage** are successful in the same way but an additional factor is the protection afforded

the chondrocytes by the matrix. With bone and artery it doesn't really matter if the grafts die because they can still provide a framework for host cells to colonize.

Kidney grafts

Hundreds of thousands of kidneys have been transplanted worldwide and with improvement in patient management there is a high survival rate. In the long term (1 year or more), the desirability of matching at the HLA-A, -B and -DR loci becomes apparent, although the effect is not overwhelming (Figure 16.18).

Patients are already partially immunosuppressed at the time of transplantation because uremia causes a degree of immunological nonresponsiveness. The **combination** of two or three immunosuppressive agents, for example a calcineurin inhibitor such as cyclosporine, azathioprine (now often replaced with mycophenolate mofetil) and a glucocorticosteroid such as prednisolone has been the mainstay for long-term

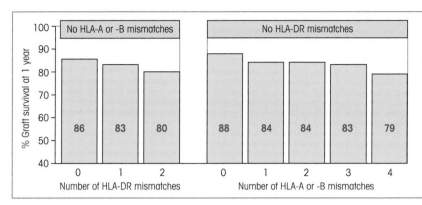

Figure 16.18. First cadaveric kidney graft survival in Europe

for the period January 1993 to December 1997 ($n = 12584$) on the basis of mismatches for HLA-A, -B and -DR. There is a significant influence of matching, $p < 0.001$, for both sets of data. (Data kindly supplied by Guido Persijn and Jacqueline Smits of the Eurotransplant International Foundation.)

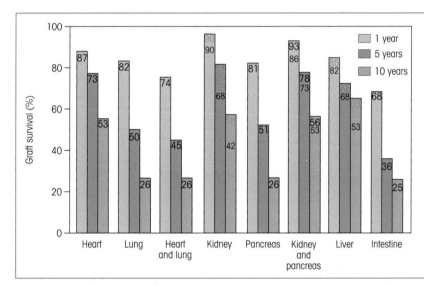

Figure 16.19. Graft survival rates for primary transplants performed in the USA.

For kidney and for liver transplants the higher figure is for transplants from living donors, the lower value the more common situation of organs from deceased donors. In the case of combined kidney and pancreas transplants, the higher value is for survival of the transplanted kidney and the lower value for the transplanted pancreas. Survival rates for repeat transplants of all organs are generally somewhat lower. (Based on data from the 2008 annual report of the Organ Procurement and Transplantation Network http://optn.transplant.hrsa.gov)

management of kidney grafts (Figure 16.11). The synergy between cyclosporine and rapamycin is also exploited to beneficial effect. These drugs are initially given at a relatively high dose, the induction phase, for the first few months following transplantation when the anti-donor immune response is at its most vigorous, and then at reduced concentrations for the subsequent maintenance phase that is usually required throughout life. If kidney function is poor during a rejection crisis, renal dialysis can be used. As mentioned above, there is active interest in the possibility of xenografting. When transplantation is performed because of immune complex-induced glomerulonephritis, the immunosuppressive treatment used may help to prevent a similar lesion developing in the grafted kidney. Patients with glomerular basement membrane antibodies (e.g. Goodpasture's syndrome) are likely to destroy their renal transplants unless first treated with plasmapheresis and immunosuppressive drugs.

Heart transplants

The overall 1-year organ survival figure for heart transplants has moved up to over 85% (Figure 16.19), helped considerably by the introduction of combination immunosuppressive

therapy of the type mentioned above. Aside from the rejection problem, it is likely that the number of patients who would benefit from cardiac replacement is much greater than the number dying with adequately healthy hearts. More attention will have to be given to the possibility of xenogeneic grafts and mechanical substitutes.

Liver transplants

Survival rates for orthotopic (in the normal or usual position) liver grafts are just slightly lower than those achieved with heart transplants (Figure 16.19). The hepatotrophic capacity of tacrolimus is an added bonus that makes it the preferred drug for liver transplantation. Rejection crises are dealt with by high-dose steroids and, if this proves ineffective, antilymphocyte globulin. The use of a totally synthetic colloidal hydroxyethyl starch solution, containing lactobionate as a substitute for chloride, allows livers to be preserved for 24 hours or more and has revolutionized the logistics of liver transplantation. To improve the prognosis of patients with primary hepatic or bile duct malignancies, which were considered to be inoperable, transplantation of organ clusters with liver as the central organ has been designed, e.g. liver and pancreas, or liver, pancreas, stomach and small bowel or even colon. Nonetheless, the outcome is not very favorable in that up to three-quarters of the patients transplanted for hepatic cancer have recurrence of their tumor within 1 year. For the future we must look forward to the creation of autologous liver from adult cells when tissue engineering techniques have been developed sufficiently.

Experience with liver grafting between pigs revealed an unexpected finding. Many of the animals retained the grafted organs in a healthy state for many months without any form of immunosuppression and enjoyed a state of unresponsiveness to grafts of skin or kidney from the same donor. True tolerance is induced by the donor-type intrahepatic hematopoietic stem cells and immature dendritic cells (see above) and possibly also by the liver parenchyma itself, known to produce copious amounts of soluble MHC class I.

Work is in progress on the transfer of isolated hepatocytes attached to collagen-coated microcarriers injected i.p. for the correction of isolated deficiencies such as albumin synthesis. This attractive approach has much wider application as a general vehicle for gene therapy.

Hematopoietic stem cell grafts

Patients with certain immunodeficiency disorders and aplastic anemia are obvious candidates for treatment with **pluripotent hematopoietic stem cells** (HSC) isolated from bone marrow, peripheral blood or cord blood; so, too, are patients with leukemia, lymphoma, myeloma and metastatic breast cancer treated radically with intensive chemotherapy and possibly whole-body irradiation in attempts to eradicate the neoplastic cells, as will be discussed in the next chapter.

Bone marrow contains not only HSCs but also mesenchymal stem cells that can give rise to cartilage, tendons and bone; after expansion in culture by a factor of 5–10 times, they provide an excellent treatment for children with osteogenesis imperfecta, a genetic disorder in which the osteoblasts produce defective type I collagen with resulting osteopenia and severe bony deformities. Favorable results have been obtained with stem cell transplantation *in utero* for severe combined immunodeficiency (SCID) using populations from paternal bone marrow enriched for the stem cell marker, CD34. From the practical standpoint, it has been recognized that cord blood contains sufficient hematopoietic stem cells for bone marrow replacement, but what is even more convenient is to use cytokines such as granulocyte colony-stimulating factor (G-CSF) to mobilize donor stem cells out of the bone marrow to increase the number of peripheral blood stem cells (PBSCs). Transplantation with either autologous (involving re-infusion of CD34+ cells taken prior to myeloablative therapy) or allogeneic PBSCs results in a more rapid recovery in neutrophil and platelet numbers than that seen following bone marrow transplantation, and in many centers is rapidly replacing bone marrow as the source of such cells. Allogeneic cells can exhibit a graft-versus-tumor effect, although this needs to be weighed against the risk of graft-versus-host (g.v.h.) disease (see below).

Hematopoietic stem cell transplantation is also increasingly being explored as a mechanism of inducing tolerance to donor antigens in solid organ transplantation by creating a state of chimerism in the recipient, which would then lead to deletion or inactivation of the relevant alloreactive lymphocytes.

Graft-versus-host disease results from allogeneic T-cells in the graft

GVH disease resulting from the recognition of recipient antigens by allogeneic T-cells in the bone marrow or peripheral blood-derived inoculum represents a serious, sometimes fatal, complication, and the incidence of GVH disease is reduced if T-cells are first depleted with a cytotoxic cocktail of anti-T-cell monoclonals.

It is fondly hoped that successful engraftment and avoidance of GVH reactions following allogeneic cell transplantation will be achieved in the clinic by strategies such as co-stimulatory blockade (Figure 16.13) without a requirement for cytoablative treatment of graft or recipient. Until then, successful results are more likely with highly compatible donors, particularly if fatal GVH reactions are to be avoided, and here siblings offer the best chance of finding a matched donor. Undoubtedly, non-HLA minor transplantation antigens are important and are more difficult to match. Acute GVH disease occurring within the first 100 days following infusion of allogeneic cells primarily affects the skin, liver and gastrointestinal tract. Current therapy uses steroids such as prednisolone in combination with either cyclosporine or tacrolimus, but inclusion of methotrexate in this regimen is said to improve efficacy. Chronic GVH disease (i.e. later than 100 days) has a relatively good prognosis if limited to skin and liver, but if multiple organs are involved, clinically resembling progressive systemic sclerosis, the outcome is poor. Patients are treated with cyclosporine and prednisolone. The pathogenesis of GVH disease may initially involve secretion of IL-1, TNF and IFNγ from damaged host tissue, with both donor and recipient dendritic cells activating donor Th1 cells to secrete IL-2 and more IFNγ. The host is attacked by donor cytotoxic T-cells and NK cells using both the Fas–FasL and the perforin/granzyme B pathways to induce apoptotic cell death, with production of TNF also putting the boot in. There is hope that Treg cells can be harnessed to limit this process, and experiments in animal models are in progress to evaluate the efficacy of such approaches. In one such model, mice treated with anti-IL21 monoclonal antibody had reduced GVH disease mortality that was associated with an increase in Foxp3+ inducible Treg cells in the lamina propria of the colon. Thus blockade of IL-21 *in vivo* led to the induction of Tregs in preference to IL-21-induced Th1 and Th17 cell differentiation.

Other organs and tissues

It is to be expected that improvement in techniques of control of the rejection process will encourage transplantation in several other areas, for example in type 1 diabetes where the number of transplants recorded is rising rapidly. The current 5-year organ-survival rate is around 75% for simultaneous transplantation of pancreas and kidney (Figure 16.19). Transplantation with isolated islet cells is a more attractive option that avoids the need for major surgery and appears to require less immunosuppression than that required following transplantation of a pancreas. Collagenase is injected into the pancreatic duct in a brain dead donor and the recovered islets purified by density gradient centrifugation. These are then infused into the hepatic portal vein of the recipient from where they lodge in the liver sinusoids. Recently, the procedure has been sucessfully extended to using islets isolated from a fragment of pancreas removed from a living donor. The benefits of islet cell transplantation as an alternative to insulin injections do, of course, need to be weighed against the risks of the immunosuppression that is required.

The 5-year graft survival rate of 45–50% for lung and simultaneous heart–lung is improving but is still less than satisfactory (Figure 16.19). Transplantation of intestine is also in need of improvement, with 5-year graft survival currently at 36% (Figure 16.19). One also looks forward to the day when the successful transplantation of skin for lethal burns becomes more commonplace. The grafting of **neural tissues** has the potential to benefit patients with neurodegenerative conditions such as Parkinson's disease, Huntington's disease and stroke. Indeed, the transplantation of human fetal mesencephalic tissue into the brain of patients with Parkinson's disease has shown that dopaminergic neurons from such tissue can integrate into the brain's neuronal circuits. Some patients were able to discontinue treatment with L-dopa for a period of several years. However, such transplantation is far from routine and the results from clinical trials have been very mixed. As already mentioned (p. 437), researchers are turning to stem cells as a source of neurons, although the optimal growth factors and culture conditions required to generate particular types of neurons require further evaluation.

Infertility, including that resulting from medical intervention such as cytotoxic therapy of cancer patients, is of great concern. It is therefore gratifying to hear of the successful pregnancy outcomes of females who have received ovarian transplants. Cryopreservation of sperm is a successful strategy in the management of adult male cancer sufferers to protect the sperm from mutagenic cancer treatment. This is not available to prepubertal boys, but an alternative for them is cryopreservation of their spermatogonial stem cells for reintroduction post-treatment, as the Sertoli cells that support differentiation into mature spermatozoa will function normally. There is a potential for identifying and correcting genetic defects in the spermatogonia before their reintroduction, but ethical committees fight shy of this sort of "Frankenstein" tinkering. More acceptably, in cases of male infertility due to dysfunctional Sertoli cells, it should be possible to develop mature spermatids by culture of the spermatogonia with Sertoli cells derived from a normal individual.

Coronary bypass surgery involves autografting with the saphenous vein from the leg, the internal mammary arteries or the radial artery from the arm. The blood vessel is grafted onto the heart to bypass a blocked or damaged coronary artery. Vascular grafts in other areas of the body can employ synthetic blood vessels, made of materials such as Dacron or polytetrafluoroethylene (PTFE), autografts or, very rarely, allografts. Work proceeds on the generation of engineered blood vessels, for example by using human stem cells grown on biodegradable fibronectin-coated polymer scaffolds in the presence of appropriate mediators such as vascular endothelial growth factor.

The fetus is a potential allograft

A consequence of polymorphism in an outbred population is that mother and fetus will almost certainly have different MHCs. In the human hemochorial placenta, maternal blood with immunocompetent lymphocytes circulates in contact with the fetal trophoblast and we have to explain how the fetus avoids allograft rejection, despite the development of an immunological response in a proportion of mothers as evidenced by the appearance of anti-HLA antibodies and cytotoxic lymphocytes. In fact, prior sensitization with a skin graft fails to affect a pregnancy, showing that trophoblast cells are immunologically protected; indeed, they are resistant to most cytotoxic mechanisms although potentially susceptible to IL-2-activated NK cells. Some of the many speculations that have been aired on this subject are summarized in Figure 16.20.

Undoubtedly, the most important factor is the well-documented lack of both conventional class I and class II MHC antigens on the placental syncytiotrophoblast and cytotrophoblast that protects the fetus from allogeneic attack. These fundamental changes in the regulation of MHC genes also lead to the unique expression of the nonclassical HLA-E, -F and -G proteins on the extravillous cytotrophoblast. These molecules, which show very limited polymorphism (9, 21 and 46 genomic sequence variants had been described for HLA-E, -F and -G, respectively, by October 2010 compared with 1381, 1927 and 960 alleles for HLA-A, -B and -C, respectively [see Figure 16.9]), may protect the trophoblast from killing by uterine endometrial NK cells that would normally attack cells lacking MHC class I molecules (cf. p. 96). Maternal IgG antipaternal MHC is found in 20% of first pregnancies and this figure rises to 75–80% in multiparous women. Some of these antibodies cross-react with HLA-G, but the vulnerability of the trophoblast cells to complement is blocked by the presence on their surface of the control proteins that inactivate C3 convertase (cf. p. 372). Mice in which the gene for the Crry complement regulatory protein has been knocked out develop placental inflammation and fetal loss. Immunohistochemical analysis revealed a deposition of complement components in the placenta of these mice, but if they were bred with mice in which complement component C3 has been knocked out then

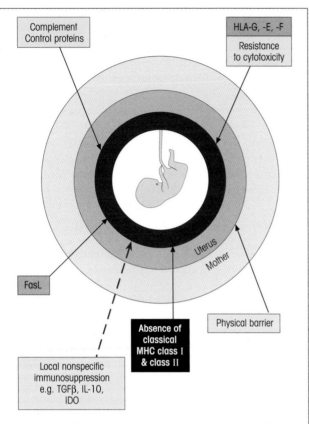

Figure 16.20. Mechanisms postulated to account for the survival of the fetus as an allograft in the mother.

IDO, indoleamine 2,3-dioxygenase.

the detrimental effect of the absence of Crry was abrogated. This clearly indicates a role for inhibition of complement activation as one of the mechanisms that helps maintain the semi-allogeneic fetus, at least in mice. The presence of Fas-ligand at the trophoblast maternal–fetal interface may contribute towards limiting immunological aggression towards the fetus, although the fact that *gld* mice that lack FasL and *lpr* mice that lack Fas give birth to live offspring suggests that this mechanism is not essential for the maintenance of pregnancy. Suppression of T-cell, B-cell and NK cell activity also occurs through the generation of toxic tryptophan metabolites by the catabolic enzyme indoleamine 2,3-dioxygenase, which is present in trophoblast cells and macrophages.

Cytokines seem to have a complex role in postimplantation pregnancy given the production of growth factors such as CSF-1 and GM-CSF, which have a trophic influence on the placenta, and of transforming growth factor-β (TGFβ), which could help to damp down any activation of NK cells by potentially abortive events such as intrauterine exposure to lipopolysaccharide (LPS) or to interferons. Indeed, production of immunosuppresive IL-10 and TGFβ by regulatory T-cells may play a central role in limiting any immunological attack on the fetus. Cells bearing the hallmark of naturally occurring regulatory T-cells, i.e. CD4$^+$CD25$^+$CTLA-4$^+$GITR$^+$FoxP3$^+$ cells, are present in increased numbers, both in the circulation and in the decidua, during the first and second trimester of human pregnancy. The absence of such T-regulatory cells has been shown to result in immunologically mediated rejection of the fetus in mice.

Graft rejection is an immunological reaction
- It shows specificity, the second set response is brisk, it is mediated by lymphocytes and antibodies specific for the graft are formed.

Genetic control of transplantation antigens
- In each vertebrate species there is a *m*ajor *h*istocompatibility *c*omplex (MHC) that is responsible for provoking the most intense graft reactions.
- Parental MHC antigens are codominantly expressed on cell surfaces.
- Siblings have a 1:4 chance of identity with respect to MHC.

Other consequences of MHC incompatibility
- Class II MHC molecules provoke a proliferative mixed lymphocyte reaction when genetically dissimilar lymphocytes interact.
- Class II differences are largely responsible for the reaction of tolerated grafted lymphocytes against host antigen (graft-versus-host [GVH] reaction).

Mechanisms of graft rejection
- Preformed antibodies cause hyperacute rejection within minutes.
- CD8 and CD4 lymphocytes, Ig and complement all play a role in the acute rejection that can occur several days after transplantation.
- The strength of allograft rejection is due to the surprisingly large number of allospecific precursor cells that directly recognize allo-MHC (the direct pathway); later rejection increasingly involves allogeneic peptides presented by self-MHC (the indirect pathway).
- Chronic rejection can occur months or years after the transplant and may involve lymphocytes, phagocytes, antibody and/or complement.

Prevention of graft rejection

- Rejection can be minimized by cross-matching donor and graft for ABO and MHC tissue types. Individual MHC antigens are typed by serological or molecular genetic techniques. HLA-DR, -A and -B are the most important to match.
- Agents producing general immunosuppression such as antimitotic drugs (e.g. azathioprine), anti-inflammatory steroids and anti-lymphocyte monoclonals can block graft rejection. Cyclosporine, tacrolimus and rapamycin represent T-cell-specific drugs; complexes of cyclosporine and tacrolimus, with their cellular ligands (cyclophilin A and FKBP, respectively), block calcineurin, a phosphatase that activates the IL-2 transcription factor NFAT, while rapamycin (which also complexes with FKBP) inhibits the TOR kinase involved in cell proliferation.
- Antigen-specific depression through tolerance induction can be achieved with injection of allogeneic bone marrow with co-stimulatory blockade by anti-CD154 (CD40L) plus a CTLA-4–Ig fusion protein. Dendritic cell precursors can also induce tolerance through antigen presentation in the absence of B7 co-stimulators.

Xenografting

- Strategies are being developed to prevent hyperacute rejection of pig grafts in humans due to reaction of natural antibodies in the host with galactose α-1,3-galactose epitopes on pig cells and acute vascular rejection by acquired antibodies produced by the xenogeneic antibody response.

Stem cell therapy

- Stem cells can be isolated from various adult tissues and have the potential to provide material for autografts.
- Introduction of transcription factors into adult cells can be used to generate induced pluripotent stem cells.

Clinical experience in grafting

- Cornea and cartilage grafts are avascular, produce local immunosuppressive factors and are comparatively well tolerated.

- Kidney grafting gives excellent results and has been the most widespread, although immunosuppression must normally continue throughout life.
- High success rates are also being achieved with heart and liver transplants particularly helped by the use of cyclosporine. Lung is less successful. Isolated islets cells from the pancreas are increasingly being used for the treatment of patients with type 1 diabetes.
- HSC grafts for immunodeficiency and aplastic anemia are accepted from matched siblings, but it is difficult to avoid GVH disease with allogeneic HSCs without first purging T-cells in the graft or preferably by inducing tolerance using co-stimulatory blockade. HSCs isolated from peripheral blood following mobilization of these cells from the bone marrow using G-CSF can be used instead of bone marrow.
- Transplantation of neural tissue has met with some success in patients with Parkinson's disease.
- Attempts at engineering tissues such as the trachea are increasingly successful.

The fetus as an allograft

- Differences between MHC of mother and fetus imply that, as a potential graft, the fetus must be protected against transplantation attack by the mother.
- A major defense mechanism is the lack of classical class I and II MHC antigens at the maternal-fetal interface.
- The placenta expresses the nonclassical MHC class I proteins, HLA-G, HLA-E and HLA-F, which may act to inhibit cytotoxicity by maternal NK cells.
- The trophoblast cells bear surface complement regulatory proteins that break down C3 convertase and so block any complement-mediated damage.
- Local production of IL-10 and TGFβ by CD4$^+$CD25$^+$Foxp3$^+$ regulatory T-cells, tryptophan degradation by indoleamine 2,3-dioxygenase, and the presence of FasL may all contribute towards the suppression of unwanted reactions.

FURTHER READING

Al-Khaldi A. & Robbins R.C. (2006) New directions in cardiac transplantation. *Annual Review of Medicine* **57**, 455–471.

Austen K.F., Burakoff S.J., Rosen F.S. & Strom T.B. (eds.) (2001) *Therapeutic Immunology*, 2nd edn. Blackwell Science, Oxford.

Cornell L.D., Smith R.N. & Colvin R.B. (2008) Kidney transplantation: mechanisms of rejection and acceptance. *Annual Review of Pathology* **3**, 189–220.

Kaplan B., Burkhart, G., Lakkis F.G. & Morris R. (eds.) (2011) *Immunotherapy in Transplantation: Principles and Practice*. Wiley-Blackwell, Oxford.

Kiskinis E. & Eggan K. (2010) Progress toward the clinical application of patient-specific pluripotent stem cells. *The Journal of Clinical Investigation* **120**, 51–59.

Prabhakaran S., Humar A. & Matas A.J. (2008) Immunosuppression: use in transplantation. In *Encyclopedia of Life Sciences* John Wiley & Sons, Ltd., Chichester. DOI: 10.1002/9780470015902.a0001242.pub2

Sayegh M.H. & Carpenter C.B. (2004) Transplantation 50 years later—progress, challenges, and promises. *New England Journal of Medicine* **351**, 2761–2766.

Shimabukuro-Vornhagen A., Hallek M.J., Storb R.F. & von Bergwelt-Baildon M.S. (2009) The role of B-cells in the pathogenesis of graft-versus-host disease. *Blood* **114**, 4919–4927.

Starzl T.E. (2004) Chimerism and tolerance in transplantation. *Proceedings of the National Academy of Sciences of the USA* **101**, 14607–14614.

Trowsdale J. & Betz A.G. (2006) Mother's little helpers: mechanisms of maternal-fetal tolerance. *Nature Immunology* **7**, 241–246.

Turka L.A. & Lechler R.I. (2009) Towards the identification of biomarkers of transplantation tolerance. *Nature Reviews Immunology* **9**, 521–526.

Now visit **www.roitt.com** to test yourself on this chapter.

CHAPTER 17
Tumor immunology

Key Topics

Just to Recap...

In earlier chapters we have discussed how the immune system becomes activated in response to infectious agents and mounts an appropriate response, via a combination of innate and adaptive components. Central to the initiation of a robust immune response is the detection of nonself, initially in the form of pathogen-associated molecular patterns (PAMPs) that are sensed through binding to either soluble or cell-borne pattern recognition receptors (PRRs) on macrophages, dendritic cells and other cells of the immune system. PAMP-mediated activation of dendritic cells triggers their maturation and consequent migration to lymph nodes where they carry out a critical function as antigen-presenting cells, enabling T-cells to respond to nonself determinants in the form of foreign peptides. Productively activated T-cells further differentiate to effector cells, coordinating B-cell responses, macrophage activation, cytotoxic cell killing in addition to other functions. In this way, the innate and adaptive arms of the immune system work cooperatively to identify and confront microorganisms. The immune system has evolved to discriminate self from nonself based upon the pragmatic principle that anything recognized as nonself may be dangerous and therefore warrants expulsion from the body. In the relentless pursuit of nonself our well-meaning immune systems sometimes work against us, rejection of transplanted organs being a case in point, but there are also situations where self may give serious cause for concern; cancer being the pre-eminent example of this.

Introduction

As we shall see in this chapter, a major problem with cancer is that the immune system has little to work with in terms of recognizing such entities as potentially

Roitt's Essential Immunology, Twelfth Edition. Peter J. Delves, Seamus J. Martin, Dennis R. Burton, Ivan M. Roitt.
© 2011 Peter J. Delves, Seamus J. Martin, Dennis R. Burton, Ivan M. Roitt. Published 2011 by Blackwell Publishing Ltd.

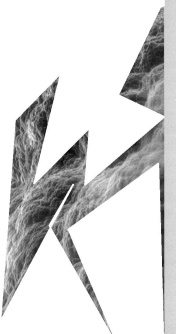

Introduction *(Continued)*

dangerous—in large measure due to the preoccupation of the immune system with recognition of nonself—and for this reason immune responses to tumors are typically modest. This has probably much to do with the lack of PAMPs that are normally required to get robust immune responses off the ground, but can also be due to manipulation of the immune system by the tumor. Indeed, there is a growing body of evidence that tumors frequently recruit macrophages as well as other innate immune cells and "re-educate" such cells towards a wound-healing phenotype for the purposes of supporting tumor growth and survival. Before we get into the reasons why transformed (i.e. cancerous) cell populations are not readily recognized and disposed of by the immune system, we will first take a look at the factors that influence the development of cancer.

Cellular transformation and cancer

Cancer is not a single disease but represents a wide spectrum of conditions caused by a failure of the controls that normally govern cell proliferation, differentiation and cell survival. Cancers can either be **benign**, where the cancer fails to spread to other tissues, or **malignant**, where the cancer is invasive and spreads to other tissues within the body. Cells that undergo **malignant transformation** escape normal growth controls, invade surrounding tissue, and may ultimately migrate to other sites in the body to establish secondary tumors.

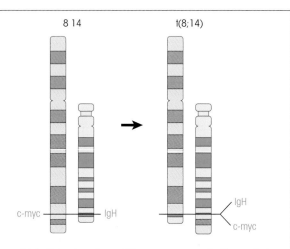

Figure 17.1. Translocation of the c-*myc* gene to the μ chain locus in Burkitt's lymphoma.

Burkitt's lymphoma is a B-cell neoplasia with a relatively high incidence among African children in whom there is an association with the EBV; in most cases studied, the c-*myc* gene, located on chromosome 8 band q24, is joined by a reciprocal translocation event to the μ heavy chain gene on chromosome 14 band q32, as depicted above. It is suggested that the normal mechanisms that downregulate c-*myc* can no longer work on the translocated gene and so the cell is held in the cycling mode. Less frequently, c-*myc* translocates to the site of the κ (chromosome 2) or λ (chromosome 22) loci.

While early theories on the nature of cancer proposed that abnormal cellular growths were caused by infectious agents, such as viruses, these theories were gradually supplanted by the idea that cancer was caused by **mutagens**; agents that provoke genetic mutation. It is now well accepted that the majority of carcinogens (i.e. cancer-causing agents) act through provoking **DNA damage** either directly or indirectly. Such damage can be relatively subtle, resulting in point mutations that alter a single amino acid in the protein encoded by the affected gene, or more dramatic, provoking translocation of whole chromosomal segments from one chromosome to another (Figure 17.1).

The results of such mutagenic events are generally of little consequence, as the DNA damage will either be repaired or the cell will be killed off via apoptosis. In a small minority of cases however, mutagenic events can produce cells with properties that enable them to disobey the rules that normally govern cellular behavior in multi-cellular organisms. But this doesn't happen overnight, as the barriers to malignant transformation are formidable. It is important to stress **that cancers almost never arise from single genetic lesions but rather progress in a series of steps from a normal untransformed state to a fully transformed one** (Figure 17.2); frequently, the acquisition of previous mutations will predispose towards acquiring additional mutations by generating DNA instability. This progression is facilitated through the stepwise and random acquisition of a series of mutations that cooperate to produce the cancerous state. Because of the distinct selection pressures operating in different tissues, different combinations of mutations are seen in cancers arising from different tissue types. In addition, although some of the same key genes (such as *P53*, *RAS*, *MYC*, *PTEN*, *RB*) are frequently mutated in a majority of cancers, these mutations can be accompanied by a whole range of additional mutations that can be relatively unique to an individual tumor.

Cellular transformation is a multi-step process

Cellular transformation is a multi-step process involving a combination of genetic lesions affecting genes that regulate,

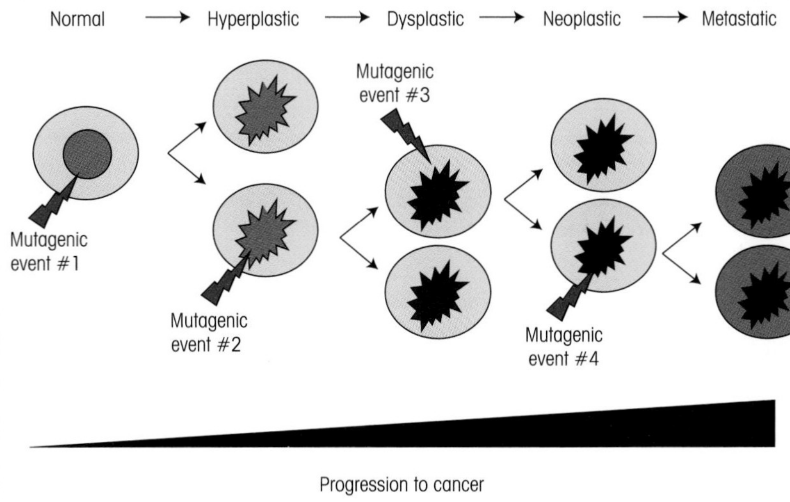

Figure 17.2. Cancer development is a multi-step process.

Cancers rarely arise from single mutations but occur as a result of the acquisition of a series of mutations that progressively transform a normal cell to a progressively more abnormal malignant one. At each step in the progression, transformed cells acquire characteristics (e.g. the ability to grow independent of growth factors, resistance to apoptosis, ability to invade surrounding tissues) that endow them with a competitive advantage over neighboring cells.

amongst other things, cell cycle entry, cell cycle exit and cell death (apoptosis). Cancer is often associated with **activating mutations** in genes that promote cell proliferation, such as *MYC* and *RAS*, which results in increased activity, stability or expression of the protein products of these genes. Such genes, which in their hyperactive state promote the development of cancer, are called **oncogenes**. In tandem with this, **inactivating mutations** or **dominant-interfering mutations** (i.e. mutations that generate a protein that has lost its normal function and is also capable of inhibiting the activity of any remaining wild-type protein) in genes that promote cell cycle arrest or apoptosis of damaged cells, *P53* and *RB* being prime examples, are frequently observed. The latter genes are called **tumor suppressor genes** because, in their wild type form, the products of such genes act to oppose the development of cancer. Deregulated expression of genes involved in the control of programmed cell death (such as *BCL-2* or *ABL*) is also a common feature of many malignancies.

Thus, **cancer arises as a consequence of a combination of gene mutations** that affect oncogenes and tumor suppressor genes and is a relatively low probability event as a consequence. Indeed, considering the literally trillions of cells an average human produces in their lifetime, our bodies are remarkably well adapted to limit the production of cells that manage to escape the normal controls that govern cell proliferation. That said, given the almost 80 year lifespan of an average human, cancer does eventually occur in a significant percentage of individuals. Let us now look at some of the factors that affect the incidence of cancer development.

Cancer incidence varies between tissues

Cancers can arise from practically any tissue in the body but are most commonly found to occur in epithelia—the sheets of cells that form the upper layer of the skin and that line the walls of cavities and tubes within the body. Cancers that arise from epithelia are called **carcinomas** and these tumors are responsible for more than 80% of all cancer-related deaths in the Western world.

The latter fact is probably related to two factors: first, epithelia are at the highest risk of exposure to cancer-causing agents (**carcinogens**) because these cells line the surfaces of the body that are in direct contact with the environment (e.g. skin, lungs, mouth, esophagus, stomach, intestine, urinary tract, cervix) that is a major source of carcinogens, which can be either chemical, physical or biological in nature. The other major factor governing the high probability of cancer arising in epithelium is due to the high replacement rate of epithelial cells, as a consequence of damage or infection, which means that such cells are constantly dividing. Cancers arise more frequently in tissues that exhibit a high rate of mitosis probably because these cells are already dividing at a relatively high rate and the barriers to cell division are lower than in nondividing (i.e. post-mitotic) tissues. Because dividing cells need to replicate their genomes, a process that can itself be a source of mutation due to errors made by DNA polymerase, such cells can be a source of genetic instability.

The remaining malignant tumors arise from non-epithelial tissues throughout the body. Those that arise from the various connective tissues, called **sarcomas**, account for 1% of the tumors encountered in cancer clinics. The second group of tumors of non-epithelial origin arise from the various cell types that constitute the blood-forming (i.e. hematopoietic) tissues and include the cells of the immune system. Such tumors, called **hematopoietic malignancies**, include the **leukaemias and lymphomas** and these account for approximately 17% of cancer-related deaths. The final group of non-epithelial tumors arise from various components of the central (i.e. brain) and peripheral nervous systems (i.e. spinal cord and outlying nerve tissue) and are termed **neuroectodermal tumors**. These account for approximately 2.5% of cancer-related deaths.

Depending on their tissue of origin and transformation stage, cancers may grow slowly, or rather rapidly, they may be poorly metastatic or highly aggressive, some cancers are relatively responsive to therapy, while others are refractory and refuse to give in to even the most protracted assaults. Cancer therapy typically involves surgery (for solid tumors) followed by cytotoxic drugs or radiation, either alone or in combination, to kill the errant cells while sparing as many normal (nonmalignant) cells as possible. It is the latter consideration that typically sets a limit on how much radiation or cytotoxic drug can be used in the hope of eradicating the tumor burden.

Mutagenic agents, including viruses, can provoke cellular transformation

As discussed earlier, cancer most frequently arises as a result of mutations that affect genes that govern the rates of mitosis, apoptosis and other cellular functions. Practically all carcinogens are mutagenic agents, that is, agents that cause gene mutations. Thus, tissues that commonly experience the highest levels of exposure to carcinogens are also at the highest risk of mutation. Because epithelial tissues are continually exposed to substances that may contain carcinogens (e.g. the air we breathe, the food we eat, the liquids we drink, the viruses we encounter) it follows that cells in these tissues are at the highest risk of acquiring mutations that may result in cancer. However, because of DNA damage detection and repair mechanisms, as well as mechanisms to limit the ability of abnormal cells to replicate (including the simple elimination of these cells by apoptosis, as well as induction of a non-replicating state called **senescence**) it is important to note that the vast majority of mutations do not result in cancer. However, when cancers do arise, they are most commonly found in epithelial tissues because, as mentioned above, these are at the greatest risk of damage or infection.

Viruses are also capable of causing cancer through insertion into the genome of their hosts. This can result in cancer in two different ways: first, the viral genome may carry a gene that enables the host cell to escape the normal controls placed upon it that restrict cell division and/or limit its lifespan, and second, the virus may integrate its genome close to a host gene that regulates proliferation and/or apoptosis and this can result in the aberrant expression of such genes.

Cell-intrinsic mechanisms of tumor suppression

Because uncontrolled growth of cells is such a potentially destructive force, there are a number of cell-intrinsic "fail-safe" systems that serve to curb the likelihood of cellular transformation occurring (Figure 17.3). These systems come into play when abnormal signals are generated within cells and typically "punish" such cells either through depriving them of the ability to divide (transiently in some cases or permanently in others) or through killing such cells outright. We shall now take a look at some of these natural cancer-restraining mechanisms.

Growth factors are essential for cell division

One of the most important limits on proliferation is that all cells typically require signals from other cells (i.e. growth factors) to permit cell division to occur. Therefore, for a tumor to develop, cells must acquire a continuous supply of growth factors, or become independent of the need for growth factor signaling. Tumors typically achieve this through mutations that either amplify the expression of growth factor receptors (that can lead to constitutive activation of the receptor), through acquiring the ability to produce their own growth factors (i.e. autocrine stimulation), or through mutation of key signal

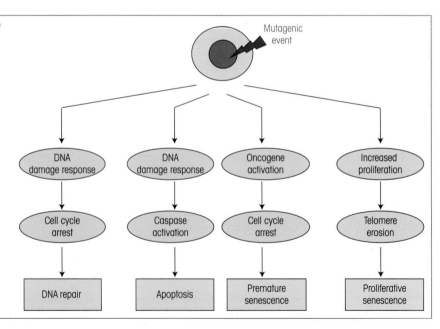

Figure 17.3. Cell-intrinsic mechanisms of tumor suppression.

Mutation normally activates a range of fail-safe measures that result either in DNA repair, cell cycle arrest, apoptosis or senescence of the affected cell. Such measures ensure that the vast majority of mutations do not progress to cancer.

transduction proteins in growth factor signaling cascades. A good example of the latter is Ras, which is found in mutant form in ~30% of human cancers. Ras mutations that offer tumors a proliferative advantage are typically gain-of-function mutations that produce a constitutively hyperactive Ras protein, thereby mimicking the action of continuous growth factor receptor stimulation. Many other oncogenic events act in a similar manner, uncoupling the normal requirement for growth factor receptor stimulation for cell division to take place. Fortunately, when such oncogenic events do occur, they frequently do not result in continuous proliferation as excessive growth signals are frequently sensed as abnormal and lead to **premature cellular senescence**, a state where cells become permanently arrested and are incapable of further division (Figure 17.3). Oncogene-induced premature senescence is mediated, in part, through upregulation of cyclin-dependent kinase inhibitors, proteins that can interfere with the key enzymes involved in coordinating cell division.

Telomere shortening acts as a barrier to cellular transformation

All cells have a limited number of cell divisions they are capable of undertaking, and this has been dubbed "the Hayflick limit" after the scientist who first described this phenomenon. This is due to problems with replicating the extreme tips of chromosomes (called telomeres), which progressively shorten with each round of cell division. Telomere shortening is not a problem for a good number of cell divisions (~45–50 or so) because telomeres are composed of noncoding repetitive DNA that seems to be there for the purposes of protecting the coding regions of chromosomes. However, there comes a point at which telomeres have become so eroded that chromosomal ends begin to fuse together and at this point cells cease to be able to divide, irrespective of whether they are receiving sufficient growth factor or downstream signals. Such cells are said to have entered **proliferative senescence** or to have reached their Hayflick limit and this acts as a natural barrier to the development of tumors (Figure 17.3). Where tumors do manage to overcome the Hayflick limit, this appears to be due to the re-activation of telomerase, an enzyme that is capable of repairing the ends of telomeres but is not normally expressed in differentiated cells.

Tumor suppressor proteins monitor cell division

The products of **tumor suppressor genes**, such as p53 and pRb, act as another barrier to transformation. These gene products are involved in signaling networks that monitor the integrity of the genome, as well as confirming that the correct proliferative signals have been received before permitting entry into the cell cycle. In the event of DNA damage or aberrant mitogenic signals, the p53 and pRb tumor suppressor proteins can halt the cell cycle, which is either followed by DNA repair and cell cycle re-entry, permanent cell cycle arrest (senescence) or cell death via apoptosis (Figure 17.3; see also Videoclip 2).

Notwithstanding the various natural barriers to transformation, as discussed above, cancers clearly do occur as a result of cells managing to overcome these failsafe measures due to a series of acquired mutations. However, without the above countermeasures, cancer would undoubtedly be much more common than it already is. For example, individuals that are born with a single mutated *P53* allele (Li–Fraumeni syndrome) have a greatly increased lifetime risk of developing cancer, with some individuals developing several types of cancer concurrently. Similarly, inherited *RB* mutations also greatly increase the probability of developing certain tumors, such as retinoblastoma of the eye, a cancer from which this gene derives its name.

The cancer problem from an immune perspective

Many tumors appear to escape the attentions of the immune system, a fact that has been an ongoing source of frustration for many immunologists who still nurture hope that there must be some way of galvanizing the immune system into action in such cases. Let us first acknowledge that advances in immunology have paved the way for a generation of new, highly targeted, cancer therapies involving humanized monoclonal antibodies specific for particular cell surface determinants expressed on certain cancers. And such passive immunotherapies work extremely effectively in many cases, a topic that is discussed at length towards the end of this chapter. However, it must be said that progress has been much more modest in terms of finding ways of harnessing the power of the immune system to recognize and kill a tumor in the way it can recognize and repel most infectious agents.

In many ways, this is not all that surprising because cancers are not infectious agents and therefore lack the molecular signatures that normally enable the immune system to recognize that something is amiss. This appears to be the nub of the problem. Cancers either fail to attract the serious attention of the immune system, or generate an environment that is generally tolerogenic towards the tumor. This tolerogenic state can either be passive, or can be maintained through the secretion of a variety factors by the tumor that actively maintain this state. Let us look at some of the issues.

Cancers lack PAMPs and contain few nonself determinants

The largely invisible nature of cancers, from the immune systems point of view, relates mainly to the fact that **cancers represent self** and are therefore devoid of PAMPs that are normally required for the initiation of effective immune responses. Because cancers are typically initiated by environmental factors (e.g. DNA-damaging agents and radiation) and typically do not have an infectious component, they usually fail to attract the attentions of the immune system in the way that PAMP-containing microorganisms do. As we shall see later in this chapter, the exception to this general rule applies

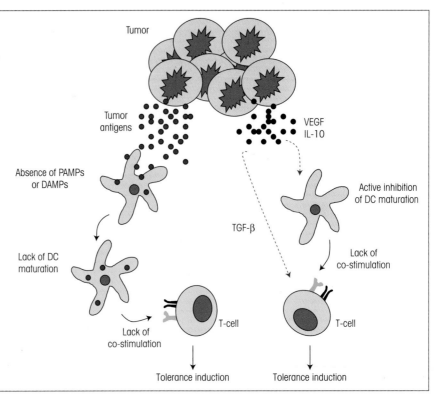

Figure 17.4. Lack of T-cell co-stimulation results in tolerance to tumor antigens.

T-cell tolerance to tumor antigens can either occur passively, due to the lack of PAMPs or DAMPs in the tumor environment to promote DC maturation and proper co-stimulation, or actively, due to the secretion of factors (such as IL-10, VEGF, and TGFβ) by the tumor that actively inhibit DC maturation or T-cell function.

to cancers that are initiated by viruses, which represent a minority of cases.

Lack of co-stimulation can tolerize towards tumor antigens

Allied to the problem of the absence of nonself determinants is the fact that cells of the adaptive immune system do not typically enter tissues unless recruited there by cells of the innate immune system as a consequence of PAMP-initiated inflammatory responses. Therefore, even if a tumor does express one or more molecules not normally expressed in the body (e.g. due to a mutation that creates a new amino acid sequence), an adaptive immune response is unlikely to be initiated unless this molecule is somehow presented to the adaptive immune system in the context of the appropriate co-stimulation. This brings us back to the issue of PAMPs. Recall, that tissue-resident dendritic cells (DCs) are immature and do not migrate to lymph nodes to present antigen unless activated by a PAMP or another source of pattern recognition receptor stimulation. Therefore, a neoantigen generated by a tumor is likely to be ignored by the immune system unless presented by a mature DC; otherwise tolerization to this antigen will occur (Figure 17.4). Tolerance induction in the latter situation occurs by default, but there is also evidence that tumors often actively tolerize DCs in the vicinity through the secretion of IL-10 and VEGF, as well as factors such as TGFβ that can suppress T-cell activation, proliferation and differentiation (Figure 17.4). Thus, much of the failure of the adaptive immune system to

engage with tumors can be explained by either T-cell apathy or tolerance.

Inflammatory responses can enhance tumor growth

This is not to say that tumors are invisible to the immune system. Indeed, tumors are frequently heavily infiltrated by tumor-associated macrophages and neutrophils but, paradoxically, such cells are often actively recruited by the tumor and can promote tumor proliferation and progression. The paradoxical effect of inflammation on the growth of tumors is frequently related to the production of inflammatory cytokines and chemokines (such as IL-1, IL-6 and IL-8), by the tumor itself. These inflammatory mediators can recruit neutrophils and macrophages, which in turn produce cytokines and other inflammatory mediators that promote proliferation of the tumor as well as the growth of new blood vessels (angiogenesis) that are required for rapidly proliferating cells. As if this were not already bad enough, there is increasing evidence that tumor-associated inflammatory cells, especially macrophages, can even promote the progression to malignancy and metastasis through the production of reactive oxygen and nitrogen species that can provoke DNA damage and thus generate additional mutations. Indeed, macrophage density correlates with a poor prognosis in approximately 80% of cancers and there is now much evidence that tumors frequently "re-educate" macrophages, through the provision of anti-inflammatory cytokines (such as IL-10 and TGFβ) to support rather than fight the tumor. Thus, tumors can manipulate cells of the immune system for their own ends, which further contributes to the difficulty of developing tumor immunity.

However, the situation is not completely hopeless, as there are instances where productive immune responses to tumors do appear to be capable of promoting tumor eradication. Furthermore, in situations where tumors maintain an inflammatory environment for their own ends, it may be possible to attack such tumors using neutralizing antibodies against the particular cytokines driving tumor growth and maintaining an adequate blood supply. In addition, existing anti-inflammatory drugs can also have utility in these situations.

Tumor antigens and immune surveillance

Immunologists have long nurtured the view that there must be ways in which the immune system can be harnessed to repel transformed cells, akin to the way in which the immune system rejects transplanted tissue with remarkable efficiency. The ability to reject transplants of tissue may be traced back a long way down the evolutionary tree—back even as far as the annelid worms. Long before the studies on the involvement of self-*major histocompatibility complex* (MHC) in immunological responses, Lewis Thomas suggested that the allograft rejection mechanism represented a means by which the body's cells could be kept under **immunological surveillance** so that altered cells with neoplastic potential could be identified and summarily eliminated. For this to operate, cancer cells must display some new discriminating structure that can be recognized by the immune system; such molecules are frequently referred to as **tumor antigens**.

For the immune system to mount an effective anti-tumor response, at a minimum, the tumor must make its presence known by expressing molecules that are not normally found within the body, or conversely, by failing to express a molecule that is normally present on healthy cells (Figure 17.5). A good example of the latter is the class I MHC molecules that are displayed on the surface of practically all nucleated cells; failure to express MHC molecules is one of the criteria used by NK cells to select target cells for attack (see p. 95), and as a result NK cells may play an important role in immune surveillance. The ideal tumor antigen would be expressed by cells of the tumor, but not by normal cells, and would be required for tumor growth or maintenance, thereby preventing the tumor from losing expression of this antigen through immune-driven selection. It might also be acceptable to target antigens that are highly expressed by the tumor but are also expressed by a restricted-range of normal nontransformed cells, depending on whether the potential damage to normal tissue can be kept within an acceptable range. However, few of the tumor antigens identified to date fit this ideal profile; for the most part tumor proteins represent nonmutated proteins or other molecules that are aberrantly expressed by the tumor. Other tumor antigens represent mutant forms of proteins that appear due to the **genomic instability** that contributed to the formation

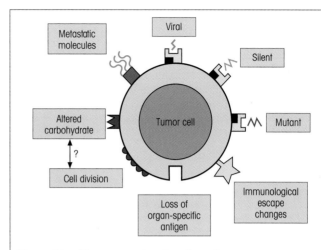

Figure 17.5. Tumor-associated surface changes.

of the tumor in the first instance. Many of the latter antigens will be specific to the tumor of a particular individual and will not be shared between individuals, thereby making it difficult to select candidate antigens that are likely to have widespread utility.

Identification of tumor antigens

A number of strategies have been used to identify tumor antigens. A tried and tested approach involves immunizing mice with tumor cells to generate panels of monoclonal antibodies that are subsequently tested for their ability to discriminate between untransformed and transformed cells from the same cell lineage. This type of approach has had limited success in identifying *bona fide* tumor antigens, but has frequently led to the identification of cell surface molecules that are overexpressed or post-translationally modified on particular tumor cell types.

A classic example is the **human epidermal growth factor receptor 2** (**HER2**), which is amplified in 15–20% of breast cancers and confers increased aggressiveness on such tumors (Figure 17.6). HER2 (also called Neu) was originally discovered by Robert Weinberg and colleagues using genetic screening techniques to search for transforming oncogenes. Transfection of cDNA derived from a chemically transformed cell line resulted in the identification of the HER2/Neu oncogene, which is related to the epidermal growth factor receptor (EGFR). HER2 was subsequently discovered to be amplified in a subset of breast cancers and to be important for the maintenance of such tumors as ablation of HER2 expression in such cases led to cessation of proliferation followed by apoptosis. Antibodies targeting this receptor are effective in the treatment of the subset of breast cancers that overexpress HER2, particularly if used in combination with standard chemotherapeutic drugs such as doxorubicin and paclitaxel. The observation that certain tumors express abnormal amounts of certain cell surface molecules has proved to be very useful

Figure 17.6. Amplification of the HER2/ Neu oncogene can lead to increased proliferation and progression to malignancy.

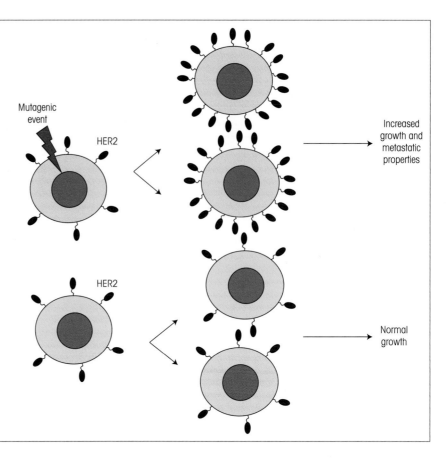

as several of these molecules have formed the basis of mono-clonal antibody-based therapies that have proved to be effective against several types of cancer (discussed later in this chapter).

In a similar vein to the use of antibodies as probes, single chain Fv phage libraries have also been used to probe tumor cell surfaces for the presence of differentially expressed antigens as well as tumor-specific antigens, with some success.

Another approach involves isolating tumor-reactive T-cells from peripheral blood or tumor tissue of cancer patients and using these cells to screen autologous target cells transfected with genes from a tumor-derived cDNA library (Figure 17.7). Expansion of T-cells in response to cells transfected with a particular cDNA identifies the protein encoded by this cDNA as a candidate tumor antigen. An alternative approach uses peptides eluted from tumor-derived MHC molecules to pulse APCs to test for their ability to elicit responses from tumor-reactive lymphocytes. Peptides eliciting positive responses in such assays can be subsequently identified by purification and sequencing; not exactly a technically simple approach but feasible nonetheless.

Yet another strategy, **serological analysis of recombinant cDNA expression libraries** (SEREX), uses diluted antiserum from cancer patients to screen for antibodies that react against proteins expressed by cDNA libraries generated from cancer tissue (Figure 17.8). This approach is predicated upon the assumption that anti-tumor antibodies are indicative of T-helper cells specific for such antigens. More than 1500

immunogenic proteins, which are all candidate tumor antigens, have been isolated using this method. So there is no shortage of candidates. But it is important to note that *in vitro* recognition assays may not select ideal or valid tumor antigens; validation of candidate tumor antigens is clearly essential, as proteins found to be immunogenic *in vitro* may exhibit little potency *in vivo*. These problems aside, it is clear that tumor antigens do indeed exist and some examples will now be discussed.

Virally encoded antigens

As alluded to earlier, a substantial minority of tumors (~10–15%) arise through infection with **oncogenic viruses**, Epstein–Barr virus (EBV) in lymphomas, *h*uman *T*-cell *l*eukemia *v*irus-1 (HTLV-1) in leukemia, human papilloma virus (HPV) in cervical cancers, hepatitis B (HBV) and C (HCV) viruses in hepatocellular carcinoma and Kaposi's associated sarcoma virus (KSHV). Some of these viruses contain genes homologous with **cellular oncogenes**, which encode factors that can override the normal controls that regulate cell division and cell death (apoptosis). Expression of these genes therefore can lead to malignant transformation. However, some other viruses, such as hepatitis B virus, can greatly increase the relative risk of developing cancer, by as much as 100-fold, in a manner that appears to be unrelated to direct mutagenic effects of the virus but rather due to the chronic

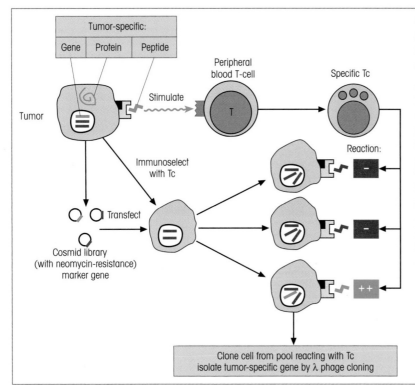

Figure 17.7. Identification of tumor-specific gene using tumor-specific cytotoxic T-cell (Tc) clones derived from mixed tumor–lymphocyte culture.

A cosmid library incorporating the tumor DNA is transfected into an antigen-negative cell line derived from the wild-type tumor by immunoselection with the Tc. Small pools of transfected cells are tested against the Tc. A positive pool is cloned by limiting dilution and the tumor-specific gene (*MAGE-1*) cloned from the antigen-positive well(s). (Based on van der Bruggen P. *et al.* (1991) *Science* **254**, 1643. Copyright © 1991 by the AAAS.) The original **MAGE-1** belongs to a family of 12 genes. Further melanoma-specific genes, including *MART-1*, *gp100* and *tyrosinase*, have been discovered.

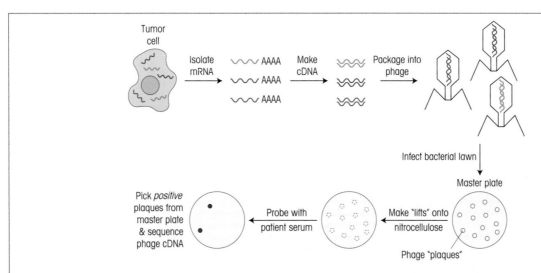

Figure 17.8. Identification of tumor antigens by serological identification of antigens expressed by recombinant cloning (SEREX).

In the SEREX method, mRNA isolated from tumor biopsies is used to construct cDNA expression libraries that are then packaged into bacteriophage. A bacterial lawn is then infected with the phage library under conditions that permit expression of the tumor-derived proteins. Replica "lifts" of the bacterial lawn are made using nitrocellulose membranes and these are then probed with diluted antisera from the cancer patient. Bacterial colonies expressing tumor-derived proteins that are detected by antibodies within the patient serum can then be identified by isolating the phage from the relevant colony and sequencing the cDNA harbored within this phage.

inflammation provoked by the virus. This raises an interesting point, which we will discuss at some length in a later section, which is that persistent immune responses can frequently promote rather than suppress tumor development. Evidence is now accumulating to suggest that protracted inflammatory responses can act as a driver of malignant transformation and—where inflammation occurs after a tumor has already become established—can also nurture tumor growth through the production of inflammatory cytokines.

Virus-derived peptides associated with MHC on the surface of the tumor cell behave as powerful transplantation antigens that generate haplotype-specific cytotoxic T-cells (Tc). All tumors induced by a given virus should carry the same surface antigen, irrespective of their cellular origin, so that immunization with any one of these tumors would confer resistance to subsequent challenge with the others provided that there were no artful mutations by the virus (Milestone 17.1). Unfortunately, viruses are not innately friendly. However, the recent develop-

⦿ Milestone 17.1—Tumors Can Induce Immune Responses

The first convincing evidence for tumor-associated antigens came from the work of Prehn and Main who demonstrated quite clearly that **chemically induced cancers** can induce immune responses to themselves but not to other tumors produced by the same carcinogen (Figure M17.1.1a). Tumors induced by **oncogenic viruses** are different in that processed viral peptides are present on the surface of all neoplastic cells bearing the viral genome so that Tc cells raised to one tumor will cross-react with all others produced by the same virus (Figure M17.1.1b).

Dramatic advances were made by Boon and colleagues. First, they showed that random mutagenesis of transplantable tumors, i.e. tumors that can be passaged within a pure mouse

strain without provoking rejection, can give rise to mutant progeny with strong transplantation antigens. As a result they could not be grown in syngeneic animals with a normal immune system; accordingly they were referred to as **tum-** variants. Boon's team developed a powerful technology (cf. Figure 17.7) that enabled them to use Tc clones specific for the tum- variant to screen cosmid clones for the mutant gene. These two breakthroughs, the recognition that mutation in tumors can generate strong transplantation reactions, and the development of the technique for identifying the relevant antigens with Tc cells, heralded really profound developments in tumor immunology and put it firmly on the map as a key area for cancer research.

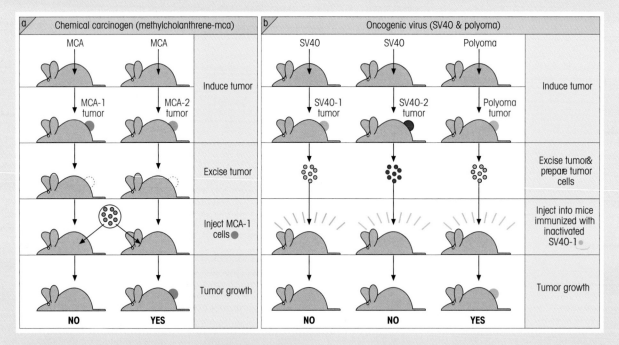

Figure M17.1.1. The specificity of immunity induced by tumors. (a) A chemically induced tumor MCA-1 can induce resistance to an implant of itself but not to a tumor produced in a syngeneic mouse by the same carcinogen. Thus each tumor has an individual antigen, now thought to be a processed mutant endogenous protein complexed with a heat-shock protein. More recent data suggest that, if immunized animals are challenged with much lower numbers of tumor cells, a greater degree of cross-protection between tumors may be observed, which has been ascribed to a 44 kDa oncofetal antigen, possibly an immature version of a laminin receptor protein. (b) Tumors produced by a given oncogenic virus immunize against tumors produced in syngeneic mice by the same but not other viruses. Thus tumors produced by an oncogenic virus share a common antigen.

ment of an effective vaccine that is highly protective against HPV infection and associated cancer (predominantly cervical cancer in women), as well as genital warts, is a good illustration of the fact that the immune system can be harnessed to ward off at least some malignancies. We will discuss this example in more detail later in this chapter (p. 463).

Expression of normally silent genes

The dysregulated uncontrolled cell division of the cancer cell creates a milieu in which the products of normally silent genes may be expressed. Sometimes these encode differentiation antigens normally associated with an earlier developmental stage. Thus tumors derived from the same cell type are often found to express such **oncofetal antigens** that are also present on embryonic cells. Examples would be α-fetoprotein in hepatic carcinoma and carcinoembryonic antigen (CEA) in cancer of the intestine. Certain monoclonal antibodies also react with tumors of neural crest origin and fetal melanocytes. Another monoclonal antibody defines the SSEA-1 antigen found on a variety of human tumors and early mouse embryos but absent from adult cells with the exception of human granulocytes and monocytes.

But the exciting quantum leap forward stems from the original observation that cytosolic viral nucleoprotein could provide a target for Tc cells by appearing on the cell surface as a processed peptide associated with MHC class I (cf. p. 122). This established the general principle that the intracellular proteins that are not destined to be positioned in the surface plasma membrane can still signal their presence to T-cells in the outer world by the processed peptide–MHC mechanism. Cytotoxic T-cells specific for tumor cells, obtained from mixed cultures of peripheral blood cells with tumor, can be used to establish the identity of the antigen employing the strategy described in Figure 17.7. By something of a *tour de force* a gene

encoding a melanoma antigen, MAGE-1, was identified. It belongs to a family of 12 genes, 6 of which are expressed in a significant proportion of melanomas as well as head and neck tumors, nonsmall cell lung cancers and bladder carcinomas. MAGE-1 is *not* expressed in normal tissues except for germ-line cells in testis and gives rise to antigenic T-cell epitopes that, in the light of the absence of class I MHC on the testis cells, must be considered tumor-specific. This exciting research reveals the tumor-specific antigen as an expression of a normally silent gene.

Mutant antigens

The seminal work on tum- mutants (Milestone 17.1) has persuaded us that single point mutations in oncogenes can account for the large diversity of antigens found on carcinogen-induced tumors. The specific immunity provoked by chemically induced tumors can be elicited by **heat-shock protein** 70 (hsp70) and hsp90 isolated from the tumor cells, but their immunogenicity is lost when the associated low-molecular-weight peptides are removed. These peptides could, however, stimulate the specific CD8 cytotoxic T-cell clones generated by the tumors, and three possible mechanisms have been advanced to account for the enhancement of tumor immune responses by hsps. First, they can act as "danger" signals by activating antigen-presenting cells. Second, necrotic tumor cells expressing the hsps can transfer hsp–peptide complexes to host antigen-presenting cells where they can cross-prime cytotoxic CD8 T-cells through the MHC class I endogenous presentation pathway. And last, the hsps may influence the capacity of the tumor cell itself to process and present endogenous mutated and, of course, "silent" antigens as targets for specific T-cells (Figure 17.9).

There is considerable evidence for the production of mutated peptides in human tumors. The gene encoding cell cycle checkpoint protein, p53, is a hotspot for mutation in

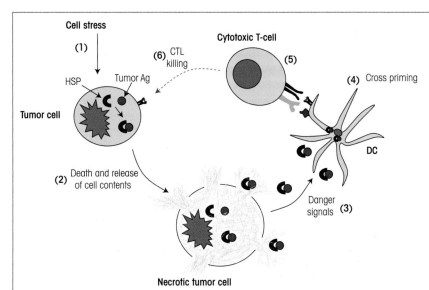

Figure 17.9. The role of heat-shock proteins (hsps) in tumor immunogenicity.

(1) Stress factors upregulate hsps that can form complexes with processed tumor antigen (Ag) and increase surface presentation of antigenic peptide by MHC class I. (2) They can also lead to necrosis and release of hsp–peptide complexes, which (3) can act as stimulatory danger signals to dendritic antigen-presenting cells and penetrate the cytoplasm, where (4) they can enter the MHC class I processing pathway by so-called cross-priming. (5) CD8 resting T-cells become activated and (6) kill the tumor cells. CTL, cytotoxic T-lymphocytes. (Based on Wells A.D. & Malkowsky M. (2000) *Immunology Today* **21**, 129.)

numerous cancers. The mutant forms of p53 that are frequently found in tumors represent loss-of-function mutants that fail to arrest division of cells that have suffered DNA damage; such damage would normally trigger cell cycle arrest or apoptosis of the afflicted cell. The oncogenic human *ras* genes differ from their normal counterparts by point mutations usually leading to single amino acid substitutions in positions 12, 13 or 61. Such mutations generate constitutively active forms of Ras that promote increased rates of cell division through activation of the MAPK pathway (see p. 211), and have been recorded in 40% of human colorectal cancers and in more than 90% of pancreatic carcinomas, as well as other malignancies. The mutated ras peptide can induce proliferative T-cell lines *in vitro*.

Changes in carbohydrate structure

The chaotic internal control of metabolism within neoplastic cells often leads to the presentation of abnormal carbohydrate structures on the cell surface. Sometimes one sees blocked synthesis, e.g. deletion of blood group A. In other cases there may be enhanced synthesis of structures absent in progenitor cells: thus some gastrointestinal cancers express the Lewis Le^a antigen in individuals who are Le(a$^-$,b$^-$) and others produce extended chains bearing dimeric Le^a or Le(a,b).

Abnormal mucin synthesis can have immunological consequences. Consider the mucins of pancreatic and breast tissue. These consist of a polypeptide core of 20-amino acid tandem repeats with truly abundant O-linked carbohydrate chains. A monoclonal antibody SM-3 directed to the core polypeptide reacts poorly with normal tissue where the epitope is masked by glycosylation, but well with breast and pancreatic carcinomas possessing shorter and fewer O-linked chains. Tc cells specific for tumor mucins are not MHC restricted and the slightly heretical suggestion has been made that the T-cell receptors (TCRs) are binding multivalently to closely spaced SM-3 epitopes on unprocessed mucins; alternatively, and closer to the party line, recognition is by γδ cells.

Molecules related to metastatic potential

Changes in surface carbohydrates can have a dramatic effect on malignancy. For example, colonic cancers expressing sialyl Le^x have a poor prognosis and higher propensity to metastasize. Lung cancer patients whose tumors showed deletion of blood group A had a much worse prognosis than those with continuous A; the finding that patients expressing H/Le^y/Le^b also had a poorer prognosis than antigen-negative subjects is consistent with this observation.

The role of **CD44** (HERMES/Pgp-1) in cell trafficking, based on its interaction with vascular endothelium, has afforded it some prominence in the facilitation of metastatic spread. CD44 occurs in several isoforms with a varying number of exons between the transmembrane and common N-terminus. Normal epithelium expresses the CD44H isoform with hyaluran-binding domains, but lacking the intervening v1–v10

exons; expression of certain of these exons on tumors is indicative of a growth advantage, as they are present with higher frequency on more advanced cancers. Stable transfection of a nonmetastatic tumor with a CD44 cDNA clone encompassing exons v6 and v7 induced the ability to form metastatic tumors—a most striking effect. Further, injection of a monoclonal anti-CD44 v6 prevented the formation of lymph node metastases. Exons v6 and v10 have now been shown to bind blood group H and chondroitin 4-sulfate, respectively, and the latest hypothesis is that these carbohydrates can bind to CD44H on endothelium and thence homotypically to each other so generating a metastatic nidus.

Changes have quite frequently been observed in the expression of class I MHC molecules. For example, oncogenic transformation of cells infected with adenovirus 12 is associated with highly reduced class I as a consequence of very low levels of TAP-1 and TAP-2 mRNA. Mutation frequently leads to diminished or absent class I expression linked in most cases to increased metastatic potential, presumably reflecting decreased vulnerability to T-cells but not NK cells. In breast cancer, for example, around 60% of metastatic tumors lack class I.

Spontaneous immune responses to tumors

Immune surveillance against strongly immunogenic tumors

When present, many of the antigens discussed in the previous section can provoke immune responses in experimental animals that lead to resistance against tumor growth, but they vary tremendously in their efficiency. Powerful antigens associated with tumors induced by oncogenic viruses or ultraviolet light generate strong resistance, while the transplantation antigens on chemically induced tumors (Milestone 17.1) are weaker and somewhat variable; disappointingly, tumors that arise spontaneously in animals produce little or no response. The **immune surveillance theory** would predict that there should be more tumors in individuals whose adaptive immune systems are suppressed. This undoubtedly seems to be the case for **strongly immunogenic tumors**. There is a considerable increase in skin cancer in immunosuppressed patients living in high sunshine regions north of Brisbane and, in general, transplant recipients on immunosuppressive drugs are unduly susceptible to skin cancers, largely associated with papilloma virus, and EBV-positive lymphomas. The EBV-related Burkitt's lymphomas crop up with undue frequency in regions infested with malarial infection, known to compromise the efficacy of the immune system. Likewise, the lymphomas that arise in children with T-cell deficiency linked to Wiskott–Aldrich syndrome or ataxia telangiectasia express *EBV* genes; they show unusually restricted expression of EBV latent proteins that are the major potential target epitopes for immune recognition, while cellular adhesion molecules, such as *inter*cellular *a*dhesion *m*olecule-1 (ICAM-1) and *l*ymphocyte *f*unction-*a*ssociated molecule-3

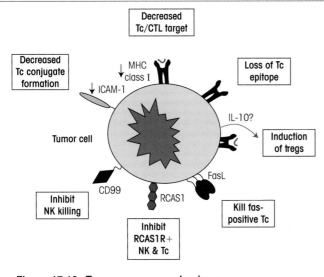

Figure 17.10. Tumor escape mechanisms.

(LFA-3), which mediate conjugate formation with Tc cells, cannot be detected on their surface (Figure 17.10). Knowing that most normal individuals have highly efficient EBV-specific Tc cells, this must be telling us that only by downregulating appropriate surface molecules can the lymphoma cells escape even the limited T-cell surveillance operating in these patients.

These examples aside, it must be acknowledged that the incidence of **spontaneous** tumor formation in mice lacking T- and B-lymphocytes is not substantially higher than in those with intact immune systems; the same is also true for immunodeficient humans. Such observations weaken arguments that adaptive immune responses have a significant role to play in cancer prevention. Nonetheless, while normal adaptive immune responses may be insufficient to deal with the establishment of many tumors, this does not necessarily mean that the immune system cannot be manipulated to deliver an effective response.

A role for innate immunity?

There is an uncommon flurry of serious interest in **natural killer (NK)** cells. It is generally accepted that they subserve a function as the earliest cellular effector mechanism against dissemination of blood-borne metastases. Let's look at the evidence. Patients with advanced metastatic disease often have abnormal NK activity and low levels appear to predict subsequent metastases. In experimental animals, removal of NK cells from mice with surgically resected B16 melanoma resulted in uncontrolled metastatic disease and death. Acute ethanol intoxication in rats boosted the number of metastases from an NK-sensitive tumor 10-fold, but had no effect on an NK-resistant cancer, hinting at a possible underlying cause for the association between alcoholism, infectious disease and malignancies. (Those who enjoy the odd bacchanalian splurge should not be too upset—be comforted by the beneficial effect in heart disease, but no excesses please!) Powerful evidence

implicating these cells in protection against cancer is provided by beige mice that congenitally lack NK cells. They die with spontaneous tumors earlier than their nondeficient +/bg littermates, and the incidence of radiation-induced leukemia is reduced by prior injection of cloned isogeneic NK cells that could be suppressing preleukemic cells. Note, however, that tumors induced chemically or with murine leukemia virus were handled normally.

Resting NK cells are spontaneously cytolytic for certain, but by no means all, tumor targets; cells activated by IL-2 and possibly by IL-12 and IL-18 display a wider lethality. As described earlier in Chapter 4, recognition of the surface structures on the target cell involves various activating and inhibitory receptors, but it is important to re-emphasize that recognition of class I imparts a **negative inactivating** signal to the NK cell. Conversely, this implies that downregulation of MHC class I, which tumors employ as a strategy to escape Tc cells (Figure 17.10), would make them **more susceptible to NK attack**. The tumor cells can fight back by expressing CD99, which downregulates NK CD16, and the growth inhibitor RCAS1 (receptor-binding cancer antigen expressed on SiSo cells), which induces apoptosis in NK as well as in Tc cells (Figure 17.10). It is not clear whether surface FasL, which can repel attack by the Fas-positive cytolytic T-cells, is also effective against NK cells, but the relative resistance of tumor cells to apoptosis must be innately protective.

Divisions are surfacing in the NK ranks. The NK cells, which remarkably constitute up to 50% of the liver-associated lymphocytes in humans, have a higher level of expression of IL-2 receptor and adhesion molecules such as integrins compared with NK cells in peripheral blood. They are precursors of a subset of activated adherent NK cells (A-NK) that adhere rapidly to solid surfaces under the influence of IL-2 and are distinguished from their nonadherent counterparts by their superiority in entering solid tumors and in prolonging survival following adoptive transfer with IL-2 into animal models of tumor growth or metastasis. The nonadherent NK variety is better at killing antibody-coated cancer cells through antibody-dependent cellular cytotoxicity (ADCC), mediated by their CD16 FcγRIII receptor.

Be kind to your NK cells. Really late nights that involve major curtailment of slow-wave sleep lead to drastic falls in NK cells and levels of IL-2, quite apart from bleary eyes.

Tumor escape mechanisms

Strong supporting evidence for a role for the immune system in surveillance against transformed cells comes from observations that tumors employ a range of strategies to evade and manipulate the immune system. Indeed, it could be said that tumors are positively brimming with various **immunological escape mechanisms** (Figure 17.10) and thus they resemble successful infections. We have already referred to the fact that downregulation of HLA class I molecules to make the tumor a less attractive target for cytolytic T-cells is a favorite ploy. This is a common feature of breast cancer metastases, and this is true also of cervical carcinoma where, prognostically, loss of HLA-B44 in premalignant lesions is an indicator of tumor progression. Rather than lose expression of all class I molecules and risk attracting the attentions of NK cells, tumors may lose just the expression of class I alleles that are capable of presenting antigenic peptides to T-cells.

Immunoediting weeds out immunogenic cells

As we have noted earlier in this chapter, many tumors are also not particularly immunogenic to begin with, possibly because strongly immunogenic tumors may be readily weeded out and fail to develop to the point that they become clinically significant. In this way, the immune system may exert a Darwinian selective pressure for cancer-causing mutations that are largely immunologically silent: a process that has been termed **immunoediting**. Subtle point mutations in oncogenes, such as *RAS*, that have profound effects on the function of the protein products of such genes and contribute to transformation, may completely fail to create any new epitopes that would result in immune attack. In a similar vein, complete loss of expression of important tumor suppressor genes, such as *P53 or RB*, through nonsense mutations would also fail to create any new epitopes.

Tolerization against tumor antigens due to the absence of co-stimulation

Loss of tumor antigen epitopes, where they do arise, represents another escape mechanism and mutations in an oncogenic virus itself can increase its tumorigenic potential. Thus the frequent association of a high-risk variant of human papilloma virus with cervical tumors in HLA-B7 individuals is attributed to the loss of a T-cell epitope that would otherwise generate a protective B7-mediated cytolytic response. As outlined earlier, there is also an increasing appreciation that tumors may create a microenvironment where **active tolerization** of tumor-infiltrating lymphocytes occurs through failure of DCs to express the appropriate co-stimulatory molecules. Recall that DCs that deliver antigen in the absence of proper co-stimulation, in the form of CD28 ligands, render T-cells anergic (Figure 17.4). As we have discussed earlier in this chapter, but it is a point worth reiterating, one reason why DCs in the vicinity of tumors may fail to become activated may be due to the absence of PAMPs or DAMPS that can upregulate co-stimulatory molecules on DCs that encounter these signals (Figure 17.4). We have already noted that **DCs do not exist in a state of perpetual activation** and are unable to provide proper co-stimulation unless they encounter appropriate molecules that possess DC-activating properties. In the context of infection, DC-activating molecules (Toll-like receptor ligands) are derived from the infectious agent and are usually structures that are shared by many pathogens but not found in the host. However, tumors that release endogenous danger signals (DAMPs) may

fail to tolerize DCs and become subject to effective immune attack that may result in tumor rejection or persistence through selection of immune escape mutants (Figure 17.11). Conversely, tumors that fail to release DAMPs may be simply regarded as self and may fail to elicit significant immune responses.

There are also other reasons why the immune system may become tolerant to a tumor. For example, many solid tumors secrete large amounts of angiogenic factors such as **vascular endothelial cell growth factor** (VEGF) that promote the development of the new blood vessels that tumors need. Evidence also suggests that VEGF can suppress the maturation of dendritic cells (DCs) and these immature or partially differentiated DCs may tolerize to antigens that they find within the vicinity of the tumor.

Tumor counterattack mechanisms

Tumors can also decrease their vulnerability to cytotoxic T-cell attack by expression of surface FasL (cf. p. 247) and a growth inhibitory molecule, RCAS1, which react with T-cells bearing their corresponding receptors and stop them in their tracks. As we have already noted earlier, tumors have also frequently been found to secrete other immunosuppressive factors such as TGFβ and IL-10 (Figure 17.4). Such factors may help to keep burgeoning immune responses at bay by inducing suppressor or regulatory T-cell populations that inhibit responses to the tumor. Natural regulatory T-cells (Tregs) that normally guard against the development of autoimmunity may also hamper robust T-cell responses against tumors. It should also be borne in mind that internal defects in the cell death machinery, that facilitated the establishment of the tumor in the first instance, may also render such cells resistant to the best efforts of cytotoxic T-cells and NK cells to eradicate them. The very existence of such "Houdini" mechanisms builds a case in favor of the notion that the adaptive immune system has a significant role in suppressing tumor growth and provides hope that this can be exploited in the clinic.

Cancers that express neoantigens of **low immunogenicity** do not come creeping out of the woodwork when patients are radically immunosuppressed and, although T-cell responses can often be rescued from tumor-infiltrating lymphocytes or relatively high numbers of tumor-specific CD8 T-cells may be detected by the peptide–HLA tetramer technique in peripheral blood, they may be functionally deficient due perhaps to suppression by local IL-10 and TGFβ. Mutation of p53 and its overexpression are very common events in human cancer and are often associated with the production of antibodies; but while these could prove to have a diagnostic utility, it is most unlikely that they are of benefit to the patient, the current view being that *cell-mediated* responses are crucial to the attack against internal antigens expressed in solid tumors. Reluctantly, one has to accept the view that, with tumors of weak immunogenicity, we are dealing with low-key reactions that clearly play little role in curbing the neoplastic process. That is not to say

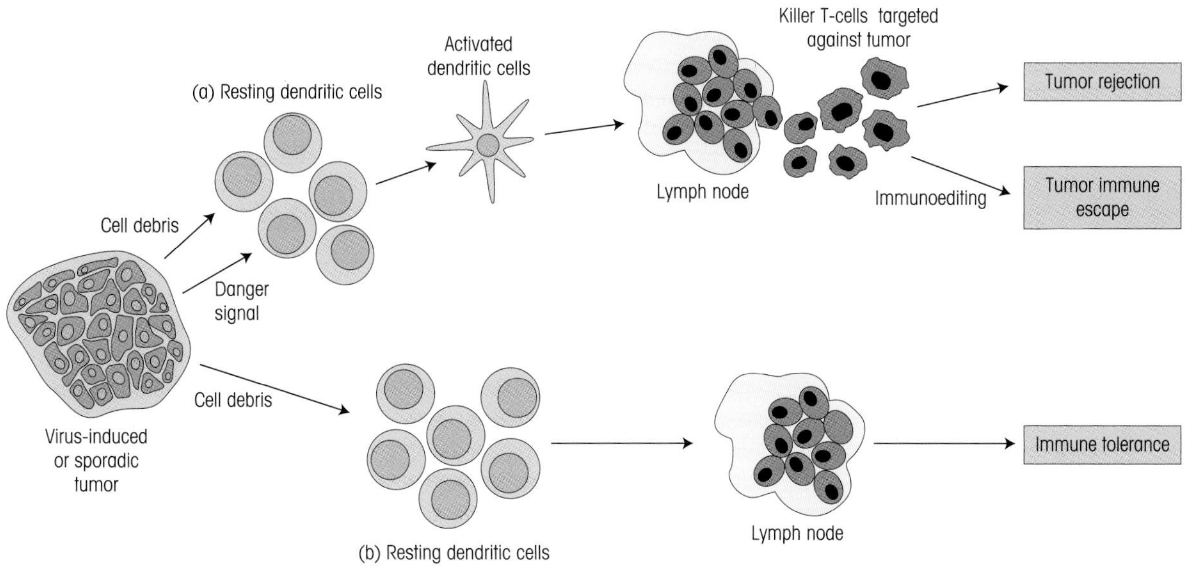

Figure 17.11. Danger signals may dictate whether dendritic cells prime for T-cell responses or induce tolerance to tumors.

Growing tumors typically shed material from dead or dying cells and this debris is picked up by local dendritic cells (DCs) that transport it to the local lymph nodes for presentation to T-cells. (a) Where the tumor is shedding molecules ("danger signals") that are capable of activating DCs, maturation of the DC occurs and these cells are capable of eliciting robust immune responses from appropriate T-cells. Such tumors may then become subject to immune attack by the activated T-cells resulting either in rejection of the tumor, or "immunoediting" of the tumor to eliminate only the cells presenting the antigen that initiated the response. (b) In the absence of signals that activate DCs, resting DCs that encounter tumor-derived material fail to become activated and any T-cells such DCs subsequently encounter may become tolerant to tumor-derived antigens presented by such DCs. (Based on Melief J.M. (2005) *Nature* **437**, 41.)

that these "weak" antigens cannot be exploited for therapeutic purposes, as we shall soon see.

Immune responses can paradoxically enhance tumor growth

Although we tend to think of immune responses in purely destructive terms—probably not unreasonably when one considers that much of the early stages of an immune response is preoccupied with detecting and eliminating nonself entities—a significant and often overlooked function of the immune system is to restore normal tissue integrity after an infection has been resolved by promoting wound healing. To this end, macrophages and other innate immune cells secrete growth factors and other mediators that can stimulate proliferation of local tissue and endothelium for the purposes of replacing cells that were killed during the acute stages of infection. There is now much evidence that tumors, through recruitment and "re-education" of inflammatory cells to a more wound healing phenotype, can harness the growth-stimulating properties of such cells to subvert the actions of the innate immune system.

For example, TNFα production in the tumor microenvironment can stimulate TNF receptor positive tumor cells leading to activation of the NFκB transcription factor, which can have two major consequences. One the one hand, NFκB can promote expression of additional cytokines, such as IL-1 and IL-6, which can have autocrine growth-promoting effects on the tumor. On the other hand, NFκB activation can also lead to expression of multiple apoptosis-inhibitory molecules within the tumor that may render such cells more difficult to kill. Either way, the tumor benefits from the combined effects of TNFα exposure. In such situations, treatment with neutralizing anti-TNF antibodies may be of therapeutic benefit. Similarly, inhibitors of NFκB are also under evaluation as potential chemotherapeutic drugs.

Infection and inflammation can enhance tumor initiation, promotion and progression

Aside from the tumor escape mechanisms detailed in the previous section, there is now considerable evidence that infection and its downstream consequences—the inflammatory response—can promote tumor development as well as progression. Initial evidence for a role for infection as a factor that can influence tumor growth came from studies that noted that post-operative infections in cancer patients frequently led to rapid growth of previously dormant metastases (i.e. secondary tumors) after surgical resection of the primary tumor mass. This was subsequently confirmed by LPS treatment of tumor-bearing mice, which showed that this had a significant growth enhancing effect on the tumor as well promoting the establishment of metastases. It is now well accepted that **chronic infection and inflammation are among the most important epigenetic and environmental factors that can influence the establishment and progression of certain tumors**. For example, there is a significant association between long-term alcohol abuse—which leads to inflammation of the liver and pancreatic tissues—and cancers of the same organs. Similarly, inflammatory bowel disease is associated with an increased risk of colon cancer; chronic viral hepatitis is associated with liver cancer; *Helicobacter pylori* infection is associated with gastric cancer; asbestos and silica exposure are associated with persistent lung inflammation and lung cancer.

TLR expression on tumors can enhance tumor growth and survival

We have already encountered the role of Toll-like receptors and their important role in immunity particularly in the initial stages of the immune response (see Chapter 1). TLRs are predominantly expressed on cells of the innate immune system, such as macrophages, dendritic cells, mast cells and NK cells, although B-cells as well as endothelial cells also utilize these receptors in several contexts. TLR stimulation by pathogen-derived molecular patterns can lead to the secretion of several cytokines and recruitment of inflammatory cells such as neutrophils and additional macrophages from monocyte precursors. However, recent evidence also suggests that tumors may harness the positive effects of TLR stimulation to promote growth and survival. Several tumor cell types have been found to express TLRs and evidence is accumulating to suggest that stimulation of these receptors on tumor cells can promote tumor proliferation and survival

via autocrine signaling. This is due to TLR engagement being a potent NFκB-activation stimulus (see Figure 1.7). NFκB activation can help the tumor in at least two ways. First, by upregulating the expression of anti-apoptotic gene products, such as members of the Bcl-2 family, this can make the tumor more resilient to the oxygen and nutrient deprivation that frequently occur in the tumor environment. Second, by promoting the production of cytokines such as IL-1 and IL-6 that can have mitogenic effects on certain cell types, tumors may produce their own growth-promoting factors. The presence of microbial factors, as a source of TLR ligands, can therefore have positive benefits for TLR-expressing tumors, which is just one way in which persistent infection can drive tumor progression.

An inflammatory environment can foster mutation

Chronic infection can also influence tumorigenesis in additional ways, with cytokine and reactive oxygen production by inflammatory cells recruited to the site of infection also capable of promoting tumor initiation and progression. Inflammatory cells, especially activated macrophages, can cause DNA damage through the production of reactive oxygen and nitrogen species and thus generate mutations that can lead to cellular transformation (Figure 17.12). Should this occur on an occasional basis, it is tolerable and can be viewed as one of the downsides of having a robust immune system. Moreover, cells with DNA damage can be dealt with through DNA repair, elimination via apoptosis, or one of the other cell-intrinsic mechanisms of tumor suppression, as we discussed earlier in this chapter (Figure 17.3). However, if an inflammatory response is allowed to smolder for months or years on end, as happens in chronic colitis and viral hepatitis for example, the inflammatory response can greatly increase the risk of malignant transformation through the generation of genetic instability at the site of inflammation (Figure 17.12).

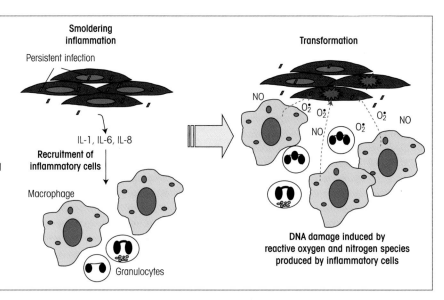

Figure 17.12. Chronic inflammation can promote malignant transformation.

Persistent, smoldering inflammation can lead to genetic instability through recruitment of macrophages and other innate immune cells that are capable of provoking DNA damage through the production of reactive oxygen and nitrogen species. Persistent DNA damage can result in the generation of mutations that can lead to cellular transformation.

Certain oncogenic mutations can drive the production of proinflammatory cytokines and chemokines

A substantial proportion of tumors carry mutations in Ras or its downstream target B-Raf that render these proteins constitutively active. Constitutively active Ras or B-Raf lead to activation of the MEK and ERK kinases downstream, which has the effect of activating a battery of transcription factors that can promote cell division. Among the targets of these transcription factors are the genes for IL-6 and IL-8 and, as a consequence, tumors carrying gain-of-function mutations in Ras and B-Raf frequently express these cytokines. If such an event were detrimental to the tumor, one would expect that clonal variants would emerge where the expression of IL-6 and IL-8 was silenced. However, it appears instead that secretion of such cytokines can enhances tumor growth in a number of ways, as we have already alluded to earlier. One possibility is that IL-6 could have autocrine growth and survival-promoting effects on the tumor itself, acting to enhance cell division or lead to the expression of anti-apoptotic proteins (Figure 17.13). Another is that IL-6 acts in a paracrine fashion on surrounding stromal cells to promote angiogenesis, thereby enhancing blood supply to the tumor. Indeed, evidence for the latter scenario has been found in mouse models where growth of chemical-induced skin tumors was impaired in *IL-6* knockout mice and this was related to the effects of IL-6 on nearby endothelial cells, rather than on the tumor itself. Use of *IL-6* knockout mice has also provided clear evidence that these animals are resistant to the development of malignant myeloma, a malignancy affecting the B-cell lineage. Furthermore, certain IL-6 promoter polymorphisms, which result in the production of higher levels of this cytokine, have been found to correlate with a poorer prognosis in breast cancer.

Similarly, tumor-derived IL-8 has been found to promote infiltration of tumors by neutrophils and macrophages that, as discussed earlier, can promote tumor growth through the production of other proinflammatory cytokines such as IL-1 and TNF as well as by secreting matrix metalloproteases that can remodel the extracellular matrix and promote tumor spread (Figure 17.13). Activity of inflammatory cells also led to increased recruitment of endothelial cells and promoted angiogenesis. Use of neutralizing anti-IL-8 antibodies in Ras-induced tumor models led to a marked reduction in tumor growth with greatly increased tumor necrosis apparent.

Although the fact that tumors can deliberately recruit cells of the innate immune system by secreting chemokines and pro-inflammatory cytokines is pretty ominous, it does suggest that one way of attacking such tumors may be through neutralizing such factors with appropriate monoclonal antibodies, as such antibodies are now available and have been approved for use in other conditions such as psoriasis.

Approaches to cancer immunotherapy

Although immune surveillance seems to operate only against strongly immunogenic tumors, the identification of a range of tumor antigens is a positive step forward (Table 17.1), and has set the stage for exploring how these antigens may be exploited to harness the patient's own immune system in the fight against cancer. On one point all are agreed: if immunotherapy is to succeed, it is essential that the tumor load should first be reduced by surgery, irradiation or chemotherapy, as not only is it unreasonable to expect the immune system to cope with a large tumor mass, but considerable amounts of antigen released by shedding would tend to prevent the generation of any significant response in some cases due to the stimulation of regulatory T-cells. This leaves the small secondary deposits as the proper target for immunotherapy.

So what type of immune response is required for tumor destruction? Studies in mouse models, as well as cancer patients, over the past decade or so suggest that a number of criteria need to be fulfilled in order to obtain killing of tumor cells in sufficient numbers to positively impact on the course of disease.

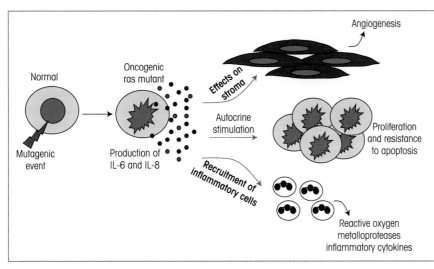

Figure 17.13. Activating Ras mutations can lead to proinflammatory effects.

Oncogenic Ras and B-Raf mutations may lead to the production of proinflammatory cytokines, such as IL-6 and IL-8, that can have diverse pro-survival and growth-promoting effects on tumors as shown.

Table 17.1. Potential tumor antigens for immunotherapy. (Reproduced with permission from Fong L. & Engleman E.G. (2000) Dendritic cells in cancer immunotherapy. *Annual Review of Immunology* **18**, 245.)

Antigen	Malignancy
Tumor specific	
Immunoglobulin V-region	B-cell non-Hodgkin's lymphoma, multiple myeloma
TCR V-region	T-cell non-Hodgkin's lymphoma
Mutant p21/ras	Pancreatic, colon, lung cancer
Mutant p53	Colorectal, lung, bladder, head and neck cancer
Developmental	
p210/bcr-abl fusion product	Chronic myelogenous leukemia, acute lymphoblastic leukemia
MART-1/Melan A	Melanoma
MAGE-1, MAGE-3	Melanoma, colorectal, lung, gastric cancers
GAGE family	Melanoma
Telomerase	Various
Viral	
Human papilloma virus	Cervical, penile cancer
Epstein–Barr virus	Burkitt's lymphoma, nasopharyngeal carcinoma, post-transplant lymphoproliferative disorders
Tissue specific	
Tyrosinase	Melanoma
gp100	Melanoma
Prostatic acid phosphatase	Prostate cancer
Prostate-specific antigen	Prostate cancer
Prostate-specific membrane antigen	Prostate cancer
Thyroglobulin	Thyroid cancer
α-Fetoprotein	Liver cancer
Overexpressed	
HER2	Breast and lung cancers
Carcinoembryonic antigen	Colorectal, lung, breast cancer
Muc-1	Colorectal, pancreatic, ovarian, lung cancer

First, sufficient numbers of T-cells with highly avid recognition of tumor antigens must be generated. Then, these cells must be able to traffic to the site of the tumor and invade the stroma (supporting cells) associated with the tumor. Finally, these lymphocytes should become activated at the site of the tumor and be capable of engaging the tumor with cytotoxic granules

or cytokines such as TNF. Experience to date suggests that fulfilling all of these criteria poses an immense challenge and that immunotherapy is unlikely to offer any "magic bullet" cures. More realistically, immunological manipulations, in tandem with conventional chemo- and radiotherapy, are likely to be the way forward.

Antigen-independent cytokine therapy

The first clear indication that manipulation of the immune system could be beneficial came from studies that utilized antigen-independent strategies to nonspecifically boost the immune response to the tumor. Cytokines such as IL-2, IFN and TNF have pleiotrophic effects on the immune system and some of these have shown promise in animal models as well as in clinical settings. Systemic toxicity has limited the utility of TNF that exhibits rapid and severe hepatotoxicity in animal models and is therefore of limited use in cancer therapy.

Interleukin treatment

High doses of IL-2 have been administered to patients with metastatic melanoma or kidney cancer, and at least partial tumor regression was observed in 15–20% of patients, with some patients displaying complete regression. The beneficial effects of high doses of IL-2 may be due to stimulation of pre-existing tumor-responsive T-cells or due to NK activation. On activation by IL-2 or IL-12, NK cells are capable of killing a variety of fresh tumor cells *in vitro* and, on the basis of studies on mice with mammary glands carrying the *HER2/neu* oncogene, it would not be unreasonable to conduct a trial of systematic IL-12 treatment in cancer patients with minimum residual disease in an attempt to prevent recurrence and to inhibit incipient metastases. Because of the promising results seen upon IL-2 administration, many subsequent tumor vaccine trials have been conducted in combination with this cytokine.

Interferon therapy

In trials using IFNα and IFNβ, a 10–15% objective response rate was seen in patients with renal carcinoma, melanoma and myeloma, an approximate 20% response rate among patients with Kaposi's sarcoma, about 40% positive responders in patients with various lymphomas and a remarkable response rate of 80–90% among patients with hairy cell leukemia and mycosis fungoides.

With regard to the mechanisms of the antitumor effects, in certain tumors IFNs may serve primarily as antiproliferative agents; in others, the activation of NK cells and macrophages may be important, while augmenting the expression of class I MHC molecules may make the tumors more susceptible to control by immune effector mechanisms. In some circumstances the antiviral effect could be contributory.

For diseases like renal cell cancer and hairy cell leukemia, IFNs have induced responses in a significantly higher proportion of patients than have conventional therapies. However, in the wider setting, most investigators consider that their role will be in combination therapy, e.g. with active immunotherapy or with various chemotherapeutic agents where synergistic action has been observed in murine tumor systems. IFNα and β synergize with IFNγ and the latter synergizes with TNF. IFNα acts as a radiation sensitizer and its ability to increase the expression of estrogen receptors on cultured breast cancer cells suggests the possibility of combining IFN with anti-estrogens in this disease.

Colony-stimulating factors

Normal cell development proceeds from an immature stem cell with the capacity for unlimited self-renewal, through committed progenitors, to the final lineage-specific differentiated cells with little or no potential for self-renewal. Therapy aimed at inducing tumor cell differentiation is founded on the idea that the induction of cell maturation decreases and possibly abrogates the capacity of the malignant clone to divide. Along these lines, GM-CSF has been shown to enhance the differentiation, decrease the self-renewal capacity and suppress the leukemogenicity of murine myeloid leukemias. Recombinant human products are now undergoing trials.

It is over 100 years since the physician Coley gave his name to the mixture of microbial products termed **Coley's toxin**. This concoction certainly livens up the innate immune system and does produce remission in a minority of patients. The suggestion has been made that these beneficial effects are due to the release of TNF as the vascular endothelium of tumors is unduly susceptible to damage by this cytokine and hemorrhagic necrosis is readily induced. It is questionable whether the critical levels of TNF are reached in the human as these would be very toxic, although one study involving perfusion of an isolated limb with TNF, IFNγ and melphalan provoked lesions in the tumor endothelium without affecting the normal vasculature. Opinion is coming round to the view that the Coley phenomenon may be linked more to boosting a pre-existing weak antitumor immunity.

Stimulation of cell-mediated immune responses

The current dogma is that T-cells rather than antibodies are capable of savaging solid tumors, particularly those expressing processed intracellular antigens on their surface, and, as the majority are MHC class II negative, it looks as though we are aiming at essentially CD8 cytotoxic T-cell responses, although CD4 T-cells can be involved in protective reactions against tumor-associated vasculature and are required for persistence of CD8 T-cells.

Vaccination with viral antigens

Based on the observation that certain forms of cancer (e.g. lymphoma, cervical carcinoma, hepatocellular carcinoma) are caused by oncogenic viruses, attempts are being made to prepare suitable vaccines against these viruses. Viruses associated with cancer include *Epstein–Barr virus* (EBV), HPV, *hepatitis B virus* (HBV), *hepatitis C virus* (HCV), *human T-cell leukemia virus-1* (HTLV-1) and *Kaposi's associated sarcoma virus* (KSHV). Vaccines against several of these viruses have been in development for some years now but progress has been hampered by the poor immunogenicity of many of the vaccine candidates tested. Happily, some of these vaccines have now made it through clinical trials and we have entered the era of vaccination against several forms of cancer.

Worldwide, chronic hepatitis B infection is responsible for 80% of all liver cancer, a major cause of mortality. Although the first HBV vaccine became available in 1981, this vaccine was based upon inactivated pooled plasma from infected donors and was discontinued in 1990 due to the development of a safer, more effective, vaccine based on a recombinant subunit approach. The HBV vaccine contains a recombinant form of one of the viral envelope proteins, hepatitis B surface antigen (HBsAg). Immunization generates strong neutralizing antibodies against HbsAg and vaccination of newborns has led to a marked decrease in rates of liver cancer. Attempts to develop a vaccine against the related HCV virus have met with little success thus far, despite several clinical trials in recent years. Vaccines based upon recombinant proteins, peptides, DNA encoding viral proteins are all at various stages of development.

A very recent example of a successful vaccination strategy against a virus-induced cancer is represented by the recent approval of two different prophylactic vaccines targeting HPV, the major cause of cervical carcinoma in women. HPV is endemic in the human population, with ~50% of women becoming HPV-positive by 24 years of age, and is responsible for the development of the majority of cervical carcinomas in women, as well as genital, anal and penile warts. Globally, cervical cancer is the second most common cause of cancer in women and each year almost 50% of women that are diagnosed with cervical cancer (~500 000 worldwide) die from it.

The search for a HPV vaccine started in the late 1980s and culminated in the approval of the first preventative HPV vaccine in 2006. An additional preventive HPV vaccine was also approved for human use a year later. These vaccines have proved to be highly effective against the development of cervical cancer in women. Both vaccines are composed of recombinant L1 protein, one of the two HPV nucleocapsid proteins, derived from the commonest HPV genotypes: HPV type 16 and 18, which are responsible for almost 70% of cervical cancers. The L1 nucleocapsid protein assembles into virus-like particles, which are morphologically identical to HPV virions but are obviously noninfectious, and produces a robust neutralizing antibody response that provides protection from HPV infection via mucosal and epithelial surfaces.

HPV vaccination should ideally take place before infection has occurred, which in practice means before sexual activity has begun. Although this has not been investigated

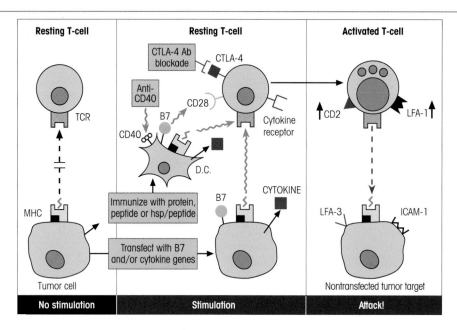

Figure 17.14. Immunotherapy by transfection with co-stimulatory molecules.

The tumor can only stimulate the resting T-cell with the co-stimulatory help of B7–1 and -2 and/or cytokines such as GM-CSF, γ-interferon and various interleukins, IL-2, -4 and -7. CTLA-4 blockade enhances immunogenicity. Alternatively, the T-cell can be stimulated directly by tumor antigens presented by dendritic cells (DCs) that can themselves be activated by cross-linking their surface CD40 with antibody (see below). Once activated, the T-cell with upregulated accessory molecules can now attack the original tumor lacking co-stimulators.

to date, it is possible that HPV vaccines may well prove to have some benefit in the early, pre-cancerous, dysplastic stages of cervical cancer progression, i.e. after infection has occurred.

Work is also in progress to develop a vaccine against Epstein-Barr virus (EBV), which is responsible for the development of Burkitt's lymphoma as well as nasopharyngeal carcinoma, one of the most common cancers in China. The major site of EBV infection is the oropharyngeal cavity with transmission occurring via oral contact, hence the name "kissing disease." The major EBV surface glycoprotein gp350/220 is the main target of EBV neutralizing antibodies and several vaccine candidates based on gp350/220 have been developed but generally need strong adjuvants to elicit decent immunity. Phase II clinical trials of one of these EBV candidate vaccines are under way.

Immunization with whole tumor cells

A variety of approaches utilizing both autologous and allogeneic whole tumor cell preparations have been tried in an effort to awaken antitumor responses. This has the advantage that we do not necessarily have to know the identity of the antigen concerned. The disadvantage is that the majority of tumors are weakly immunogenic, and do not present antigen effectively and so cannot overcome the **barrier to activation of *resting***

T-cells. Remember, the surface MHC–peptide complex on its own is not enough; co-stimulation with molecules such as B7.1 and B7.2 and possibly certain cytokines is required to push the G0 T-cell into active proliferation and differentiation. Once we get to this stage, however, **the activated T-cell no longer requires the accessory co-stimulation** to react with its target, for which it has a greatly increased avidity due to upregulation of accessory binding molecules such as CD2 and LFA-1 (cf. p. 215; Figure 17.14). Whole cell immunization approaches have been largely unsuccessful in human clinical trials, possibly because of the very limited quantity of antigenic molecules present in whole cells where the majority of proteins present are nonimmunogenic.

When proper co-stimulation is provided encouraging results have been reported, at least in animal models. Vaccination with B7-transfected murine melanoma generated CD8+ cytolytic effectors that protected against subsequent tumor challenge; in other words, transfection enabled the melanoma cells to present their own antigens efficiently, while the untransfected cells were vulnerable targets for the cytotoxic T-cells so produced. A further telling observation was that an irradiated nonimmunogenic melanoma line that had been transfected with a retroviral vector carrying the *GM-CSF* gene stimulated potent and specific antitumor immunity, almost certainly by enhancing the differentiation and activation of host antigen-presenting cells.

A less sophisticated but more convenient approach ultimately utilizing similar mechanisms involves the administration of the irradiated melanoma cells together with BCG that, by generating a plethora of inflammatory cytokines, increases the efficiency of presentation of tumor antigens derived from necrotic cells. In a large-scale study of over 1500 patients, 26% of vaccinees were alive at 5 years compared with only 6% of those treated with the best available conventional therapy. It would be exciting to suppose that in the future we might expose a tumor surgically and then transfect it *in situ* by firing gold particles (cf. p. 179) bearing appropriate gene constructs such as B7, IFNγ (to upregulate MHC class I and II), GM-CSF, IL-2, and so on (Figure 17.14). There is a real risk of inducing autoimmune responses to cryptic epitopes shared with other normal tissues that the prudent investigator will not overlook.

Therapy with subunit vaccines

The variety of potential tumor antigens thus far identified (Table 17.1) has spawned a considerable investment in clinical therapeutic trials using peptides as vaccines. Because of the pioneering work in characterizing melanoma-specific antigens, this tumor has been the focus of numerous studies that exploit to the full the academic background to modern immunology. Encouraging results in terms of clinical benefit, linked to the generation of cytolytic T-cells (CTLs), have been obtained following vaccination with peptides complexed with heat-shock proteins or modified at class I anchor residues to improve MHC binding. Such peptides have been delivered either alone, using recombinant viruses (fowlpox, adenovirus, vaccinia), or as naked DNA, along with adjuvant. The inclusion of accessory factors, such as IL-2 or GM-CSF, and **CTLA-4 blockade** can be crucial for success. Potentially tolerogenic peptide vaccines can be converted into strong primers for CTL responses by triggering CD40 with a cross-linking antibody that can substitute for T-cell help in the direct activation of CTLs (Figure 17.15). Anti-CD40 treatment alone was also shown to partially protect mice bearing *CD40-negative* lymphoma cells, an effect attributed to the activation of endogenous dendritic antigen-presenting cells (cf. Figure 17.14). However, although some promising indications of immune responses to tumors have been recorded using such approaches, a recent evaluation of multiple vaccine-based clinical trials involving 440 patients, mainly suffering from melanoma, produced an objective response rate of only 2.6%. This disappointingly poor statistic is rather sobering and suggests that we still have some way to go before optimism is warranted. It would be premature to write-off vaccination approaches at this stage, however, as it should be borne in mind that all of the clinical trials that have been carried out using such vaccines have been conducted in patients with advanced disease. Moreover, all standard therapies have, more often than not, also failed in such individuals. Vaccination with tumor antigens may prove to be more successful where early diagnosis has occurred, or where a genetic

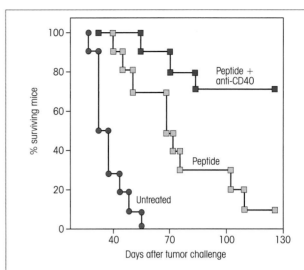

Figure 17.15. CD40 ligation enhances the protective effect of a peptide vaccine against a pre-existing tumor.

Six days after injection of human papilloma virus-16 (HPV16)-transformed syngeneic cells, mice were immunized with the HPV16-E7 peptide in incomplete Freund's adjuvant with or without an anti-CD40 monoclonal, or left untreated. (Data from Diehl L. *et al.* (1999) *Nature Medicine* **5**, 774, reproduced with permission.)

predisposition towards a familial form of cancer exists, as a preventative measure against tumor development.

Enhancing immunoreactivity of existing tumor infiltrating lymphocytes

As mentioned earlier, tumors frequently exhibit the presence of infiltrating lymphocytes that appear anergic. One means of reactivating such cells may be to neutralize signals that serve to dampen TCR triggering, CTLA-4 being a prime example. Recall from Chapter 8 that CTLA-4 can inhibit TCR co-stimulation by raising the threshold for successful TCR activation, as a result of competing for CD80/CD86 molecules on the DC. Thus, blockade of CTLA-4 interaction with its ligands may boost the capacity of tumor infiltrating lymphocytes to get on with the job of attacking the tumor and this is currently under exploration in cancer patients.

A related strategy involves inhibiting members of the c-Cbl ubiquitin ligase family that have been implicated in desensitizing the T-cell receptor to peptide-MHC stimulation. Recall from Chapter 8 that Cbl-b-deficient naive T-cells do not have a requirement for CD28-dependent co-stimulation for productive activation. This appears to be due to the role of Cbl-b in suppressing certain TCR-initiated signals under normal circumstances, thereby raising the threshold for T-cell activation. Thus, strategies aimed at selectively inhibiting Cbl-b in tumor-infiltrating T-cells may sufficiently lower their threshold for activation, such that productive immune responses now ensue without recourse to co-stimulation.

Figure 17.16. Improving the efficacy of adoptive cell transfer-based immunotherapy.

A variety of strategies are being employed to enhance the efficacy of adoptive therapy using *ex vivo* expanded T-cells. (a) Tumor-reactive T-cells (dark blue) from the patient are stimulated *in vitro* with APCs. To enhance stimulation of tumor-reactive T-cells antigen-presenting cells (APCs) can be transfected with genes encoding tumor antigens. (b) Selection of tumor-reactive T-cell clones or lines can be enhanced using peptide–MHC tetramers or bispecific antibodies to stimulate specific T-cell precursors. (c,d) Tumor-specific cells are then expanded in IL-2 followed by (e) intravenous infusion of tumor-specific T-cells into the patient. (f) Successful persistence of the transferred T-cells may be enhanced by prior depletion of host lymphocytes and/or administration of homeostatic cytokines (IL-2, IL-15, IL-21) post-infusion. (Based upon Riddell S.R. (2004) *Journal of Experimental Medicine* **200**, 1533.)

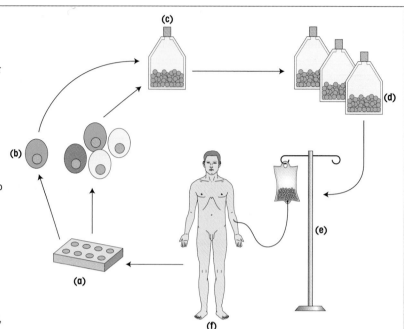

Adoptive T-cell transfer

Adoptive cell transfer (ACT) with large numbers of *ex vivo* expanded T-cells may overcome some of the barriers to effective therapy seen with conventional vaccination approaches (Figure 17.16). It may even be possible to genetically engineer the adoptively transferred cells to constitutively express cytokines such as IL-2 or GM-CSF to boost their activity. The generation of cytotoxic T-cell effectors *ex vivo* has the potential to uncover responses that are not evident in an environment where tumor-derived inhibitory factors, or T-regulatory cells, may be present. The typical approach involves isolating T-cells from patients and these are then expanded *in vitro* in the presence of high concentrations of IL-2 (Figure 17.16). To maximize the chances of expanding rare tumor-reactive T-cell precursors, mature DCs expressing co-stimulatory signals along with a source of tumor antigen are now in common use. Over a period of 2–3 weeks 1000-fold expansion of T-cells can be achieved. These *in vitro* expanded CD8 T-cells are then transferred back to the patient (up to 10^{11} cells per individual!) but can rapidly disappear if the tumor burden is high. Administration of IL-2 *in vivo* or co-transfer of CD4 T-cells can improve CD8 T-cell survival; **the presence of CD4 T-cells appears to be crucial for persistence of CD8 T-cells** and optimal cytotoxic effector function. The failure of vaccination approaches using predominantly class I-based peptides may be due to the lack of CD4 T-cell expansion and this should be perhaps borne in mind for future studies. ACT of *in vitro* expanded lymphocytes into lymphodepleted hosts can result in up to 75% of circulating T-cells with antitumor activity, way beyond the levels seen with peptide vaccines. Although the numbers of individuals that have received such ACT-based therapy are

still low, very impressive objective response rates of 40–50% have been reported in lymphodepleted melanoma patients, with persistence of transferred cells for up to 4 months. Clearly some risks must be borne in mind when transferring such large numbers of activated lymphocytes into a patient, not least the possibility of generating autoimmunity to tissues other than the tumor. Careful selection of tumor antigens to favor those that are not expressed, or are minimally expressed, on tissues other than the tumor is clearly essential in these situations.

There are some indications that lymphocyte-mediated tumor eradication may be simply a numbers game. While peptide vaccination approaches can increase circulating tumor-reactive cells five- to ten-fold, this pales in comparison with observations that up to 40% of circulating CD8 T-cells are reactive against EBV in patients with infectious mononucleosis. Early indications suggest that ACT is capable of achieving such impressive numbers of specific T-cells, especially when combined with prior lymphodepletion. The lymphopenic environment may be favorable as this may free-up space in the lymphoid compartment for the incoming T-cells and create less competition for homeostatic cytokines such as IL-7 and IL-15. Another advantage of this approach is that depletion of recipient lymphocytes can remove suppressor/regulatory T-cells that are suspected to play a significant part in damping down antitumor responses in the first place.

NK cell therapy

We have already alluded to the possible importance of NK cells in tumor surveillance and tumor killing, so it is natural to consider that *in vivo* expansion or adoptive transfer of large

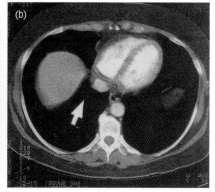

Figure 17.17. Clinical response to autologous vaccine utilizing dendritic cells pulsed with idiotype from a B-cell lymphoma.

Computed tomography scans through patient's chest: (a) prevaccine and (b) 10 months after completion of three vaccine treatments. The arrow in (a) points to a paracardiac mass. All sites of disease had resolved and the patient remained in remission 24 months after beginning treatment. (Photography kindly supplied by Professor R. Levy from the article by Hsu F.J. *et al.* (1996) *Nature Medicine* **2**, 52; reproduced by kind permission of Nature America Inc.)

numbers of activated NKs may also be of clinical benefit. NK-based therapies are somewhat lagging behind T-cell-based approaches although they are not being overlooked. Clinical trials on cancer patients have assessed the effects of daily subcutaneous administration of low-dose IL-2, following high-dose cytotoxic chemotherapy, for its effects on NK cell numbers and activation status in these individuals. While NK cell expansion was seen, these cells did not appear to be maximally cytotoxic, perhaps because of inhibitory NK receptors finding the appropriate ligands on the tumor. More recent attempts involved using NK cells from related **haploidentical donors** to treat poor prognosis patients with acute myeloblastic leukemia. The idea here is to achieve a partial mismatch between the donor NKs and the recipient that may provoke NK activation and greater tumor kill as a result. Expansion and persistence of the donor NK cells was observed after high-dose immunosuppression of recipients and complete remission in five out of 19 patients was achieved—encouraging signs indeed.

Dendritic cell therapy

The sheer power of the **dendritic cell (DC)** for the initiation of T-cell responses has been the focus of an ever-burgeoning series of immunotherapeutic strategies that have elicited tumor-specific protective immune responses via injection of isolated DC loaded with tumor lysates or tumor antigens or peptides derived from them. Considerable success has been achieved in animal models and increasingly with human patients (Figure 17.17). The copious numbers of DCs needed for each patient's individual therapy are obtained by expansion of CD34-positive precursors in bone marrow by culture with GM-CSF, IL-4 and TNF, and sometimes with extra goodies such as stem cell factor (SCF) and Fms-like tyrosine kinase 3 (Flt3)-ligand. CD14-positive monocytes from peripheral blood are easier to access, and generate DC in the presence of GM-CSF plus IL-4; however, they need additional maturation with TNFα that increases cost and the chance of bacterial contamination. Another approach is to expand the DCs *in vivo* by administration of Flt3-ligand. The circulating blood DCs increase in number 10–30-fold and can be harvested by leukopheresis.

Some general points may be made. First, where peptides are used to load the DC, sequences that bind strongly to a given MHC class I haplotype must be identified; sequences will vary between patients with different haplotypes and they may not include potential CD4 helper epitopes. Recombinant proteins will overcome most of these difficulties, and a mixture should be even better as it should recruit more CTLs and be more able to "ride out" any new tumor antigen mutations. However, proteins taken up by DCs are relatively inefficient at "cross-priming" CD8 CTLs through the class I processing pathway, although several tactics are being explored to circumvent this problem: they include conjugation to an HIV-tat "transporter" peptide that increases class I presentation 100-fold and transfection with RNA and recombinant vectors such as fowlpox. Second, the procedure is cumbersome and costly but, if it becomes common, it will be streamlined and, anyway, the costs must be set against the expenses of conventional therapy and the immeasurable benefit to the patient. Third, why does the administration of small numbers of antigen-pulsed DCs induce specific T-cell responses and tumor regression in patients in whom both the antigen and DCs are already plentiful? As we discussed earlier in this chapter, the suggestion has been made that DCs in or near malignant tissues may be defective or immature, perhaps due to vascular endothelium growth factor (VEGF) or IL-10 secretion by the tumor that may arrest DC maturation to generate immature "tolerogenic" DCs. Such immature DCs may smother tumor-reactive T-cell responses at birth rather than nurture them. Along these lines, recent evidence suggests that melanoma tumors secreting the CCL21 chemokine recruit CD4+CD25+Foxp3+ regulatory T-cells, shifting the tumor environment to a tolerogenic as opposed to an immunogenic one. Alternatively, immature DCs that capture antigen in the vicinity of a tumor, in the absence of appropriate Toll receptor ligands (PAMPs) or danger signals (DAMPs), may simply not function as effective antigen-presenting cells (Figure 17.4). It will certainly be interesting to see whether direct treatment of patients with Flt3-ligand plus accessory cytokines or intratumoral transfection with MIP-3α (CCL20) (cf. p. 235), which attracts immature DCs, can initiate an antitumor response through maturation and activation of endogenous DCs.

Vaccination against neovascularization

Solid tumors are composed of malignant cells as well as a variety of nonmalignant cell types, collectively called stromal cells, such as endothelial cells and fibroblasts. Because solid tumors cannot grow to any appreciable size without a blood supply, tumors stimulate the production of new blood vessels by secreting angiogenic factors, such as VEGF, that stimulate endothelial cell proliferation. Because growing tumors are highly reliant on their blood supply, attacking the tumor vasculature by targeting antigens selectively expressed on these blood vessels may deprive the tumor of oxygen and nutrients, provoking regression one would hope. VEGF, one of a family of angiogenic factors, exerts its effects through interaction with its cognate receptor, VEGF-R2 (also known as KDR in humans and Flk-1 in the mouse), which provides signals that promote proliferation, survival and motility of endothelial cells. Antibodies directed against VEGF-R2, or indeed VEGF itself, can block tumor angiogenesis in murine tumor models but translation into the clinic has been hampered due to problems relating to delivery of sufficient amounts of these agents to fully block VEGF-R2 activity. An alternative strategy involves **breaking immune tolerance** to VEGF-R2-positive endothelial cells by pulsing *in vitro* generated DCs with soluble VEGF-R2 followed by transferring these cells back into the animal. A major advantage of this approach is that the tumor endothelium, unlike the tumor itself, is genetically stable as it represents nontransformed tissue, and this makes it unlikely that mutant cells will arise that have lost VEGF-R2 expression. This strategy has been reported to generate VEGF-R2-specific neutralizing antibody as well as cytotoxic T-cells capable of effectively destroying endothelial cells.

Treatment of leukemia

Radical cytoablative treatment of leukemia patients using radiochemotherapy will destroy bone marrow stem cells. These can be removed prior to treatment, purged of any leukemic cells with cytotoxic antibodies, and reinfused subsequently to "rescue" the patient (Figure 17.18). However, not all leukemic cells are eliminated by this treatment, and a more effective strategy is transplantation of *allogeneic* bone marrow from rea-

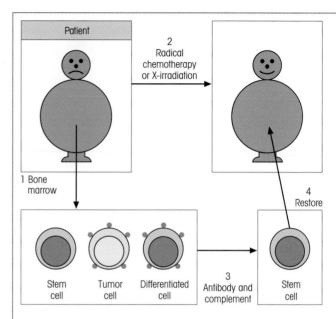

Figure 17.18. Treatment of leukemias by autologous bone marrow rescue.

By using cytotoxic antibodies to a differentiation antigen (●) present on leukemic cells and even on other normal differentiated cells, but absent from stem cells, it is possible to obtain a tumor-free population of the latter that can be used to restore hematopoietic function in patients subsequently treated radically to destroy the leukemic cells. Another angle is positive selection of stem cells utilizing the CD34 marker.

sonably MHC-compatible donors that exerts an important, albeit not completely understood, graft-versus-leukemia effect. Purging the bone marrow of T-cells to prevent graft-versus-host (GVH) disease, which is a serious complication of such transplants, would at the same time remove the prized antileukemic activity—a dilemma. "Suicide gene therapy" could provide a solution as illustrated in Figure 17.19. Stem cells from the T-cell-purged allogeneic bone marrow are given together with donor T-cells transfected with herpes simplex virus thymidine kinase. The T-cells provide factors that facilitate engraftment, defense against viral infection and the graft-versus-leukemia action at a time when the recipient patient will have a low tumor burden. With time, as GVH disease develops, the dividing aggressor donor T-cells can be switched off by administration of ganciclovir through the mechanism explained in the legend to Figure 17.19.

An alternative that avoids GVH disease altogether is to inject the purged bone marrow together with an allogeneic cytotoxic T-cell clone specific for a leukemia-associated peptide presented by the MHC allele of the prospective recipient patient. This usually works because the residues on the MHC helices that contact the T-cell receptor are relatively conserved (unlike those within the groove), so that the allo-T-cells can recognize the MHC–peptide complex from the leukemia. Potential targets are cyclin-D1 and mdm-2 that are overexpressed in tumor cells and, in leukemic cells in particular,

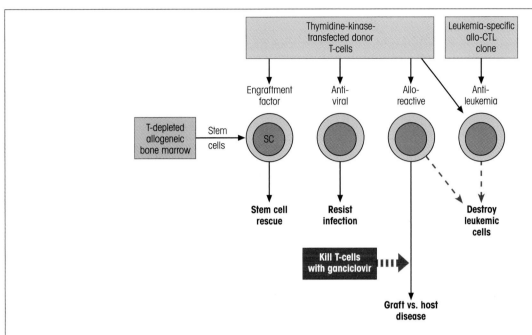

Figure 17.19. Treatment of leukemia with allogeneic bone marrow transfer.

T-depleted allogeneic marrow provides the stem cells to "rescue" the patient treated with cytoablative therapy. T-cells from the donor, transfected with thymidine kinase (TK), help engraftment, provide protection against infection and eliminate residual tumor cells by a graft-versus-leukemia effect. The alloreactive cells eventually produce graft-versus-host disease and can be eliminated by administration of ganciclovir. This is converted by the TK into a nucleoside analog that ultimately becomes toxic for dividing cells. The alternative shown is to destroy leukemic cells by supplementing purged allogeneic marrow with a leukemia peptide-specific CTL clone produced in third party T-cells. (Based on articles by Cohen J.L., Boyer O. & Klatzmann D. (1999) *Immunology Today* **20**, 172; and Stauss H.J. (1999) *Immunology Today* **20**, 180.)

the transcription factors WT-1 and GATA1 and the differentiation antigens myeloperoxidase and CD68, which are expressed exclusively in hematopoietic cells and are likely to have established tolerance in the patient but not in the allogeneic CTL donor (who will have been exposed to different processed peptides) (cf. p. 428). A rather masterful development would be to transfect the recipient with the genes encoding the T-cell receptor of the allo-CTL clone.

Passive immunotherapy with monoclonal antibodies

After many false dawns, monoclonal antibodies are finally delivering on their early promise and some of the most promising results from immunotherapeutic approaches to cancer treatment have been achieved with humanized monoclonal antibodies. As detailed earlier (see Chapter 6), early attempts to use mouse monoclonal antibodies for therapeutic purposes were severely hampered by strong immune responses against the foreign sequences within the mouse antibody, the so-called *h*uman *a*nti-*m*ouse *a*ntibody (HAMA) response. Furthermore, mouse antibodies frequently failed to activate desirable cytotoxic actions against the tumor, such as complement activation and ADCC. These early difficulties have now been overcome with the result that numerous "humanized" monoclonal antibodies (see Chapter 6 for further details of how antibodies can be engineered in various ways) have now entered clinical trials and 12 monoclonal antibodies targeting cell surface receptors have been approved for therapeutic use in cancer (Table 17.2). Earlier in this chapter we discussed the example of HER2 (human epidermal growth factor receptor 2; also called Neu or erb-B2), a member of the epidermal growth factor receptor family, and its overexpression in a subset of breast cancers (Figure 17.6). This discovery led to the development of monoclonal antibodies targeting HER2 (Herceptin), which proved to be effective against tumors overexpressing this antigen, leading to the approval of Herceptin® for cancer therapy in 1998. Following on from this success, antibodies directed against a variety of other cell surface molecules, such as CD20, EGF receptor and VEGF have been approved for therapeutic use and a raft of others are currently in the clinical pipeline. Moreover, the NIH clinical trials website currently lists more than 1600 clinical trials, either ongoing or completed, involving monoclonal antibodies targeting various cell surface antigens in cancer. Thus, it is very likely that we will see the introduction of numerous additional monoclonal antibodies to clinical practice in the coming years, either as stand alone therapeutic agents, or as adjuncts to conventional chemotherapy.

HER2-directed antibodies appear to work through disrupting growth-promoting signals propagated via this EGF family receptor. Although HER2 does not appear to bind to EGF directly (a ligand for this receptor has yet to be identified), it

Table 17.2. Selected mAbs approved or in late-stage clinical trials for cancer therapy. (From data of Adams G.P. & Weiner L.M. (2005) *Nature Biotechnology* **23**, 1147.)

Target antigen	Format	Indication	Status
HER2/neu	unconjugated	Breast cancer	Approved for therapeutic use
CD20	Unconjugated	Lymphoma	Approved for therapeutic use
CD20	^{90}Y- and ^{131}I-conjugates	Lymphoma	Approved for therapeutic use
EGF receptor	unconjugated	Colorectal cancer & head & neck cancer	Approved for therapeutic use
VEGF	unconjugated	Colorectal & lung cancer	Approved for therapeutic use
CD52	unconjugated	Chronic lymphocytic leukemia	Approved for therapeutic use
CD33	drug-conjugate	Acute Myelogenous leukemia	Approved for therapeutic use
DNA-associated	^{131}I-conjugate	Advanced lung cancer	Approved for therapeutic use
GD2	unconjugated	Neuroblastoma	In late-stage clinical trials
CTLA-4	unconjugated	Melanoma	In late-stage clinical trials
MHC class II	unconjugated	Non-Hodgkin's lymphoma	In late-stage clinical trials

is capable of forming heterodimers with other members of the same receptor family that do bind EGF. Thus, antibodies targeting the HER2 receptor presumably interfere with EGF-dependent growth factor signaling, as well as spontaneous HER2 signals that are generated as a result of its elevated surface expression, thereby provoking growth arrest rather than death of HER2-positive tumors. However, through use of mice lacking Fcγ receptors, a major role for ADCC responses mediated by NK cells has also been implicated in the mode of action of Herceptin.

In general, antibodies reacting with antigens on the surface of tumor cells can also protect the host by complement-mediated opsonization and lysis (modified by host complement regulatory proteins) and through recruitment of macrophage and NK ADCC function by engagement of FcγRIII receptors, although for macrophages this is partially countered by inhibitory FcγRII signals. These FcR-bearing cells serve not only as cytotoxic effectors but also as multivalent surfaces that hyper-cross-link antibody-coated target cells so providing, in many cases, a transmembrane signal that leads to apoptosis or premature exit from the cell cycle. This effect appears to sensitize neoplastic cells to irradiation and DNA-damaging chemotherapy and holds out the exciting prospect of novel synergistic treatments whose efficacy may be enhanced by the increased immunogenicity of the dying cells.

Immunologists have long been entranced by the idea of eliminating tumor cells by specific antibody linked to a killer molecule and there is a truly impressive array of ingenious initiatives. It is axiomatic that multimeric fragments bind much more avidly than monomeric fragments due principally to the lower off-rates (cf. p. 119), and that constructs in the 60–120 kDa range are optimal for targeting solid tumors—too large and penetration is difficult, too small and kidney secretion is excessively fast. Monovalent fragments include Fv, scFv

selected by antigen from phage libraries (cf. p. 146) and V$_H$ domains based on the large CDR loops of the camel and llama heavy chain antibodies. For polymers we have bivalent and bispecific (think about the difference) diabodies (cf. p. 148), trivalent and trispecific triabodies, even tetrabodies, and Fabs have been linked into dimers or trimers.

Therapeutic immunoconjugates

While antibody alone is sometimes effective, immunoconjugates are where the most exciting developments have been made, particularly with respect to solid tumors. Therapeutic immunoconjugates consist of a tumor-targeting antibody linked with a toxic effector component, which can either be a radioisotope, a toxin or a small drug molecule. Initial attempts to treat tumors with such immunoconjugates proved disappointing, mainly because the cytotoxic payloads conjugated to the mAbs were conventional chemotherapeutic drugs (such as doxorubicin) that are not sufficiently toxic when delivered in small doses. Dosimetry studies using **radioimmunoconjugates** indicate that very modest amounts, between 0.01% and 0.001% of the administered antibody per gram of solid tumor, actually reach the tumor site. So, if the initial dose delivered to the patient is 10 micromolar, which would be a pretty high dose of most cytotoxic compounds, and less than 0.01% of this dose is actually delivered to the tumor, this effectively means that the effector drug or toxin has to work in the picomolar range. The nature of the problem can be grasped when one considers that many conventional chemotherapeutics are effective in the micromolar or high nanomolar range.

This limitation prompted a search for much more toxic molecules to act as conjugates and toxins seemed to fit the bill initially. Protein toxins such as pseudomonas exotoxin and diphtheria toxin are highly toxic *in vitro* and display activity in animal models, but they also proved to be highly immunogenic in humans and rapidly induce neutralizing antibody responses that limit their efficacy and the ability to administer repeated doses: a problem known as the *h*uman *a*nti-*t*oxin *a*ntibody (HATA) response. In some cases, practically 100% of patients developed HATA responses by their second treatment with a toxin immunoconjugate. Quite apart from HATA, another disadvantage of **immunotoxin conjugates** is a syndrome that appears to result from nonspecific toxin-induced damage to endothelium, called **vascular leak syndrome**, which also reduces the maximum tolerated doses of such conjugates that can be used. However, where patients are severely immunosuppressed, in the case of hematologic malignancies for example, immunotoxin conjugates are of benefit; very impressive complete remission rates approaching 70% have been recorded for patients with hairy cell leukaemia using an anti-CD22–pseudomonas toxin conjugate.

Another approach that has been pursued for several years now aims to exploit the cytotoxic properties of radionuclides, such as iodine-131 and yttrium-90, to irradiate the tumor in a highly precise manner. Several clinical trials have been conducted with such radioimmunoconjugates, and while there have been some notable successes, ^{90}Y- and ^{131}I-labeled anti-CD20 conjugates for non-Hodgkin's lymphoma for example, the results have been generally disappointing. It has proved difficult to achieve therapeutic efficacy with many radioimmunoconjugates without exceeding the **maximum tolerated dose**, and side-effects such as myeloablation are frequently seen. Attempts have been made to reduce these nonspecific toxic effects by using α particle emitters, such as astatine-211, that have much shorter path lengths than β-emitters that reduces collateral damage to other cells. Such manipulations have the desired effect, with up to 1000-fold higher absorbed dose ratios in target organs with α-emitters relative to their β-emitter counterparts. But every silver lining has a cloud, or so it seems; the α particle radioimmunoconjugates have half-lives ranging from 60 minutes to a few hours or so, making them impractical for routine clinical use.

The search for toxic molecules in the high picomolar range eventually paid off with the discovery of inhibitors of tubulin polymerization such as auristatin and molecules that cause DNA double-stranded breaks such as calicheamicin and esperamicin. One very attractive feature of these agents is that conjugation of the drug to the antibody frequently converts it into a **pro-drug** that requires removal from the antibody to regain activity. Because the linker between drug and antibody is stable in the blood, the conjugate exhibits virtually no toxicity until it becomes bound and internalized by an antigen-positive target cell. Many such **drug immunoconjugates** are currently in clinical trials or have been approved for a range of cancers, including: acute myeloid leukemia (anti-CD33–calicheamycin), colorectal and pancreatic cancer (anti-CanAg–DM1), small cell lung carcinoma (anti-CD56–DM1) and several other malignancies (anti-HER2/Neu–DM1). Consider-

able effort is also underway to develop even more potent cytotoxic compounds for the preparation of drug immunoconjugates. Because of their stability, potency and clinical utility, small drug immunoconjugates are likely to rule the roost within a short time.

Attack on the tumor blood supply

For solid tumors, the focus is upon two main targets. The first would be **minimal residual micrometastases in the bone marrow** that occur in one-third to one-half of patients with epithelial cancer after curative radical treatment of the primary lesion. The second would be the **reactive tissue evoked by the malignant process**, such as stromal fibroblasts expressing the F19 glycoprotein and newly formed blood vessels.

As we discussed earlier, tumors generally cannot grow beyond 1 mm in diameter without the support of blood vessels that the tumor promotes formation of by secreting angiogenic factors such as VEGF. New blood vessels are biochemically and structurally different from normal resting blood vessels and so provide differential targets for therapeutic monoclonal antibodies, even though the cancer cells themselves in a solid tumor are less vulnerable to antibodies directed to specific antigens on their surface. Thus, receptors for VEGF and Eph, oncofetal fibronectin, matrix metalloproteases MMP-2 and MMP-9 and the pericyte markers aminopeptidase A and the NG2 proteoglycan are all highly and selectively expressed in vasculature undergoing angiogenesis. Consequently, considerable effort has been expended in the direction of angiogenesis inhibitors such as humanized monoclonal antibodies against VEGF and its main receptor VEGF-R2.

A noteworthy maneuver, which is unexpectedly successful, is to identify peptides that home specifically to the endothelial cells of certain tumors by injecting peptide phage libraries *in vivo*. One of the panel of peptide motifs that has emerged from this probing strategy includes RGD in the cyclic peptide CDCRGDCFC, a selective binder of the $\alpha_V\beta_3$- and $\alpha_V\beta_5$-integrins known to be upregulated in angiogenic tumor endothelial cells. For therapeutic exploitation, these peptides can be linked to appropriate drugs, such as doxorubicin, or a pro-apoptotic peptide. Overall, there are undoubtedly a substantial number of targets for the "magic bullets."

Inhibition of the production of proinflammatory cytokines in the tumor environment

Based on the observation that production of proinflammatory cytokines by tumor-associated macrophages and fibroblasts can frequently be beneficial for the tumor, there may be instances in which neutralizing antibodies towards IL-6 and TNF, as well as other proinflammatory cytokines may have beneficial effects in terms of reducing the blood supply and the stromal support network in the vicinity of the tumor. Studies in mice have shown that neutralizing antibodies against TNF, as well as NFκB inhibitors can have protective effects in colon and breast cancer models.

Cellular transformation

- Cancer is typically caused by genetic lesions that affect genes that promote proliferation in tandem with lesions that interfere with the elimination of cells through apoptosis.
- Cancer is not a single disease and represents a wide spectrum of conditions caused by a failure of the controls that normally govern cell proliferation, differentiation and cell survival.
- Cellular transformation is a multi-step process and involves the acquisition of a series of mutations in oncogenes and tumor suppressor genes that cooperate to achieve the fully transformed state.
- Cancer incidence varies between tissues.
- Mutagenic agents, including viruses, promote cellular transformation.

A variety of cell-intrinsic mechanisms of tumor suppression exist

- The requirement for growth factors normally prevents uncontrolled growth.
- Telomere shortening acts as a barrier to cellular transformation.
- Tumor suppressor proteins monitor cell division and can deploy a range of countermeasures upon detection of DNA damage or aberrant mitogenic signaling, including: DNA repair, premature cellular senescence or apoptosis.

The cancer problem from an immune perspective

- Transformed cells are not usually highly immunogenic are therefore not recognized by cells of the immune system.
- Cancers lack PAMPs and contain few nonself determinants.
- Lack of T-cell co-stimulation can tolerize to tumor antigens.
- Inflammatory cytokines can enhance tumor growth.

Tumor antigens

- Many candidate tumor antigens have now been identified but most are specific to an individual tumor and are not shared between individuals.
- Processed peptides derived from oncogenic viruses are powerful MHC-associated transplantation antigens.
- Some tumors express genes that are silent in normal tissues: sometimes they have been expressed previously in embryonic life (oncofetal antigens).
- Many tumors express weak antigens associated with point mutations in oncogenes such as *ras* and *p53*. Peptides presented by heat-shock proteins 70 and 90 represent the unique chemically induced tumor

antigens. The surface Ig on chronic lymphocytic leukemia (CLL) cells is a unique tumor-specific antigen.
- Dysregulation of tumor cells frequently causes structural abnormalities in surface carbohydrate structures.
- The v6 and v10 exons of CD44 are intimately involved with metastatic potential. Loss of blood group A determinants leads to a poor prognosis.

Immune response to tumors

- T-cells generally mount effective surveillance against tumors associated with oncogenic viruses or UV induction that are strongly immunogenic.
- More weakly immunogenic tumors are not controlled by T-cell surveillance, although sometimes low-grade responses are evoked.
- NK cells probably play a role in containing tumor growth and metastases. They can attack MHC class I-negative tumor cells because the class I molecule imparts a negative inactivation signal to NK cells. The A-NK subset, which expresses high levels of adhesion molecules, is more cytolytic for fresh tumor cells.
- Tumors utilize a variety of mechanisms to escape host immune responses that suggests that the immune system exerts selective pressure on tumors.

Infection and inflammation can enhance tumor initiation, promotion and progression

- TLR expression on tumors can enhance tumor growth and survival through harnessing NFκB-dependent upregulation of anti-apoptotic proteins that can make tumors resistant to stress. TLR-driven NFκB activation can also lead to the production of cytokines, such as IL-1 and IL-6, which can have autocrine growth-promoting effects.
- An inflammatory environment can foster mutation through the production of reactive oxygen and nitrogen species that can provoke DNA damage and generate mutations that drive cellular transformation.
- Certain oncogenic mutations can promote the production of pro-inflammatory cytokines and chemokines, thereby recruiting cells of the innate immune system that can enhance tumor proliferation, the growth of new blood vessels (angiogenesis) and tumor spread.

Approaches to cancer immunotherapy

- Immunotherapy is only likely to work after a tumor mass has been debulked.
- Innate immune mechanisms can be harnessed. High concentrations of IL-2 can enhance responses to

malignant melanoma and other tumors, systemic IL-12 may be effective against minimal residual disease. IFNγ and IFNβ are very effective in the T-cell disorders, hairy cell leukemia and mycosis fungoides, less so but still significant in Kaposi's sarcoma and various lymphomas; they may be used in synergy with other therapies. GM-CSF enhances proliferation and decreases leukemogenicity of murine myeloid leukemias.

■ Cancer vaccines based on oncogenic viral proteins are likely to be effective and will provide a prophylactic measure against virus-induced cancers, such as cervical cancer.

■ Weakly immunogenic tumors provoke anticancer responses if given with an adjuvant, such as BCG, or if transfected with co-stimulatory molecules, such as B7 and cytokines IFNγ, IL-2, -4 and -7.

■ CD8 CTLs are favored for the attack on solid tumors, and CD4 T helper cells are likely to be required for persistence and optimal effector function of CD8 T-cells.

■ A variety of potential tumor antigens have been identified and intense effort is being expended in the investigation of peptides as subunit vaccines. Their immunogenicity can be enhanced by complexing with heat-shock proteins and by accessory factors such as GM-CSF, CTLA-4 blockade and anti-CD40 stimulation.

■ Clinical trials using peptide-based vaccines have been disappointing but adoptive cell transfer-based immunotherapy using *in vitro* expanded CD8 T-cells has shown more promise.

■ Powerful immunogens have been created by pulsing dendritic antigen-presenting cells with peptides from melanoma antigens and framework regions of CLL Ig.

■ A graft-versus-leukemia effect is achieved by allogeneic CTLs or by allogeneic bone marrow transplantation with measures to limit graft-versus-host disease.

■ Monoclonal antibodies conjugated to drugs, toxins or radiolabels can target tumor cells or antigens on new blood vessels or the reactive stromal fibroblasts associated with malignancy. Impressive, therapeutic results have been obtained with antibodies to CD20 in B-cell lymphoma, CD33 in myeloid leukemia, anti-MUC-1 in ovarian cancer and c-erbB2 overexpressed on breast cancers. Bifunctional antibodies can bring effectors such as NK and Tc close to the tumor target.

FURTHER READING

Ancrile B.B., O'Hayer KM. & Counter C.M. (2008) Oncogenic *Ras*-induced expression of cytokines: a new target of anti-cancer therapeutics. *Molecular Interventions* **8**, 22–27.

Banchereau J. & Palucka A.K. (2005) Dendritic cells as therapeutic vaccines against cancer. *Nature Reviews Immunology* **5**, 296–306.

Begent R.H.J. *et al.* (1996) Clinical evidence of efficient tumor targeting based on single-chain Fv antibody selected from a combinatorial library. *Nature Medicine* **2**, 979–984.

Chen R., Alvero A.B., Silasi D.A., Steffensen K.D. & Mor G. (2008) Cancers take their Toll—the function and regulation of Toll-like receptors in cancer cells. *Oncogene* **27**, 225–233.

Finn O.J. (2008) Tumor immunology top 10 list. *Immunological Reviews* **222**, 5–8.

Ho W.Y. *et al.* (2003) Adoptive immunotherapy: engineering T-cell responses as biologic weapons for tumor mass destruction. *Cancer Cell* **3**, 431–437.

Kahn J.A. (2009) HPV vaccination for the prevention of cervical intraepithelial neoplasia. *New England Journal of Medicine* **361**, 271–278.

Karin M., Lawrence T. & Nizet V. (2006) Innate immunity gone awry: linking microbial infections to chronic inflammation and cancer. *Cell* **124**, 823–835.

Lake R.A. & Robinson B.W.S. (2005) Immunotherapy and chemotherapy: a practical partnership. *Nature Reviews Cancer* **5**, 397–405.

Lin W.W. & Karin M. (2007) A cytokine-mediated link between innate immunity, inflammation, and cancer. *Journal of Clinical Investigation* **117**, 1175–1183.

Loo D.T. & Mather J.P. (2008) Antibody-based identification of cell surface antigens: targets for cancer therapy. *Current Opinion in Pharmacology* **8**, 627–631.

Muranski P. & Restifo N.P. (2009) Adoptive immunotherapy of cancer using CD4⁺ T cells. *Current Opinion in Immunology* **21**, 200–208.

Murphy A. *et al.* (2005) Gene modification strategies to induce tumor immunity. *Immunity* **22**, 403–414.

Payne G. (2003) Progress in immunoconjugate cancer therapeutics. *Cancer Cell* **3**, 207–212.

Rafii S. (2002) Vaccination against tumor neovascularization: promise and reality. *Cancer Cell* **2**, 429–431.

Rabinovich G.A., Gabrilovich D. & Sotomayor E.M. (2007) Immunosuppressive strategies that are mediated by tumor cells. *Annual Review of Immunology* **25**, 267–296.

Reichert J.M. & Valge-Archer, V.E. (2007) Development trends for monoclonal antibody cancer therapeutics. *Nature Reviews Drug Discovery* **6**, 349–356.

Rosenberg S.A., Yang J.C. & Restifo N.P. (2004) Cancer immunotherapy: moving beyond current vaccines. *Nature Medicine* **10**, 909–915.

Ruoslahti E. & Rajotte D. (2000) An address system in the vasculature of normal tissues and tumors. *Annual Review of Immunology* **18**, 813–827.

Smyth M.J. Godfrey D.I. & Trapani J.A. (2001) A fresh look at tumor immunosurveillance and immunotherapy. *Nature Immunology* **2**, 293–299.

Srivastava P.K. (2000) Immunotherapy of human cancer: lessons from mice. *Nature Immunology* **1**, 363–366.

Zou W. (2005) Immunosuppressive networks in the tumor environment and their therapeutic relevance. *Nature Reviews Cancer* **5**, 263–274.

Now visit **www.roitt.com** to test yourself on this chapter.

CHAPTER 18
Autoimmune diseases

Key Topics

Just to Recap...

Although most immune responses are beneficial in that they recruit antibodies, complement, phagocytic cells, lymphocytes and so forth in order to eliminate infectious pathogens, sometimes immunity is inadvertently directed against antigens that do not pose a threat. The word hypersensitivity is often used to describe such reactions. They include tissue damaging responses to what should be innocuous environmental antigens, as seen in allergy, and the rejection of foreign tissue introduced into the body by the procedure of transplantation. It is clear that the diversity-generating mechanisms involved in recombination of the V(D)J antigen receptor genes of lymphocytes have the potential to give rise to specific recognition of almost any antigen. One downside of this flexibility is that some of the antigen receptors that are produced are able to recognize our own body components—self antigens. Usually autoreactive cells that are potentially pathogenic (e.g. those with high affinity receptors) are either "weeded out" by the central and peripheral tolerance mechanisms, resulting in clonal deletion and clonal anergy, or restrained by regulatory T-cells.

Introduction

In all individuals there is a degree of recognition of self. Indeed, T-cells are required to be positively selected in the thymus for recognition of **self MHC** (p. 291). Furthermore self-reactive B-cells, and self peptide + self MHC reactive

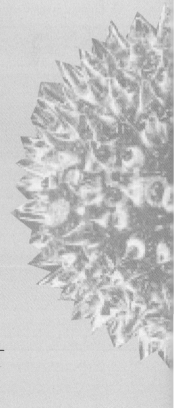

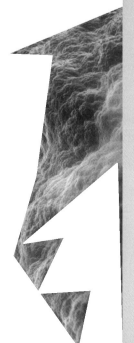

Roitt's Essential Immunology, Twelfth Edition. Peter J. Delves, Seamus J. Martin, Dennis R. Burton, Ivan M. Roitt.

Introduction (*Continued*)

T-cells, are detectable in the circulation of all individuals, as are **autoantibodies** (i.e. antibodies capable of reacting with self components). In people without autoimmune disease the latter are predominantly low affinity IgM autoantibodies, often produced by CD5+ B-1 cells as part of the "natural" antibody spectrum (p. 298). The term **autoimmune disease** is applied when **autoimmunity** results in **pathology**. Nonpathological autoimmunity may in fact assist in the removal of worn-out or damaged cells and molecules. Thus, a low level of autoimmunity seems to be the norm and generally does not result in pathology. However, if immunological tolerance fails to eliminate or control pathogenic self-reactive lymphocytes then autoimmune disease arises.

The spectrum of autoimmune disease

A substantial minority of individuals, estimated to be 5–8% of the population, do however develop autoimmune disease. Once they occur, most of these diseases then remain for life. Whilst some are relatively mild in nature, quite a few are associated with significant morbidity and mortality.

It is not in fact always clear whether a particular clinical entity is in fact an "autoimmune disease" or a disease whose prime cause is not an autoimmune attack but which, nonetheless, is associated with autoimmune phenomenon (Table 18.1). We will discuss some such diseases, including psoriasis and atherosclerosis, later in this chapter. There are also a number of autoinflammatory diseases such as the hereditary periodic fever syndromes (p. 372) characterized by an **absence** of high-titer autoantibodies or autoantigen-specific T-cells. Such conditions are due to malfunction of innate immune system components and therefore do not depend upon the breakdown of the specific immunological toler-

ance, which is so closely involved in the classical autoimmune diseases.

In the conventional autoimmune diseases the tissue distribution of the **autoantigen** to a large extent determines whether the disease is "**organ-specific**" or "**nonorgan-specific**." **Hashimoto's disease** is an example where the antigens that are recognized are pretty much restricted to a single organ, in this case the thyroid (Figure 18.1a). There is a specific lesion in this endocrine gland involving infiltration by mononuclear cells (lymphocytes, macrophages and plasma cells), destruction of thyroid epithelial cells, and germinal center formation accompanied by the production of circulating antibodies that are specific for thyroid antigens (Milestone 18.1). In some other disorders, however, the lesion tends to be localized to a single organ even though the antibodies are nonorgan-specific. A good example would be **primary biliary cirrhosis** where the small bile ductule is the main target of inflammatory cell infiltration but the serum antibodies present—mainly mitochondrial—are not liver-specific.

Table 18.1. Classification criteria for autoimmune diseases. Not all these criteria will necessarily need to be fulfilled, as clearly if will often not be possible to demonstrate transfer of disease with autoreactive serum and/or autoreactive lymphocytes in humans.

Indications that a disease is autoimmune

Presence of high titer autoantibodies and/or autoreactive lymphocytes *in vivo*

Autoantibody binding and/or T-cell reactivity to autoantigen *in vitro*

Transfer of disease with autoreactive serum and/or autoreactive lymphocytes

Immunopathology consistent with autoimmune-mediated processes

Beneficial effect of immunosuppressive interventions

Exclusion of other possible causes of disease

MHC association

Animal model mirroring the human disease

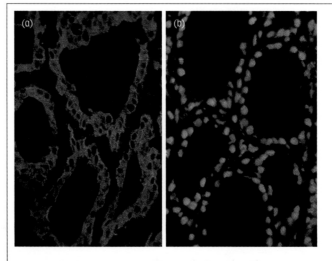

Figure 18.1. Fluorescent antibody studies in autoimmune diseases.

(a) Thyroid peroxidase antibodies staining cytoplasm of thyroid epithelial cells. (b) Diffuse nuclear staining on a thyroid section obtained with nucleoprotein antibodies from a patient with systemic lupus erythematosus. (Kindly provided by F. Bottazzo.)

⚲ Milestone 18.1—The Discovery of Thyroid Autoimmunity

Over a century ago Sergei Metalnikoff, in 1900, reported that some male animals were able to produce antibodies that recognized their own spermatozoa. However, these antibodies were not pathogenic and the view of the highly respected Paul Ehrlich that the body would not produce harmful anti-self immune responses (a situation he referred to as "horror autotoxicus") was at that time widely accepted. However, reports followed of self immunity to erythrocytes (Donath and Landsteiner, 1904) and lens (Krusius, 1910). In the early 1930s Thomas Rivers and his colleagues developed the experimental allergic encephalomyelitis (EAE) model and provided evidence that immune cells can attack the brain. Nonetheless, during the first half of the twentieth century there was a general air of skepticism regarding the idea that disease could arise as a result of autoimmunity. However, during the 1940s more reports of what seemed to be autoimmune pathology were published. Eventually any remaining skeptics were won over in 1956 when, remarkably, three major papers from the far corners of the globe established a link between autoimmunity and pathology in the thyroid.

Noel Rose and Ernest Witebsky in Boston [USA] immunized rabbits with rabbit thyroid extract in complete Freund's adjuvant. To what one might hazard was Witebsky's dismay and Rose's delight, this procedure resulted in the production of thyroid autoantibodies and chronic inflammatory destruction of the thyroid gland architecture (Figure M18.1.1a,b).

Having noted the fall in serum γ-globulin that followed removal of the goiter in Hashimoto's thyroiditis and the similarity of the histology (Figure M18.1.1c) to that of Rose and Witebsky's rabbits, Ivan Roitt, Deborah Doniach and Peter Campbell in London (UK) tested the hypothesis that the plasma cells in the gland might be making an autoantibody to a thyroid component, so causing the tissue damage and chronic inflammatory response. Sure enough, the sera of the first patients tested had precipitating antibodies to an autoantigen in normal thyroid extracts that was soon identified as thyroglobulin (Figure M18.1.2).

Finally, in Dunedin [New Zealand], Duncan Adams and Herbert Purves were seeking a circulating factor that might be responsible for the hyperthyroidism of Graves' disease. They injected patient's serum into guinea-pigs whose thyroids had been prelabeled with ^{131}I, and followed the release of radiolabeled material from the gland with time. Whereas the natural pituitary thyroid-stimulating hormone (TSH) produced a peak in serum radioactivity some 4 hours or so after injection of the test animal, serum from Graves' disease patients had a prolonged stimulatory effect (Figure M18.1.3). The so-called *long-acting thyroid stimulator* (LATS) was ultimately shown to be an IgG mimicking TSH through its reaction with the TSH receptor but differing in its time-course of action, largely due to its longer half-life in the circulation.

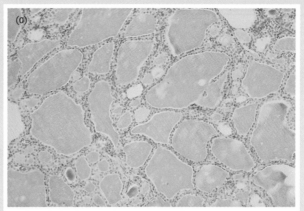
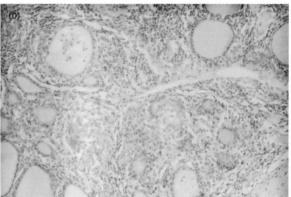
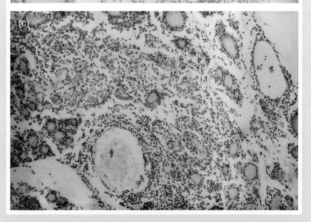

Figure M18.1.1. Experimental autoimmune thyroiditis.

(a) The follicular architecture of the normal thyroid.
(b) Thyroiditis produced by immunization with rat thyroid extract in complete Freund's adjuvant; the invading chronic inflammatory cells have destroyed the follicular structure. (Based on the experiments of Rose N.R. & Witebsky E. (1956) *Journal of Immunology* **76**, 417–427.) (c) Similarity of lesions in spontaneous human autoimmune disease to those induced in the experimental model.

Milestone 18.1—(Continued)

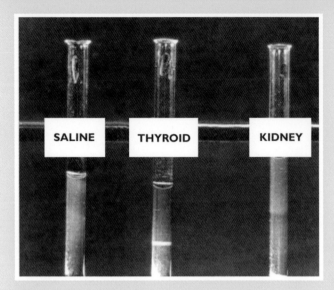

Figure M18.1.2. Thyroid autoantibodies in the serum of a patient with Hashimoto's disease demonstrated by precipitation in agar.

Test serum is incorporated in agar in the bottom of the tube; the middle layer contains agar only, while the autoantigen is present in the top layer. As serum antibody and thyroid autoantigen diffuse towards each other, they form a zone of opaque precipitate in the middle layer. Saline and kidney extract controls are negative. (Based on Roitt I.M., Doniach D., Campbell P.N. & Hudson R.V. (1956) *Lancet* **ii**, 820–821.)

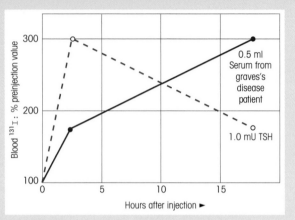

Figure M18.1.3. The long-acting thyroid stimulator in Graves' disease.

Injection of TSH causes a rapid release of ^{131}I from the prelabeled animal thyroid in contrast to the prolonged release that follows injection of serum from a Graves' disease patient. (Based on Adams D.D. & Purves H.D. (1956) *Proceedings of the University of Otago Medical School* **34**, 11–12.)

The nonorgan-specific autoimmune diseases, as their name suggests, are systemic in nature and often have a rheumatological component. **Systemic lupus erythematosus (SLE)** is an excellent example where anti-nuclear antibodies (ANA) are present that react with the nucleus of all cell types (Figure 18.1b) and the lesions are not confined to any one organ. Pathological changes are widespread and are seen in the skin (the "lupus" butterfly rash on the face is characteristic), kidney glomeruli, joints, serous membranes, blood cells and blood vessels.

Some of the most prevalent autoimmune diseases, and their associated autoantibodies, are listed in Table 18.2. Much of our understanding of autoimmune disease, and the development of new and effective therapies, have arisen from the study of animal models (Table 18.3).

Overlap of autoimmune disorders

There is a tendency for more than one autoimmune disorder to occur in the same individual and when this happens the association is often, but by no means always, between diseases within the same region of the organ-specific or nonorganspecific autoimmune spectrum. Thus patients with Hashimoto's thyroiditis have a much higher incidence of pernicious anemia than would be expected in a random population matched for age and sex (10% as against 0.2%). Conversely, both Hashimoto's thyroiditis and Graves' disease of the thyroid are diagnosed in pernicious anemia patients with an unexpectedly high frequency. Other associations are seen between Addison's disease (an autoimmune disease affecting the adrenal gland) and autoimmune thyroid disease and so on.

There is an even greater overlap in serological findings. Thirty percent of patients with autoimmune thyroid disease also have readily detectable parietal cell antibodies (which are found in patients with pernicious anemia) in their serum. It should be stressed that these are not cross-reacting antibodies. The thyroid-specific antibodies will not react with stomach and vice versa. When a serum reacts with both organs it means that two populations of antibodies are present, one with specificity for thyroid and the other for stomach.

Systemic autoimmune disease such as SLE is clinically associated with a number of other disorders including rheumatoid arthritis (RA) and Sjögren's syndrome. Antinuclear

Table 18.2. The major autoimmune diseases. This list includes only those diseases for which there is strong evidence that the primary cause of the pathology is an autoimmune attack. Other diseases which may also be autoimmune, but for which the pathological contribution of autoimmunity requires further investigation, are discussed later (p. 500).

Disease	Prevalence (%)	Characteristic autoantibodies
Graves' disease	1.12	TSH receptor (stimulatory)
Rheumatoid arthritis	0.92	Citrullinated proteins, IgG Fc
Hashimoto's disease	0.55	Thyroid peroxidase, thyroglobulin
Sjögren's syndrome	0.37	SS-A, SS-B
Pernicious anemia	0.15	Intrinsic factor
Multiple sclerosis	0.14	Myelin basic protein
Ankylosing spondylitis	0.13	Multiple connective tissue & skeletal proteins
Type 1 diabetes	0.12	Glutamic acid decarboxylase 65, insulin, IA-2
SLE	0.08	dsDNA, Sm, U1RNP, SS-A, SS-B, histones

Table 18.3. Spontaneous and induced animal models of autoimmune disease. A few examples from amongst the large number of such models CFA, Complete Freund's adjuvant.

Animal model	Human equivalent
Spontaneous	
Nonobese diabetic mouse (NOD)	Type 1 diabetes
Obese strain chicken	Hashimoto's disease
HLA-B27 transgenic rat	Ankylosing spondylitis
NZB mouse	Autoimmune hemolytic anemia
NZB × NZW F1	SLE
MRL/*lpr* mouse	SLE
Induced (by injection of antigens)	
Experimental autoimmune thyroiditis (EAT). Thyroglobulin in CFA into mice	Hashimoto's disease
Experimental autoimmune encephalomyelitis (EAE). Myelin basic protein in CFA into mice	Multiple sclerosis
Adjuvant arthritis. *Mycobacterium tuberculosis* in CFA into rats	Rheumatoid arthritis
Collagen-induced arthritis. Rat type II collagen in CFA into mice	Rheumatoid arthritis
Autoimmune hemolytic anemia. Rat RBC into mice	Autoimmune hemolytic anemia

antibodies and anti-IgG (rheumatoid factor) are a general feature.

What causes autoimmune disease?

Genetic factors

Autoimmune phenomena tend to aggregate in certain families. For example, the first degree relatives (siblings, parents and children) of patients with Hashimoto's disease show a high incidence of thyroid autoantibodies and of overt and subclinical thyroiditis. Parallel studies have disclosed similar relationships in the families of pernicious anemia patients, in that gastric parietal cell antibodies are prevalent in the relatives who develop achlorhydria (absent or low hypochloric acid in gastric secretions) and atrophic gastritis. Turning to SLE, a sibling of a patient with this disease is 20 times more likely to develop

lupus compared to the population as a whole. Figure 18.2 shows a multiplex family with type 1 diabetes in which the disease is linked to a particular serologically defined HLA haplotype (see below).

These familial relationships could be ascribed to environmental factors such as infective microorganisms, but there is powerful evidence that genetic components are involved. The data on **twins** is unequivocal. When Graves' disease or type 1 (insulin-dependent) diabetes occurs in twins, there is a far greater **concordance rate** (i.e. both twins affected) in identical than in nonidentical twins. Second, lines of animals have been bred that spontaneously develop autoimmune disease (Table 18.3). In other words, **the autoimmunity is genetically programed**. There is an obese strain of chickens with autoimmune thyroiditis, the nonobese diabetic (NOD) mouse modeling human type 1 diabetes and the New Zealand Black (NZB) strain succumbing to autoimmune hemolytic anemia. The

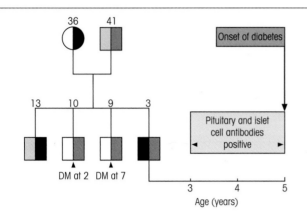

Figure 18.2. HLA haplotype linkage and onset of type 1 diabetes (DM).

Haplotypes: ☐ A3, B14, DR6; ■ A3, B7, DR4; ▨ A28, B51, DR4; and ▦ A2, B62, C3, DR4. Disease is linked to possession of the A2, B62, C3, DR4 haplotype. The 3-year-old brother had antibodies to the islet cell surface for 2 years before developing frank diabetes indicative of the lengthy pathological process preceding disease. (Data provided by G.F. Bottazzo.)

Table 18.4. Association of HLA with autoimmune disease. Relative risk refers to the chance of developing the disease compared to an individual who lacks the allele, and are for typical studies in white populations. These will often be different in other ethnic groups.

Disease	HLA allele	Relative risk
Class II associated		
Hashimoto's disease	DR5	3.2
Graves' disease	DR3	3.7
Type 1 diabetes	DQ8	14
	DQ2 + DQ8	20
	DQ6	0.2
Addison's disease	DR3	6.3
Rheumatoid arthritis	DR4	5.8
Sjögren's syndrome	DR3	9.7
Multiple sclerosis	DR2	3
Class I associated		
Ankylosing spondylitis	B27	87.4
Myasthenia gravis	B8	3

hybrid of NZB with another strain, the New Zealand White (B × W hybrid), actually develops antinuclear antibodies including anti-double-stranded DNA (anti-dsDNA) and a fatal immune complex-induced glomerulonephritis, key features of human SLE.

By far the vast majority of autoimmune diseases involve multiple susceptibility genes in each patient, i.e. they are **polygenic**. There are a few incredibly rare instances where an inherited mutation in the *Foxp3* (resulting in IPEX, *i*mmune dysregulation, *p*olyendocrinopathy, *e*nteropathy, *X*-linked syndrome), *AIRE* (causing autoimmune polyendocrine syndrome-1) or either *Fas* or *Fas ligand* (autoimmune lympho-proliferative syndrome) genes are alone responsible. Such diseases are therefore also classed as primary immunodeficiencies and have already been mentioned in Chapter 14 (p. 378). Some idea of the much greater genetic complexity of conventional autoimmune diseases has been gained from genome-wide searches for susceptibility genes. This approach has so far identified the involvement of around 20 gene loci for type 1 diabetes in NOD mice and some 25 or so for murine SLE. Generally speaking, in both mice and humans, each gene alone confers only a small increased risk. It is the **combination** of these genes that results in a substantially enhanced chance of developing autoimmune disease.

The strongest genetic associations with autoimmune diseases is linkage to the **major histocompatibility complex (MHC)**: HLA in humans and H-2 in mice. Of the many examples in humans are the increased risk of type 1 diabetes for DQ8 individuals, and the higher incidence of DR3 in Addison's disease and of DR4 in RA (Table 18.4). It should be

noted that such associations vary with ethnicity, as an example HLA-B27 shows an unusually strong linkage to ankylosing spondylitis and is present in 95% of white patients but in only 50% of African-American patients with this disease.

The use of antibodies to define MHC specificities is an informative approach, but with the improved precision gained by using gene sequencing it has become apparent that there is huge variation within each of the antibody-defined alleles. The naming of HLA alleles can therefore get quite complicated. However a standardized nomenclature was widely adopted in 2010 and a very clear and detailed explanation can be found at http://hla.alleles.org/nomenclature. Thus, again using HLA-B27 as an example, the accumulation of sequence data from different individuals quickly led to an appreciation that there are many different variants of HLA-B27, conferring differing degrees of susceptibility. Just to take three examples: the HLA-B*27:04 allelic variant is more strongly associated with ankylosing spondylitis than is HLA-B*27:05, whilst the HLA-B*27:06 allele shows only very weak or no association. As more data is accumulated, the precise variants that constitute disease susceptibility genes are becoming clearer. Some of the MHC associations that are seen are due to linkage disequilibrium with a disease susceptibility gene inherited *en bloc* with the

MHC variant. However, it is often the case that it is the MHC gene itself that leads to an increased or decreased risk of developing a particular autoimmune disease. Even a single amino acid difference in the peptide-binding groove can have a profound impact on the spectrum of both self and foreign peptides that are presented. Thus, an aspartic acid at amino acid residue position 57 in the HLA-DQ β chain confers resistance, whereas an alanine, valine or serine at this position confers susceptibility, to type 1 diabetes. The close relationship to MHC is not altogether unexpected given that, as we shall see, autoimmune diseases are T-cell dependent and most T-cell responses are MHC restricted.

Amongst the plethora of non-MHC-linked loci are genes encoding autoantigens (e.g. TSH receptor, insulin), pattern recognition receptors (e.g. NOD2), cytokines (e.g. IL-2, IL-12, IL-21) and their receptors (e.g. IL-2R, IL-7R and IL-23R), co-stimulatory molecules (e.g. CD40), signaling molecules (e.g. BLK, TRAF1) and transcription factors (e.g. STAT4). Polymorphisms in such genes enhance susceptibility or lead to resistance in otherwise predisposed subjects, and some have the potential to alter the balance of Th1/Th2/Th17/Treg subsets. Any polymorphism identified in more than one autoimmune disease is particularly noteworthy, a good example being *CTLA-4*, linked to a number of conditions including type 1 diabetes, Graves' disease and RA. Variants of *PTPN22* have also been implicated in susceptibility to these and several other autoimmune diseases. Given that both the cell surface CTLA-4 and the PTPN22 intracellular tyrosine phosphatase are involved in inhibiting T-cell co-stimulation, it is perhaps unsurprising that defects in their expression or function could contribute toward to development of normally suppressed autoimmune responses.

Unraveling such complex polygenic conditions is a very tough assignment. If we may take SLE as archetypal, genetic analysis of the predisposition to disease is most compatible with a threshold liability model requiring additive and/or epistatic (suppressing the function of another gene) contributions of multiple susceptibility genes probably linked to different stages of disease pathogenesis (Figure 18.3).

Hormonal influences

Whether or not one is of the XX or XY genotype has a profound effect on many aspects of life! This includes a general trend for autoimmune disease to occur more frequently in women than in men (Figure 18.4) probably due, in essence, to differences in hormonal patterns. Indeed, collectively, 75% of autoimmune disease is found in females and most commonly arises during the childbearing years. The most striking gender bias is seen in SLE where, during this time of their life, women are 10 times more likely to develop this disease than men. However, this drops to only a 2.5-fold excess following the menopause. There is a suggestion that higher estrogen levels are found in patients compared with controls. Knocking out the estrogen receptor α chain in the NZB × NZW model

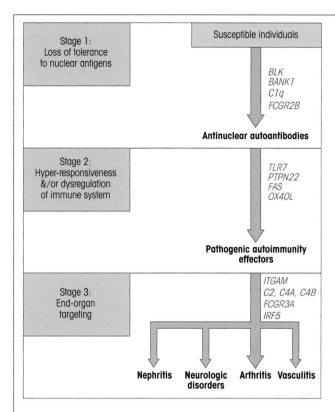

Figure 18.3. Possible stages in development of SLE in susceptible individuals.

An estimated 20–50 genes have been implicated in human SLE from genome-wide association studies, some examples of which are shown in red. BLK, B-lymphoid tyrosine kinase; BANK1, B-cell scaffold protein with ankyrin repeats-1; IRF5, Interferon regulatory factor-5. ITGAM encodes the integrin α_M component of the CR3 complement receptor, FCGR2B encodes FcγRIIb and FCGR3A encodes FcγRIIIa.

lowers autoantibody levels, decreases the severity of glomerulonephritis and increases survival (Figure 18.5).

Pregnancy is often associated with amelioration of autoimmune disease severity, for example in rheumatoid arthritis (RA), and there is sometimes a striking relapse after giving birth, a time at which there are drastic changes in hormones such as prolactin, not forgetting the loss of the placenta. Certainly a general quietening down of immune responses in order to prevent immunological rejection of the fetus (p. 441) would be consistent with some degree of remission of an autoimmune disease during pregnancy. However, there needs to be a degree of caution in making any generalized statement here because some autoimmune diseases, such as lupus, can actually get worse during pregnancy. It may be that the relative contribution of the various T-cell subsets to different types of autoimmune disease, and changes in these subsets during pregnancy, go some way to explaining these apparently opposite affects.

In Chapter 10, we dwelt on the importance of the neuro-endocrine immune feedback encompassing the cytokine–hypothalamic–pituitary–adrenal control circuit. Abnormalities in this feedback loop have now been revealed in several autoimmune disorders. Rheumatoid arthritis patients with ongoing chronic inflammation have normal levels of circulating cortisol despite the presence of inflammatory cytokines that would normally be expected to stimulate increased secretion of this adrenal hormone. The Obese strain (OS) chicken and several strains of lupus mice also show blunted IL-1-induced corticosteroid responses.

Does the environment contribute?

Twin studies

Concordance rates reported in the literature tend to vary somewhat from study to study, but consistently re-enforce the fact that although there is a strong genetic contribution, inherited genes are not the whole story. Thus, even the relatively high 65% or so concordance rates that are reported for the development of type 1 diabetes in identical twins followed throughout life indicates very clearly that noninherited factors must also be involved. This is not necessarily all due to environment as, although monozygotic twins have identical germline immunoglobulin and T-cell receptor (TCR) genes, the processes of diversification of receptors and of internal anti-idiotype interactions are so complex that the resulting receptor repertoires will be extremely variable and unlikely to be identical. Nonetheless, in many other autoimmune diseases, including Graves' disease and SLE, reported concordance rates in identical twins are only of the order 20–25%, leaving much room

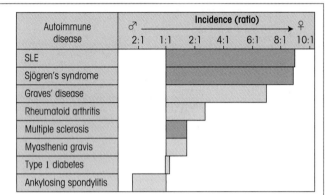

Figure 18.4. Increased incidence of autoimmune disease in females.

Ankylosing spondylitis is one of very few autoimmune diseases that bucks the trend and is more common in males than females.

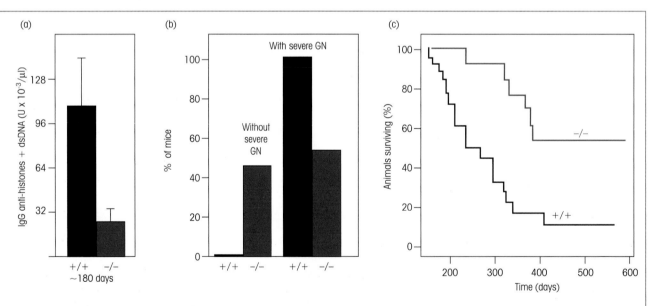

Figure 18.5. Estrogen receptor α-chain (ERα) knockout inhibits autoantibodies and nephritis, and prolongs lifespan in murine lupus.

Female NZB × NZW F$_1$ mice bearing homozygous deletion (–/–) of the estrogen receptor α-chain: (a) develop lower levels of IgG autoantibodies to a histones/dsDNA mixture; (b) exhibit a reduced incidence of severe glomerulonephritis (GN) compared with ERα$^{+/+}$ mice siblings; and (c) have an increased lifespan. (Based on data from Bynoté K.K. *et al.* (2008) *Genes and Immunity* **9**, 137–152.)

for other contributory factors. Although the genetics of autoimmune disease is at least partly worked out, the nongenetic influences are relatively poorly understood—particularly in the human.

Diet

What environmental agents can we identify? Well, diet could be one although there is scant evidence so far. Fish oils containing omega-3 polyunsaturated fatty acids (PUFAs) have anti-inflammatory activity and, in some studies, have been shown to be beneficial for patients with RA. However, a recent meta-analysis (i.e. combining the results of several studies) concluded that much larger trials are needed before any firm conclusions can be reached regarding dietary influences in this disease. There is some evidence that iodine supplementation in iodine-deficient populations can lead to an increase in thyroid autoimmune disease.

Drugs

Although many autoimmune diseases have been linked in case reports to a wide range of drugs, the most firmly established example is **drug-induced lupus**. Procainamide and quinidine (both used to treat cardiac arrhythmia) and hydralazine (an antihypertensive drug) are most often implicated in this disease that shares many features with SLE, although the specificity of the anti-DNA tends to be towards the single-stranded form rather than double-stranded DNA (dsDNA) and patients tend to have more joint and less neurological and kidney involvement.

Noninfectious environmental agents

Sunshine is an undisputed trigger of the skin lesions in SLE. Necrosis and apoptosis of keratinocytes resulting from the detrimental effects of sunlight leads to the release of nuclear autoantigens; in the case of apoptosis these are associated with the cell surface blebs that characteristically appear in this type of cell death. The situation is not helped by the defective phagocytosis seen in this disease, resulting in reduced clearance of apoptotic debris. UV-irradiation also stimulates production of both CCL and CXCL chemokines by skin epithelial cells, resulting in recruitment of T-cells and dendritic cells into the inflammatory lesion.

Occupational exposure to a number of agents has been linked to the development of autoimmune disease. Particularly convincing associations are silica exposure with SLE, RA and scleroderma. Solvents have been implicated in, for example, multiple sclerosis, and pesticides with RA. Cigarette smoking increases the risk of RA and of Hashimoto's and Graves' diseases. The mechanisms remain unclear.

Infection

The finger of suspicion is often pointed in the direction of an infectious microorganism, and there is indeed substantial evidence in animal models that infection can play an important role in the development of autoimmune disease. However, there is only one clear-cut example in humans: acute rheumatic fever following infection with group A *Streptococcus*. In 3–4% of untreated patients, usually children, who develop a sore throat due to *S. pyogenes* infection there is a resulting polyarthritis, carditis and chorea (i.e. joint and heart inflammation together with involuntary movement). The link to the infection lies in the fact that the streptococcal M protein shares structural homology with cardiac myosin—a clear situation of molecular mimicry. Despite numerous other proposals of microbial involvement in the precipitation of autoimmune disease in genetically susceptible individuals, such links are still at the level of speculation due to a lack of definitive evidence. In most cases of human autoimmune disease, the problem regarding the identification of putative infectious agents is the long latency period that makes it difficult to track down the initiating event (cf. Figure 18.2) and, secondly, viable organisms usually cannot be isolated from the affected tissues. Nonetheless the clear evidence of microbial influences in animal models is sufficiently compelling to suggest that the hunt to link pathogens to human autoimmune diseases is worth pursuing.

Further complexity is injected by the knowledge that environmental microbes may sometimes **protect** against spontaneous autoimmune disease. The incidence of diabetes is greatly increased if NOD mice are kept in specific pathogen-free conditions, while Sendai virus inhibits the development of arthritis in the MRL/*lpr* mouse model of SLE. The extraordinary variation in incidence of diabetes in NOD colonies bred in a wide variety of different animal houses (Figure 18.6) testifies to the dramatic influence of environmental flora on the expression of autoimmune disease.

Mechanisms in autoimmune disease

Although innate responses play important roles in the development and maintenance of autoimmune disease, at the most fundamental level pathogenic autoimmunity represents a breakdown in specific immunological tolerance. Given that tolerance is a mechanism that applies only to lymphocytes, the contribution of the adaptive response is blindingly obvious. Note also that we state "breakdown" in tolerance. It may be that in some cases there is a failure to establish tolerance in the first place, but given that autoimmune diseases often do not arise until early middle age or beyond it would seem that tolerance is initially operating effectively but that in genetically predisposed individuals an accumulation of environmental influences, and possibly mutations, eventually leads to uncontrolled pathogenic anti-self responses. Whether or not the response is driven by self antigen, foreign antigen, by superantigens or other polyclonal activators, or by anti-idiotypes is not always entirely clear. It is also worth bearing in mind that a seemingly identical autoimmune disease may arise due to different sets of circumstances in individual patients.

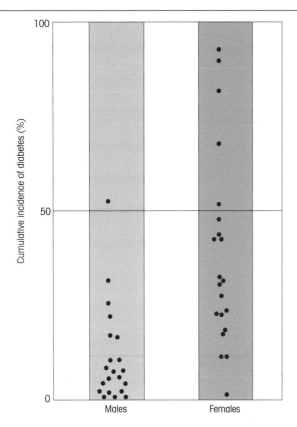

Figure 18.6. The incidence of spontaneous diabetes in geographically dispersed colonies of NOD mice at 20 weeks of age.

Each point represents a single colony. The extreme spread of values is not attributable to genetic drift to any significant extent. The lower incidence in males is particularly evident. (Data adapted from Pozzilli P., Signore A., Williams A.J.K. & Beales P.E. (1993) *Immunology Today* **14**, 193–196.)

Tolerance is not absolute

Of the various tolerance mechanisms employed by the immune system, only apoptosis leads to a loss of antigen-specific lymphocytes. Although high affinity B-cells will be tolerized by apoptosis, particularly to autoantigens that circulate at high concentration, this most extreme way of dealing with unruly lymphocytes is largely targeted at T-cells during negative selection in the thymus. Receptor editing (p. 92) can eliminate autoreactive B-cells through continued V(D)J recombination. Those self-reactive B-cells that are present in the periphery usually do not pose a problem due to a lack of cognate T-cell help (see Figure 11.16). However, for autoantigens that are not expressed at an adequate level in the thymus (p. 293) self-reactive T-cells will be available. Processing of an autoantigen will lead to certain (dominant) peptides being preferentially expressed on antigen-presenting cells (APCs) while others (cryptic) only appear in the MHC groove in very low concentrations which, although capable of expanding their cognate T-cells in the context of thymic positive selection (cf. p. 291),

may nonetheless fail to provide a sufficiently powerful signal for negative selection of these cells. As a consequence, autoreactive T-cells specific for **cryptic epitopes** will survive in the repertoire that will therefore be biased towards weak self-reactivity.

Autoantigen-driven responses

The Obese strain (OS) chicken is unlikely to appear on the menu of your local restaurant, but is of interest because it spontaneously develops IgG autoantibodies to thyroglobulin and a chronic inflammatory antithyroid response that destroys the gland so causing hypothyroidism. If the source of antigen is removed by neonatal thyroidectomy, no autoantibodies are formed. Injection of these animals with normal thyroglobulin then induces antibodies. Thyroidectomy of OS chickens with established thyroiditis is followed by a dramatic fall in antibody titer. Conclusions: the spontaneous antithyroglobulin immunity is initiated and maintained by autoantigen from the thyroid gland. Furthermore, as the response is completely T-cell dependent, we can infer that both B- and T-cells are driven by thyroglobulin in this model.

As usual, human disease is a tougher nut to crack and one has to rely on more indirect evidence. T-cell lines have been established from Graves' disease glands and it has been possible to show direct stimulation by whole thyroid cells. Removal of the putative antigen source by thyroidectomy of Hashimoto's disease patients is followed by a fall in serum γ-globulins, one of the clues that led to the discovery of thyroid autoimmunity (cf. Milestone 18.1); incidentally, this accords well with the data from OS chickens quoted above. The production of high affinity IgG autoantibodies accompanied by somatic hypermutation in patients with thyroid autoimmune disease is powerful evidence for the selection of B-cells by antigen in a T-dependent response. The reason for this, simply, is that high affinity IgG antibodies only arise through mutation and selection by antigen within germinal centers (cf. p. 248). More indirect, but equally convincing, is the argument that antibodies are regularly formed against a cluster of epitopes on a single autoantigen or of autoantigens within a single organ (e.g. thyroglobulin plus thyroid peroxidase, or different constituents of the nucleosome). It is difficult to propose a hypothesis which does not depend finally on stimulation by antigen. T-cells are critical for such responses as depletion of CD4 T-cells in a number of animal models abrogates autoantibody production.

The visibility of autoantigens to the immune system

For a few body constituents (e.g. sperm, lens and heart) the antigens are completely **sequestered** (hidden) from the immune system and therefore no degree of immunological tolerance is established. This does not pose a problem unless a mishap (e.g. physical trauma) causes release of the antigen into the circulation with subsequent activation of self-reactive lym-

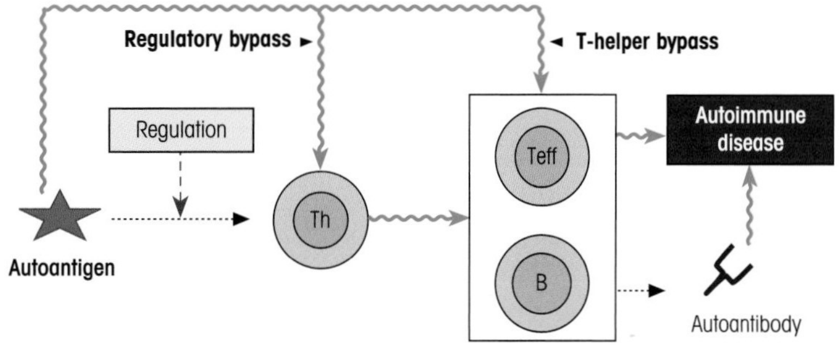

Figure 18.7. Autoimmunity arises through bypass of the control of autoreactivity.

The constraints on the stimulation of self-reactive helper T-cells by autoantigen can be circumvented either through bypassing the helper cell or by disturbance of the regulatory mechanisms.

phocytes. Even here, in general, the experience has been that injection of *unmodified* extracts of those tissues concerned in the organ-specific autoimmune disorders does not readily elicit antibody formation. In fact, in the majority of cases—e.g. red cells in autoimmune hemolytic anemia, ribonucleoprotein (RNP) and nucleosome components present as blebs on the surface of apoptotic cells in SLE, and surface receptors in many cases of organ-specific autoimmunity—the autoantigens are readily accessible to circulating lymphocytes.

Presumably, antigens present at adequate concentrations in the extracellular fluid will be processed by professional APCs, but for autoantigens associated with cells, the derivative peptides will only interact "meaningfully" with specific T-cells if there are appropriate MHC surface molecules, if the concentration of processed peptide associated with them is significant and, for resting T-cells, if co-stimulatory signals can be given. As we shall see, these are important constraints.

The message then is that we are all sitting on a minefield of self-reactive cells, with potential access to their respective autoantigens. However as autoimmune disease only occurs in a minority of the population the body must possess homeostatic mechanisms to prevent such self-reactive cells being triggered under normal circumstances. Accepting its limitations, Figure 18.7 provides a framework for us to examine ways in which these mechanisms may be circumvented to allow autoimmunity to develop. It is assumed that the key to the system is control of the autoreactive T-helper cell as the evidence heavily favors the T-dependence of virtually all autoimmune responses; thus, interaction between the T-cell and MHC-associated peptide becomes the core consideration. We start with the assumption that these cells are normally unresponsive because of clonal deletion, clonal anergy, T-suppression or inadequate autoantigen presentation. Immediately, one could conceive of an *abnormal* degree of responsiveness to self-antigens as a result of relatively low intrathymic expression of a particular molecule (cf. p. 295). Abnormalities in the signaling pathways affecting the thresholds for positive and negative selection in the thymus would

also affect subsequent responsiveness to peripheral autoantigens. So might defects in apoptotic cell death.

Obtaining T-cell help for autoantigen-specific B-cells

Allison and Weigle argued independently that, if autoreactive T-cells are tolerized and thereby unable to collaborate with B-cells to generate autoantibodies (Figures 18.8a), provision of new carrier determinants (i.e. helper T-cell epitopes) to which no self-tolerance had been established would provide a "T-cell bypass." In other words, help could now be given for autoreactive B-cells even though the autoreactive T-cells were absent, leading to autoantibody production (Figure 18.8b).

Modification of the autoantigen

A new carrier could arise through post-translational modification to the molecule (Figure 18.8b.1), seen for example in the citrullination (a post-translational arginine modification) of vimentin, fibrinogen, collagen type II and α-enolase in RA. Modification can also be achieved through combination with a drug (Figure 18.8b.3). In one example of many, the autoimmune hemolytic anemia associated with administration of α-methyldopa might be attributable to modification of the red cell surface in such a way as to provide a carrier for stimulating B-cells that recognize the rhesus antigen. This is normally regarded as a "weak" antigen and would be less likely to induce B-cell tolerance than the "stronger" antigens present on the erythrocyte.

Molecular mimicry of T-cell epitopes

B-cell epitopes present on a microbial antigen may cross-react, due to molecular mimicry, with an epitope on a human autoantigen. However, because the microbial antigen and the self antigen are only partially similar there will be no T-cell tolerance to sequences on other parts of the microbial antigen. Thus, T-cells to these sequences will be present and can provide

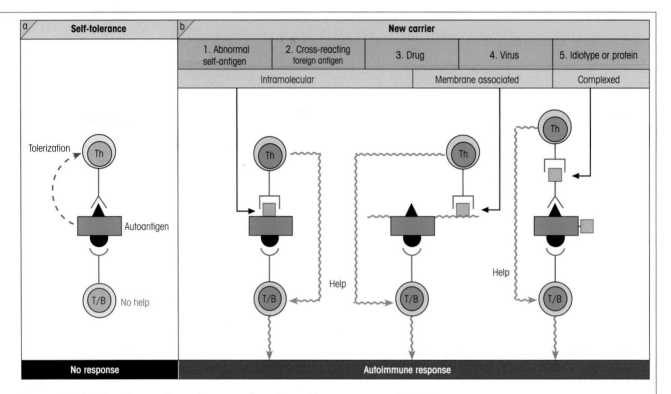

Figure 18.8. T-helper bypass through new carrier epitope (▨) generates autoimmunity.

For simplicity, processing for MHC association has been omitted from the diagram, but is elaborated in Figure 18.9. (a) The pivotal autoreactive T-helper is unresponsive either through tolerance or inability to see a cryptic epitope. (b) Different mechanisms providing a new carrier epitope.

help for B-cells that recognize the cross-reactive epitope (Figure 18.8b.2). The mechanism is spelt out in more detail in Figure 18.9a. We have already mentioned that in rheumatic fever antibodies produced to the *Streptococcus* also react with heart. Another example is the envelope proteins of *Yersinia enterolytica*, which share epitopes with the thyroid-stimulating hormone (TSH) receptor.

The drawback of this B-cell epitope cross-reaction model is that once the cross-reacting agent is eliminated from the body the T-cell epitope will no longer be present. However, the infecting agent may also mimic an autoantigen by producing a **cross-reacting T-cell epitope** on professional APCs that can prime the T-cell and upregulate its adhesion molecules. The T-cell now has the **avidity** to bind to and be persistently activated by the self-epitope presented on the target tissue cell provided that it is associated with the appropriate MHC molecule (Figure 18.9b). Remember the transgenic cytotoxic T-cells (Tc) that could only destroy the pancreatic β-cells bearing a viral transgene when they were **primed** by a real viral infection (cf. Figure 11.9). Recall also the tumor cells that could only be recognized by primed not resting T-cells (cf. Figure 17.14). Theoretically, the resting T-cell could also be primed in a nonantigen-specific manner by a microbial **superantigen**.

Although we have ascribed the dominant role of MHC alleles as risk factors for autoimmune diseases to their ability to present key antigenic epitopes to autoreactive T-cells, they might also operate in a quite distinct way. We may recollect that, during intrathymic ontogeny, T-cells are positively selected by weak interaction with self-peptides complexed with MHC. Now as around **50% of the class II peptides are MHC derived**, then the mature T-cells leaving the thymus will have been selected with a strong bias to weak recognition of self-MHC peptides presented by class II. There must therefore be a major pool of self-reactive T-cells vulnerable to stimulation by exogenously derived cross-reacting epitopes that mimic these MHC peptides. Just so. The sequence QKRAA (the so-called "shared epitope" sequence) lies within a polymorphic region of the DRβ chain of DR1 and certain DR4 alleles, and is also present in the dnaJ heat-shock proteins from *E. coli*, *Lactobacillus lactis* and *Brucella ovis*, as well as the Epstein–Barr virus gp110 protein. This provides an opportunity for priming of T-cells with autoreactive specificity for a processed peptide containing QKRAA presented by another HLA molecule. Thus, the sequence QKRAAVDTY of the RA susceptibility allele HLA-DRB1*04:01 is closely similar to the QKRAAYDQY of the dnaJ heat-shock protein of *E. coli* (Table 18.5), and this

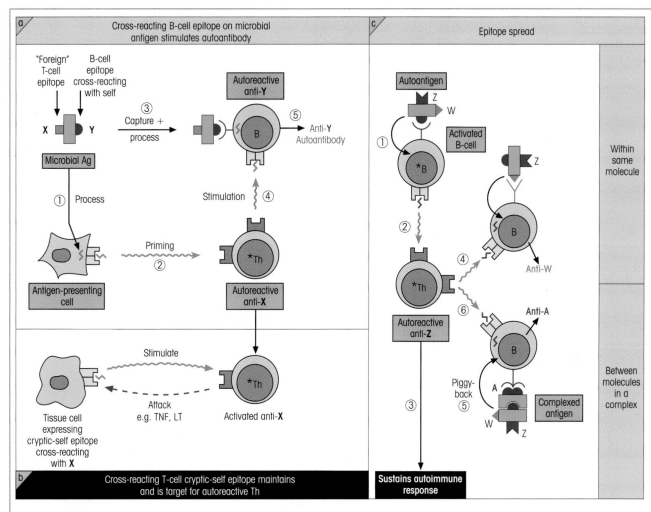

Figure 18.9. Mechanisms of microbial induction of autoimmunity and epitope spread.

(This is a complex mouthful but digestion is recommended because these ideas are crucial. The more faint-hearted may require an ice-pack and persistence, but following the numbers should help.) (a) A microbial antigen (Ag) bearing an epitope Y that cross-reacts with self and a foreign T-cell epitope X is (1) processed by an antigen-presenting cell; (2) activates the T-helper; which (3) recognizes the processed X after capture by an anti-Y B-cell; and (4) stimulates the B-cell to secrete anti-Y autoantibody. (b) The *activated* anti-X T-helper, as distinct from the *resting* cell, may recognize and be stimulated by a cross-reacting cryptic T-cell epitope expressed by a tissue cell. This stimulation will maintain the autoimmune response even after elimination of the microbe, because of the persistence of the self-epitope. The tissue expressing the epitope will also be a target for immunological attack. Note also that a T-helper primed nonspecifically by a polyclonal superantigen activator could also

fulfil the same function of responding to a cryptic epitope. (c) If the autoantigen is soluble or capable of uptake and processing after capture by the activated autoreactive B-cell (1) (either from (a) or through nonspecific polyclonal activation), a new epitope can be presented on the B-cell class II which now stimulates an autoreactive (anti-Z) T-helper (2), which can then sustain an autoimmune response entirely through autoantigen stimulation (3). It can also produce epitope spread within the same molecule through helping a B-cell which captures the autoantigen through a new epitope W (4), or to another component in an intermolecular complex such as nucleosomal histone–DNA or idiotype-positive (Id⁺) anti-DNA–DNA which is "piggy-backed" into the B-cell (5). Processed antigen is presented by the B-cell to the T-helper (6); in the cases cited, specific for histone or Id, respectively. *Denotes activation.

Table 18.5. Molecular mimicry. Some examples of homologies between microbes and body components as potential cross-reacting T-cell epitopes.

Disease	Microbial molecule		Sequence
Rheumatoid arthritis	Microbe:	*Escherichia coli*	QKRAAVDTY
	Self:	HLA-DRB1*04:01	QKRAAYDQY
Multiple sclerosis	Microbe:	Epstein–Barr virus	VYHFVKKHV
	Self:	Myelin basic protein	VVHFFKNIV
Multiple sclerosis	Microbe:	*Chlamydia pneumoniae*	YGCLLPRNPRTEDQN
	Self:	Myelin basic protein	YGSLPQKSQRTQDEN
Type 1 diabetes	Microbe:	Hepatitis C virus	AAARRWAC
	Self:	Glutamic acid decarboxylase 65	AAARKAAC
Myasthenia gravis	Microbe:	Polio virus	TKESRGTT
	Self:	Acetylcholine receptor	IKESRGTK
Rheumatic fever	Microbe:	*Streptococcus pyogenes*	LTDQNKNLTTEN
	Self:	Cardiac myosin	LTSQRAKLQTEN

peptide presented by DQ causes proliferation of synovial T-cells from RA patients.

In fact, a large number of microbial peptide sequences with varying degrees of homology with human proteins have been identified (Table 18.5), although it should be emphasized at this stage that they only provide clues for further study. The mere existence of homology provides no evidence that infection with that organism will necessarily lead to autoimmunity because everything depends on several contingencies, including the manner in which the proteins are processed by the APCs.

"Piggy-back" T-cell epitopes and epitope spread

One membrane component may provide help for the immune response to another (associative recognition). In the context of autoimmunity, a new helper determinant may arise through drug modification as mentioned above, or through the insertion of viral antigen into the membrane of an infected cell (cf. Figure 18.8b.4). That this can promote a reaction to a pre-existing cell component is clear from the studies in which infection of a tumor with influenza virus elicited resistance to uninfected tumor cells. In a comparable fashion, T-cell help can be provided for a molecule such as DNA, which cannot itself form a T-cell epitope, by complexing with a T-dependent carrier, in this example a histone, or an anti-DNA idiotype to which T-cells were sensitized. For this mechanism to work, the helper component must still be physically attached to the fragment bearing the B-cell epitope. When this is recognized by the B-cell receptor, the helper component will be "piggybacked" into the B-cell, processed and presented as an epitope for recognition by T-cells (Figure 18.9c). By the same token, the autoimmune response can spread to other epitopes on the same molecule.

Idiotype bypass mechanisms

Lymphocytes with specificity for exogenous antigens could be connected to autoreactive lymphocytes through idiotype network connections (Figure 18.10), particularly as some autoimmune diseases are characterized by major cross-reactive idiotypes. T-helpers with specificity for the idiotype on a lymphocyte receptor can be instrumental in the stimulation of the idiotype-bearing cell. Thus, it is conceivable that an environmental agent such as a parasite or virus could trigger antibody carrying a cross-reactive idiotype which happened to be shared with the receptor of an autoreactive T- or B-cell, and thereby provoke an autoimmune response.

Polyclonal activation

Microbes often display adjuvant properties through their possession of polyclonal lymphocyte activators such as bacterial endotoxins. The variety of autoantibodies detected in cases with infectious mononucleosis must surely be attributable to the polyclonal activation of B-cells by the Epstein–Barr virus (EBV). Nevertheless, it is difficult to see how a pan-specific polyclonal activation could give rise to the patterns of autoantibodies characteristic of the different autoimmune disorders without the operation of some antigen-directing factor. We have already hinted at scenarios in which polyclonally activated B- or T-cells might contribute to a sustained autoimmune response (see legend to Figure 18.9b,c).

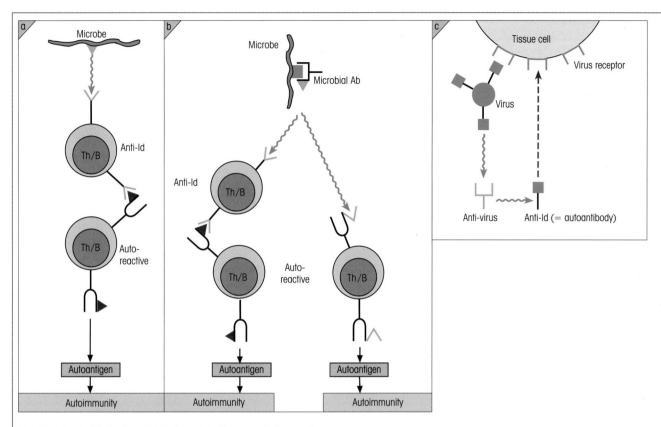

Figure 18.10. Idiotypic mechanisms leading to autoimmunity.

(a) Microbial antigen cross-reacts with autoreactive lymphocyte Id. (b) Microbial antibodies either share Ids with, or are anti-Id to, autoreactive lymphocytes. (c) Anti-virus generates anti-Id that is autoantibody to viral receptor.

Regulatory defects

It should be emphasized that these T-helper bypass mechanisms for the induction of autoimmunity do not by themselves ensure the continuation of the response, as normal animals have been shown to be capable of damping down autoantibody production through CD4 regulatory T-cell interactions as, for example, in the case of red cell autoantibodies induced in mice by injection of rat erythrocytes (Figure 18.11). When regulatory T-cell activity is impaired by low doses of cyclophosphamide, or if strains like the SJL, which have prematurely aging regulators are used, induced autoimmunity is prolonged and more severe. Much work has focused on the CD4⁺CD25⁺Foxp3⁺ regulatory T-cell (cf. Figure 10.12) that has been shown to suppress many different autoimmune phenomena. However, cellular control mechanisms are never straightforward and it is important to appreciate that CD25⁻ T-cells have proved to be effective in controlling T-cell mediated disease in certain circumstances. Interestingly, TGFβ can convert these CD4⁺, CD25⁻, Foxp3⁻ cells to the CD4⁺, CD25⁺, Foxp3⁺ Tr1 phenotype (cf. Figure 10.12) characteristic of the mucosal regulatory cells that mediate oral tolerance; they produce IL-10 on activation and promote the differentiation

of T-cells that secrete TGFβ (Th3) and skew responses towards the Th2-type pole. Yet another player in the field is the NKT-cell that is deficient in NOD mice, but can prevent the development of diabetes if transferred from F1(BALB/c × NOD) donors. Patients with a variety of autoimmune diseases have been reported to have reduced numbers or function of this cell type (Figure 18.12). Fascinatingly, the compromised regulatory T-cell function seen in RA patients normalizes after successful therapy with anti-TNF monoclonals (Figure 18.13).

Do abnormalities in apoptotic mechanisms also contribute to these regulatory defects? T- and B-cells of NOD mice are resistant to apoptosis, as are lymphocytes of the MRL/*lpr* lupus mouse strain that has a *fas* gene mutation. This mutation produces the characteristic lymphoproliferation, and possibly failure to limit the expansion of self-reactive T- and B-cell clones by apoptosis. The *gld* lupus model complements this situation with mutations in the *fas ligand*.

Attention has also focused on yet another facet of immune regulation, namely the regulatory IgG receptor on B-cells whose function is feedback control through surface immune complex signaling (cf. p. 264). Dysfunction in the FcγRIIB B-cell receptor in lupus-prone mice can be corrected by retroviral transduction of a normal gene (Figure 18.14).

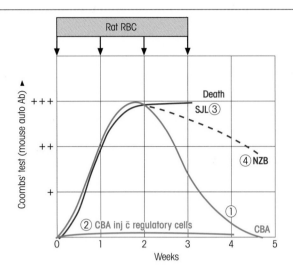

Figure 18.11. Regulation of self-reactivity.

When CBA strain mice (1) are injected with **rat** red cells, autoantibodies are produced by this **cross-reacting** antigen (see Figure 18.9a) that coat the host **mouse** erythrocytes and are detected by the Coombs' antiglobulin test (see p. 407). Despite repeated injections of rat erythrocytes, the autoantibody response is switched off by the expansion of CD4 mouse red cell-specific regulatory cells that do not affect antibody production to the heterologous erythrocyte determinants. When these regulatory cells are injected into naive CBA mice (2), rat red cells cannot induce autoantibodies. The SJL strain (3), in that suppressor activity declines rapidly with age, is unable to regulate the autoimmune response and develops particularly severe disease. The response is also prolonged in the autoimmune NZB strain (4). (Based on data of Cooke A. & Hutchings P., e.g. (1984) *Immunology* **51**, 489–492.)

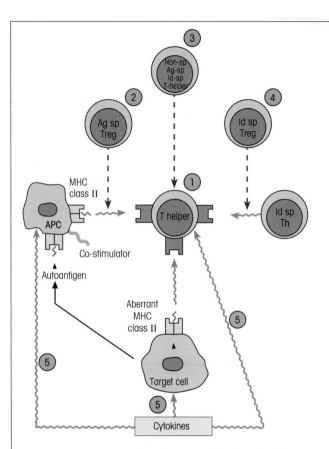

Figure 18.12. Bypass of regulatory mechanisms leads to triggering of autoreactive T-helper cells.

Through defects in (1) tolerizability or ability to respond to or induce T-regulators (Treg); or expression of (2) antigen-specific (Ag-sp), (3) hsp and other nonspecific (Non-sp), or (4) idiotype-specific (Id-sp) T-regulators; or (5) through imbalance of the cytokine network, producing derepression of class II genes with inappropriate cellular expression of class II and presentation of antigen on target cell, stimulation of antigen-presenting cell (APC), and possible activation of anergic T-helper.

We have previously drawn attention to the distinctive properties of the B-1 population with respect to its propensity to synthesize IgM autoantibodies and its possible intimate relationship to the setting up of the regulatory idiotype network (cf. p. 298), and one must seriously entertain the hypothesis that unregulated activity by these cells could be responsible for certain autoimmune disorders. In humans, a high proportion of B-1 cells make IgM rheumatoid factors (anti-Fcγ) and anti-DNA using germline genes.

Aberrant expression of MHC class II

Normally, only professional antigen-presenters such as dendritic cells express MHC class II molecules. Therefore the majority of organ-specific autoantigens usually appear on the surface of the cells of the target organ in the context of class I (present on all nucleated cells) but not class II. Thus the autoantigens cannot be presented to T-helpers by the tissue cells that are therefore immunologically silent. Pujol-Borrell, Bottazzo and colleagues reasoned that, if the class II genes were somehow derepressed and class II molecules were now synthe-

sized, they would endow these cells with the ability to present peptides to CD4⁺ T-cells (Figure 18.12). Indeed, they were able to show that human thyroid cells in tissue culture can be persuaded to express HLA-DR (class II) molecules on their surface after stimulation with γ-interferon (IFNγ). Inappropriate class II expression has also been reported on the bile ductules in primary biliary cirrhosis and on endothelial cells and some β-cells in the pancreas of type I diabetics.

Whether aberrant expression of class II on these cells through activation by something like virally induced IFN is responsible for *initiating* the autoimmune process by priming autoreactive T-helpers, or whether reaction with *already activated* T-cells induces class II by release of IFNγ and makes the cell a more attractive target for provoking subsequent tissue damage, is still an unresolved issue. However, transfection of

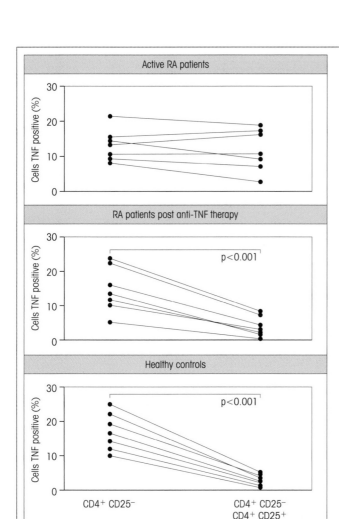

Figure 18.13. Reversal of compromised regulatory T-cell function in rheumatoid arthritis (RA) patients by anti-TNF therapy.

CD4+CD25− cells isolated from peripheral blood were stimulated with a mixture of anti-CD3 and anti-CD28 alone or after adding back the CD4+CD25+ regulatory T-cells. Activation of the T-cells was assessed by staining for intracellular TNF. The lines join values for individual patients after adding back regulatory CD4+CD25+ T-cells. The Tregs were dysfunctional in active RA but were able to suppress activation of the CD25− population after successful anti-TNF therapy. (Data from Ehrenstein M.R. *et al.* (2004) *Journal of Experimental Medicine* **200**, 277–285.)

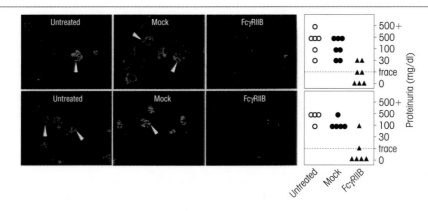

Figure 18.14. Retroviral transduction of the regulatory IgG receptor on B-cells (FcγRIIB) in spontaneous lupus prone mice.

Six months after receiving FcγRIIB retroviral-transduced bone marrow, immune complex deposition is reduced and kidney function is improved in NZM2410 (top row) and BXSB (bottom row) lupus prone mice. Kidney sections were examined for the presence of IgG complexes with direct immunofluorescence (×40). Arrowheads indicate subendothelial complexes indicative of active lupus. (Excerpted with permission from McGaha T.L., Sorrentino B. & Ravetch J.V. (2005) *Science* **307**, 590–593. Copyright 2005 AAAS.)

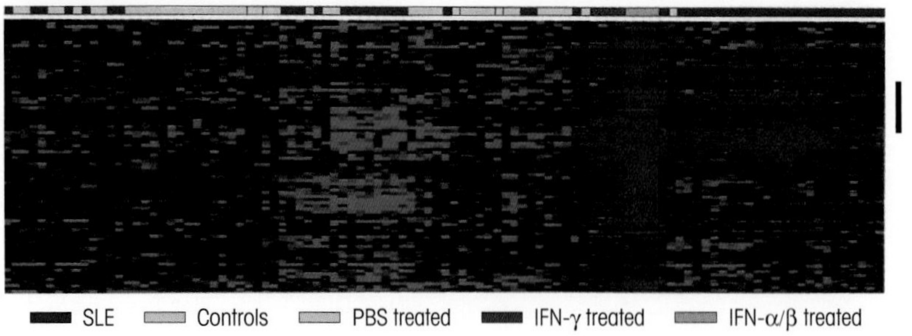

Figure 18.15. The IFNα signature in a major subset of SLE patients.

Expression patterns of IFN-induced genes in the blood of lupus patients and controls (red = highly expressed). The black bar indicates 22 of the IFN-upregulated genes that delineate the "signature pattern." (Reproduced from Baechler E.C., Gregersen P.K. & Behrens T.W. (2004) *Current Opinion in Immunology* **16**, 801–807; with permission of the authors and publishers.)

mice with the class II *H-2A* genes linked to the insulin promoter led to expression of class II on the β-islet cells of the pancreas but did *not* induce autoimmunity. Lack of B7 co-stimulatory molecules seems to be responsible for the failure of these class II-positive β-cells to activate naive T-cells, a job that may have to be left to the professional APCs.

Cytokine imbalance may induce autoimmunity

By contrast, transfection with the *IFNγ* gene on the insulin promoter under the same circumstances produced a local inflammatory reaction in the pancreas with aberrant expression of class II *and* diabetes; this must have been a result of autoimmunity as a normal pancreas grafted into the same animal suffered a similar fate. This situation implies that unregulated cytokine production producing a local inflammatory reaction can initiate autoimmunity, probably by enhancing the presentation of islet antigen by recruiting and activating dendritic cells, by increasing the concentration of processed intracellular autoantigen available to them, and by increasing their avidity for naive T-cells through upregulation of adhesion molecules; perhaps previously anergic cells may be made responsive to antigen (Figure 18.12). Once primed, the T-cells can now interact with the islet β-cells that will be displaying increased amounts of class II and adhesion molecules for T-cells on their surface.

This all seems very straightforward but, although other proinflammatory cytokines, IL-12 and TNF as well as IFNγ, can promote the induction of organ-specific autoimmune disease at an early time by priming pathogenic Th1 responses, late expression of the same cytokines can drive the terminal differentiation and death of autoreactive T-cells. Thus some spontaneous models of autoimmune disease can be corrected by the injection of cytokines: IL-1 cures the diabetes of NOD mice, *tumor necrosis factor* (TNF) prevents the onset of SLE symptoms in NZB × W hybrids and *transforming growth factor-β* (TGFβ) is known to protect against collagen-induced arthritis and relapsing *experimental autoimmune encephalo-*

myelitis (EAE). The pleiotropic effects of the cytokines on different cell types involved at different stages in these diseases, and their positive and negative networking interactions with each other, add some uncertainty to the analysis and prediction of these complex events. Turning to human disorders, a window on cytokine activity in SLE has been provided by analysis showing expression of a number of genes known to be upregulated by interferon-α (Figure 18.15) and elevated levels of the cytokine that correlate with more severe disease.

Pathogenic effects of humoral autoantibody

We should now look at the evidence that helps to uncover the mechanisms by which autoimmunity, however it arises, plays a **primary pathogenic role** in the production of tissue lesions within the group of diseases labeled as "autoimmune." Let us look first at autoantibody effectors.

Blood cells

The erythrocyte antibodies play a dominant role in the destruction of red cells in **autoimmune hemolytic anemia**. Normal red cells coated with autoantibody eluted from Coombs' positive erythrocytes (cf. Figure 15.17) have a shortened half-life after reinjection into the normal subject, essentially as a result of their adherence to Fcγ receptors on phagocytic cells in the spleen.

Lymphopenia occurring in patients with systemic lupus erythematosus and rheumatoid arthritis (RA) may be a direct result of antibody, as nonagglutinating antibodies coating the white cells have been reported in such cases.

Platelet antibodies are apparently responsible for **idiopathic thrombocytopenic purpura** (ITP). IgG from a patient's serum when given to a normal individual causes a depression of platelet counts and the active component can be absorbed out with platelets. The transient neonatal thrombocytopenia that may be seen in infants of mothers with ITP is explicable in terms of transplacental passage of IgG antibodies to the child.

The primary **antiphospholipid syndrome** is characterized by recurrent venous and arterial thromboembolic phenomena, recurrent fetal loss, thrombocytopenia and cardiolipin antibodies. Passive transfer of such antibodies into mice is fairly devastating, resulting in lower fecundity rates and recurrent fetal loss. The effect seems to be mediated through reaction of the autoantibodies with a complex of cardiolipin and β_2-glycoprotein 1 that inhibits triggering of the coagulation cascade. The placental trophoblast is a primary target of these antibodies as the villous cytotrophoblast is one of the few cell types that externalizes phosphatidyl serine during development.

Surface receptors

Thyroid

Under certain circumstances antibodies to the surface of a cell may stimulate rather than destroy (cf. "stimulatory hypersensitivity"; Chapter 15). This is certainly the case in **Graves'**

disease (Basedow's disease) where a direct link with autoimmunity came with the discovery by Adams and Purves of thyroid-stimulating activity in the serum of these patients (Milestone 18.1), ultimately shown to be due to the presence of antibodies to TSH receptors (TSHRs), which mimic the effect of TSH (Figure 18.16a). Both operate through the adenyl cyclase system and produce similar changes in ultrastructural morphology in the thyroid cell. Under constant stimulation by the autoantibody an enlarged thyroid (referred to as a **goiter**) results, leading to **hyperthyroidism** (an overactive thyroid). This hyperthyroidism is often accompanied by exophthalmos (where the eyes bulge out from the orbit) that is probably due to inflammation caused by the fact that the TSHR is also expressed on orbital fibroblasts. It is one of nature's "passive transfer experiments" that links TSHR antibodies most directly with the pathogenesis of Graves' disease. When thyroid-stimulating antibodies from a pregnant female cross the placenta, they cause the production of neonatal hyperthyroidism (neonatal thyrotoxicosis) (Figure 18.17). This is essentially a transient form of Graves' disease in the offspring, except that in this case it is caused by maternal antibody rather

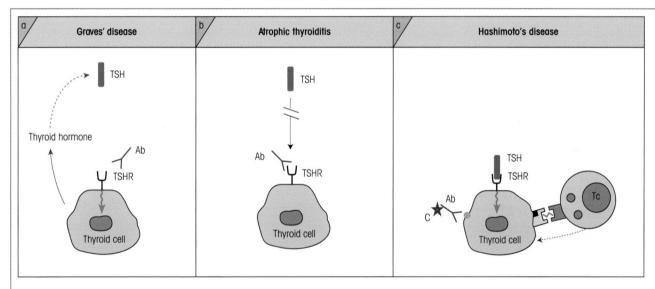

Figure 18.16. Thyroid autoimmune dieases.

The three major types of thyroid autoimmune disease are illustrated. (a) In Graves' disease autoantibodies bind to the thyroid-stimulating hormone receptor (TSHR) on thyroid epithelial cells. These antibodies act as agonists and mimic the effect of TSH. The autoantibodies are continuously produced from plasma cells and therefore their production is not directly affected by the levels of thyroid hormone, unlike the levels of TSH that are subject to a negative feedback loop and therefore decrease when adequate levels of thyroid hormone are produced. Constant activation of the thyroid cells by the stimulatory autoantibody results in hyperthyroidism. (b) In atrophic thyroiditis (primary myxedema) autoantibodies are also produced to the TSH receptor but bind to different epitopes to

those found in Graves' disease and act as antagonists rather the agonists. Their ability to block access of TSH to the TSHR results in hypothyroidism. (c) The autoantibodies in Hashimoto's disease are predominantly directed against thyroid peroxidase and thyroglobulin. The thyroid cells can be attacked by cytotoxic T-cells recognizing peptides derived from these autoantigens and/or by complement-fixing antibodies directed to intact autoantigen. Alhough TSH is able to bind to the TSH receptor and stimulate the thyroid cells the destruction of the thyroid by the autoimmune attack results in hypothyroidism. These diseases most likely form a spectrum of autoimmune thyroid conditions with some Hashimoto's disease patients also possesing either stimulatory or inhibitory anti-TSHR.

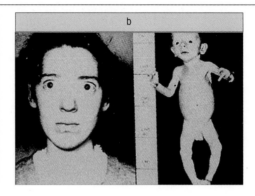

Figure 18.17. Neonatal thyrotoxicosis.

(a) The autoantibodies that stimulate the thyroid through the TSH receptors are IgG and cross the placenta. (b) The thyrotoxic mother therefore gives birth to a baby with thyroid hyperactivity that spontaneously resolves as the mother's IgG is catabolized. (Photograph courtesy of A. MacGregor.)

than autoantibody and is thus not an "autoimmune" disease in the infant. IgG has a half life of around 3 weeks and therefore the neonatal disease resolves after a few weeks as the maternal IgG is catabolized. Also remember, though, that the class switching to IgG that has occurred in the mother required T-cell assistance and therefore, although antibody in this instance seems quite clearly to be the effector in both the mother and the child, the primary defect in the immune response may well lie elsewhere.

By contrast, sera from patients with **atrophic thyroiditis** (primary myxedema) contain antibodies capable of blocking the stimulation by TSH (Figure 18.16b), resulting in **hypothyroidism** (an underactive thyroid). In **Hashimoto's disease** there is a destructive thyroiditis, with damage thought to be caused by thyroid-infiltrating CD8+ cytotoxic T-cells and also possibly by complement-fixing IgG autoantibodies (Figure 18.16c), again leading to hypothyroidism. The exact relationship between atrophic thyroiditis and Hashimoto's disease is not entirely clear but it is thought they may represent two ends of a spectrum of autoimmune thyroiditis.

Muscle and nerve

The transient muscle weakness seen in a small proportion of babies born to mothers with **myasthenia gravis** would, as in Graves' disease, be compatible with the transplacental passage of an IgG. In this case the antibody would be capable of inhibiting neuromuscular transmission. Strong support for this view is afforded by the consistent finding of antibodies to muscle acetylcholine receptors (AChRs) in myasthenics and the depletion of these receptors within the motor endplates. In addition, myasthenic symptoms can be induced in animals by injection of monoclonal antibodies to AChR or by active immunization with the purified receptors themselves. Nonetheless, the majority of babies with myasthenic mothers do not display muscle disease and, as appears to be the case in other transient neonatal

diseases caused by maternal antibody, this relates largely to the levels of autoantibodies present in the mother.

Neuromuscular defects can also be elicited in mice injected with serum from patients with the **Lambert–Eaton** syndrome containing antibodies to presynaptic calcium channels. Autoantibodies to sodium channels that cross-react with campylobacter bacilli have been identified in **Guillain–Barré syndrome**, a self-resolving peripheral polyneuritis.

Stomach

The underlying histopathological lesion in **pernicious anemia** is an atrophic gastritis in which a chronic inflammatory mononuclear invasion is associated with degeneration of secretory glands and failure to produce gastric acid. The development of achlorhydria is almost certainly accelerated by the inhibitory action of antibodies to the gastric proton pump, an H^+/K^+-dependent ATPase.

Other tissues

Gut

Some patients with **autoimmune atrophic gastritis** diagnosed by achlorhydria and parietal cell antibodies just meander on year after year without developing the vitamin B_{12} deficiency that precipitates **pernicious anemia**. It is probable that autoimmune destruction is roughly balanced by regeneration of mucosal cells, an explanation that could account for the observation that high doses of steroids may restore gastric function in certain patients with pernicious anemia. However, the balance would be upset were the patient now to produce antibodies to intrinsic factor in the lumen of the gastrointestinal tract; these would neutralize the small amount of intrinsic factor still available and the body would move into negative balance for vitamin B_{12}. The symptoms of vitamin B_{12} deficiency, pernicious anemia and sometimes subacute degeneration of the spinal cord, would then appear some considerable time later as the liver stores became exhausted

The normally acquired tolerance to dietary proteins seems to break down in **celiac disease** (p. 417) where T-cell sensitivity to wheat gluten in the small intestine can be demonstrated. As gluten can bind strongly to the extracellular matrix protein, endomysium, the uptake of the complex by IgA B-cells specific for endomysium might "piggy-back" the gluten into the B-cell for processing and presentation on MHC class II to gluten-specific T-helpers (cf. Figure 18.9). Stimulation of the B-cell would now follow with secretion of the IgA anti-endomysial autoantibodies that are exclusive to patients with celiac disease. Despite the presence of these autoantibodies, the dietary trigger means that this disease is considered to be a type IV hypersensitivity rather than a *bone fide* autoimmune disease.

Skin

An antibody pathogenesis for **pemphigus vulgaris** is favored by the correlation between disease severity and the titre of autoantibodies against desmoglein 3 (a member of the cadherin family of Ca^{2+}-dependent adhesion molecules) present at the cell-cell junctions of squamous epithelial cells. Likewise, antibodies to desmoglein 1 are thought to mediate the blistering of the epidermis in **pemphigus foliaceus**.

Sperm

In some **infertile males**, agglutinating antibodies cause aggregation of the spermatozoa and interfere with their penetration into the cervical mucus.

Glomerular basement membrane (GBM)

With immunological kidney disease, the experimental models preceded the finding of parallel lesions in the human. Injection of cross-reacting heterologous GBM preparations in complete Freund's adjuvant produces glomerulonephritis in sheep and other experimental animals. Antibodies to GBM can be picked up by immunofluorescent staining with anti-IgG of biopsies from nephritic animals. The antibodies are largely, if not completely, absorbed out by the kidney *in vivo* and can passively transfer the disease to another animal of the same species.

An entirely analogous situation occurs in humans in certain cases of glomerulonephritis, particularly those associated with lung hemorrhage (**Goodpasture's syndrome**). Kidney biopsy from the patient shows *linear* deposition of IgG and C3 along the basement membrane of the glomerular capillaries (see Figure 15.18a). Lerner and his colleagues eluted the GBM antibody from a diseased kidney and injected it into a squirrel monkey. The antibody rapidly fixed to the GBM of the recipient animal and produced a fatal nephritis. It is hard to escape the conclusion that the lesion in the human was the direct result of attack on the GBM by these complement-fixing antibodies. The lung changes in Goodpasture's syndrome are attributable to cross-reaction with some of the GBM antibodies.

Heart

Neonatal lupus erythematosus is the most common cause of permanent **congenital complete heart block**. Almost all cases have been associated with high maternal titers of anti-La/SS-B or anti-Ro/SS-A. The mother's heart is unaffected. The key observation was that anti-Ro bound to neonatal rather than adult cardiac tissue and altered the transmembrane action potential by inhibiting repolarization. IgG anti-Ro reaches the fetal circulation by transplacental passage but, although maternal and fetal hearts are exposed to the autoantibody, only the latter is affected. Anti-La also binds to affected fetal hearts reacting with laminin in the basement membrane.

Pathogenic effects of complexes with autoantigens

Systemic lupus erythematosus

Where autoantibodies are formed against soluble components to which they have continual access, complexes are formed that can give rise to type III hypersensitivity reactions, especially when defects in the early classical complement components prevent effective clearance. Thus, although homozygous complement deficiency is a rare cause of SLE, the archetypal immune complex disorder, it represents the most powerful disease susceptibility genotype so far identified; more than 80% of cases with homozygous C1q and C4 deficiency have SLE. Up to one-half of the patients carry autoantibodies to the collagenous portion of C1q, but in truth there are a rich variety of different autoantigens in lupus (cf. Table 18.2), some of them constituents of the nucleosome (cf. Figure 18.1b), with the most characteristic being **double-stranded DNA** (dsDNA). Anti-dsDNA is enriched in cryoglobulins and acid eluates of renal tissue from patients with lupus nephritis where it can be identified, in complexes containing complement, by immunofluorescent staining of kidney biopsies from patients with evidence of renal dysfunction. The staining pattern with a fluorescent anti-IgG or anti-C3 is punctate or "lumpy-bumpy" as once described (see Figure 15.18b), in marked contrast with the linear pattern caused by the GBM antibodies in Goodpasture's syndrome (Figure 15.18a). The complexes grow in size to become large aggregates visible in the electron microscope as amorphous humps on both sides of the GBM (Figure 18.18). During the active phase of the disease, serum complement levels fall as components are affected by immune aggregates in the kidney and circulation. Deposition of complexes is widespread as the name implies and, although 40% of patients eventually develop kidney lesions, the corresponding figures for organ involvement are 98% for skin (Figure 18.19), 98% for joints/muscle, 64% for lung, 60% for blood, 60% for brain and 20% for heart.

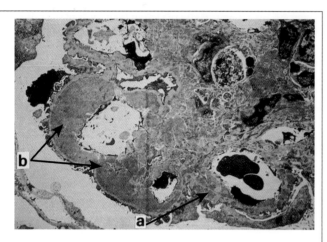

Figure 18.18. Renal biopsy of an SLE patient with severe immune complex glomerulonephritis and proteinuria.

Electron micrograph showing irregular thickening of glomerular capillary walls by subepithelial complexes (a) and subendothelial complexes (b). The mesangial region shows abundant (probably phagocytosed) complexes. (Courtesy of A. Leatham.)

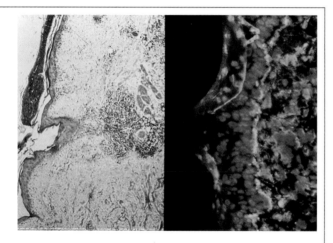

Figure 18.19. The "lupus band" in SLE.

Left—section of skin showing slight thickening of the dermo-epidermal junction with underlying scattered inflammatory cells and a major inflammatory focus in the deeper layers. Low power, hematoxylin and eosin (H&E) staining. *Right*—green fluorescence staining of a skin biopsy at higher power showing deposition of complexes containing IgG (anti-C3 gives the same picture) on the basement membrane at the dermoepidermal junction. (Kindly provided by D. Isenberg.)

Spontaneous production of anti-dsDNA is also a dominant feature of the animal models of SLE such as NZB × W and MRL/lpr mice, which involve fatal immune complex disease. The high affinity and IgG class of these antibodies, and the amelioration of symptoms and reduction of renal glomerular immune complexes by treatment of NZB × W mice with

DNase I or anti-CD4, provide convincing evidence for a T-dependent antigen-driven complex-mediated pathology. But as DNA itself is not a thymus-dependent antigen and the SLE autoantibodies include a cluster directed to the physically linked antigens constituting the nucleosome, one might envisage a "piggy-back" mechanism of the type portrayed in Figure 18.9. Knowing that nucleosome "blebs" appear that contain fragments of chromatin (DNA plus histones) on the surface of apoptotic cells and that a spontaneous expansion of nucleosome-specific T-cell populations precedes the clinical onset of SLE, a likely scenario is as follows. Nucleosome material is captured on the surface receptors of anti-DNA B-cells and internalized, followed by presentation of processed histone peptide–MHC class II complex to the histone-specific T-helper cells, and clonal proliferation of DNA antibody-forming cells (Figure 18.20). Complexes of anti-DNA with circulating nucleosome material are demonstrable, and these will bind through the histone to extracellular heparan sulfate where they can accumulate and damage end-organ targets such as the kidney glomerulus.

Rheumatoid arthritis

Morphological evidence for immunological activity

The joint changes in RA are in essence produced by the dysregulated and invasive growth of the synovial cells developing into what is referred to as a **pannus** that overlays and destroys cartilage and bone (Figure 18.21a–e). The synovial membrane that surrounds and maintains the joint space becomes intensely cellular as a result of considerable immunological hyperreactivity, as evidenced by large numbers of T-cells, mostly CD4, in various stages of activation, usually associated with dendritic cells and macrophages (Figure 18.21f); plasma cells are frequently observed and sometimes even secondary follicles with germinal centers are present as though the synovium had become an active lymph node (Figure 18.21g–j). There is widespread expression of surface HLA-DR (class II); T- and B-cells, dendritic and synovial lining cells and macrophages are all positive, indicative of some pretty lively action (Figure 18.21k). This fiery immunological reactivity provides an intense stimulus to the synovial lining cells that transform into the invasive pannus thereby bringing about joint erosion through the release of destructive mediators. Granulomatous rheumatoid nodules may also develop (Figure 18.21l,m).

IgG autosensitization and immune complex formation

Autoantibodies to the IgG Fc region (Figure 18.22a), known as **rheumatoid factors**, are a feature of the disease, being demonstrable in virtually all patients with RA. The majority have IgG or IgM rheumatoid factors. We must take into account a strange and unique feature of IgG rheumatoid factors; because they are both antigen and antibody at the same

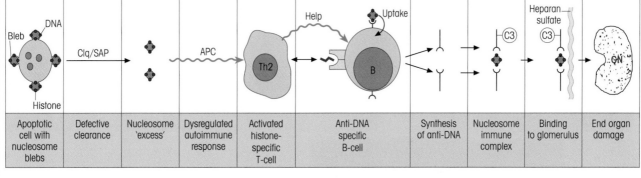

Figure 18.20. Conceivable pathogenetic pathway leading to end-organ damage in SLE.

Nucleosomes derived from apoptotic cells can stimulate anti-DNA production by a "piggy-back" mechanism in susceptible hosts. The resulting complexes bind to heparan sulfate in the glomerular basement membrane where they induce glomerulonephritis. The high incidence of lupus in C1q deficient individuals and the susceptibility of lupus patients to skin rashes on exposure to UV in sunlight, that induces apoptosis in skin cells, are well known. APC, antigen-presenting cell; GN, glomerulonephritis; SAP, serum amyloid precursor.

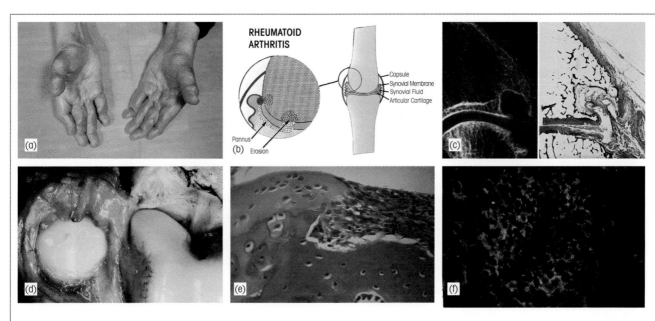

Figure 18.21. Rheumatoid arthritis (RA).

(a) Hands of a patient with chronic RA showing classical swan-neck deformities. (b) Diagrammatic representation of a diarthrodial joint showing bone and cartilagenous erosions beneath the synovial membrane-derived pannus. (c) Proximal interphalangeal joint depicting marked bony erosion and marginal erosion of the cartilage. (d) Early pannus of granulation tissue growing over the patella. (e) Histology of pannus showing clear erosion of bone and cartilage at the cellular margin. (f) Rheumatoid synovium showing class II-positive antigen-presenting cells (green) in intimate contact with CD4+ T-cells (orange).

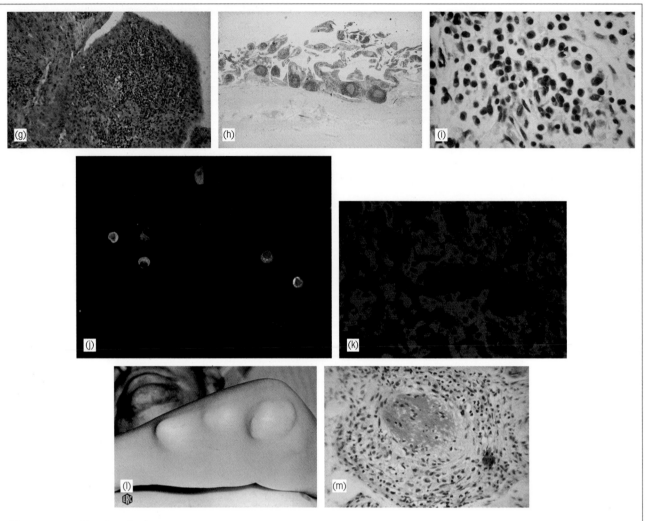

Figure 18.21. (*Continued*)

(g) Chronic inflammatory cells in the deep layers of the synovium in RA. (h) A hypervillous synovium revealing well-formed secondary follicles with germinal centers (relatively rare occurrence). (i) A high power view of an area of diseased synovium showing collections of classical plasma cells. (j) Plasma cells isolated from a patient's synovial tissue stained simultaneously for IgM (with fluorescein-labeled F(ab′)₂ anti-μ) and rheumatoid factor (with rhodamine-labeled aggregated Fcγ). Two of the four IgM-positive plasma cells appear to be synthesizing rheumatoid factors. (k) Rheumatoid synovium showing large numbers of cells stained by anti-HLA-DR (anti-class II) antibodies. (l) Large rheumatoid nodules on the forearm. (m) Granulomatous appearance of the rheumatoid nodule with central necrotic area surrounded by epithelioid cells, macrophages and scattered lymphocytes. Plasma cells making rheumatoid factor are often demonstrable and the lesion probably represents a response to the formation of insoluble anti-IgG complexes. (Kindly given by: D. Isenberg (a); L.E. Glynn (c–e, g–i); G. Janossy (f, k); and P. Youinou and P. Lydyard (j).)

time they are capable of **self-association** (Figure 18.22b) to form what are in effect "hermaphroditic" immune complexes. IgG aggregates can be detected in the synovial tissues and in the joint fluid where they give rise to typical acute inflammatory reactions with fluid exudates.

The percentage of Fcγ sugars completely lacking galactose in the IgG of RA patients is nearly always higher than in the controls. It is well established that pregnant women with RA have a remission of their disease as they approach term, but an exacerbation postpartum; as the arthritis remits, the agalacto-IgG values fall but, as the disease worsens after birth, agalacto-IgG becomes abnormal again suggesting intimate involvement with the disease process.

The production of tissue damage

As explained in the legend to Figure 18.22, the immune complexes can be stabilized by the multivalent Fcγ-binding

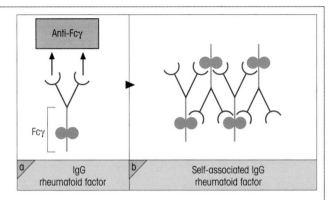

Figure 18.22. Self-associated complexes of IgG rheumatoid factor.

(a,b) Although of relatively low affinity, the strength of binding is boosted by the "bonus effect" of the mutual attachment and, furthermore, such complexes in the joint may be stabilized by IgM rheumatoid factor (IgM anti-Fcγ) and C1q which have polyvalent binding sites for IgG.

molecules, IgM rheumatoid factor and C1q, and when present in the joint space they may provoke an influx of neutrophils leading to the release of *r*eactive *o*xygen *i*ntermediates (ROIs) and lysosomal enzymes. These include neutral proteases and collagenase that can **damage the articular cartilage** by breaking down proteoglycans and collagen fibrils. More damage results if the complexes are adherent to the cartilage, as the neutrophil binds but is unable to internalize them ("frustrated phagocytosis"); as a result, the lysosomal hydrolases are released extracellularly into the space between the cell and the cartilage where they are protected from enzyme inhibitors such as α₂-macroglobulin.

The aggregates may also stimulate the macrophage-like cells of the synovial lining, either directly through their surface receptors or indirectly through phagocytosis and resistance to intracellular digestion. At this point we should acknowledge that the release of cytokines such as TNF and GM-CSF from activated T-cells (see below) provides further potent macrophage stimulation. The activated synovial cells grow out as pannus over the cartilage (Figure 18.21d) and, at the margin of this advancing tissue, breakdown can be seen (Figure 18.21e), almost certainly as a result of the release of enzymes, ROIs and especially of IL-1, IL-6 and TNF. Activated macrophages also secrete plasminogen activator and the plasmin formed as a consequence activates a latent collagenase produced by synovial cells. The secreted products of the stimulated macrophage can influence chondrocytes (the cells that secrete and maintain the cartilage) to exacerbate **cartilage breakdown**, and osteoclasts to bring about **bone resorption** that is a further complication of severe disease (Figure 18.21c).

T-cell-mediated hypersensitivity as a pathogenic factor in autoimmune disease

Arthritis again

In rheumatoid artritis the chronically inflamed synovium is densely crowded with activated T-cells and their critical role in the disease process is emphasized by the beneficial effects of cyclosporine and anti-CD4 treatments. High levels of IL-15 within the synovial membrane can recruit and activate T-cells whose secretion of cytokines and ability to induce macrophage synthesis of TNF and further IL-15 drives pannus development with consequent erosion of cartilage and bone (Figure 18.21e). Chondrocytes themselves may also be disease targets.

The antigenic history of **reactive arthritis** is more amenable to study as it is triggered by an infection either of the urogenital tract by *Chlamydia trachomatis* or of the enteric tract with *Yersinia*, *Salmonella*, *Shigella* or *Campylobacter*. All these microbes are either obligate or facultative intracellular bacteria and so may escape the immune system by hiding inside cells. However, we may be dealing with molecular mimicry. Natural infection of mice with *Salmonella typhimurium* generates CD8 cytotoxic T-cells that recognize an immunodominant epitope of the GroEL molecule presented by the class Ib Qa-1 and cross-react with a peptide from mouse hsp60, so permitting a reaction with stressed macrophages. In humans, HLA-B27 individuals are particularly at risk of developing reactive arthritis and the importance of the microbial component is emphasized by experiments on mice bearing an HLA-B27 transgene; if reared in a germ-free environment, lesions are restricted to the skin, but in the microbiological wilderness of the normal animal house, the skin, gut and joints are all affected. Why, as in RA, are the joints targeted and what does B27 do? Only one in 300 of the T-cells in the reactive arthritis synovium is CD8 and therefore class I restricted. It could be that a cross-reactive B27 sequence functions as a cryptic epitope perpetuating a gentle microbial stimulus with an amplifying autoimmune response.

Another rheumatological condition closely associated with HLA-B27 is **ankylosing spondylitis** (AS). It is only recently that autoantibodies have been described in this condition, with specificity for a range of connective & skeletal tissue proteins. The beneficial effects of anti-TNF therapy indicate an important role for this cytokine in disease pathogenesis. Despite the very strong class I association, studies in the HLA-B27 transgenic rat, a model for human AS, indicate the CD8⁺ cytotoxic T-cells do not play a role in disease pathogenesis. Rather, the tendency of HLA-B27 molecules to misfold in the endoplasmic reticulum, and subsequently dimerise, leads to an unfolded protein stress response resulting in excessive production of IL-23 by Th17 cells following pattern recognition receptor activation. Polymorphisms of the IL-23 receptor gene are associated with the development of AS in humans.

Organ-specific endocrine disease

Hashimoto's disease

The inflammatory infiltrate in Hashimoto's thyroiditis (see Figure M18.1.1c) represents a T-cell-mediated hypersensitivity. The demonstration of class II molecules on patients' thyroid epithelial cells and the presence of antigen-specific Th1 cells in the thyroid implicate the involvement of these cells. Destruction of the thyroid epithelial cells may involve engagement of Fas on their surface with subsequent induction of apoptosis.

We must turn to the animal models for further evidence, albeit indirect. Removal of T-cells in the Obese strain (OS) chicken prevents the spontaneous development of thyroiditis and, at the target cell level, the threshold for induction of MHC class II on OS thyroid epithelial cells by IFNγ is far lower than that reported for normal thyroid cells, further reinforcing the notion that a thyroid abnormality is a contributory factor to the susceptibility phenotype. Another model, in which thyroiditis is induced by thyroglobulin in complete Freund's adjuvant (see Figure M18.1.1b), can be transferred to naïve histocompatible recipients with CD4+ T-cell clones specific for peptides containing thyroxine.

Type 1 diabetes

Just as in autoimmune thyroiditis, type 1 diabetes involves chronic inflammatory infiltration and destruction of the specific tissue, in this case the insulin-producing β-cells of the pancreatic islets of Langerhans. The delay in onset of disease achieved by early treatment with cyclosporine, at levels that have little effect on antibody production, points an accusing finger at effector T-cells as the agents of destruction, as this drug targets T-cell cytokine synthesis so specifically. *In vitro* T-cell responses to islet cell antigens including glutamic acid decarboxylase (GAD) directly reflect the risk of progression to clinical diabetes. The strength of the risk factors associated with certain HLA-DQ alleles also has a strong whiff of T-cell action.

To obtain further insight into the cellular siege and destruction of the islet β-cells, one has to look to the **nonobese diabetic (NOD) mouse** that spontaneously develops diabetic disease closely resembling human type 1 diabetes in its range of autoimmune responses and the association of islet breakdown with a chronic infiltration by T-cells and macrophages (Figure 18.23). Many of the T-cells infiltrating the islets in diabetic mice have a Th1-type cytokine profile and can transfer disease to NOD recipients congenic for the severe combined immunodeficiency (*SCID*) mutation. However, increases in Th17-derived IL-21 resulting from NOD-associated polymorphisms in the binding site for the Sp1 transcription factor in the promoter region of the *IL-21* gene are also strongly implicated.

Up to 50% of the infiltrating T-cells isolated from pre-diabetic NOD islets are insulin-specific and can transfer disease to young NOD mice. However, GAD-specific T-cells can also be recovered and these too are diabetogenic.

GAD in the central and peripheral nervous system produces γ-aminobutyric acid (GABA), a major inhibitory neurotransmitter, from glutamine. Autoantibodies to GAD are seen not only in type I diabetes, but also in **stiff man syndrome** where the GABA-ergic pathways controlling motor neuron activity are defective. The antibodies cannot be pathogenic because GAD is present on the inner surface of the plasma membrane, but T-cells could be. How the brain as distinct from the pancreatic islet could be specifically targeted is a conundrum but 30% of patients do develop type 1 diabetes.

Multiple sclerosis (MS)

The idea that MS could be an autoimmune disease has for long been proposed due to its morphological resemblance to *e*xperimental *a*utoimmune *e*ncephalomyelitis (EAE, originally described by the alternative name experimental autoallergic encephalomyelitis). This demyelinating disease is produced by immunization with myelin, usually *m*yelin *b*asic *p*rotein (MBP) in complete Freund's, leading to motor paralysis (Figure 18.24). T-cell clones specific for MBP will transfer disease but this can be exacerbated by injection of a monoclonal antibody to Theiler's virus, a murine encephalomyelitis virus, cross-reacting with an epitope on myelin and oligodendrocytes. Presumably the T-cell incites a local inflammation affecting the endothelial cells at the blood–brain barrier that opens the gate for antibody to penetrate the brain tissue.

In humans the serologically defined white DR2 phenotype (DRB1*15:01, DQA1*01:02, DQB1*06:02) is strongly associated with susceptibility to MS. Furthermore, at least 37% of activated T-cells responsive to IL-2/4 in cerebrospinal fluid are specific for myelin components, compared with a figure of 5% for subjects with other neurological disturbances. These hints that we are dealing with an autoimmune disease is strengthened by the observation that a Leu-Arg-Gly amino acid sequence motif found in around 40% of TCR Vβ5.2 N(D)N rearrangements in T-cells from MS lesions is present in a Vβ5.2 clone from an MS patient cytotoxic towards targets containing the MBP 89–106 peptide. One is greatly encouraged to continue with attempts to induce tolerance.

Some other diseases with autoimmune activity

Attacks on the vasculature

The characteristic feature of **Wegener's granulomatosis** is a necrotizing granulomatous vasculitis associated with the presence of antineutrophil cytoplasmic antibodies (cANCA, Figure 18.25). Although these autoantibodies are directed to the intracellular protease III in the primary granules of the neutrophil, TNF priming of these cells causes translocation of the protease to the cell surface. The autoantibody then activates the cell causing degranulation with the release of various proteolytic enzymes, and the generation of reactive oxygen

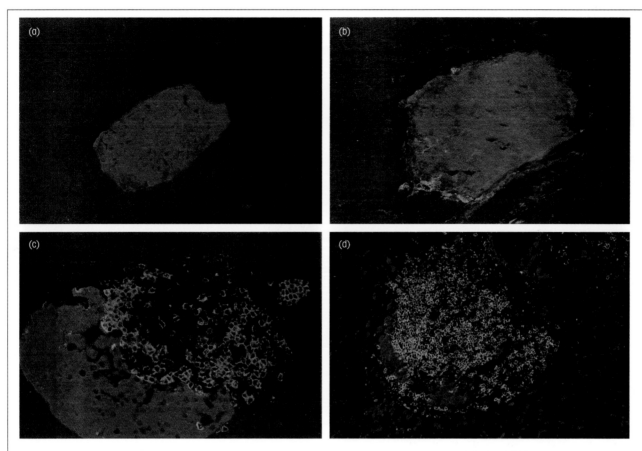

Figure 18.23. Destruction of pancreatic islet β-cells by infiltrating T-cells in the nonobese diabetic (NOD) mouse.

(a) Normal intact islet. (b) Early peri-islet infiltration. (c) Penetration of the islet by infiltrating T-cells. (d) Almost complete destruction of insulin-producing cells with replacement by invading T-cells. Insulin stained by rhodamine-conjugated antibodies and T-cells by fluoresceinated anti-CD3. (Data reproduced from Quartey-Papafio R. *et al.* (1995) *Journal of Immunology* **154**, 5567–5575; photographs kindly provided by J. Phillips.)

*i*ntermediates (ROIs), which together damage the blood vessel endothelium thereby accounting for the vasculitic lesions.

Giant cell arteritis (sometimes referred to as temporal arteritis because the temporal artery is often involved) is a vasculitis of large- and medium-sized arteries affecting around 1 in 500 individuals over the age of 50. It gets its name from the presence of multinucleate giant cells which result from the fusion of macrophages. The dendritic cells, macrophages and CD4+ T-cells in the lesion are thought to be central to the pathogenesis. Putative autoantigens are presented by the dendritic cells to Th1 cells whose copious production of IFNγ leads the macrophages to secrete IL-1β and IL-6. Reactive oxygen intermediates and matrix metalloproteases are also produced by the activated macrophages resulting in vessel damage. In addition, IFNγ stimulates the giant cells to produce vascular endothelial growth factor (VEGF) that promotes the growth of capillaries, and the interferon also causes both giant cells and conventional macrophages to secrete platelet-derived growth factor (PDGF) leading to proliferation of the intimal

cells that form the inner lining of the blood vessel. The antigen is elusive but the disease is strongly associated with HLA-DR4 and is exquisitely sensitive to high-dose steroids.

Scleroderma, also known as **systemic sclerosis**, is divided into two major subgroups, limited cutaneous scleroderma where, as the name suggests, lesions are generally restricted to the skin, and diffuse cutaneous scleroderma where internal organs are also damaged. Both forms are characterized by increased deposition of collagen and other matrix components, causing extensive fibrosis of the skin and internal organs centered around small arteries and microvasculature, eventually producing capillary occlusion. The pathogenesis is poorly understood, but the presence of centromere, nucleolar and topoisomerase-1 (Scl-70) autoantibodies suggests some major intrusion by autoimmune elements, and the lesions are infiltrated by T- and B-cells, macrophages and mast cells. The T-cells are mostly of the Th2 phenotype, and B-cells may contribute to the production of TGFβ and IL-6. Mutations in the fibrillin-1 gene coding for an extracellular matrix protein

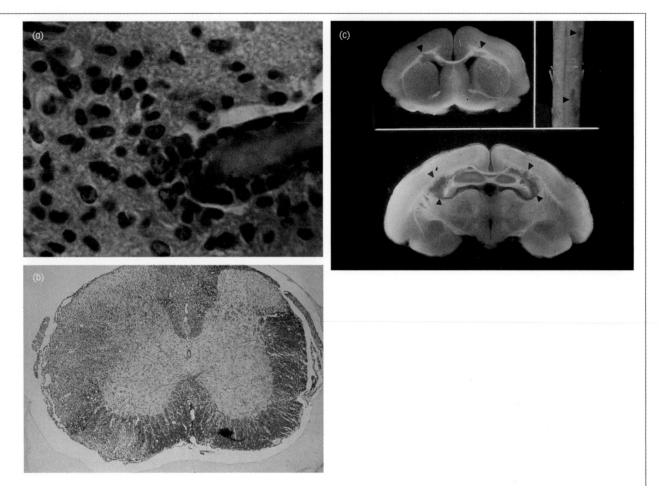

Figure 18.24. Experimental autoimmune encephalomyelitis (EAE), a demyelinating model for multiple sclerosis induced by immunization with brain antigens in complete Freund's adjuvant (CFA).

(a) Early lesion of EAE in the rat at 9 days after immunization with rat spinal cord homogenate in CFA. The lesion in brain white matter, which is probably a few hours old, shows perivenous infiltration of lymphocytes and monocytes (a pure mononuclear inflammation) with cells invading the nervous parenchyma. Myelin is not stained. (b) Lumbar spinal cord of rat with chronic EAE after immunization with myelin proteolipid protein. Large demyelinating lesions in dorsal columns, in both left (large) and right (small) columns, as well as on lower left. Also gray matter involved with ongoing inflammation, in particular affecting left dorsal horn. Normal myelin is stained brown. (c) Chronic relapsing EAE in guinea-pig. Large demyelinated plaques in brain white matter (arrows) closely similar to plaques of multiple sclerosis. (Legend and slides provided by B. Waksman; (b) originally from Trotter and (c) from Lassmann and Wisniewski.)

might play an important role by increasing the deposition of polymers of this protein that are known to activate the pro-fibrotic activity of TGFβ.

Atherosclerotic plaques are focal lesions in large elastic and muscular arteries. The plaques cause intimal thickening and are composed of a subendothelial fibrous cap of collagen and matrix-rich connective tissue, foam cells (lipid-filled macrophages) and proliferating smooth muscle cells. Rupture of a plaque leads to thrombosis. T-cells, mostly of the Th1 phenotype, B-cells, macrophages, dendritic cells, mast cells and neutrophils are all present in the lesion. This has led to the idea that atherosclerosis may be an autoimmune disease. The lead candidate autoantigens are low density lipoprotein (LDL), heat-shock protein (hsp) and β₂-glycoprotein-1. Macrophage scavenger receptors take up oxidized LDL, including the highly proinflammatory adducts malondialdehyde and 4-hydroxynonenal aldehyde, and may then present these autoantigens to the T-cells. Furthermore, immune complexes that contain IgG, oxidized LDL and β₂ glycoprotein-1 are thought to be pro-atherogenic. Also of note is that immunization with mycobacterial hsp65 elicits atherosclerotic lesions at sites subject to major hemodynamic stress, and a cholesterol-rich diet makes them worse. Antibodies and Th1 cells are produced that react with human hps60 (Figure 18.26) due to its substantial sequence homology with mycobacterial hsp65. With a prevalence of 1.7% in the USA, atherosclerosis would

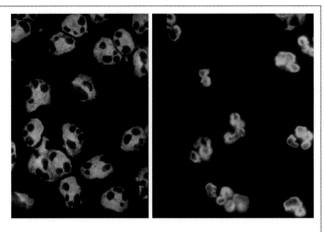

Figure 18.25. Antineutrophil cytoplasmic antibodies (ANCA).

Left—cytoplasmic cANCA diffuse staining specific for protease III in Wegener's granulomatosis; *right*—perinuclear p-ANCA staining by myeloperoxidase antibodies in periarteritis nodosa. Fixed neutrophils are treated first with patient's serum then fluorescein-conjugated anti-human Ig. (Kindly provided by G. Cambridge.)

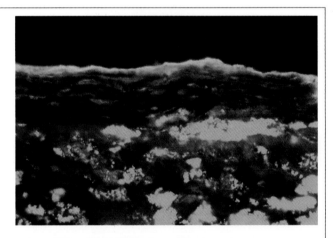

Figure 18.26. Expression of heat-shock protein 60 in an early human arteriosclerotic lesion.

Frozen, unfixed, 4-µm thick section of a fatty streak (=early lesion) of a human carotid artery stained in indirect immunofluorescence with a monoclonal antibody to heat-shock protein 60 and a fluorescein-labeled secondary antibody. A strong reaction with endothelial cells as well as cells infiltrating the intima, including foam cells, is evident. (Original magnification ×400.) (Photograph kindly provided by G. Wick.)

rank as almost the most common autoimmune disease if it were to be generally accepted as such.

Possible autoimmune diseases of the skin

We have already mentioned quite a few autoimmune diseases with skin involvement, including the fibrosis seen in sclero-

derma and the characteristic butterfly rash in systemic lupus erythematosus. Pretibial myxedema is seen in some patients with Graves' disease, and skin blistering occurs in both pemphigus vulgaris and pemphigus foliaceus. The evidence that these various conditions represent autoimmune diseases is pretty strong. However, there are other diseases affecting skin, which may also turn out to be autoimmune. Thus, although it is currently unclear whether the chronic inflammation in **psoriasis**, a condition affecting around 2% of the population, is driven by an infectious agent, by autoantigen, or by a response to stressed or damaged cells, a profound immunological involvement seems beyond doubt. If an autoimmune pathology is confirmed, then psoriasis will go straight to the top of the "hit parade" in Table 18.2. Immunological meddling is underscored by dendritic cell and T-cell infiltration of the psoriatic plaques, with the $\alpha_1\beta_1$ integrin on the T-cells binding to type IV collagen in the epidermal basement membrane. Many of these T-cells are of the Th17 subset and secrete IL-17A and IL-22, the latter cytokine known to be a potent inducer of keratinocyte proliferation. The therapeutic effectiveness of antibodies against either TNF or against the shared p40 component of the heterodimeric IL-12 and IL-23 cytokines only serves to re-enforce the immunological contribution to this disease.

An autoimmune component has also been proposed for the skin depigmentation seen in **vitiligo**. This disease, it should be pointed out, has an increased incidence in patients with known autoimmune disorders, particularly Graves' disease. The presence of autoreactive T-cells and antibodies against melanocytes certainly arouses one's suspicions. Of particular interest is the discovery of blocking autoantibodies against the melanin-concentrating hormone receptor 1, although a direct role in pathogenesis is yet to be established.

Measurement of autoantibodies

Some of the tests employed in the detection of autoantibodies are illustrated in Figures 6.8, 6.29, 6.30 and 18.1. Serum autoantibodies frequently provide valuable diagnostic markers. Screening of the serum can be carried out by immunofluorescence on frozen tissue sections. Agglutination tests are available for rheumatoid factors and for thyroglobulin, thyroid peroxidase and red cell antibodies as well as ELISAs for antibodies to intrinsic factor, DNA, IgG, extractable nuclear antigens, and so on. Purified gene-cloned antigens in minispot array ELISAs or in addressable laser bead assays (ALBAs) are taking over and beginning to supplant the need for immunofluorescence which is time-consuming and more skilled.

Autoantibody detection tests will also prove of value in screening for people at risk, e.g. relatives of patients with autoimmune diseases such as type 1 diabetes where antibodies against GAD, IA2 and insulin are predictive of future disease onset (particularly so if all three antibodies are present). Unfortunately quite what one does to prevent the disease arising in the autoantibody–positive relatives is, at this point in time, not entirely clear.

Therapeutic options

Organ-specific autoimmunity

The majority of approaches to treatment, not unnaturally, involve manipulation of immunological responses (Figure 18.27). However, in many organ-specific diseases, metabolic control is usually sufficient, e.g. thyroxine replacement in autoimmune thyroiditis (Hashimoto's disease and atrophic thyroiditis), insulin in type 1 diabetes, vitamin B_{12} in pernicious anemia. In Graves' disease antithyroid drugs that block the action of the thyroid peroxidase required for the production of thyroid hormone can be given, or alternatively the thyroid ablated with ^{131}I or the surgical approach of subtotal thyroidectomy used. Anticholinesterase drugs are commonly used for long-term therapy in myasthenia gravis, and thymectomy is also an option with well established efficacy. Transplantation of pancreatic islets can be used for type I diabetics although with all the problems associated with any graft, i.e. shortage of donors, the need to match HLA, and the requirement for potentially harmful immunosuppressive drugs. Encapsulation of the islets to prevent allograft rejection is one approach that is being actively explored.

Based on the possibility that multiple sclerosis (MS) is virally driven, patients were treated with IFNβ; relapse rates were reduced by a third in relapsing–remitting disease and this has become a standard treatment for this form of the disease. However, there is only a modest effect on progressive disease. It is likely that IFNβ is not acting primarily as an anti-viral in MS, but rather exhibiting anti-inflammatory and immunomodulatory activities via multiple actions on T-cells. Natalizumab, a humanized monoclonal antibody against the

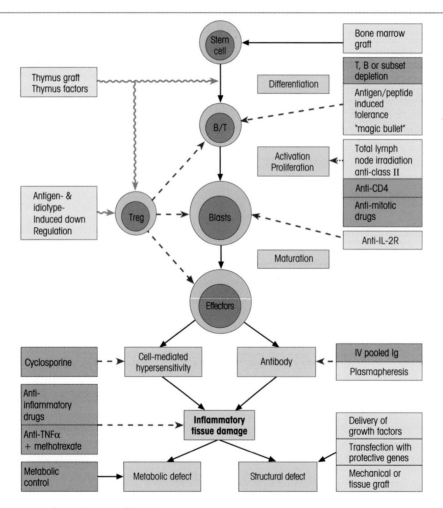

Figure 18.27. The treatment of autoimmune disease.

Current conventional treatments are in dark orange; some feasible approaches are given in lighter orange boxes. (In the case of a live graft, bottom right, the immunosuppressive therapy used may protect the tissue from the autoimmune damage that affected the organ being replaced.) IV, intravenous.

α_4-integrin, can reduce the number of relapses by two-thirds although it carries the risk of triggering progressive multifocal leukoencephalopathy, a condition that actually exacerbates myelin breakdown. It is therefore only used in those patients with relapsing–remitting MS that have failed to respond adequately to IFNβ and in patients with rapidly evolving severe relapsing-remitting disease.

Disease-modifying anti-rheumatic drugs (DMARDs)

Nonsteroidal anti-inflammatory drugs (NSAIDs) are effective in reducing inflammation but have little effect on disease progression. Patients with RA and with other autoimmune diseases respond well to high doses of steroids but there are significant adverse side effects associated with long term use. Disease-modifying anti-rheumatic drugs (DMARDs) such as methotrexate (MTX), sulfasalazine, gold salts and leflunomide can be effective. For example, the active metabolite of leflunomide inhibits *de novo* rUMP synthesis thereby leading to G_1 arrest of cycling lymphocytes.

A major advance in therapy came with the finding that neutralizing TNF with a monoclonal antibody is highly effective, so revealing the pathogenetic role of this cytokine. Following this observation three anti-TNF agents have been approved for use in RA: infliximab, a mouse–human chimeric monoclonal anti-TNF, adalimumab, a human monoclonal anti-TNF, and etanercept, a fusion protein of the extracellular ligand binding region of the TNF receptor and the Fcγ portion of IgG. Anti-TNFs can be used effectively in combination with methotrexate (Figure 18.28).

Anti-mitotic drugs

Conventional nonspecific antimitotic agents such as azathioprine, cyclophosphamide and methotrexate, usually in combination with steroids, have been used effectively in SLE, RA, chronic active hepatitis and autoimmune hemolytic anemia, for example.

In a sense, because it blocks cytokine secretion by T-cells, cyclosporine is an anti-inflammatory drug and, as cytokines like IL-2 are also obligatory for lymphocyte proliferation, cyclosporine is also an antimitotic drug. It is of proven efficacy in uveitis, early type 1 diabetes, nephrotic syndrome and psoriasis and of moderate efficacy in idiopathic thrombocytopenic purpura, SLE, polymyositis, primary biliary cirrhosis and myasthenia gravis.

High-dose IV cyclophosphamide plus adrenocorticotropic hormone (ACTH) or total lymph node irradiation through its effect on the peripheral immune system either slowed or stopped the advance of disease in approximately two-thirds of progressive multiple sclerosis (MS) patients for 1–2 years, a strong indication that the disease is mediated by immune mechanisms. This is further supported by the unfortunate finding that IFNγ exacerbates disease in the majority of patients.

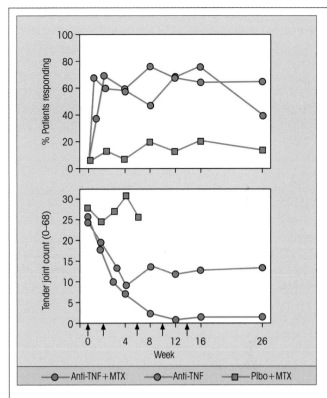

Figure 18.28. Combination of anti-TNF and methotrexate in the treatment of rheumatoid arthritis.

Top panel: Duration of response to therapy as defined by 20% Paulus criteria at three doses of monoclonal chimeric anti-TNF (infliximab) with and without methotrexate (MTX) and placebo (Plbo) plus MTX. Results shown are the proportion (%) of patients responding at weeks 1, 2, 4, 8, 12, 16 and 26. The Paulus response is achieved by 20% improvement in four out of six of the following: tender joint and swollen joint scores, duration of morning stiffness, erythrocyte sedimentation rate and a two-grade improvement in the patient's and observer's assessment of disease severity. Lower panel: Serial measurements (median values) of the tender joint count, before (day 0), during (weeks 1–14) and after (weeks 14–26) treatment. Results are included only up to the point at which ≥50% of patients remained in the trial (up to week 6 for the placebo plus MTX group). Arrows indicate the timing of infusions of infliximab at weeks 0, 2, 6, 10 and 14. Methotrexate was given weekly and virtually eradicated the production of antibodies to the human chimeric antibody. Note the normalization of defective regulatory T-cell function by this treatment (cf. Figure 18.13). (Data kindly provided by R.N. Maini, M. Feldmann, *et al.* see Maini R.N. *et al.* (1998) *Arthritis and Rheumatism* **41**, 1552–1563. Reproduced with permission from Lippincott Williams & Wilkins, MD, USA.)

Immunological control strategies

Cellular manipulation

It should one day be practical to correct any relevant defects in stem cells or in thymus processing by gene therapy, bone marrow or thymus grafting or perhaps, in the latter case, by thymic hormones. Many centers are carrying out autologous stem cell transplantation following hemato-immunoablation by cytotoxic drugs in severe cases of autoimmune disease in an attempt the "reset" the immune response. Overall, over one-third of difficult cases of SLE, scleroderma, juvenile and adult RA and so on achieve drug-free remission. Transplant-related mortality is around 5%, comparable to that seen with cancer patients.

Because T-cell signaling is so pivotal, it is the target for many strategies. Injection of monoclonal anti-MHC class II and anti-CD4 successfully fends off lupus in spontaneous mouse models. Some take the anti-IL-2 receptor approach to deplete activated T-cells, but we would like to refer back to our discussion of the long-lasting effect of *nondepleting* anti-CD4 for the induction of tolerance (Figure 16.14), particularly when reinforced by repeated exposure to antigen (cf. p. 436). Antigen reinforcement of course is an obvious continuing feature in autoimmune disease, so that anti-CD4 should be ideal as a therapy in disorders where the natural "switch-off" tolerogenic signals are still accepted by the CD4 cells. Abatacept, which has gained regulatory approval for use in RA, is a fusion protein of the extracellular domain of CTLA-4 with Fcγ. Its binding to CD80 and CD86 blocks the action of these co-stimulatory molecules, leading to T-cell anergy.

Pulsing relapsing-remitting MS patients with alemtuzumab (Campath-1H, a humanized anti-CD52) produced a brutal and surprisingly persistent reduction in T-cell numbers, with around 80% of patients having no relapses in 3 years post-treatment. This result compares with about 50% who received IFNβ. One has to balance this improvement against the side effects of alemtuzumab treatment that include precipitation of

the development of either idiopathic thrombocytopenic purpura or Graves' disease in some patients.

Now, if one takes the view that rheumatoid factor immune complexes are major players in the pathogenesis of the RA joint lesions, logic suggests the radical approach of B-cell ablation with rituximab, a mouse-human chimeric monoclonal anti-CD20, as used in the treatment of B-cell leukemia. B-cells may also play a role as antigen-presenting cells for T-cell activation, and are of course also the source of the antibodies to citrullinated peptides/proteins that are so characteristically associated with RA. Successful clinical trials have led to the licensing of rituximab for use, in combination with methotrexate, in RA patients that fail to respond adequately to anti-TNF treatment (Figure 18.29). There looks to be a good future for similar therapy in SLE, Sjögren's syndrome and dermatomyositis–polymyositis.

Manipulation of regulatory mediators

Some spontaneous models of autoimmune disease can be corrected by injection of cytokines: IL-1 cures the diabetes of NOD mice; TNF prevents the onset of SLE symptoms in NZB × W hybrids; and transforming growth factor-β1 (TGFβ1) is known to protect against collagen arthritis and relapsing EAE. Cytokine action can be blocked using specific monoclonals, soluble versions of receptors, or natural antagonists. We have already discussed the use of anti-TNFs. Other biologics targeting regulatory mediators that have been approved for the treatment of RA include anakinra, a recombinant nonglycosylated IL-1 receptor antagonist, and tocilizumab, a humanized anti-IL6 receptor. Monoclonal antibodies

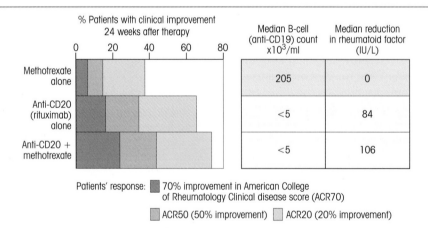

Figure 18.29. B-cell depletion therapy in patients with active rheumatoid arthritis.

Rituximab, a humanized monoclonal antibody specific for B-cell CD20, can act in combination with the anti-mitotic agents cyclophosphamide or methotrexate to produce marked amelioration of disease. (Data adapted from Edwards J.C.W. *et al.* (2004) *New England Journal of Medicine* **350**, 2572–2581.)

against IL-15, IL-17 and the shared p40 subunit of IL-12/23 are also being investigated for efficacy in RA, as are small molecule inhibitors of the p38, JAK3 and syk signal transduction kinases involved in lymphocyte activation.

Pooled normal immunoglobulin

Intravenous injection of Ig pooled from several thousand normal donors has long been used for the treatment of patients with immunodeficiencies affecting B-cells (p. 374). However, in the 1980s it was discovered that it also frequently has a beneficial effect in a number of autoimmune diseases including idiopathic thrombocytopenia, multiple sclerosis, dermatomyositis and myasthenia gravis. The inhibitory effects of $F(ab')_2$ fractions in patients with autoantibodies to procoagulant factor VIII suggest a possible role for anti-idiotypic reactions. However, in an animal model of RA (involving injection of arthritis-inducing serum from K/B × N transgenic mice into C57Bl/6 mice), administration of either biochemically-produced or recombinant Fcγ possessing 2,6-sialylated glycans reduced inflammation, possibly due to enhanced expression of the inhibitory FcγRIIb.

Manipulation by antigen

The object is to present the offending antigen in sufficient concentration and in a form that will turn off an ongoing autoimmune response. As T-cells have been accorded such a pivotal role, it is natural to devise the strategy in terms of T-cell epitopes rather than whole antigen, obviously a far more practical proposition because this reduces the problem to dealing with relatively short peptides. One strategy is to design high affinity peptide analogs (altered peptide ligands) that will bind obstinately to the appropriate MHC molecule and antagonize the response to autoantigen. As we express several different MHC molecules, this should not impair microbial defenses unduly. However, we are now talking of patients not mice and this could involve repeated very high doses of peptide, although, much in their favor, peptides are well defined chemically and *relatively* cheap to produce. Antigen-specific suppression of T-cells would be advantageous in this respect, and giving the peptide under an umbrella of anti-CD4 or using partial agonists could be feasible. Injection of an MBP peptide, particularly as a palmitoylated derivative inserted in liposomes, can block EAE and an hsp60 peptide can prevent the onset of diabetes in the NOD mouse (cf. p. 500).

We have already noted that, because the mucosal surface of the gut is exposed to a horde of powerfully immunogenic microorganisms, and as enterocytes are especially vulnerable to damage by IFNγ and TNF, it has been important for the immune defenses of the gut to evolve mechanisms that deter Th1-type responses. This objective is attained by the stimulation of regulatory cells that release cytokines such as TGFβ, IL-4 and IL-10 and suppress the unwanted responses. Thus feeding antigens should tolerize Th1 cells and this has proved to be a successful strategy for blocking EAE, as well as the type

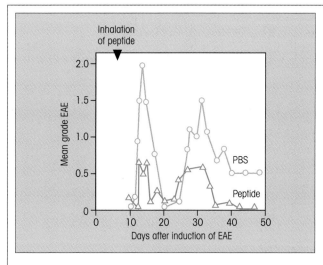

Figure 18.30. Influence of peptide inhalation on experimental autoimmune encephalomyelitis (EAE) induced with pig spinal cord in complete Freund's adjuvant.

Aerosols of the peptide were inhaled 8 days after injection of the encephalitogen. A single dose can give long-lived protection that is extended indefinitely if the mice are thymectomized. Regulation is IL-10 dependent and both Th1 and Th2 can be tolerized. Administration of a single peptide T-cell epitope can induce tolerance to other autoantigenic epitopes on the same protein (linked suppression) and to epitopes on different antigens within the nervous tissue used for immunization (bystander tolerance). PBS, phosphate-buffered saline; the peptide was an acetylated N-terminal 11-mer from myelin basic protein with lysine at position 4 substituted by alanine. (Data from Metzler B. & Wraith D.C. (1996) *Annals of the New York Academy of Science* **778**, 228–242; with permission of the publishers.)

II collagen arthritis model and the development of diabetes in NOD mice. Promising results have been obtained in clinical trials in which RA patients are fed type II chicken collagen.

The tolerogen can also be delivered by inhalation of peptide aerosols (Figure 18.30), and this could be a very attractive way of generating antigen-specific T-cell suppression in many hypersensitivity states. Induction of anergy or active suppression may contribute to different extents. Intranasal peptides have been used successfully to block collagen-induced arthritis, EAE, and the spontaneous diabetes (NOD) mouse models. Significantly, treatment can be effective even *after* induction of disease (Figure 18.30), although in established human disease this may be more difficult to achieve and might require supplementary therapy, such as anti-CD4, and preliminary reduction of primed T-cells with cyclosporine or steroids. There is no shortage of strings to pull.

Now this is really important. A single internal epitope of MBP can inhibit disease induced by the *mixture* of epitopes or antigens contained within whole myelin. In other words, a

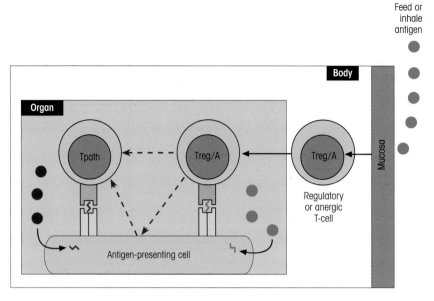

Figure 18.31. Organ-related bystander tolerance induced by feeding or inhaling an organ-related autoantigen.

Induced regulatory or anergic tolerogen-specific T-cells (Treg/A) enter the organ and inhibit pathogenic T-cells (Tpath) on the same antigen-presenting cell that processes both the tolerogen and the other organ-derived antigen recognized by the pathogenic cell.

Regulators act by production of IL-10 and TGFβ, that downregulate the Th1 cells either directly or through an intermediate effect on the antigen-presenting cell.

single epitope can induce suppression of the pathogenic T-cells specific for other epitopes on the same or other molecules provided that they are generated within the same organ or locality. We have referred to this already as **organ-related bystander tolerance**, a phenomenon best understood in terms of interactions on the same antigen-presenting cell between the regulatory cell, be it Th2 or anergic, recognizing the suppressor epitope and the pathogenic Th1-cell recognizing a **separate epitope** processed from the same or another molecule in the same organ (Figure 18.31).

- The immune system balances precariously between effective responses to environmental pathogens and regulatory control of an array of potentially suicidal responses to self-molecules.

The range of autoimmune diseases
- Five to eight percent of individuals develop autoimmune disease.
- In **organ-specific** autoimmune disease, exemplified by Hashimoto's thyroiditis, Graves' disease and type 1 diabetes, the target autoantigens and lesions are restricted to a particular organ. **In nonorgan-specific (systemic) autoimmune diseases**, such as SLE and RA, the autoantibodies have widespread reactivity and the lesions involve deposition of circulating immune complexes.
- Patients quite often develop more than one autoimmune disease.

Genetic and environmental influences
- Autoimmune diseases generally involve multiple genetic contributions, including polymorphisms associated with HLA, autoantigens, PRRs, cytokines, cytokine receptors, co-stimulatory and signaling molecules, and transcription factors.
- Seventy-five percent of autoimmune disease occurs in females, most commonly between puberty and the menopause.
- Changes in disease severity can occur during pregnancy.
- Feedback control of lymphocytes through the cytokine–hypothalamus–pituitary–adrenal loop may be defective in rheumatoid arthritis and some other autoimmune diseases.
- Twin studies reinforce the importance of genetic contributions but also indicate a strong environmental influence.

- Both microbial and nonmicrobial environmental factors are implicated.

Mechanisms
- Autoimmune disease represents a breakdown in immunological tolerance.
- Autoantigen appears to drive the response.
- Most autoantigens are readily accessible to the immune system, but a few such as lens and sperm proteins are sequestered (hidden).
- The development of high affinity mutated antibodies and immune responses to clusters of anatomically related antigens strongly imply B-cell selection of autoantigen.
- T-cells specific for self peptides usually presented at low concentrations (cryptic epitopes) may not be eliminated in the thymus.
- Abnormal modification of the autoantigen, cross-reaction with exogenous antigens or "piggy-back" recognition of T-helper epitopes can provide new epitopes for nontolerized helper T-cells.
- B-cells and T-cells can be stimulated directly by polyclonal activators such as Epstein–Barr virus or superantigens.
- Defects in Foxp3⁺ Tregs are implicated in a number of autoimmune diseases.
- De-repression of class II genes giving rise to inappropriate cellular expression of class II may help perpetuate autoimmune reactions initially primed by dendritic cells.
- Cytokine imbalances are often seen in autoimmune disease.

Pathogenic effects of humoral autoantibody
- Autoantibodies are thought to play a central role in many autoimmune diseases including autoimmune hemolytic anemia, idiopathic thrombocytopenic purpura, Graves' disease, myasthenia gravis, pernicious anemia and Goodpasture's syndrome.
- Passive transfer of disease is seen in "experiments of nature" in which transplacental passage of maternal IgG autoantibody produces a comparable but transient disorder in the fetus and neonate (e.g. Graves' disease, myasthenia gravis).
- In these diseases where antibody plays a central role, pathology can be mimicked in animal models by passive transfer of monoclonal autoantibodies.

Pathogenic effects of complexes with autoantigens
- Immune complexes, usually with bound complement, appear in the kidneys, skin and joints of patients with SLE, associated with lesions in the corresponding organs.
- Most patients with RA produce autoantibodies to IgG (rheumatoid factors) that self-associate to form complexes.
- These give rise to acute inflammation in the joint space and stimulate the synovial lining cells to grow as a **pannus**, which **produces erosions in the underlying cartilage and bone** through the release of IL-1, IL-6, TNF, collagenase, neutral protease and reactive oxygen intermediates.

T-cell-mediated hypersensitivity as a pathogenic factor
- Suppression of disease by cyclosporine or anti-CD4 treatment is strong evidence for T-cell involvement. So is an HLA-linked risk factor.
- There is a prevailing view that organ-specific inflammatory lesions are caused by autoreactive pathogenic Th1 and/or Th17 cells.
- Activated T-cells are abundant in the rheumatoid synovium and their production of TNF and IL-15 complements the immune complex stimulus for pannus formation.
- Thyroid epithelial cells often express MHC class II in autoimmune thyroid disease and Th1 cells infiltrate the gland.
- That autoimmunity can cause thyroiditis is further shown by the deliberate induction of disease in rodents through immunization with thyroid antigens in complete Freund's adjuvant.
- The onset of type 1 diabetes is delayed by cyclosporine, and HLA-DQ risk factors are prominent.
- Th1 cells from diseased NOD mice, which mimic the human disorder in histopathology and autoimmunity, can produce typical pancreatic lesions in young mice of the same strain. IL-21 from Th17 cells may also play an important role.
- That autoimmunity plays a central role in MS is suggested by the similarity to experimental autoimmune encephalomyelitis, a demyelinating disease induced by immunization of rodents with myelin in complete Freund's adjuvant. Approximately one-third of the IL-2 or IL-4 activatable T-cells in the CSF of MS patients are specific for myelin and the HLA-DR2 phenotype is a strong risk factor.

Some other diseases with an autoimmune component
- Immunologically mediated vascular lesions are of central importance in Wegener's granulomatosis, giant cell arteritis, scleroderma and atherosclerosis.

- Pemphigus and vitiligo may also be autoimmune diseases.

Measurement of autoantibodies
- A wide range of serum autoantibodies provide valuable diagnostic markers.
- Solid-phase ELISA tests, increasingly in the form of microarrays, are used for the detection of antibodies.
- Immunofluorescent screening can be carried out on sections of normal tissue.
- Agglutination tests for rheumatoid factors and addressable laser bead assays are amongst other commonly employed diagnostic tests.
- Autoantibody screening can predict future occurrence of autoimmune disease in the close relatives of type 1 diabetics.

Treatment of autoimmune disorders
- Therapy involves metabolic control and the use of anti-inflammatory and immunosuppressive drugs.
- Striking success in RA has been achieved by therapy with anti-TNF.
- A whole variety of potential immunological control therapies are under intensive investigation. These include wholesale B- and T-cell depletion and attempts to induce antigen-specific tolerance.
- Restoring defective Treg activity could potentially be of great benefit.
- Organ-related bystander tolerance means that single epitopes can induce suppression of pathogenic cells within an organ reacting to other epitopes on the same or other antigens.

FURTHER READING

Bugatti S., Codullo V., Caporali R. & Montecucco C. (2007) B cells in rheumatoid arthritis. *Autoimmunity Reviews* **7**, 137–142.

Chapel M., Haeney M., Misbah S. & Snowden N. (2006) *Essentials of Clinical Immunology*, 5th edn. Blackwell Publishing, Oxford.

Cunningham M.W. (2009) Molecular mimicry. In *Encyclopedia of Life Sciences*. John Wiley & Sons, Ltd, Chichester http://www.els.net/ DOI: 10.1002/9780470015902.a0000958.pub2

Eizirik D.L., Colli M.L. & Ortis F. (2009) The role of inflammation in insulitis and β-cell loss in type 1 diabetes. *Nature Reviews Endocrinology* **5**, 219–226.

Guilherme L. & Kalil J. (2010) Rheumatic fever and rheumatic heart disease: cellular mechanisms leading to autoimmune reactivity and disease. *Journal of Clinical Immunology* **30**, 17–23.

Marsh S.G. *et al.* (2010) Nomenclature for factors of the HLA system, 2010. *Tissue Antigens* **75**, 291–455.

Masters S.L., Simon A., Aksentijevich I. & Kastner D.L. (2009) Horror autoinflammaticus: the molecular pathophysiology of autoinflammatory disease. *Annual Review of Immunology* **27**, 621–668.

Nestle F.O., Kaplan D.H. & Barker J. (2009) Psoriasis. *The New England Journal of Medicine* **361**, 496–509.

Oh S., Rankin A.L. & Caton A.J. (2010) CD4+CD25+ regulatory T cells in autoimmune arthritis. *Immunological Reviews* **233**, 97–111.

Pascual V., Chaussabel D. & Banchereau J. (2010) A genomic approach to human autoimmune diseases. *Annual Review of Immunology* **28**, 535–571.

Rahman A. & Isenberg D.A. (2008) Systemic lupus erythematosus. *The New England Journal of Medicine* **358**, 929–939.

Rose N.R. & Mackay I.R. (eds.) (2006) *The Autoimmune Diseases*, 4th edn. Elsevier, Oxford.

Tha-In T. *et al.* (2008) Modulation of the cellular immune system by intravenous immunoglobulin. *Trends in Immunology* **29**, 608–615.

Zenewicz L.A., Abraham C., Flavell R.A. & Cho J.H. (2010) Unraveling the genetics of autoimmunity. *Cell* **140**, 791–797.

Now visit **www.roitt.com** to test yourself on this chapter.

Glossary

acquired immune response: Immunity mediated by lymphocytes and characterized by antigen-specificity and memory.

acute phase proteins: Serum proteins, mostly produced in the liver, that rapidly change in concentration (some increase, some decrease) during the initiation of an inflammatory response.

addressin: Cell adhesion molecule present on the luminal surface of blood and lymph vessel endothelium, and recognized by homing molecules that direct leukocytes to tissues with the appropriate "address."

adjuvant: Any substance that nonspecifically enhances the immune response to antigen.

affinity (intrinsic affinity): The strength of binding (affinity constant) between a receptor (e.g. one antigen-binding site on an antibody) and a ligand (e.g. epitope on an antigen).

affinity chromatography: The use of immobilized antibody (or antigen) to select specific antigen (or antibody) from a mixture. The purified ligand is then released by disrupting the antibody–antigen interaction, for example by changing the pH.

allele: Variants of a polymorphic gene at a given genetic locus.

allelic exclusion: The phenomenon whereby, following successful rearrangement of one allele of an antigen receptor gene, rearrangement of the other parental allele is suppressed.

allergen: An antigen that causes allergy.

allergy: IgE-mediated hypersensitivity, e.g. asthma, eczema, hayfever and food allergy.

allogeneic: Refers to the genetic differences between individuals of the same species.

allograft: Tissue or organ graft between allogeneic individuals.

allotype: An allelic variant of an antigen that, because it is not present in all individuals, may be immunogenic in members of the same species that have a different version of the allele.

alternative pathway (of complement activation): Activation pathway involving complement components C3, factor B, factor D and properdin that, in the presence of a stabilizing activator surface such as microbial polysaccharide, generates the alternative pathway C3 convertase C3bBb.

anaphylatoxin: A substance (e.g. C3a, C4a or C5a) capable of directly triggering mast cell degranulation.

anaphylaxis: An often fatal hypersensitivity reaction, triggered by IgE or anaphylatoxin-mediated mast cell degranulation, leading to anaphylactic shock due to vasodilatation and smooth muscle contraction.

anergy: Potentially reversible specific immunological tolerance in which the lymphocyte becomes functionally nonresponsive.

antibody-dependent cellular cytotoxicity (ADCC): A cytotoxic reaction in which an antibody-coated target cell is directly killed by an Fc receptor-bearing leukocyte, e.g. NK cell, macrophage or neutrophil.

antigen: Any molecule capable of being recognized by an antibody or T-cell receptor.

antigen-presenting cell (APC): A term most commonly used when referring to cells that present processed antigenic peptide and MHC class II molecules to the T-cell receptor on CD4$^+$ T-cells, e.g. dendritic cells, macrophages, B-cells. Note, however, that most types of cell are able to present antigenic peptides with MHC class I to CD8$^+$ T-cells, e.g. as occurs with virally infected cells.

antigenic determinant: A cluster of epitopes (*see* epitope).

apoptosis: A form of programed cell death, characterized by endonuclease digestion of DNA.

atopic allergy: IgE-mediated hypersensitivity, i.e. asthma, eczema, hayfever and food allergy.

autologous: From the same individual.

avidity (functional affinity): The binding strength between two molecules (e.g. antibody and antigen) taking into account the valency of the interaction. Thus the avidity will always be equal to or greater than the intrinsic affinity (*see* affinity).

Roitt's Essential Immunology, Twelfth Edition. Peter J. Delves, Seamus J. Martin, Dennis R. Burton, Ivan M. Roitt.
© 2011 Peter J. Delves, Seamus J. Martin, Dennis R. Burton, Ivan M. Roitt. Published 2011 by Blackwell Publishing Ltd.

β₂-microglobulin: A 12-kDa protein, not itself encoded within the MHC, but forming part of the structure of MHC class I-encoded molecules.

B-1/B-2-cells: The two major subpopulations of B-lymphocytes. B-1-cells bear high levels of surface IgM, lower levels of surface IgD, are CD43⁺, CD23⁻ and most express the cell surface antigen CD5; they are self-renewing, and frequently secrete high levels of antibody, which binds to a range of antigens ("polyspecificity") with a relatively low affinity. The majority of B-cells, however, are B-2 that express low levels of surface IgM, higher levels of surface IgD, do not express CD5, and are CD43⁻, CD23⁺; they are directly generated from precursors in the bone marrow, and secrete highly specific antibody.

basophil: A type of granulocyte found in the blood and resembling the tissue mast cell.

BCG (bacille Calmette–Guérin): Attenuated *Mycobacterium tuberculosis* used both as a specific vaccine for tuberculosis and as an adjuvant.

biolistics: The use of small particles, e.g. colloidal gold, as a vehicle for carrying agents (drugs, nucleic acid, etc.) into a cell. Following coating with the desired agent(s), the particles are fired into the dermis of the recipient using a helium-powered gun.

bispecific antibody: An artificially produced hybrid antibody in which each of the two antigen-binding arms is specific for a different antigenic epitope. Such antibodies, which can be produced either by chemical cross-linkage or by recombinant DNA techniques, can be used to link together two different antigens or cells, e.g. a cytotoxic T-cell and a tumor cell.

bursa of Fabricius: A primary lymphoid organ in avian species, located at the cloacal-hind gut junction; it is the site of B-cell maturation.

capping: An active process whereby cross-linking of cell surface molecules (e.g. by antibody) leads to aggregation and subsequent migration of the molecules to one pole of the cell.

caspases: A family of cysteine proteases involved in generating apoptosis.

carrier: Any molecule that when conjugated to a nonimmunogenic molecule (e.g. a hapten) makes the latter immunogenic by providing epitopes for helper T-cells which the hapten lacks.

CD antigen: Cluster of differentiation designation assigned to leukocyte cell surface molecules that are identified by a given group of monoclonal antibodies.

CD3: A trimeric complex of γ, δ and ε chains that together with a ζζ homodimer or ζη heterodimer acts as a signal transducing unit for the T-cell receptor.

CD4: Cell surface glycoprotein, usually on helper T-cells, that recognizes MHC class II molecules on antigen-presenting cells.

CD8: Cell surface glycoprotein, usually on cytotoxic T-cells, that recognizes MHC class I molecules on target cells.

cell-mediated immunity (CMI): Refers to T-cell-mediated immune responses.

central memory: Immunological memory that is dependent on CCR7⁺ T-cells that, under the influence of chemokines, travel to secondary lymphoid organs where they give rise to CCR7⁻ effector memory T-cells.

central tolerance: Specific immunological tolerance due to the induction of lymphocyte apoptosis or anergy within the primary lymphoid organs (bone marrow in the case of B-cell tolerance and the thymus for T-cells).

chemokines: A family of structurally related cytokines that selectively induce chemotaxis and activation of leukocytes. They also play important roles in lymphoid organ development, cell compartmentalization within lymphoid tissues, Th1/Th2 development, angiogenesis and wound healing.

chemotaxis: Movement of cells up a concentration gradient of chemotactic factors.

chimeric: Composite of genetically distinct individuals, e.g. following an allogeneic bone marrow graft.

citrullination: The enzymatic conversion, by peptidyl arginine deiminase, of an arginine in a protein to a citrulline.

class switching: The process by which a B-cell changes the class but not specificity of a given antibody it produces, e.g. switching from an IgM to an IgG antibody.

class switch recombination: The recombination of immunoglobulin heavy chain constant region gene segments, e.g. switching from Cμ and Cδ to Cγ1 to convert an IgM (and IgD) antibody into an IgG1 antibody.

classical pathway (of complement activation)**:** Activation pathway involving complement components C1, C2 and C4 that, following fixation of C1q, e.g. by antigen–antibody complexes, produces the classical pathway C3 convertase C4b2a.

clonal deletion: A process by which contact with antigen (e.g. self antigen) at an early stage of lymphocyte differentiation leads to cell death by apoptosis.

clonal selection: The selection and activation by antigen of a lymphocyte bearing a complementary receptor, which then proliferates to form an expanded clone.

clone: Identical cells derived from a single progenitor.

colony-stimulating factors (CSF): Factors that permit the proliferation and differentiation of hematopoietic cells.

combinatorial diversity: That component of antibody and T-cell receptor (TCR) diversity that is generated by the recombination of variable (V), diversity (D, for immunoglobulin heavy chains, and for TCR β and α chains) and joining (J) gene segments.

complement: A group of serum proteins, some of which act in an enzymatic cascade, producing effector molecules involved in inflammation (C3a, C5a), phagocytosis (C3b), and cell lysis (C5b–9).

complementarity determining regions (CDR): The hypervariable amino acid sequences within antibody and T-cell receptor variable regions that interact with complementary amino acids on the antigen or peptide–MHC complex.

ConA (concanavalin A): A T-cell mitogen.

congenic: Animals that only differ only at a single genetic locus.

conjugate: Covalently linked complex of two or more molecules (e.g. fluorescein conjugated to antibody).

convergent evolution: Independent evolution of similarity between molecules or between species.

Coombs' test: Diagnostic test using anti-immunoglobulin to agglutinate antibody-coated erythrocytes.

cortex: Outer (peripheral) layer of an organ.

C-reactive protein: An acute phase protein that is able to bind to the surface of microorganisms where it functions as a stimulator of the classical pathway of complement activation, and as an opsonin for phagocytosis.

cyclophospha-mide: Cytotoxic drug used as an immunosuppressive.

cyclosporine: A T-cell-specific immunosuppressive drug used to prevent graft rejection.

cytokines: Low-molecular-weight proteins that stimulate or inhibit the differentiation, proliferation or function of immune cells.

cytophilic: Binds to cells.

cytotoxic: Kills cells.

cytotoxic T-lymphocyte (CTL, Tc): T-cells (usually CD8$^+$) that kill target cells following recognition of foreign peptide–MHC molecules on the target cell membrane.

danger-associated molecular pattern (DAMP): A structure or molecule produced by necrotic cells and which provides danger signals to activate the immune response following tissue damage.

defensins: A family of small basic antimicrobial peptides, produced by both animals and plants.

delayed-type hypersensitivity (DTH): A hypersensitivity reaction occurring within 48–72 hours and mediated by cytokine release from sensitized T-cells.

dendritic cell (DC): Refers to an interdigitating dendritic cell that is MHC class II-positive and presents processed antigens to T-cells in the T-cell areas of secondary lymphoid tissues. (NB:a different cell type to follicular dendritic cells).

differential splicing: The utilization and splicing of different exons from a primary RNA transcript in order to generate different mRNA sequences.

differentiation antigen: A cell surface molecule expressed at a particular stage of development or on cells of a given lineage.

DiGeorge syndrome: Immunodeficiency caused by a congenital failure in thymic development resulting in a lack of mature functional T-cells.

diversity (D) gene segments: Found in the immunoglobulin heavy chain gene and T-cell receptor β- and δ-gene loci between the V- and J-gene segments. Encode part of the third hypervariable region (CDR3) in these antigen receptor chains.

domain: a structural element of a polypeptide.

edema: Swelling caused by accumulation of fluid in the tissues.

effector cells: Cells that carry out an immune function, e.g. cytokine release, cytotoxicity.

ELISA (enzyme-linked immunosorbent assay): Assay for detection or quantitation of an antibody or antigen using a ligand (e.g. an anti-immunoglobulin) conjugated to an enzyme that changes the color of a substrate.

endocytosis: Cellular ingestion of macromolecules by invagination of plasma membrane to produce an intracellular vesicle that encloses the ingested material.

endogenous: From within.

endosomes: Intracellular smooth surfaced vesicles in which endocytosed material passes on its way to the lysosomes.

endotoxin: Pathogenic cell wall-associated lipopolysaccharides of Gram-negative bacteria.

eosinophil: A class of granulocyte, the granules of which contain toxic cationic proteins.

epitope: That part of an antigen recognized by an antigen receptor (*see* antigenic determinant).

Epstein–Barr virus (EBV): The virus responsible for infectious mononucleosis and Burkitt's lymphoma. Can be used to immortalize human B-cells *in vitro*.

equivalence: The ratio of antibody to antigen at which immunoprecipitation of the reactants is virtually complete.

erythema: The redness produced during inflammation due to erythrocytes entering tissue spaces.

erythropoiesis: Erythrocyte production.

exotoxin: Pathogenic protein secreted by bacteria.

exudate: The extravascular fluid (containing proteins and cellular debris) that accumulates during inflammation.

Fab: Monovalent antigen-binding fragment obtained following papain digestion of immunoglobulin. Consists of an intact light chain and the N-terminal V_H and C_H1 domains of the heavy chain.

F(ab′)₂: Bivalent antigen-binding fragment obtained following pepsin digestion of immunoglobulin. Consists of both light chains and the N-terminal part of both heavy chains linked by disulfide bonds.

Fas: A member of the TNF receptor gene family. Engagement of Fas (CD95) on the surface of the cell by the Fas ligand (CD178) present on cytotoxic cells, can trigger apoptosis in the Fas-bearing target cell.

Fc: Crystallizable, nonantigen-binding fragment of an immunoglobulin molecule obtained following papain digestion. Consists of the C-terminal portion of both heavy chains that is responsible for binding to Fc receptors and C1q.

Fc receptors: Cell surface receptors that bind the Fc portion of particular immunoglobulin classes.

fibroblast: Connective tissue cell that produces collagen and plays an important part in wound healing.

fluorescein isothiocyanate (FITC): Green fluorescent dye used to "tag" antibodies for use in immunofluorescence.

fluorescent antibody: An antibody conjugated to a fluorescent dye such as FITC.

foam cell: Macrophages that have engulfed low density lipoproteins. They are characteristically present in atherosclerotic plaques.

follicular dendritic cell: MHC class II-negative Fc receptor-positive dendritic cells that bear immune complexes on their surface and are involved in the stimulation of B-cells and maintenance of B-cell memory in germinal centres. (N.B. a different cell type to interdigitating dendritic cells).

follicular helper T-cell: Subset of helper T-cells that direct B-cell development, class switch recombination and survival within germinal centers.

Foxp3: A transcription factor present in the nucleus of most regulatory T-cells.

framework regions: The relatively conserved amino acid sequences that flank the hypervariable regions in immunoglobulin and T-cell receptor variable regions and maintain a common overall structure for all V-region domains.

Freund's adjuvant: Complete Freund's adjuvant is an emulsion of aqueous antigen in mineral oil that contains heat-killed mycobacteria. Incomplete Freund's adjuvant lacks the mycobacteria.

Fv: The variable region fragment of an antibody heavy or light chain.

γ-globulin: The serum proteins, mostly immunoglobulins, which have the greatest mobility towards the cathode during electrophoresis.

germline: The arrangement of the genetic material as transmitted through the gametes.

germinal center: Discrete areas within secondary lymphoid tissues where B-cell maturation and memory development occur.

giant cell: Large multinucleate cell derived from fused macrophages and often present in granulomas.

glomerulonephritis: Inflammation of renal glomerular capillary loops, often resulting from immune complex deposition.

graft versus host (GVH) reaction: Reaction occurring when T-lymphocytes present in a graft recognize and attack host cells.

granulocyte: Myeloid cells containing cytoplasmic granules (i.e. neutrophils, eosinophils and basophils).

granuloma: A tissue nodule containing proliferating lymphocytes, fibroblasts, and giant cells and epithelioid cells (both derived from activated macrophages), which forms due to inflammation in response to chronic infection or persistence of antigen in the tissues.

granzymes: Serine esterases present in the granules of cytotoxic T-lymphocytes and NK cells. They induce apoptosis in the target cell that they enter through perforin channels inserted into the target cell membrane by the cytotoxic cell.

gut-associated lymphoid tissue (GALT): Includes Peyer's patches, appendix and solitary lymphoid nodules in the submucosa.

H-2: The mouse major histocompatibility complex (MHC).

haplotype: The set of allelic variants present at a given genetic region.

hapten: A low-molecular-weight molecule that is recognized by preformed antibody but is not itself immunogenic unless conjugated to a "carrier" molecule that provides epitopes recognized by helper T-cells.

helper T-lymphocyte (Th): A subclass of T-cells that provide help (in the form of cytokines and/or cognate interactions) necessary for the expression of effector function by other cells in the immune system.

hemagglutinin: Any molecule that agglutinates erythrocytes.

hematopoiesis: The production of erythrocytes, leukocytes and platelets.

hematopoietic stem cells: Self-renewing stem cells that are capable of giving rise to all of the formed elements of the blood (i.e. leukocytes, erythrocytes and platelets).

heterozygous: Possessing different alleles at a given locus on the two homologous chromosomes.

high endothelial venule (HEV): Capillary venule composed of specialized endothelial cells allowing migration of lymphocytes into lymphoid organs.

hinge region: Amino acids between the Fab and Fc regions of immunoglobulin that permit flexibility of the molecule.

histamine: Vasoactive amine present in basophil and mast cell granules that, following degranulation, causes increased vascular permeability and smooth muscle contraction.

HLA (*h*uman *l*eukocyte *a*ntigen): The human major histocompatibility complex (MHC).

homing receptors: Cell surface molecules that direct leukocytes to specific locations in the body.

homozygous: Possessing the same allele at a given locus on the two homologous chromosomes.

humanized antibody: A genetically engineered monoclonal antibody of nonhuman origin in which all but the antigen-binding CDR sequences have been replaced with sequences derived from human antibodies. This procedure is carried out to minimize the immunogenicity of therapeutic monoclonal antibodies.

humoral: Pertaining to extracellular fluid such as plasma and lymph. The term humoral immunity is used to denote antibody-mediated immune responses.

hybridoma: Hybrid cell line obtained by fusing a lymphoid tumor cell with a lymphocyte that then has both the immortality of the tumor cell and the effector function (e.g. monoclonal antibody secretion) of the lymphocyte.

hypersensitivity: Excessive immune response that leads to undesirable consequences, e.g. tissue or organ damage.

hypervariable regions: Those amino acid sequences within the immunoglobulin and T-cell receptor variable regions that show the greatest variability and contribute most to the antigen or peptide–MHC binding site.

idiotope: An epitope made up of amino acids within the variable region of an antibody or T-cell receptor that reacts with an anti-idiotope.

idiotype: The complete set of idiotopes in the variable region of an antibody or T-cell receptor that react with an anti-idiotypic serum.

idiotype network: A regulatory network based on interactions of idiotypes and anti-idiotypes present on antibodies and T-cell receptors.

immune complex: Complex of antibody bound to antigen that may also contain complement components.

immunoadsorption: Method for removal of antibody or antigen by allowing it to bind to solid phase antigen or antibody.

immunofluorescence: Technique for detection of cell- or tissue-associated antigens by the use of a fluorescently tagged ligand (e.g. an anti-immunoglobulin conjugated to fluorescein isothiocyanate).

immunogen: Any substance that elicits an immune response. Whilst all immunogens are antigens, not all antigens are immunogens (*see* hapten).

immunoglobulin superfamily: Large family of proteins characterized by possession of "immunoglobulin-type" domains of approximately 110 amino acids folded into two β-pleated sheets. Members include immunoglobulins, T-cell receptors and MHC molecules.

immunological synapse: A contact point between the T-cell and antigen-presenting cell that is generated by reorganization and clustering of cell surface molecules in lipid rafts. The synapse facilitates interactions between TCR and MHC, costimulatory and adhesion molecules, thereby potentiating the TCR-mediated activation signal.

immunotoxin: A biochemical conjugate, or recombinant fusion protein, consisting of an immune targeting molecule such as an antibody or antibody fragment together with a cytotoxic molecule.

inflammasome: A multi-protein cytoplasmic complex that promotes inflammation by converting the IL-1β precursor into active IL-1β, and additionally by stimulating the generation of IL-18.

inflammation: The tissue response to trauma, characterized by increased blood flow and entry of leukocytes into the tissues, resulting in swelling, redness, elevated temperature and pain.

innate immunity: Immunity that is not intrinsically affected by prior contact with antigen, i.e. all aspects of immunity not directly mediated by lymphocytes.

integrins: A family of heterodimeric cell adhesion molecules.

interdigitating dendritic cell: MHC class II-positive antigen-presenting dendritic cell found in T-cell areas of lymph nodes and spleen. (NB:a different cell type to follicular dendritic cells).

interferons (IFN): IFNα and IFNβ (type I interferons) can be induced in most cell types, whereas IFNγ (type II interferon) is produced by T-lymphocytes. All three types induce an antiviral state in cells and IFNγ additionally acts in the regulation of immune responses.

interleukins (IL): Designation for some of the cytokines secreted by leukocytes.

internal image: An epitope on an anti-idiotype that binds in a way that structurally and functionally mimics the antigen.

invariant chain: A polypeptide that binds MHC class II molecules in the endoplasmic reticulum, directs them to the late endosomal compartment and prevents premature association with self peptides.

Ir (immune response) genes: The genes, including those within the MHC, that together determine the overall level of immune response to a given antigen.

isotype: An antibody constant region structure present in all normal individuals, i.e. antibody class or subclass.

ITAM: *I*mmunoreceptor *t*yrosine-based *a*ctivation *m*otifs are amino acid consensus sequences recognized by src-family tyrosine kinases. These motifs are found in the cytoplasmic domains of several signaling molecules including the signal transduction units of lymphocyte antigen receptors and of Fc receptors.

ITIM: *I*mmunoreceptor *t*yrosine-based *i*nhibitory *m*otifs present in the cytoplasmic domains of certain cell surface molecules, e.g. FcγRIIB, inhibitory NK cell receptors, and that mediate inhibitory signals.

J chain: A molecule that forms part of the structure of pentameric IgM and dimeric IgA.

joining (J) gene segments: Found in the immunoglobulin and T-cell receptor gene loci and, upon gene rearrangement, encode part of the third hypervariable region (CDR3) of the antigen receptors.

junctional diversity: Diversity of the splice junctions in the recombined variable (V), diversity (D, for immunoglobulin heavy chains, and for TCR β and δ chains) and joining (J) gene segments of antibody and T-cell receptor (TCR) genes.

K (killer) cell: A generic term for any leukocyte that mediates antibody-dependent cellular cytotoxicity (ADCC).

kinins: A family of polypeptides released during inflammatory responses and that increase vascular permeability and smooth muscle contraction.

KIRs: *K*iller cell *i*mmunoglobulin-like *r*eceptors found on NK cells, some γδ and some αβ T-cells. KIRs recognize MHC class I molecules and, like the C-type lectin receptors also found on these cells, can either inhibit or activate the killer cells. If ITIM sequences are present in their cytoplasmic domain they are inhibitory. KIRs lacking ITIMs can associate with ITAM-containing adaptor molecules, in which case they can activate the NK cell or T-cell.

knockout: The use of homologous genetic recombination in embryonal stem cells to replace a functional gene with a defective copy of the gene. The animals that are produced by this technique can be bred to homozygosity, thus allowing the generation of a null phenotype for that gene product.

Kuppfer cells: Fixed tissue macrophages lining the blood sinuses in the liver.

lamina propria: The connective tissue underlying the epithelium at mucosal sites.

Langerhans' cell: Fc receptor and MHC class II-positive antigen-presenting dendritic cell found in the skin.

large granular lymphocyte (LGL): Leukocytes (most are not actually true lymphocytes) that contain cytoplasmic granules and function as natural killer (NK) and killer (K) cells. Activated CD8⁺ cytotoxic T-lymphocytes (Tc) also assume an LGL morphology.

lectins: A family of proteins that bind specific sugars on glycoproteins and glycolipids. Some plant lectins are mitogenic (e.g. PHA, ConA).

leukocyte: White blood cells, which include neutrophils, basophils, eosinophils, lymphocytes, NK cells and monocytes.

leukotrienes: Metabolic products of arachidonic acid that promote inflammatory processes (e.g. chemotaxis, increased vascular permeability) and are produced by a variety of cell types including mast cells, basophils and macrophages.

ligand: General term for a molecule recognized by a binding structure such as a receptor.

linkage disequilibrium: The occurrence of two alleles being inherited together at a greater frequency than that expected from the product of their individual frequencies.

lipid raft: Cholesterol- and glycosphingolipid-rich membrane subdomain in which molecules involved in cellular activation become concentrated.

lipopolysaccha-ride (LPS): Endotoxin derived from Gram-negative bacterial cell walls that has inflammatory and mitogenic actions.

lymph: The tissue fluid that drains into and through the lymphatic system.

lymphadenopathy: Enlarged lymph nodes.

lymphotoxin (also called TNFβ): A T-cell-derived cytokine that is cytotoxic for certain tumor cells and also has immunoregulatory functions.

lysosomes: Membrane-bound cytoplasmic organelles containing hydrolytic enzymes involved in the digestion of phagocytosed material.

lysozyme: Anti-bacterial enzyme present in phagocytic cell granules, tears and saliva, which digests peptidoglycans in bacterial cell walls.

macrophage: Large phagocytic cell, derived from the blood monocyte, which also functions as an antigen-presenting cell and can mediate ADCC.

mannose binding lectin (mannose binding protein): A member of the collectin family of calcium-dependent lectins, and an acute phase protein. It functions as a stimulator of the lectin pathway of complement activation, and as an opsonin for phagocytosis by binding to mannose, a sugar residue usually found in an exposed form only on the surface of microorganisms.

marginal zone: The outer area of the splenic periarteriolar lymphoid sheath (PALS) that is rich in B-cells, particularly those responding to thymus-independent antigens.

margination: Leukocyte adhesion to the endothelium of blood vessels in the early phase of an acute inflammatory reaction.

mast cell: A tissue cell with abundant granules that resembles the blood basophil. Both these cell types bear high affinity Fc receptors for IgE, which when crosslinked by IgE and antigen cause degranulation and the release of a number of mediators including histamine and leukotrienes.

medulla: Inner (central) region of an organ.

megakaryocyte: A bone marrow precursor of platelets.

membrane attack complex (MAC): Complex of complement components C5b–C9 that inserts as a pore into the membrane of target cells leading to cell lysis or apoptosis.

memory (immunological): A characteristic of the acquired immune response of lymphocytes whereby a second encounter with a given antigen produces a secondary immune response; faster, greater and longer lasting than the primary immune response.

memory cells: Clonally expanded T- and B-cells produced during a primary immune response and that are "primed" to mediate a secondary immune response to the original antigen.

MHC (major histocompatibility complex): A genetic region encoding molecules involved in antigen presentation to T-cells. Class I MHC molecules are present on virtually all nucleated cells and are encoded mainly by the H-2K, -D and -L loci in mice and by HLA-A, -B and -C in man, whilst class II MHC molecules are expressed on antigen-presenting cells (primarily dendritic cells, macrophages and B-cells) and are encoded by H-2A and -E in mice and HLA-DR, -DQ and -DP in man. Allelic differences are associated with the most intense graft rejection within a species.

MHC restriction: The necessity that T-cells recognize processed antigen only when presented by MHC molecules of the original haplotype associated with T-cell priming.

minor histocom-patibility antigens: Non-MHC-encoded processed peptides derived from the allogeneic products of polymorphic gene loci. In association with

MHC-encoded molecules they contribute to graft rejection, albeit not usually as severe as that due to MHC mismatch.

mitogen: A substance that nonspecifically induces lymphocyte proliferation.

mixed lymphocyte reaction (MLR): A T-cell proliferative response induced by cells expressing allogeneic MHC.

monoclonal antibody: Homogeneous antibody derived from a single B-cell clone and therefore all bearing identical antigen-binding sites and isotype.

monocyte: Mononuclear phagocyte found in blood and that is the precursor of the tissue macrophage.

mononuclear phagocyte system: A system comprising blood monocytes and tissue macrophages.

mucosa-associated lymphoid tissue (MALT): Lymphoid tissue present in the surface mucosa of the respiratory, gastrointestinal and genitourinary tracts.

multiple myeloma: Plasma cell malignancy resulting in high levels of monoclonal immunoglobulin in serum and of free light chains (Bence Jones protein) in urine.

murine: Pertaining to mice.

myeloma protein: Monoclonal antibody secreted by myeloma cells.

naive lymphocyte: A mature T- or B-cell that has not yet been activated by initial encounter with antigen.

negative selection: Deletion by apoptosis in the thymus of T-cells that recognize self peptides presented by self MHC molecules, thus preventing the development of autoimmune T-cells. Negative selection of developing B-cells also occurs if they encounter high levels of self antigen in the bone marrow.

neutrophil: The major circulating phagocytic polymorphonuclear granulocyte. Enters tissues early in an inflammatory response and is also able to mediate antibody-dependent cellular cytotoxicity (ADCC).

NK (natural killer) cell: Large granular leukocyte that does not rearrange nor express either immunoglobulin or T-cell-receptor genes but is able to recognize and destroy certain tumor and virally infected cells in an MHC and antibody-independent manner. Also able to mediate ADCC.

NKT cell: NK1.1$^+$ lymphoid cells with a morphology and granule content intermediate between T-cells and NK cells. They express low levels of $\alpha\beta$ TCR with an invariant α chain and very restricted β chain specificity, recognize lipid and glycolipid antigens presented by the nonclassical MHC-like molecule CD1d, and are potent producers of IL-4 and IFNγ.

nude mouse: Mouse that is T-cell deficient due to a homozygous gene defect (*nu/nu*) resulting in the absence of a thymus (and also lack of body hair).

N-nucleotides: Nontemplated nucleotides added to the junctions between antibody (and T-cell receptor) variable (V), diversity (D) and joining (J) gene segments during gene rearrangement.

Nod-like receptor: A family of cytoplasmic pattern recognition receptors involved in sensing the presence of pathogens.

oligoclonal: A few different clones, or the product of a few different clones.

oncofetal antigen: Antigen whose expression is normally restricted to the fetus but that may be expressed during malignancy in adults.

opsonin: Substance, e.g. antibody or C3b, which enhances phagocytosis by promoting adhesion of the antigen to the phagocyte.

opsonization: Coating of antigen with opsonin to enhance phagocytosis.

PAF (platelet activating factor): An alkyl phospholipid released by a variety of cell types including mast cells and basophils, which has immunoregulatory effects on lymphocytes and monocytes/macrophages as well as causing platelet aggregation and degranulation.

paracortex: The part of an organ (e.g. lymph node) that lies between the cortex and the medulla.

pathogen-associated molecular pattern (PAMP): Molecules such as lipopolysaccharide, peptidoglycan, lipoteichoic acids and mannans, which are widely expressed by microbial pathogens as repetitive motifs but are not present on host tissues. They are therefore utilized by the pattern recognition receptors (PRRs) of the immune system to distinguish pathogens from self antigens.

pattern recognition receptor (PRR): Cell-associated or soluble receptors that enable the immune system to detect pathogen-associated molecular patterns (PAMPs) and danger-associated molecular patterns (DAMPs). Amongst the large number of different PRRs are the mannose receptor (CD206), macrophage scavenger receptor (CD204) and the Toll-like receptors.

perforin: Molecule produced by cytotoxic T-cells and NK cells that, like complement component C9, polymerizes to form a pore in the membrane of the target cell leading to cell death.

periarteriolar lymphoid sheath (PALS): The lymphoid tissue that forms the white pulp of the spleen.

peripheral tolerance: Specific immunological tolerance occurring outside of the primary lymphoid organs.

Peyer's patches: Part of the gut associated lymphoid tissue (GALT) and found as distinct lymphoid nodules mainly in the small intestine.

PHA (phytohemagglutinin): A plant lectin that acts as a T-cell mitogen.

phage antibody library: A collection of cloned antibody variable region gene sequences that can be expressed as Fab or scFv fusion proteins with bacteriophage coat proteins. These can be displayed on the surface of the phages. The gene encoding a monoclonal recombinant antibody is enclosed in the phage particle and can be selected from the library by binding of the phage to specific antigen.

phagocyte: Cells, including monocytes/macrophages and neutrophils, which are specialized for the engulfment of cellular and particulate matter.

phagolysosome: Intracellular vacuole where killing and digestion of phagocytosed material occurs following the fusion of a phagosome with a lysosome.

phagosome: Intracellular vacuole produced following invagination of the cell membrane around phagocytosed material.

phorbol myristate acetate (PMA): A mitogenic phorbol ester that directly stimulates protein kinase C and acts as a tumor promoter.

plaque forming cell (PFC): Antibody-secreting plasma cell detected *in vitro* by its ability to produce a "plaque" of lysed antigen-sensitized erythrocytes in the presence of complement.

plasma cell: Terminally differentiated B-lymphocyte that actively secretes large amounts of antibody.

pluripotent stem cell: A cell that has the potential to differentiate into many different cell types.

P-nucleotides: Palindromic nucleotide sequences generated at the junctions between antibody (and T-cell receptor) variable (V), diversity (D) and joining (J) gene segments during gene rearrangement.

pokeweed mitogen (PWM): A plant lectin that is a T-cell dependent B-cell mitogen.

polyclonal: Many different clones, or the product of many different clones, e.g. polyclonal antiserum.

poly-Ig receptor: A receptor molecule that specifically binds J-chain containing polymeric Ig, i.e. dimeric secretory IgA and pentameric IgM, and transports it across mucosal epithelium.

polymorphic: Highly variable in structure or sequence.

positive selection: The selection of those developing T-cells in the thymus that are able to recognize self MHC molecules. This occurs by preventing apoptosis in these cells.

precipitin: Precipitate of antibody and multivalent antigen due to the formation of high molecular weight complexes.

primary immune response: The relatively weak immune response that occurs upon the first encounter of naive lymphocytes with a given antigen.

primary lymphoid organs: The sites at which immunocompetent lymphocytes develop, i.e. bone marrow and thymus in mammals.

prime: The process of giving an initial sensitization to antigen.

prostaglandins: Acidic lipids derived from arachidonic acid that are able to increase vascular permeability, mediate fever, and can both stimulate and inhibit immunological responses.

proteasome: Cytoplasmic proteolytic enzyme complex involved in antigen processing to generate peptides for association with MHC.

protein A: *Staphylococcus aureus* cell wall protein that binds to the Fc region of IgG.

protein tyrosine kinases: Enzymes that are able to phosphorylate proteins on tyrosines, and often act in a cascade-like fashion in the signal transduction systems of cells.

Qa antigens: "Nonclassical" MHC class I molecules of mice.

radioimmunoconjugate: A biochemical conjugate consisting of an immune targeting molecule such as an antibody or antibody fragment together with a cytotoxic radionuclide.

recombination signal sequence (RSS): Conserved heptamer (7-nucleotide)-nonamer (9-nucleotide) sequences, separated by a 12 or 23 base spacer, which occur 3′ of variable gene segments, 5′ and 3′ of diversity gene segments, and 5′ of joining gene segments, in both immunoglobulin and T-cell receptor genes. They function as recognition sequences for the recombinase enzymes that mediate the gene rearrangement process involved in the generation of lymphocyte antigen receptor diversity.

regulatory idiotope: An antibody or T-cell receptor idiotope capable of regulating immune responses via interaction with lymphocytes bearing complementary idiotopes (anti-idiotopes).

regulatory T-cell: T-cells, mostly CD4+, that suppress the functional activity of lymphocytes and dendritic cells.

respiratory burst: The increased oxidative metabolism that occurs in phagocytic cells following activation.

reticuloendothelial system (RES): A rather old term for the network of phagocytes and endothelial cells throughout the body.

rheumatoid factor: IgM, IgG and IgA autoantibodies to the Fc region of IgG.

rosette: Particles or cells bound to the surface of a lymphocyte (e.g. sheep erythrocytes around a human T-cell).

scavenger receptors: Cell surface receptors, for example on phagocytic cells, that recognize cells or molecules that require clearance from the body.

scFv: A single chain molecule composed of the variable regions of an antibody heavy and light chain joined together by a flexible linker.

SCID (*severe combined immunodeficiency*): Immunodeficiency affecting both T- and B-lymphocytes.

secondary immune response: The qualitatively and quantitatively improved immune response that occurs upon the second encounter of primed lymphocytes with a given antigen.

secretory component: Proteolytic cleavage product of the poly-Ig receptor that remains associated with dimeric IgA in sero-mucus secretions.

secretory IgA: Dimeric IgA found in sero-mucus secretions.

somatic hypermutation: The enhanced occurence of point mutations in the recombined immunoglobulin variable region V(D)J genes that occurs following antigenic stimulation and acts as a mechanism for increasing antibody diversity and affinity.

stem cell: Multipotential cell from which differentiated cells derive.

stochastic: A process involving at least some element of randomness.

superantigen: An antigen that reacts with all the lymphocytes belonging to a particular T-cell receptor or immunoglobulin V region family, and that therefore stimulates (or deletes) a much larger number of cells than does conventional antigen.

surface plasmon resonance: A technique based upon changes in the angle of reflected light that occur upon ligand binding to an immobilized target molecule on a biosensor chip. This permits the observation of protein–protein interactions (such as antibody binding to an antigen) in "real-time," i.e. by continuous monitoring of the association and dissociation of the reversible reaction.

switch sequences: Highly conserved repetitive sequences that mediate class switching in the immunoglobulin heavy chain gene locus.

syngeneic: Genetically identical, e.g. a fully inbred strain of mice.

systemic: Throughout the body.

TAP: The *t*ransporters associated with *a*ntigen *p*rocessing (TAP-1 and TAP-2) are molecules that carry antigenic peptides from the cytoplasm into the lumen of the endoplasmic reticulum for incorporation into MHC class I molecules.

T-cell receptor (TCR): The heterodimeric antigen receptor of the T-lymphocyte exists in two alternative forms, consisting of α and β chains, or γ and δ chains. The $\alpha\beta$ TCR recognizes peptide fragments of protein antigens presented by MHC molecules on cell surfaces. The function of the $\gamma\delta$ TCR is less clearly defined but it can often recognize native proteins on the cell surface.

T-dependent antigen: An antigen that requires helper T-cells in order to elicit an antibody response.

T-independent antigen: An antigen that is able to elicit an antibody response in the absence of T-cells.

thymocyte: Developing T-cell in the thymus.

titer: Measure of the relative "strength" (a combination of amount and avidity) of an antibody or antiserum, usually given as the highest dilution that is still operationally detectable in, for example, an ELISA.

tolerance: Specific immunological unresponsiveness.

tolerogen: An antigen used to induce tolerance. Often depends more on the circumstances of administration (e.g. route and concentration) than on any inherent property of the molecule.

Toll-like receptors (TLRs): A family of pattern recognition receptors involved in the detection of structures associated with pathogens or damaged host tissues.

toxoid: Chemically or physically modified toxin that is no longer harmful but retains immunogenicity.

tumor antigens: Antigens whose expression is associated with tumor cells.

tumor necrosis factor (TNF, also called TNFα): Together with the related cytokine lymphotoxin (TNFβ), was originally named for its cytotoxic effect on certain tumor cells, but also has important inflammatory and immunoregulatory functions.

variable (*V*) gene segments: Genes that rearrange together with *D* (diversity) and *J* (joining) gene segments in order to encode the variable region amino acid sequences of immunoglobulins and T-cell receptors.

vascular addressins: Cell adhesion molecules present on the luminal surface of blood and lymph vessel endothelium recognized by homing molecules that direct leukocytes to tissues with the appropriate "address."

vasoactive amines: Substances including histamine and 5-hydroxytryptamine that increase vascular permeability and smooth muscle contraction.

xenogeneic: Genetic differences between species.

xenograft: A tissue or organ graft between individuals of different species.

Index

Page numbers in *italics* indicate figures; those in **bold** indicate tables.

---

human herpesvirus 8
    K3 protein *333*
    viral FLICE inhibitory protein 333
human leukocyte antigen *see* HLA
human leukocyte Fc receptors *see* Fc
        receptors
human monoclonal antibodies 145–6
human orthopoxvirus, interleukin-18
        binding protein 332
human papillomavirus, vaccines **359**, 455,
        463–4
humoral mechanisms 23–6, 33
    against parasites 336–8
    see also antibodies
hybridoma technology 57, 143–5, 179,
        183, 515
    T-cells 170
hydrogen bonding *120*
hydrogen peroxide 13
hydrophobic surfaces, thermodynamics
        119, *120*
hydrophobic transmembrane regions 81
hydroxyl radicals 13
hygiene hypothesis 403
hyperacute graft rejection **427**, 429
    xenografts 436, *437*
hyper-IgE syndrome 378
hyper-IgM syndrome 377
hypermutation, somatic 74, 92–5, 250,
        252, *253*, 520
hypersensitivity 49, 394–422, 515
    parasites 341
    see also immunopathology
hypervariable regions (CDRs) 515
    chimeric grafts 145
    epitope binding 115
    IgG 57, 59
    T-cell receptors 84–6, 88
        in ternary complexes 131–3
hypnosis 279
hypogammaglobulinemia, infants 375–6
hypothalamic–pituitary–adrenal axis 278

ICAM-1 131, 191–3, *249*, *316*
    common cold 332
    see also adhesion molecules
"iccosomes" 203
idiopathic pulmonary fibrosis 418
idiopathic thrombocytopenic purpura 408,
        492–3
idiotopes 66–8, 515
    regulatory 519
idiotypes 271–4, 281, 515
    antibodies 66–8
    bypass mechanisms 488, *489*

I domain, integrins *191*
IgA 61, *62*, 66, *69*
    class switching and 250
    FcαRI 65–6, *67*
    Fc units *63*
    mucosa 324
    protection from cholera 326
    secretory 61, *62*, 66, *69*, 324, 348, 520
    selective deficiency 375
Ig-α, B-cell receptors 82
Ig-β, B-cell receptors 82
IgD 61, *62*
    B-cell receptors 81, *82*
IgE 61, *62*, 324–5
    anaphylaxis 395, *397*
    blockade 405
    desensitization 404
    Fc receptors for 64–5
    Fc units *63*
    helminths 337
        deviation of response 341
    interaction with FcεRI 66, *67*, *397*
    radioallergosorbent test 167
    regulatory function 264
    see also hyper-IgE syndrome
IgG 54–60
    affinity *vs* abundance 162–3
    C3b bound to, bacterial opsonization
        323
    class switching and 251
    complement classical pathway 36
    divalent binding 121
    Fc units *63*
    indirect plaque techniques 177–8
    for malaria 341
    neonatal Fc receptor and 66, *69*
    regulatory function 264–5
    rheumatoid factors 496–7
    subclasses 55–7
    see also maternal IgG
IgG4 56
Ig-like receptors 96
    see also killer immunoglobulin-like
        receptors
IgM 60–1, *62*, *63*
    B-cell receptors *82*
    binding avidity 121
    class switching and 250
    complement classical pathway 36
    neonates 304
    regulatory function 264–5
    see also hyper-IgM syndrome
IgSF cytokine receptors 233
IκB (nuclear factor κB inhibitor) 12, 212
Ikaros gene *286*, 296

IL1R-associated kinase-4 (IRAK4),
        deficiency 370
IL-2 gene 212
immortalization, B-lymphocytes 143, 146,
        170
immune complexes
    detection 168
    see also under complexes
immune complex glomerulonephritis 412,
        413, 495, *496*
    kidney transplantation 439
immune complex-induced nephrotic
        syndrome, malaria 341, 412
immune complex-mediated hypersensitivity
        409–14, 420, **421**
immune dysregulation, polyendocrinopathy,
        enteropathy, X-linked (IPEX) 243,
        378
immune response
    anatomy 188–204
    deviation, parasites 341
    enhancement by immunodeficiencies
        378
    evolution 304–8, 309
    neonates 303–4, 309
    plants 304–5
    primary *45*, 519
    regulation 174–5
    secondary 44–6, 520
    tissue damage 4–6
    tumor growth enhancement 459
immune response genes (Ir genes) 275–7
immunoadsorption 515
immunoassays 156–7
    labels 167–8
    with solid-phase antigen 165–8, *169*
immunoblotting 158, *159*, *160*
immunoconjugates
    therapeutic 470–1
    see also radioimmunoconjugates
immunodeficiencies 369–93
    diagnosis 379–80
    treatment 380
    vaccination and 352–3
    see also severe combined
            immunodeficiency disorders
immunodominance
    antigens 264
    vaccine development and 357
immunoediting 458
immunofluorescence 515
immunofluorescence microscopy 150–2
immunofluorescence sandwich test *150*,
        176–7
immunogens 116–7, 142, 515